MW00769325

CURRENT THERAPY *in*
ORTHODONTICS

CURRENT THERAPY *in*
ORTHODONTICS

Ravindra Nanda, BDS, MDS, PhD
UConn Orthodontic Alumni Endowed Chair
Professor and Head
Department of Craniofacial Sciences
Chair
Division of Orthodontics
School of Dental Medicine
University of Connecticut Health Center
Farmington, Connecticut

Sunil Kapila, BDS, MS, PhD
Robert W. Browne Endowed Professor and Chair
Department of Orthodontics and Pediatric Dentistry
Program Director of Graduate Orthodontics
School of Dentistry
University of Michigan
Ann Arbor, Michigan

MOSBY

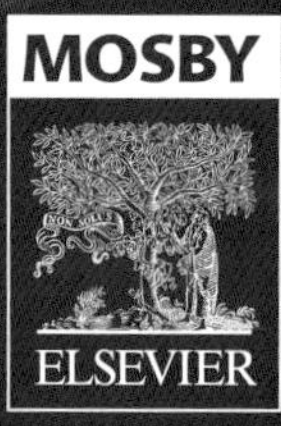

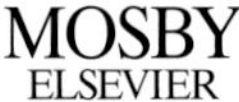

11830 Westline Industrial Drive
St. Louis, Missouri 63146

CURRENT THERAPY IN ORTHODONTICS ISBN: 978-0-323-05460-7

Notice

Neither the Publisher nor the Authors assume any responsibility for any loss or injury and/or damage to persons or property arising out of or related to any use of the material contained in this book. It is the responsibility of the treating practitioner, relying on independent expertise and knowledge of the patient, to determine the best treatment and method of application for the patient.

The Publisher

Library of Congress Cataloging-in-Publication Data

Current therapy in orthodontics / [edited by] Ravindra Nanda, Sunil Kapila.—1st ed.
p. ; cm.
Includes bibliographical references and index.
ISBN 978-0-323-05460-7 (hardcover : alk. paper) 1. Orthodontics. I. Nanda, Ravindra. II. Kapila, Sunil (Sunil D.), 1958-
[DNLM: 1. Orthodontics—methods. 2. Malocclusion—therapy. WU 400 C9765 2010]
RK521.C874 2010
617.6′43—dc22

2008047501

Vice President and Publisher: Linda Duncan
Senior Editor: John Dolan
Senior Developmental Editor: Courtney Sprehe
Publishing Services Manager: Patricia Tannian
Project Manager: Claire Kramer
Designer: Margaret Reid

Printed in China

Last digit is the print number: 9 8 7 6 5 4 3 2 1

DEDICATION

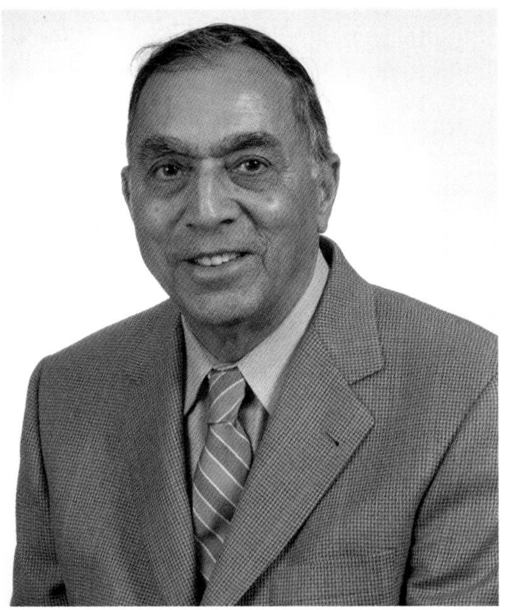

It is a matter of immense pleasure for us to dedicate this book to Dr. Ram Nanda as a small token of our appreciation and love for one of the most eminent leaders of orthodontics. For more than 50 years, Dr. Nanda has made exemplary contributions to the world of orthodontics. He has been a constant source of inspiration and a role model to several generations of orthodontists around the world. His mentorship, thought-provoking ideas, literary contributions, and scientific presentations at various levels have played a major role in the genesis of modern orthodontics and in establishing a more scientific and objective approach to this area of health sciences.

Ram joined the Government Dental College in Lahore, India, in 1945. After the partition of India he moved to Bombay (now Mumbai) and finished his dental education at the University of Bombay in 1949. In 1950 he came to the United States as a Fellow at Forsyth Dental Institute in Boston. Subsequently, he pursued and completed a doctorate in Human Growth at the University of Colorado in 1955. Ram returned to India in 1955 and served as a Professor in the Division of Orthodontics and Pedodontics at the Dental College and Hospital in Lucknow, India. Maintaining his ties with the United States, he completed his orthodontic specialty training at the Loyola University School of Dentistry from 1959 to 1961. In 1972 Ram was recruited as the founding Chair of the Division of Developmental Dentistry and Chair of the Department of Orthodontics at the University of Oklahoma, College of Dentistry. He served in this capacity until 2006.

From 1955 to 2006, Ram was actively involved in teaching the nuances of orthodontics to hundreds of graduate and undergraduate students in India, in the United States, and in numerous other countries. His exceptional ability as a team leader, coupled with his vision and hard work, helped to make the orthodontic department at the University of Oklahoma into one of the best in the country. Over the years, the department has attracted some of the best students and orthodontists from all over the world. Many of them have now matured into successful practitioners, and several hold prominent positions in academic orthodontics and in organized dentistry. Ram was also instrumental in guiding not only the orthodontic careers of both of us, but also the career of our late brother, Surender Nanda.

Ram and his wife, Pramod, celebrated their 50th wedding anniversary in 2007. They have been blessed with three children, Ruchi, an orthodontist, and Mohit and Sumit, both retinal surgeons, and eight loving grandchildren.

Ram is recognized for his many contributions to a broad range of topics in clinical orthodontics. He has presented numerous scientific lectures at both national and international meetings in topics ranging from craniofacial growth to orthodontic treatment outcomes and friction in orthodontic appliances. He has published one book, several chapters in reputed books, and more than 150 articles in peer-reviewed journals that have been well received throughout the world. During his early days in orthodontics, his work on human growth brought about a paradigm shift in the concepts related to craniofacial growth and development. He also provided valuable input in clinical orthodontics related to retention and stability, application of magnets for tooth movement, prediction of human growth, and biomaterials.

In recognition and appreciation of his tireless service, Ram has received awards and widespread acclaim from around the world, including the first Edward H. Angle Research Prize; appointment as an Endowed Professor in the Department of Orthodontics at the University of Oklahoma; the H.D. Merchant Oration Award from the Indian Orthodontic Society; the Martin Dewey Memorial Award from the Southwestern Society of Orthodontics; and his crowning achievement, honoree as the Father of Edgewise Orthodontics in India by the Indian Orthodontic Society.

Ram's numerous students, friends, and admirers have always described him as an outstanding educator, clinician, researcher, mentor, and role model and, above all, as a true gentleman. The dedication of this book in Ram's honor serves as a small token of gratitude and appreciation from all of us for his unselfish contributions to our profession.

Our sincere thanks to all the contributors who participated in this worthy project and submitted some of their finest work in honor of Dr. Ram Sarup Nanda.

Ravi Nanda
Sunil Kapila

CONTRIBUTORS

S. Jay Bowman, DMD, MSD
Adjunct Associate Professor
Saint Louis University
St. Louis, Missouri
Instructor
University of Michigan
Ann Arbor, Michigan

Lucia H.S. Cevidanes, DDS, MS, PhD
Assistant Professor
Department of Orthodontics
School of Dentistry
University of North Carolina
Chapel Hill, North Carolina

William J. Clark, BDS, DDO
Orthodontist
Fife, Scotland

R. Scott Conley, DMD
Clinical Associate Professor
Department of Orthodontics and Pediatric Dentistry
University of Michigan
Ann Arbor, Michigan

Tarisai C. Dandajena, DDS, MS, PhD
Assistant Professor
Department of Orthodontics
College of Dentistry
Assistant Professor
Department of Cell Biology
College of Medicine
University of Oklahoma Health Sciences Center
Oklahoma City, Oklahoma

Nejat Erverdi, DDS, PhD
Professor
Faculty of Dentistry
Department of Orthodontics
Marmara University
Istanbul, Turkey
Visiting Professor
Department of Orthodontics
School of Dentistry
University of Connecticut
Farmington, Connecticut

Leonard S. Fishman, DDS
Clinical Professor and Research Director
Department of Orthodontics and Temporomandibular Joint Disorders
Eastman Dental Center
University of Rochester
Rochester, New York

Julia Harfin, DDS, PhD
Chairman and Professor
Department of Orthodontics
Maimónides University
Buenos Aires, Argentina

Hong He, DDS, MDS, PhD
Chair and Associate Professor
Department of Orthodontics
School of Stomatology
Key Laboratory for Oral Biomedical Engineering
Ministry of Education
Wuhan University
Wuhan, Hubei Province, China

Haluk İşeri, DDS, PhD
Professor and Chair
Department of Orthodontics
School of Dentistry
Ankara University
Ankara, Turkey

Sunil Kapila, BDS, MS, PhD
Robert W. Browne Endowed Professor and Chair
Department of Orthodontics and Pediatric Dentistry
Program Director of Graduate Orthodontics
School of Dentistry
University of Michigan
Ann Arbor, Michigan

Hiroshi Kawamura, DDS, DDSc
Professor and Chairman
Department of Maxillofacial Surgery
Graduate School of Dentistry
Tohoku University
Sendai, Miyagi, Japan

Jin Y. Kim, DDS
Resident in Orthodontics
Department of Orthodontics
College of Dental Medicine
Columbia University
New York, New York

Gregory J. King, DMD, DMSc
Moore Riedel Professor
Department of Orthodontics
School of Dentistry
University of Washington
Seattle, Washington

Reha Kişnişci, DDS, PhD
Professor
Department of Oral and Maxillofacial Surgery
School of Dentistry
Ankara University
Ankara, Turkey

Yukio Kitafusa, DDS, PhD
Kitafusa Orthodontic Clinic
Asahi City, Chiba Prefecture, Japan

Vincent G. Kokich, DDS, MSD
Professor
Department of Orthodontics
School of Dentistry
University of Washington
Seattle, Washington

Gökmen Kurt, DDS, PhD
Assistant Professor
Faculty of Dentistry
Department of Orthodontics
University of Erciyes
Kayseri, Turkey

Harry L. Legan, DDS
Professor and Director
Department of Orthodontics
Vanderbilt University Medical Center
Nashville, Tennessee

Steven J. Lindauer, DMD, MDSc
Norborne Muir Professor and Chair
Department of Orthodontics
School of Dentistry
Virginia Commonwealth University
Richmond, Virginia

Jeremy J. Mao, DDS, PhD
Professor
Department of Orthodontics
College of Dental Medicine
University of Columbia
New York, New York

James A. McNamara, Jr., DDS, MS, PhD
Thomas M. and Doris Graber Endowed Professor
of Dentistry
Department of Orthodontics and Pediatric Dentistry
School of Dentistry
Professor of Cell and Developmental Biology
School of Medicine
University of Michigan
Ann Arbor, Michigan
Research Professor
Center for Human Growth and Development
University of Michigan
Ann Arbor, Michigan

Thomas F. Mulligan, DDS, MSD
Private Practice
Phoenix, Arizona

Hiroshi Nagasaka, DDS, DDSc
Clinical Professor
Department of Maxillofacial Surgery
Tohoku University
Sendai, Miyagi, Japan
Director
Department of Oral Surgery and Dentistry
Miyagi Children's Hospital
Sendai, Miyagi, Japan

Ravindra Nanda, BDS, MDS, PhD
UConn Orthodontic Alumni Endowed Chair
Professor and Head
Department of Craniofacial Science
Chair
Division of Orthodontics
School of Dental Medicine
University of Connecticut Health Center
Farmington, Connecticut

Peter Ngan, DMD
Professor and Chair
Department of Orthodontics
West Virginia University
Morgantown, West Virginia

Hyo-Sang Park, DDS, MSD, PhD
Department of Orthodontics
School of Dentistry
Kyungpook National University
Daegu, South Korea

Carol Pilbeam, PhD, MD
Professor of Medicine
Department of Medicine
University of Connecticut Health Center
Farmington, Connecticut

Birte Prahl-Andersen, DDS, PhD, FDSRCS (Edin)
Professor (Emeritus) and Former Chairman of the Orthodontics Department
Department of Orthodontics
Academic Centre for Dentistry
Amsterdam, The Netherlands
Visiting Professor
Faculty of Dentistry
West China College of Stomatology
Sichuan University
Chengdu, China
Honorary Professor
Padjadjaran State University
Bandung, Indonesia

William R. Proffit, DDS, PhD
Kenan Professor
Department of Orthodontics
School of Dentistry
University of North Carolina
Chapel Hill, North Carolina

Bhavna Shroff, DDS, MDentSc
Professor and Graduate Program Director
Department of Orthodontics
School of Dentistry
Virginia Commonwealth University
Richmond, Virginia

Pramod K. Sinha, DDS, BDS, MS
Affiliate Professor
Department of Orthodontics
University of Washington
Seattle, Washington
Chair
Department of Health
Dental Quality Assurance Commission
Tumwater, Washington

Anoop Sondhi, DDS, MS
Sondhi-Biggs Orthodontics
Indianapolis, Indiana

Martin Styner, PhD
Assistant Professor
Departments of Psychiatry and Computer Science
University of North Carolina
Chapel Hill, North Carolina

Junji Sugawara, DDS, DDSc
Visiting Clinical Professor
Division of Orthodontics
Department of Craniofacial Science
School of Dental Medicine
University of Connecticut
Farmington, Connecticut
Director
SAS Orthodontic Centre
Ichiban-cho Dental Office
Sendai, Miyagi, Japan

Madhur Upadhyay, BDS, MDS
Fellow
Division of Orthodontics
Department of Craniofacial Sciences
School of Dental Medicine
University of Connecticut Health Center
Farmington, Connecticut

Flavio Andres Uribe, DDS, MDentSc
Assistant Professor
Division of Orthodontics
Department of Craniofacial Sciences
School of Dental Medicine
University of Connecticut Health Center
Farmington, Connecticut

Serdar Üşümez, DDS, PhD
Associate Professor and Chairman
Faculty of Dentistry
Department of Orthodontics
University of Gaziantep
Gaziantep, Turkey

Sunil Wadhwa, DDS, PhD
Charles Burstone Assistant Professor
Department of Craniofacial Sciences
School of Dental Medicine
University of Connecticut
Farmington, Connecticut

Kazunori Yamaguchi, DDS, PhD
Professor and Chair
Division of Orofacial Functions and Orthodontics
Department of Growth and Development of Functions
Kyushu Dental College
Kitakyushu, Fukuoka, Japan

Björn U. Zachrisson, DDS, MSD, PhD
Professor II
Department of Orthodontics
University of Oslo
Oslo, Norway

Candice Zemnick, DMD, MPH, MS
Director, Predoctoral Prosthodontics
Associate Director, Maxillofacial Prosthetics
Department of Prosthodontics
College of Dental Medicine
Columbia University
New York, New York
Associate Fellow, American Academy of Maxillofacial Prosthetics

PREFACE

Current Therapy in Orthodontics is the first book of its kind to look at the ever-evolving science of orthodontics and its relation to optimal patient therapy and care. It is designed to be a clear and modern reference for orthodontists and dental practitioners and to provide access to state-of-the-art concepts in orthodontics. Leaders in the field have come together to provide the basis of contemporary orthodontics in one complete book. The detailed coverage walks the reader through diagnosis and treatment planning; the management of transverse, sagittal, and vertical discrepancies; the management of both adult and complex cases; and the application of biomedicine in orthodontic treatment.

One essential area addressed in this book is the management of adult cases. As more and more adults seek orthodontic treatment, today's orthodontic practitioner must have a good understanding of the best ways to treat the adult patient. Part III, Management of Adult and Complex Cases, concentrates on the treatment of adult patients and the problems and issues specific to them.

ORGANIZATION

Part I, Orthodontic Diagnosis and Treatment, begins by looking at the impact that orthodontic treatment can have on the patient's quality of life and a value-based health care system in Chapter 1 and then goes on to address what factors affect patient compliance and how to improve compliance in Chapter 2. Chapter 3 addresses how facial morphology and variations in development can influence the timing and methodology of clinical treatment. Chapter 4 reviews the Dental Prescale Occluzer, whereas Chapter 5 looks at how a fully automated, voxelwise, rigid registration at the cranial base and three-dimensional superimposition methods are used to evaluate displaced anatomical structures. Both Chapters 6 and 7 address brackets, starting with the process of bonding brackets (and other appliances) in Chapter 6, followed by the impact that proper bracket selection and placement can have on the final treatment outcome. Part I concludes with Chapter 8, which looks at the importance of long-term, follow-up clinical research and experience-based information on orthodontic therapy and how this should be incorporated into treatment planning.

Part II, Clinical Management of Sagittal and Vertical Discrepancies, starts with Chapter 9, which looks at the distinction between orthodontics and facial orthopedics and the different effects of these two approaches on the correction of dentofacial deformities. Chapter 10 addresses three types of functional appliances (removable, fixed, and hybrid) and how they are used in the treatment of Class II malocclusion. Chapter 11 reviews Class II combination therapy, a treatment method for Class II malocclusions that requires only a single phase of treatment and reduces the need for patient compliance. Chapter 12 addresses the best way to recognize and treat maxillary deficiency syndrome, whereas Chapter 13 looks at the prevalence, etiology, diagnosis, and treatment of Class III malocclusion. Both Chapters 14 and 15 address open bite. Chapter 14 covers the classification, mechanisms, and clinical implications of open bite, including mouth breathing, and Chapter 15 looks at the characteristics of excessive vertical skeletofacial pattern and the different mechanics for its correction. Part II finishes with Chapter 16, which addresses deep overbite, three treatment options, and the use of implants in deep bite correction.

Part III, Management of Adult and Complex Cases, begins by looking at how the periodontal condition can affect orthodontic treatment in adult patients in Chapter 17. Chapter 18 reviews a treatment approach designed by the chapter author that addresses the problem of stabilizing a diastema closure without the need for permanent retention. Chapter 19 provides an overview of continuous and segmented mechanics, introduces the concept of hybrid sectional mechanics, and uses biomechanical principles to discuss the pros and cons of each of these approaches. Chapter 20 looks at sleep apnea, including its diagnosis and various treatments. Chapter 21 looks at the importance of dental esthetics, providing a systemic method of evaluating dentofacial esthetics in a logical, interdisciplinary manner. Chapter 22 reviews the use of temporary anchorage devices during routine orthodontic therapy, and Chapter 23 looks at the development and use of microimplants. Chapter 24 addresses the skeletal anchorage system, which was developed by the chapter authors and involves the use of titanium miniplates and monocortical screws for absolute anchorage. Part III ends with Chapter 25, a look at a technique known as dentoalveolar distraction, a relatively new technique that achieves rapid tooth movement using the principles of distraction osteogenesis.

Part IV, Applications of Biomedicine to Orthodontics, concludes the book with a discussion of mechanotransduction in Chapter 26. Chapter 27 addresses orthodontic root resorption, and, finally, Chapter 28 looks at the major clinical challenges in craniofacial reconstruction, the clinical approaches to its management, and the emerging approaches in tissue engineering and stem cell biology in achieving the biologically based reconstruction of dental, oral, and craniofacial defects.

CONTRIBUTORS

A book of this nature is a product of numerous contributors, many of whom have spent their careers developing ways to advance our profession. Bringing together this distinguished group of practitioners and scholars from all over the world has resulted in a comprehensive book on contemporary orthodontics that encompasses all their experience and expertise.

NOTE FROM THE EDITORS

This book is not meant to be a compendium of every aspect of orthodontics. The idea of current therapy is to understand how today's research affects optimal patient care. It is our hope that this book will serve as a way for both the orthodontic and general practitioner to stay up to date on the latest advances and current issues in this continually evolving field.

Ravi Nanda
Sunil Kapila

ACKNOWLEDGMENTS

Our heartfelt thanks to all the contributors for participating and joining us in our recognition of Ram Nanda. Their participation was imperative to the success of this project.

Our thanks to Dr. Madhur Upadhyay for his help in editing several chapters.

Our sincere thanks to Mr. John Dolan, Senior Editor, who supported and encouraged the development of this book. This book could not have been completed without the help of Ms. Courtney Sprehe, Senior Developmental Editor, who took charge of this book from day one and brought it to fruition with her hard work.

CONTENTS

CURRENT THERAPY *in*
ORTHODONTICS

PART I

Orthodontic Diagnosis and Treatment

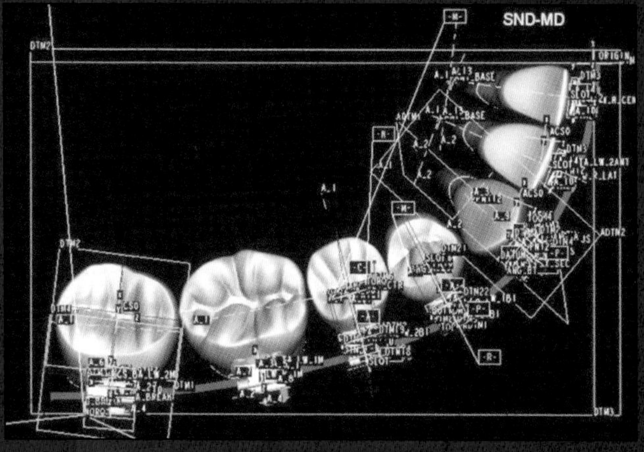

CHAPTER 1

Quality of Life as an Indicator for Orthodontic Treatment

Birte Prahl-Andersen

The world is facing an increased demand for health care and disease prevention. The consequence of this demand is increasing requests for public and private funding. To cope with this request for funds, only those needs based on sound scientific evidence should be met.

The increasing demands and rising costs require that professionals review treatment and prevention strategies to make sure that these are not the result of pressure from patients or a personal pursuit. It is imperative that endeavors undertaken by professionals increase the quality of life for specific patients and benefit the general population.

When focusing on oral health–related quality of life in relation to orthodontics, it is important to realize that for the majority of the world's population, orthodontic treatment is not a priority; their priorities are obtaining the basic necessities of life, such as food, shelter, and clothing. Additionally, research into the demand for treatment of oral conditions often uses a self-administered questionnaire, so the patient must be able to read. Therefore the only scientific data available on this issue come from the developed world.

If patients with craniofacial malformations and malocclusions need orthodontic treatment, the decision to treat should be made based on consumer values.[1,2] Generally, in a values-based health care system, decisions should be made using the knowledge from the outcomes of scientific evaluation of prevention programs and treatment methods. The main values to be addressed are evidence, need, and costs (Fig. 1-1).

EVIDENCE-BASED ORTHODONTICS

The values of "evidence" and "costs" can ethically be seen to be directed toward two different goals: *evidence-based medicine* alludes to an individual's ethics (doing everything possible for the patient), whereas *cost-effectiveness* alludes to social ethics (maximum gains in population health from a finite budget). In general, regarding evidence-based medicine and cost-effectiveness, the common concern is that the outcome measures used in clinical trials should be as relevant as possible to the patient and include the effects on quality of life. Measuring the quality of life should be based on consumer values if orthodontic treatment is to remain a part of publicly funded health care systems.

Regarding evidence-based orthodontic care (barring a few exceptions), new treatment methods and materials are often proposed without genuine interest in the experimental testing by orthodontic professionals or the industry.[3,4] Orthodontists will often change the materials they use or the treatment methods in a clinical setting without sound scientific evidence to support the change. Although available, no consistent regulatory measures are implemented to monitor the safety, costs, and efficacy of the primary process in orthodontic care.

NEED FOR ORTHODONTIC TREATMENT

The present interest in the guidelines regarding indications for orthodontic treatment is not new. Different methods for assessing the need for orthodontic treatment have been described for the last 50 years, including Handicapping Labiolingual Deviations (HLD), Treatment Priority Index (TPI), Handicapping Malocclusions, Occlusal Index (OI), and Dental Aesthetic Index (DAI). These methods are based on a comparison between irregular malocclusion and normal or ideal occlusion, as well as on the assumption that "the greater the deviation from the norm, the greater the risk for problems." Solow[5] correctly questions the validity of this

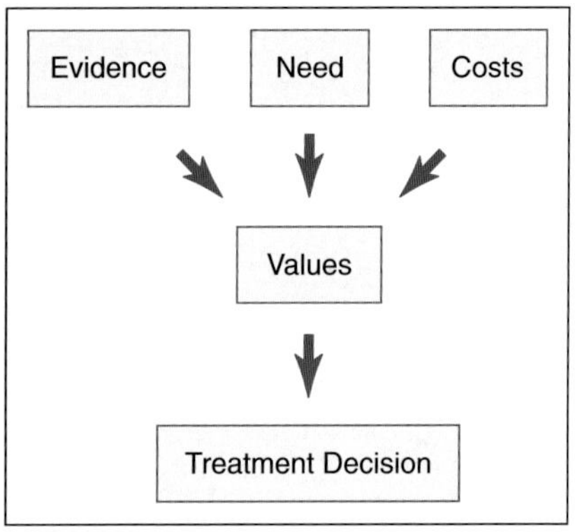

Evidence → Values ← Costs; Need → Values; Values → Treatment Decision

Fig. 1-1 Values-based health care. The values involved in treatment decisions.

assumption because the limiting values employed in the indices are arbitrary. For example, it would be impossible to demonstrate any difference in the risk involved in having an overjet just above or just below any specific millimeter limit.

The Swedish system[6] is based on a gradation of various types of malocclusions into one of four categories. A child is classified in the category covering the most severe deviation. The Index of Orthodontic Treatment Need (IOTN),[7] the Need for Orthodontic Treatment Index (NOTI),[8] and the Index of Complexity, Outcome, and Need (ICON)[9] are based on the same principles as the Swedish system. Unfortunately, these systems cannot be used internationally. A Dutch reliability and validity study concluded that the ICON needs to be adjusted for the specific Dutch perception of need for orthodontic treatment.[10] This probably holds true for other countries and cultures as well.

Assessment of individual treatment needs is a process that varies in different countries, depending on the structure of health care and orthodontic care. Ideally, patients, orthodontic professionals, and third parties should agree on a method for the distribution of financial resources. The amount of money that is available for orthodontic care per country should be balanced with the extent of orthodontic care required by the population.

In 1990 a Danish system was introduced based on health risks related to malocclusion.[11] By explicitly incorporating an assessment of the health risks, this approach differs from the other screening systems. This model addresses the following health risks:

- Risk of damage to the teeth and surrounding tissues
- Risk of functional disorders
- Risk of psychosocial stress
- Risk of late sequelae

The problem with the Danish system (in a society with an increasing demand for orthodontic treatment) is that improvement in quality of life for everyone cannot be seen as a task for public financing. It leads to questions such as, "Is it legitimate to use health resources [for persons with a] risk of psychosocial stress?"[12] and "How should body dysmorphic disorder in teenagers and adults be handled?"[13]

In Denmark, third-party financing is provided by the community orthodontic service, and 29% of all children are treated orthodontically. In Norway, with a combination of public and private financing of orthodontic care, an estimated 35% of the children are treated.[12] It seems that the "gatekeeper" function (practitioner involved in screening process) is not a problem in Scandinavia, although it may be in other European countries and in the United States, because often the gatekeeper is also the health care provider. This is an undesirable situation because it can promote the misuse of financial resources and overtreatment.

In The Netherlands a nationwide longitudinal epidemiological study showed that an increase in orthodontic care delivered between 1990 and 1996 did not improve the dental health of 20-year-old patients in terms of the prevalence of malocclusions, the demand for orthodontic treatment, and satisfaction with tooth position.[14] These findings are supported by a systematic literature search initiated by the Swedish Council on Technology Assessment in Health Care (2005).[15] A global solution to these dilemmas has not yet been presented.

The validity of "improvement in quality of life" as an indicator for orthodontic treatment must still be substantiated, but few tools for measurement of oral health–related quality of life have been developed, especially concerning children. Proper measurements of oral health–related quality of life can be used to assess both the need for and the outcome of clinical interventions from the perspective of the individual in question or the population under study.

PSYCHOSOCIAL PERSPECTIVE

In the 1980s a vast amount of research addressed the psychosocial meanings of facial appearance and malocclusion.[16-19] Social class, race, age, and gender did not seem to influence the perception of dental and facial appearance in children. Little evidence is available on how thoughts about self and social interaction change as a result of orthodontic treatment, or how long changes in self-image and possible improvement in social interaction last after treatment.[20,21]

In regard to "dental esthetic" self-perception in adults who are undergoing or have undergone orthodontic treatment,[22] the differences in results between studies may be attributed to the use of different assessment tools. Major changes over the last 40 years in the developed world have influenced attitudes toward physical appearance. These changes include the following[23]:

- Increased disposable income
- Expansion of the press and media
- The impression that looking youthful and attractive aids success in the workplace (with associated financial awards) and in a social setting
- Increased and more targeted advertising to consumers
- Possibility of correcting a condition allows people to consider the condition to be unacceptable

"Beauty is a currency system, like the gold standard, worth a lot of money. Western women have been controlled by ideals and stereotypes, beauty pornography—through advertisements and powerful market manipulation."[24] Perhaps Strauss[23] is correct when he suggests that the more a physical variation can be controlled, the less likely it is to be tolerated.

The concept of quality of life depending on the patient's views of the acceptability or nonacceptability of their appearance forces the profession to examine more closely the social and psychological processes that forge self-perception of appearance. Generic and disease-specific measures developed in the 1990s are not appropriate for use with oral or orofacial conditions and, specifically, are not appropriate for use in the study of children. Further, it is important that such measures or instruments conform to contemporary concepts of health, as well as complement the traditional clinical measures used in research and in clinical practice. As the World Health Organization (WHO) stated in 1959, health represents more than the absence of disease. Contemporary concepts of health recognize that there are positive and negative aspects of health and health outcomes, and such perceptions should be measured with valid and reliable tools.

To date, only a few questionnaires on children's oral health–related quality of life have been published.[25] These questionnaires are not generally applicable over different cultures, and the choice of questions needs adaptation. Reliability and validity testing of an improved questionnaire has been done in an international setting. When developing and testing the Child Oral Health Impact Profile (COHIP), a multistage impact approach (as described by Juniper, Guyatt, and Jaeschke[26] in 1996) was employed. Validity, reliability, interpretability, and responsiveness were all tested. The COHIP has been adopted in The Netherlands and the United States.

The tools used to measure oral health–related quality of life should focus on discrimination across health care systems and should distinguish between people with different clinical oral conditions and people with the same clinical orofacial condition but different levels of severity. The tools should work as a short, self-administered measurement instrument, and the hope is that this user-friendly format will facilitate use of these instruments in clinical practice and international research. The following domains should be addressed on the questionnaire:

- Oral symptoms
- Functional well-being
- Emotional well-being
- Peer interaction
- School and family impact

The international corporate study to develop COHIP included members from France, The Netherlands, United States, Great Britain, Canada, Hong Kong, South Africa, New Zealand, and Argentina.[27] The purpose of this study was to examine all the steps needed for the development of a questionnaire that can be used in countries with different cultures. The steps addressed included item generation, face validity, item reduction, and reliability.

In The Netherlands the study surveyed 514 schoolchildren and showed that the mean frequency scores for children with craniofacial abnormalities (responses from child and caregiver) were greater than those for children with malocclusions, and that the impact of malocclusion on quality of life was not significant (Fig. 1-2). No cultural

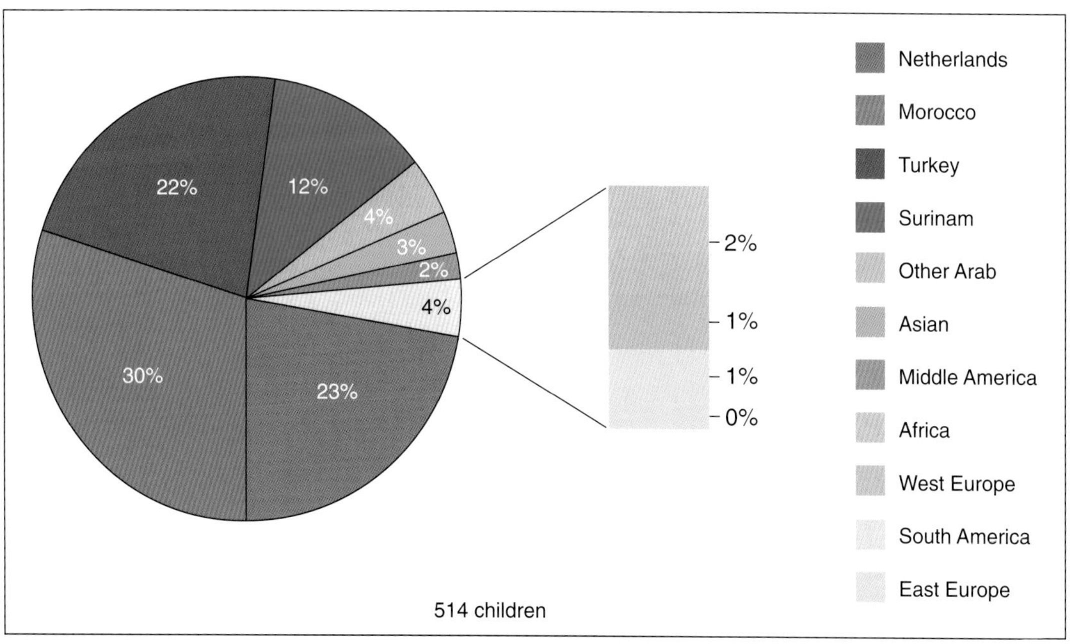

Fig. 1-2 Results from Amsterdam: nationalities of a community sample. Distribution of Amsterdam schoolchildren according to origin, as reported in study using Child Oral Health Impact Profile (COHIP); 23% of the children were "full-blooded" Dutch (both parents Dutch).

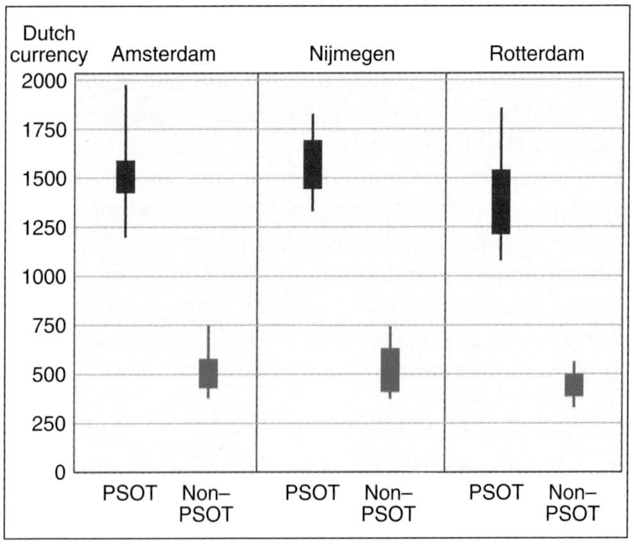

Fig. 1-3 Box-whisker plots of the direct medical costs of treating children with *(red)* or without *(blue)* presurgical orthopedic treatment (PSOT). Data collected in three Dutch cleft centers.

differences were found, and a significant difference was seen only between boys and girls, with girls affected more often than boys.[28]

The results from the United States were based on answers from 157 pediatric patients, 152 orthodontic patients, 111 craniofacial patients, and 105 from a community sample.

The results of this international study[27] can be summarized as follows:

1. COHIP demonstrated psychometric worthiness.
2. Children with craniofacial malformations showed the greatest negative impact on oral health–related quality of life.
3. Among orthodontic patients, an inverse relationship was found between the extent of overjet and quality of life.
4. Among pediatric patients, greater decay was associated with reduced quality of life.

Therefore the COHIP can be considered to be a valid and discriminating measuring instrument that can be used internationally to measure quality of life in relation to oral conditions.

Need Versus Demand

Traditionally, a distinction is made between need and demand, and differences between need and demand should not be confused. The *need* for treatment is the orthodontist's assessment of the necessity of performing treatment. *Demand* is the patient's expressed desire for treatment. The patient asks, "Will my bite be better?" or "Will my teeth last longer?" What they really want is to present the best possible face to the world.

The need for orthodontic treatment is unquestioned for children with severe craniofacial deformities and cleft lip and palate. According to the Swedish Council on Technology Assessment in Health Care, only an extreme overjet, overbite, and ectopic eruption of canines are risk factors in pediatric dental health.[15]

COSTS

No inventory of the cost-effectiveness of orthodontic care has been made and few studies on cost-effectiveness executed. A survey of the literature for evidence of cost-effectiveness of orthodontic treatment reveals deficient study designs, inconsistent treatment outcomes, small sample sizes, and publication bias (often, only positive results published).

Prospective *randomized clinical trials* (RCTs) are state of the art, but the orthodontic profession has produced only flimsy evidence with regard to cost-effectiveness of orthodontic treatments. One exception is the Dutch study on cost-effectiveness of *presurgical orthopedic treatment* (PSOT) for patients with cleft lip and palate[29] (Fig. 1-3). A drawback of RCTs is that generalization to other groups may be inappropriate because of a possible selection bias.

Generally, a "win-win-win" situation should focus on the following:

1. A "win" for patients because of the consistent evidence-based treatment outcomes, optimal information, minimal pain and discomfort, and affordable financial structure.
2. A "win" for health care professionals because of the rewards for proficiency, delivery of high-standard service, use of new validated means, and preservation of the profession.
3. A "win" for society because of the clinical accountability, increased access, cost containment, and linkage of orthodontic care to population need.

To guarantee that quality orthodontic care is accessible for those who need it and want it, a balance should be struck between real need and resources. This problem has been addressed by the Euro-Qual project, in which policy statements for quality orthodontic care, an orthodontic quality manual, and a database for orthodontics were developed with support from the European Commission[30,31] (Fig. 1-4).

In many cases the demands for treatment are dictated by the surroundings of the patients. Unfortunately, societal values focus heavily on external beauty. As stated, patients with craniofacial malformations have a 100% treatment need, and resources should be available for the treatment of these patients. Children with craniofacial malformations can seldom live up to the "beauty myth." The demand for treatment is dictated by the wish of the parents and the patient to be able to live a normal life without others staring. Patients do not need to win a beauty contest to be happy, as long as they look "normal."

As stated, values-based treatment of children with malocclusions should focus on the effect on the patient's quality of life. Evidence, need, and cost-effectiveness are the key

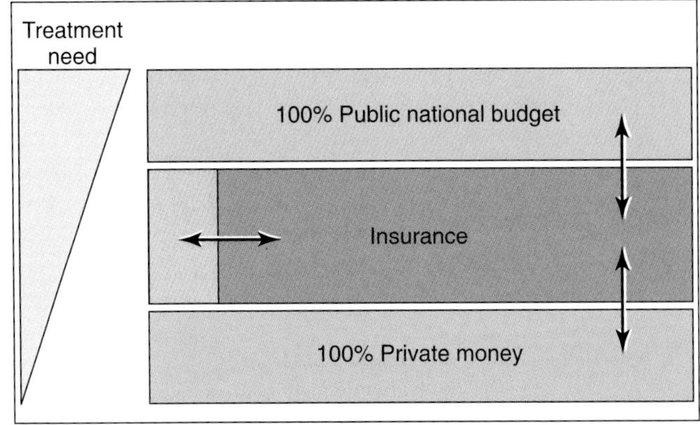

Fig. 1-4 Possible variations in the financing of orthodontic care according to available financial resources, in relation to treatment indication.

issues. "Quality of life" is a subjective notion, with different meanings for different people, and it changes over time. Efforts by the orthodontic profession should be ongoing to keep pace with changes in these issues.

CONCLUSION

Ideally, indication or need for orthodontic treatment should be dictated by its impact on dental health and the patient's quality of life. Malocclusions that impact dental health are excessive overjet, ectopic erupting canines, and severe hypodontia. If the indication for orthodontic treatment used in developed countries is dictated by the idea that the treatment will improve the patient's quality of life, it must still be substantiated. Little evidence is available to support the assumption that orthodontic treatment improves the patient's quality of life. It could be argued that in the developed world, too many patients are orthodontically treated, wasting financial resources that could be used more effectively on other health issues. Using "free market" philosophy, patients should be able to receive treatment if they have insurance coverage, in other words, if they pay for standard orthodontic treatment themselves.

Acknowledgment

Economic and social forces are creating a need for effective and efficient health care. The aim of my contribution to this book is primarily to honor an old friend. Ram Nanda visited Nijmegen in The Netherlands in 1968, and since then we have followed each other's careers through our mutual interest in growth and development. Ram and I both experienced what it means to be a foreigner in other countries, where we have given many years of our working life. The United States community has been blessed with a kind teacher and dedicated researcher for many years.

References

1. Cunningham SJ, Hunt NP: Quality of life and its importance in orthodontics, *J Orthod* 28:152-158, 2001.
2. Vig KWL, Weyant R, O'Brien K, Bennet E: Developing outcome measures in orthodontics that reflect patient and provider values, *Semin Orthod* 5:85-95, 1999.
3. O'Brien K, Wright J, Conboy F, et al: Effectiveness of early orthodontic treatment with the twin-block appliance: a multicenter, randomized, controlled trial. Part 2. Psychosocial effects, *Am J Orthod Dentofacial Orthop* 124:488-494, 2003.
4. Tulloch JFC, Philips C, Proffit WR: Benefit of early Class II treatment: progress report of a two-phase randomized clinical trial, *Am J Orthod Dentofacial Orthop* 113:62-72, 1998.
5. Solow B: Orthodontic a screening and third party financing (guest editorial), *Eur J Orthod* 17:79-83, 1995.
6. Socialstyrelsen: Anvisningar for journal foringinom folktandvardens tandregleringsvard. Kungl Medicinalstyrelsens cirkular den 21 Februari 1966. Linder-Aronson S: Orthodontics in the Swedish public dental services, *Trans Eur Orthod Soc,* 1974, pp 233-240.
7. Brook P, Shaw WC: The development of an index of orthodontic treatment priority, *Eur J Orthod* 11:309-320, 1989.
8. Espeland LV, Stenvik A, Medin L: Concern for dental appearance among young adults in a region with non-specialist orthodontic treatment, *Eur J Orthod* 15:17-25, 1993.
9. Daniels CP, Richmond S: The development of an Index of Complexity, Outcome, and Need (ICON), *J Orthod* 27:149-162, 2000.
10. Louwerse TJ, Aartman IHA, Kramer GJC, Prahl-Andersen B: The reliability and validity of the Index of Complexity, Outcome, and Need for determining treatment need in Dutch orthodontic practices, *Eur J Orthod* 28:58-64, 2006.
11. Sundhedsstyrelsen: Memorandum on orthodontic screening and indications for orthodontic treatment, Copenhagen, 1990, Danish National Board of Health.
12. Stenvik S, Torbjornson TE: Hvem gjor hva innenfor ortodontien? *Tandlagebladet* 111:6-11, 2007.
13. Hepburn S, Cunningham S: Body dysmorphic disorder in adult orthodontic patients, *Am J Orthod* 130:569-574, 2006.
14. Kieft JA, Kalsbeek H, Eijkman MAJ: Patient satisfaction of orthodontic-treated and non-treated persons, abstract 2643, 1998, International Association for Dental Research.
15. Bettavvikelser och tandreglering i ett hälsoperspektiv. En systematisk litteraturoversikt. Swedish Council on Technology Assessment in Health Care, 2005, SBU.
16. Kenealy P, Frude N, Shaw W: An evaluation of the psychological and social effects of malocclusion: some implications for dental policy making, *Soc Sci Med* 28:583-591, 1989.
17. Jenny J, Cons NC, Kohout FJ, Frazier PJ: Test of a method to determine socially acceptable occlusal conditions, *Community Dent Oral Epidemiol* 8:424-433, 1980.
18. Tesco LA, Albino JE, Cunat JJ, et al: A dental-facial attractiveness scale. Part II. Consistency of perception, *Am J Orthod* 83:44-46, 1983.
19. Albino JE, Lawrence SD, Tedesco LA: Psychological and social effect of orthodontic treatment, *J Behav Med* 17:81-98, 1994.
20. O'Brien K, Kay L, Fox D, Mandall N: Assessing oral health outcomes for orthodontics: measuring health status and quality of life, *Community Dent Health* 15:22-26, 1998.

21. De Oliveira CM, Sheiham A: Orthodontic treatment and its impact on oral health–related quality of life in Brazilian adolescents, *J Orthod* 31:20-27, 2004.
22. Bernabe E, Kresevic VD, Cabrejos SC, et al: Dental esthetic self-perception in young adults with and without previous orthodontic treatment, *Angle Orthod* 76:412-416, 2006.
23. Strauss R: Surgery, activism and aesthetics: a sociological perspective on treating facial disfigurement. In Lucker GW, Ribbens KA, McNamara JA, editors: *Psychological aspects of facial form,* Ann Arbor, Mich, 1980, Center for Human Growth and Development, pp 210-213.
24. Wolf N: *Beauty myth*, London, 1990, Vintage, Random House.
25. Jokovic A, Locker D, Stephens M, et al: Validity and reliability of a questionnaire for measuring child oral-health-related quality of life, *J Dent Res* 81:459-463, 2002.
26. Juniper EF, Guyatt GH, Jaeschcke R: How to develop and validate a new health-related quality of life instrument. In Spilker B, editor: *Quality of life and pharmacoeconomics in clinical trials,* Philadelphia, 1996, Lippincott-Raven, pp 49-56.
27. Broder HL, Jokovic A, Prahl-Andersen B, et al: Developing the Child Oral Health Impact Profile: an international study, *J Dent Res* 81:433, 2002 (special issue A).
28. Calis EM, Prahl-Andersen B, Zentner A: Oral health–related quality of life and dental aesthetics of schoolchildren in Amsterdam, *J Dent Children*, 2008 (in press).
29. Severens JL, Prahl C, Kuijpers-Jagtman AM, Prahl-Andersen B: Short-term cost-effectiveness analysis of presurgical orthopedic treatment in children with complete unilateral cleft lip and palate, *Cleft Palate Craniofac J* 35:222-226, 1998.
30. Njio BJ, Stenvik A, Ireland RS, Prahl-Andersen B, editors: European orthodontic quality manual, *Biomedical and Health Research*, vol 31, Amsterdam, 1999, IOS Press.
31. Njio BJ, Prahl-Andersen B, ter Heege G, et al, editors: Quality of orthodontic care: a concept for collaboration and responsibilities, *Biomedical and Health Research*, vol 32, Amsterdam, 2002, IOS Press.

CHAPTER 2

Patient Compliance in Orthodontic Practice

Pramod K. Sinha

Patient noncompliance can limit the effective conversion of accurate orthodontic treatment plans to excellent treatment results. Factors related to noncompliance are wide ranging.[1-3] Initially, these factors may be related to the patient's personal experiences in the dental office or the patient's perceptions based on the experiences of family or peers.[4] Patients often avoid dental treatment completely because of "dental anxiety."[5,6] Anxiety can lead to a fear of future orthodontic appointments and procedures, causing problems at the chair side for placing or applying different orthodontic appliances or procedures. Chair-side anxiety can be modified by good communication and patient education regarding procedures.[4] Once the patient overcomes this initial anxiety, the orthodontist and staff can focus on obtaining patient compliance in oral hygiene and appliance wear.

Orthodontic treatment processes require changes in established individual routines and also affect different social activities. Behavior modification to accommodate new demands placed by orthodontic techniques and appliances may involve changes that range from simple to extremely complex.[1] Decreasing the complexity of the required behavior change may lead to better compliance.[7] Also, because most patients are in the adolescent age group, they present with a unique process of changing from parental values toward acceptance of peer-group standards.[1] Not surprisingly, studies have shown better compliance in patients under age 12 years than in older groups.[8,9] Although important, this fact may not effectively predict or improve patient compliance.

This chapter discusses different factors that influence orthodontic patient compliance and provides strategies to improve compliance.

TREATMENT TECHNIQUES TO AVOID COMPLIANCE ISSUES

A variety of orthodontic treatment techniques have been devised to overcome the noncompliance barrier in the attempt to obtain good results.[9,10] Despite earlier claims by the proponents of these techniques, none is completely successful without the patient's partial or complete participation. Further, many of these so called noncompliance techniques have now reverted back to traditional methods of anchorage control, using headgear and elastics for part of the treatment period.[9]

Orthodontic anchorage control has evolved over the years, and use of bone-borne anchors is now widespread. These *temporary anchorage devices* (TADs) provide solutions to difficult situations and in some cases simplify compliance needs. Further, innovative orthodontic tools and refined treatment protocols have also improved the overall efficiency of the orthodontic treatment process. However, addressing issues of appliance breakage, elastic wear, and oral hygiene always requires discipline and compliance.

INFLUENCE OF FACIAL ESTHETICS

Perceived improvement of facial esthetics or cosmetic change may be the main reason why patients and parents seek orthodontic treatment.[1] Functional considerations do not necessarily correspond to the patient's desire for orthodontic treatment. Often, professional assessments differ from the parent's or patient's assessment of the need or severity of malocclusion or the need for orthodontic treatment. Epidemiological studies show that more than 70% of the population could benefit from orthodontic correction of occlusal functional discrepancies.[11]

Cultural and maturational differences exist in how individuals associate dentofacial attractiveness to overall esthetics and self-esteem. However, most patients view orthodontic treatment as a means to improve dentofacial esthetics.[1] Significant changes are observed daily in people's self-esteem through minor or major orthodontic correction. These positive changes can have a significant impact in people's daily lives. During orthodontic pretreatment consultation, patients frequently comment on their inhibition toward a natural smile because of the malalignment of their dentition. Therefore these positive changes (or the expected changes) may be used to motivate the patient's compliance.

A clinical "pearl" to remember is to use facial esthetic changes to motivate and sustain the patient's overall compliance.

FACTORS AFFECTING ORTHODONTIC PATIENT COMPLIANCE

During the initial treatment stages the parent's positive attitudes toward perceived changes resulting from orthodontic treatment predict patient compliance.[2] In the later stages the patient's own perception regarding treatment and outcomes directly correlates with compliance levels.[2] Patients show better compliance when they believe their actions directly lead to superior treatment results than when they believe they have no control over treatment outcomes.[2,12]

Different patient, parent, and practitioner variables have been correlated with orthodontic patient compliance. Patient variables range from different demographic factors to personality type and desire for treatment.[1-4,7,12,13] The parent's previous orthodontic experience can have a positive influence on patient compliance.[14] If an increase in fees for noncompliance occurs during orthodontic treatment, parental influence on the child's performance may influence future compliance. Studies have shown that doctor-patient rapport can significantly influence patient satisfaction and compliance.[4]

Factors found to correlate with patient compliance have not shown any particular trend. Studies have largely been inconclusive, or the results have not been reproducible. This inconsistency has forced practitioners to develop different methods for improving compliance. Depending on the practice or the patient, these methods range from punishment for poor compliance to rewards for better compliance.

Results of demographic studies may clarify some of the reasons for noncompliance but do not provide solutions to improve compliance, because practitioners cannot change these demographics for their patients. Therefore the focus of research efforts has been on areas outside the practitioner's influence or parental/patient influence. Also in this context, "prediction" may not necessarily lead to prevention. The emphasis should be on *prevention* or *improvement* of noncompliance rather than relying on demographics or predictions of expected behavior. Along with other solutions, this chapter discusses different prevention and improvement concepts that can positively affect orthodontic patient compliance.

The paradigm shift from a practitioner-centered model of patient care to a patient-centered approach is occurring in all areas of health care. In current orthodontic practice the patients and parents are more informed about their condition and treatment needs. More resources are available to obtain information on orthodontic treatment as well as the practitioner from a variety of Internet locations. This can be viewed as a positive change to disseminate information regarding orthodontic practice and patient care. The increase in parent/patient knowledge about orthodontic treatment influences day-to-day orthodontic work. Increased patient involvement has switched the traditional practitioner-centered care to a patient-centered approach.

PATIENT-CENTERED ORTHODONTIC TREATMENT

Traditionally, orthodontic treatment was prescribed by the practitioner based on defined professional standards, without considering the priorities and capabilities of the patient. Understanding this concept requires evaluation of the initial examination, diagnosis, and treatment-planning process.

During the selection of treatment techniques and appliances, the practitioner-centered plan uses tools to treat patients with the assumption of patient acceptance. Patients who fail to follow prescribed instruction are labeled as "noncompliant," often without considering that the treatment prescribed may not have taken into account the capabilities, motivations, and expectations of the individual patient. Thus, patients endure the outcome of "noncompliance" rather than considering the inability of the practitioner to understand individual patient needs and make appropriate treatment plans.

A patient-centered approach places some of the responsibility of successful patient compliance on the practitioner. In this model the practitioner prescribes treatment plans based on individual patient expectations, priorities, and most importantly the patient's capabilities.[15]

Repeated treatment progress evaluation and patient-parent consultation are key components of success in this proposed model. Orthodontic treatment planning should emphasize patient education, empowerment, and contracting procedures.

Patient Education

Patient management works better when patients understand the nature of their condition and the proposed treatment plan or procedure.[16,17] Educating patients regarding their malocclusion or condition and the means to obtain acceptable results are important measures in successfully motivating patients to succeed. In many cases, treatment is prescribed for patients who have limited understanding of their orthodontic problem and the need for certain appliances or mechanics to achieve a successful outcome. At the same time, parents may be unclear about treatment goals and mechanics. Further, the parent's ability to explain details of the condition and the necessity for different appliances to their children may be limited as well. The result is a patient who is less likely to have a successful treatment outcome because they cannot associate cause and effect. Also, in many cases, alternative strategies have not been discussed as options for patients and parents in deciding what would work for the patient.

A strong effort to educate patients regarding their condition will allow patients to make informed choices about appliance selection and limitations of the selection. As treatment progresses, the education component needs to be revisited to ensure complete understanding. This will result in individuals who take greater responsibility for their actions during orthodontic treatment.

Different demonstration tools are available to aid in the education process. Standard patient records such as study casts and photographs are excellent tools to describe the problem. A presentation customized for the patient using commercially available computer software programs is also an excellent method for explaining mechanics and appliances. The use of demonstration models allows the patient to understand different appliances. In addition, the practitioner can prepare a database of examples that can be digitally stored and used for these presentations. Another source of information is the practice's website, where information may be presented for patients and parents.

In current orthodontic practice, it is important to evaluate and explain treatment using the evidence-based literature. Although evidence is somewhat lacking in certain areas, the fundamentals of bone biology and growth serve as references for orthodontic techniques.

Patient Empowerment

Educating patients about their condition provides them with essential tools toward making informed decisions. The individual is involved in the process of selecting the best option for the necessary change. Sometimes the patient's decision conflicts with his or her best interests and also with the wishes of the parents regarding possible outcomes. In these situations, flexible treatment strategies need to be devised to succeed; a compromise may offer the best solution. In other situations, a suggestion to postpone treatment or to withdraw from seeking treatment may solve the conflict. Most often, alternatives are available and should be offered after an understanding of the limitations of different approaches. These discussions should be well documented in signed consultation reports and letters.

Contracting Procedures

Once a decision has been reached using this process, the patient is empowered and selects a treatment option from choices offered. This process obligates the patient to comply with a previously reached agreement. Continuing this process, a contract is made with the patient to reconfirm the previous choice. This approach has been successful in improving compliance in different areas of orthodontic care.[18,19]

PATIENT'S PERCEPTION OF CONTROL

Patients attribute events in their lives (e.g., progress of orthodontic treatment) to external and internal causes. *External causes* are outside their control (external locus of control), whereas *internal causes* are within their control (internal locus of control). The relationship between locus of control and orthodontic patient compliance has been studied.[2] El-Mangoury[12] found that orthodontic patients who attributed outcomes to internal causes were significantly more cooperative. Albino et al.[2] found that patients who attributed responsibility for their malocclusion, oral hygiene, and treatment externally to either chance or the orthodontist demonstrated lower compliance scores than others.

Therefore patients who attribute *internally* are better compliers than those who attribute *externally.* Patients who make fewer external attributions possess a sense of responsibility and consequently believe that their participation and cooperation facilitate treatment progress. These findings can be used clinically to improve patient compliance by initially developing a strong relationship and high level of communication with patients. Good rapport, along with patient education, can empower patients to make informed decisions about their role in improving compliance, which in turn determines the success of treatment.

SUPPORT AT HOME AND THE ORTHODONTIC OFFICE

Family support for the patient to follow prescribed instructions is necessary for successful implementation of this program. Also, continuous encouragement and feedback from the orthodontic office create a supportive environment for the patient. Patients are often required to wear cumbersome appliances that are difficult to use. If a task is suddenly introduced requiring the patient to do too much, a noncompliance problem is created from the beginning.

Consider patients who must use the reverse face-mask headgear for Class III skeletal growth modification. The headgear appears as a complicated device to the patient. This appliance must be worn over a long period for successful correction. Often a rapid palatal expander is used in combination with this appliance, which creates other challenges. The patient should first receive the expansion device for 2 weeks, followed by gradual introduction of the headgear. Initially the patient may wear the device only 2 hours, progressing to 4 hours in 3 to 4 weeks. Time should be incrementally increased to 12 to 14 hours of wear, as dictated by the treatment plan. This method of gradually introducing tasks to patients may help them in their adaptation to newer, more difficult tasks.

In addition to verbal feedback to the patient and parent, other methods include feedback by completing report cards, rewarding patients for compliant behavior, verbal praise, and regular patient-parent consultations. Visual feedback in demonstrating lack of oral hygiene using disclosing agents is also helpful. In addition, charted notations, which are highly visible to patients, can also be used to assist compliance.[20]

A survey conducted to evaluate different factors that influence orthodontic patient compliance showed that practicing orthodontists believed verbal praise and patient education were the most important methods of improving patient compliance.[21] Doctor-patient rapport and communication are key factors in the successful implementation of any plan.[4]

PATIENT REWARDS TO IMPROVE COMPLIANT BEHAVIOR

Improving patient compliance in day-to-day practice is a challenging and often complex problem. The reasons for noncompliance are difficult to diagnose and thus difficult to address.

Behavior modification using a reward program can effectively improve patient compliance to prescribed instructions. Various recommendations for establishing a reward program to motivate patients and improve compliance have been presented in orthodontic literature.[2,22-27] A University of Oklahoma study revealed the following findings regarding the use of awards as a motivating tool[28]:

- The award/reward program showed improvement in patient compliance scores in *below-average compliers,* reflected in improved oral hygiene scores. Oral hygiene improved over time when incentives were provided to patients whose hygiene scores were low at the beginning.
- *Above-average compliers* remained above average throughout the study. Below-average compliers improved with rewards but never reached the compliance levels achieved by the above-average compliers.

Therefore rewards can be a means of positive feedback to patients whose compliance was low at the outset. Combined with education and communication, rewards can result in some improvement.

DOCTOR/STAFF-PATIENT RAPPORT AND COMMUNICATION

The successful practice of orthodontics greatly depends on the interaction between orthodontist and patient. Also important is the interaction between office staff and patient. Therefore it is important to work on this aspect to improve the relationship for superior treatment outcomes, patient satisfaction, and doctor/staff satisfaction.[3,4,16,17] In a busy orthodontic practice, it is often difficult to establish a close rapport with the patient. Better doctor/staff-patient communication can result in more accurate patient information, thus improving the quality of care and compliance.

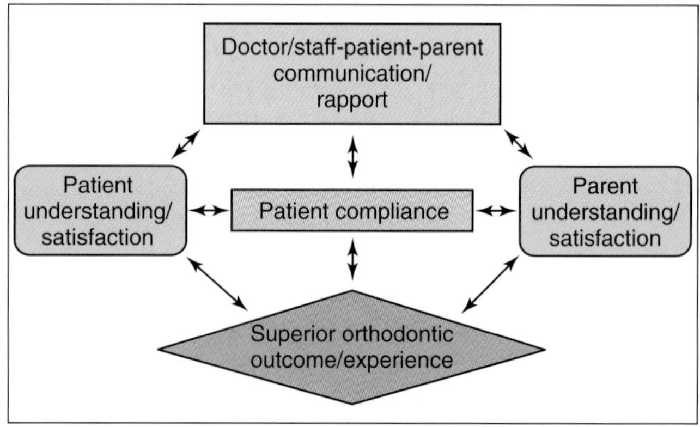

Fig. 2-1 Interrelationships among communication/rapport, satisfaction, compliance, and superior treatment outcomes in orthodontic treatment.

Physician/staff-patient relationships in orthodontics can positively influence treatment outcomes by encouraging the patient to cooperate in following prescribed instructions, as shown in different studies[3] (Fig. 2-1). The patient's perception that the orthodontist/staff paid attention and seriously considered the patient's input is significantly related to superior physician/staff-patient relationships. Also, making the patient feel welcome is a significant factor in establishing this rapport.[4]

Attention to behavioral issues can greatly enhance the rapport and can result in superior patient experiences and treatment results (see Fig. 2-1). Improving doctor/staff-patient/parent communication is an important factor in improving patient compliance, as reported by practicing orthodontists.[21]

Box 2-1 presents practical guidelines to help improve and maintain compliance.

CONCLUSION

Patient compliance/noncompliance depends on the duration, frequency, and complexity of the required behaviors. Because orthodontic treatment typically lasts 12 to 36 months, compliance levels must be sustained over this period. Demands on patient compliance increase further because compliance is required during this entire time. Also, more complex required behaviors (i.e., wearing appliances) may be difficult to maintain over a long period. Therefore it may be necessary to separate different compliance areas and individually address these with patients and parents for success in dealing with noncompliance issues. Also, continued support from the doctor and staff through communication and encouragement helps patients improve and maintain compliance.

Results of past research focusing on the prediction of patient compliance have largely been inconclusive or inconsistent. Practitioners are unable to apply these results clinically because of the largely demographic nature of the variables assessed; in most cases these demographic factors cannot be modified. Thus the focus should be on prevention and management rather than prediction of the noncompliance problem.

BOX 2-1 Guidelines for Improving and Maintaining Patient Compliance

1. The first step toward prevention of noncompliance is to understand the *patient's needs and desires.* The patient's main concern and the reasons for seeking orthodontic treatment are important. Further, once the treatment has progressed to a point where positive esthetic changes have occurred, these changes should be demonstrated to the patient and the parent. Also, progress photographs can reinforce and recruit patient compliance. Patients who experience significant satisfaction and improved self-esteem after orthodontic treatment, as well as those who are aware of positive changes, often respond better to future treatment and compliance needs. The office staff and the doctor can use this reaction as positive reinforcement and improve/maintain compliance for the duration of treatment.
2. Another necessary initial step in the process involves *patient empowerment* through education regarding their orthodontic problem, treatment options, required behaviors for the different options, and limitations of each approach.
3. The next step involves an *agreement* between the orthodontist and patient (and parent) regarding the treatment plan to be used. A clear understanding of the potential for success and the limitations of the selected approach is necessary. When the orthodontist and patient do not agree on the desired treatment goals and required behaviors, a clear understanding of the limitations should be presented and documented before initiating treatment.
4. Doctor-patient-parent *rapport* is critical in establishing a "win-win" situation that will lead to a favorable environment (see Fig. 2-1). Thus, patients believe they have participated in the treatment decisions and will be responsible to achieve mutually accepted goals.
5. A *supportive environment* at home as well as in the clinic helps patients with compliance on required behaviors. Further, it is important to provide feedback and reinforce success in performing required tasks. An "award" program or "report card" system can be effective in providing feedback and reinforcement.
6. Reinforcement of *cause and effect* regarding required behaviors to achieve success should be emphasized. The patient should be shown that significant changes related to treatment in terms of time and the finished result are in the patient's control.
7. Finally, repeated evaluation and consultation may further clarify goals, roles, and responsibilities for success.

REFERENCES

1. Albino J: Factors influencing adolescent cooperation in orthodontic treatment, *Semin Orthod* 6:214-223, 2000.
2. Albino J, Lawrence S, Lopes C, et al: Cooperation of adolescents in orthodontic treatment, *J Behav Med* 14:53-70, 1991.
3. Nanda RS, Kierl MJ: Prediction of cooperation in orthodontic treatment, *Am J Orthod Dentofacial Orthop* 102:15-21, 1992.
4. Sinha PK, Nanda RS, McNeil DW: Perceived orthodontist behaviors that predict patient satisfaction, orthodontist-patient relationship, and patient adherence in orthodontic treatment, *Am J Orthod Dentofacial Orthop* 110:370-377, 1996.
5. Heaton LJ, Carlson CR, Smith TA, et al: Predicting anxiety during dental treatment using patients' self-reports: less is more, *J Am Dent Assoc* 138:188-195, 2007.
6. Smith TA, Heaton LJ: Fear of dental care: are we making any progress? *J Am Dent Assoc* 134:1101-1108, 2003.
7. Sinha PK, Nanda RS: Improving patient compliance in orthodontic practice, *Semin Orthod* 6:237-241, 2000.
8. Weiss J, Eiser HM: Psychological timing of orthodontic treatment, *Am J Orthod* 72:198-204, 1977.
9. Bowman SJ: Class II combination therapy, *J Clin Orthod* 32:611-620, 1998.
10. Hilgers JJ: The pendulum appliance for Class II noncompliance therapy, *J Clin Orthod* 26:706-714, 1992.
11. Jago JD: Epidemiology of dental occlusion: a critical approach, *J Public Health Dent* 34:80-93, 1974.
12. El-Mangoury NH: Orthodontic cooperation, *Am J Orthod* 80:604-622, 1981.
13. Allan TK, Hodgson EW: The use of personality measures as a determinant of patient cooperation in an orthodontic practice, *Am J Orthod* 54:433-440, 1968.
14. Sinha PK: Unpublished data, 1994.
15. Rosen DS: Creating the successful adolescent patient: a practical patient-oriented approach. In McNamara JA Jr, Trotman C, editors: *Creating the compliant patient: Proceedings of the 23rd Annual Moyers Symposium,* Ann Arbor, Mich, 1996, pp 59-72.
16. Dougherty HL: Quo vadis? (guest editorial), *Am J Orthod* 87:345-346, 1985.
17. Laskin D: The doctor-patient relationship: a potential communication gap, *J Oral Surg* 37:786, 1979.
18. Rubin RM: Recognition and empowerment: an effective approach to enlisting patient cooperation, *J Clin Orthod* 29:24-26, 1995.
19. Gross AM, Schwartz CL, Kellum GD, Bishop FW: The effect of a contingency contracting procedure on patient compliance with removable retention, *J Clin Orthod* 25:307-310, 1991.
20. Knierim R: Use of stamped chart notations to enhance patient compliance, *J Clin Orthod* 26:394-395, 1992.
21. Mehra T, Nanda RS, Sinha PK: Orthodontists' assessment and management of patient compliance, *Angle Orthod* 68:115-122, 1998.
22. Gershater MM: The psychologic dimension in orthodontic diagnosis and treatment, *Am J Orthod* 54:327-338, 1968.
23. Kreit LH, Burstone C, Delman L: Patient cooperation in orthodontic treatment, *J Am Coll Dent* 35:327-332, 1968.
24. Gross AM, Samson G, Dierkes M: Patient cooperation in treatment with removable appliances: a model of patient noncompliance with treatment implications, *Am J Orthod* 87:392-397, 1985.

25. Gross AM, Bishop W, Reese D, et al: Increasing patient compliance with appointment keeping, *Am J Orthod* 92:259-260, 1985.
26. Sinclair PM: The readers' corner, *J Clin Orthod* 23:795-797, 1989.
27. Southard KA, Tolley EA, Arheart KL, et al: Application of the Millon Adolescent Personality Inventory in evaluating orthodontic compliance, *Am J Orthod Dentofacial Orthop* 100:553-561, 1991.
28. Richter DD, Nanda RS, Sinha PK, et al: Effect of behavior modification on patient compliance in orthodontics, *Angle Orthod* 68:123-132, 1998.

CHAPTER 3

Cephalomorphic and Biological Approach to Diagnosis and Treatment

Leonard S. Fishman

Without exception, every patient exhibits unique developmental variations relative to the timing, the rate, and the morphologic characteristics of craniofacial growth. This is particularly true in patients who demonstrate skeletal growth disharmony. If the clinician ignores these developmental factors and bases treatment exclusively on dental considerations, treatment and the stability of the result could be compromised.

The clinician needs to correlate both craniofacial morphological information and physiological maturational information that is unique to the patient before an individualized diagnosis and treatment plan can be established (Fig. 3-1). It is irresponsible to disregard the fact that every patient demonstrates unique developmental patterns, including the chronologic timing of maxillary and mandibular growth, variations in the rate of growth, direction and incremental increases in growth, the chronologic termination of skeletal growth, and dental and soft tissue relationships to this growth. All this information is easy to obtain in a systematic manner and is pertinent regardless of the choice of treatment mechanics. Because individuals usually exhibit consistency in maintaining basic skeletal growth patterns, and because facial growth is closely correlated with general skeletal growth, monitoring must occur during and after active treatment until a stable skeletal pattern has resulted.[1,2]

The primary purpose of this chapter is to demonstrate how variations in facial morphology and variations in maturational development influence both the timing and the methodology of clinical treatment. A series of patient examples are used to illustrate many of these factors.

CEPHALOMORPHIC EVALUATION OF FACIAL FORM

Individuals demonstrate wide variations in facial skeletal morphology. Many cephalometric analyses have been developed for the primary purpose of comparing the individual patient to so-called normative values usually derived from angular and millimetric measurements. These analyses depend on significant standardization of values, which is often poorly represented. Measurements often represent conflicting interpretations and do not rationally depict growth patterns known to exist. The generation of numbers derived manually or from a computer does not in itself make cephalometrics a science, and cephalometrics should not necessarily be considered as a science.

A more effective method of assessing skeletal, dental, and soft tissue morphological balance or imbalance is to view the lateral craniofacial radiograph "cephalomorphically," not cephalometrically. Whereby a cephalometric analysis deals with numerical measurements, a *cephalomorphic analysis* can be defined as a strictly nonnumerical approach to the evaluation of craniofacial form and balance. For reasons previously mentioned, many investigators have expressed the *negative* value of a numerical (cephalometric) approach to the diagnostic problem and have expressed the *positive* value of a cephalomorphic (nonnumerical) analysis.[3-5]

CentroGraphic Analysis[6-9]

The primary objective of the *CentroGraphic Analysis* (CGA) is to provide the clinician with the ability to evaluate facial

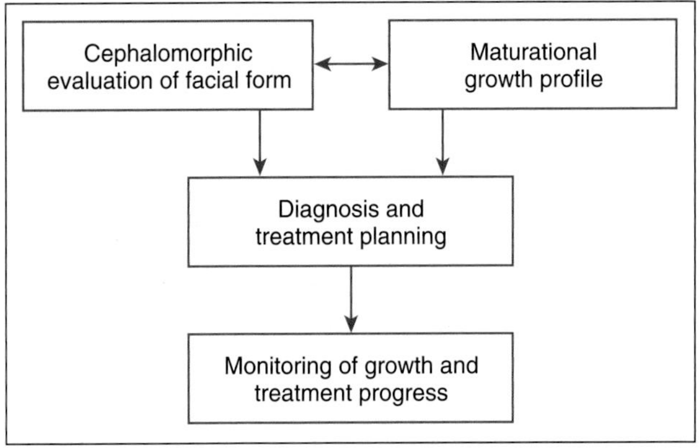

Fig. 3-1 Cephalometric and maturational diagnostic components of treatment planning.

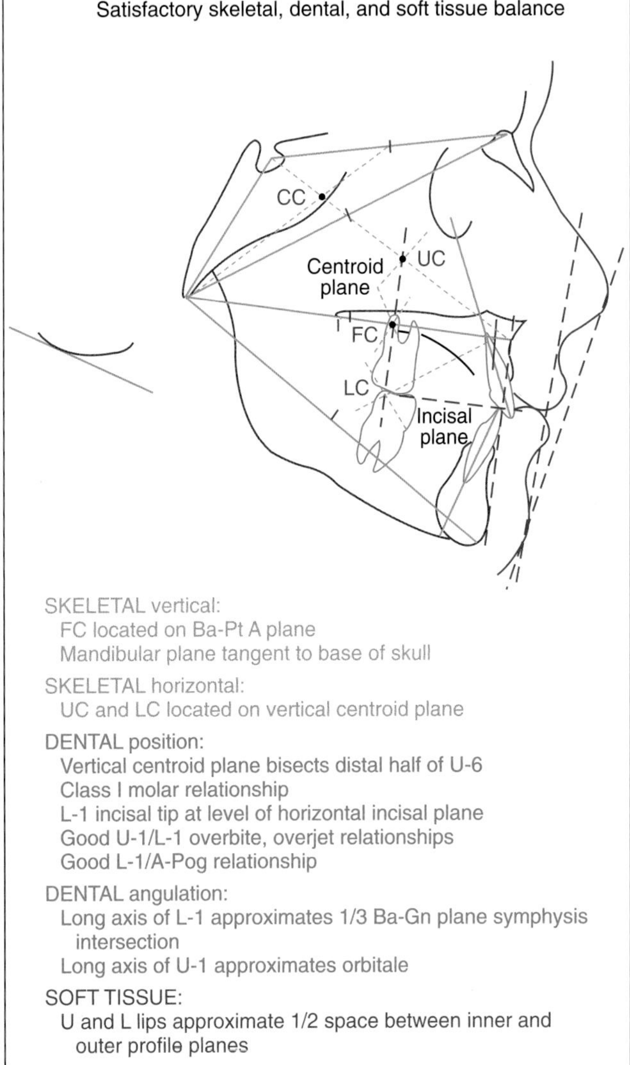

Fig. 3-2 Centrographic Analysis (CGA). Satisfactory skeletal, dental, and soft tissue balance. *CC*, Cranial Centroid; *UC*, Upper Centroid; *LC*, Lower Centroid; *FC*, Facial Centroid; *U*, upper; *L*, lower.

form graphically on an individualized basis without the need for potentially invalid numerical standards of reference (Fig. 3-2). This subjective graphic analysis is based on the principle that similar craniofacial relationships exist in all individuals, regardless of gender, race, or ethnic variation, when skeletal, dental, and soft tissue morphology is in a state of balance and harmony. The selected anatomical areas evaluated by CGA have not been selected on the basis of demonstrating any inherent mechanisms of growth. No numerical values are relevant because even subgroups of individuals do not objectively demonstrate sufficient standardization of facial form. This analysis is concerned with overall facial balance and respects the "natural variability" associated with variations relative to age, ethnicity, race, and gender.

Centroid geometry and facial form

A *centroid* can be defined as the center of mass or gravity as applied to a three-dimensional object or a two-dimensional area. As seen in Figure 3-2, one way of geometrically constructing the centroid of a triangle is by evenly dividing either two or three sides of a triangle and connecting these midpoints with the opposing vertices. The point of intersection of the planes is defined as the "centroid" of the triangle. Because all three planes intersect at exactly the same point, it becomes obvious that only two intersecting planes are required. For this reason, only four planes need to be drawn for this analysis (S-Na, Na-Ba, Ba–Pt A, and Ba-Gn) to achieve the construction of the four required centroids: Cranial, Facial, Upper, and Lower.

The *Cranial Centroid* (CC) is represented by the triangle defined by points *S* (sella), *Na* (nasion), and *Ba* (basion). The *Facial Centroid* (FC) is represented by the total facial triangle defined by points Na, Ba, and *Gn* (gnathion). The *Upper Centroid* (UC) is represented by the triangle defined by points Na, Ba, and *Pt A* (point A). The *Lower Centroid* (LC) is represented by the triangle defined by the point of intersection among the Na-Gn, Ba–Pt A, and Ba-Gn planes.

As the face increases in size with growth, the centroids demonstrate relative stability even though the skeletal triangular areas that they represent increase significantly in size. This relative positional stability of the centroids is the fundamental principle on which CGA is based. In a well-balanced face, after eruption of the first permanent molars, the upper and lower facial areas demonstrate vertical equality or minimal difference in value, as demonstrated by the longitudinal comparison of the posterior facial angles (Na-Ba–Pt A and Pt A–Ba-Gn).

Vertical skeletal evaluation of facial balance is based on the relationship of FC to the Ba–Pt A plane, which is the common border between the upper and lower facial triangles. Centroid geometry dictates that the centroid representing two equal triangles will be located on the side that is common to both triangles. In a vertically well-balanced Caucasian face, FC is located on the Ba–Pt A plane, the common border shared by both upper and lower facial triangles that represents the division between upper and lower facial heights. A vertically deficient lower face is depicted by FC being positioned above the Ba–Pt A plane. A vertically excessive lower face is depicted by FC being positioned below the Ba–Pt A plane. Excessive vertical mandibular growth is also depicted by the mandibular plane being positioned more superiorly within the base of the skull instead of tangent to it.

Horizontal skeletal evaluation of facial balance is based on the relationships of UC and LC to the vertical *Centroid Plane* (CP), which is constructed perpendicular to the Ba–Pt A plane through FC. In a horizontally well-balanced face, UC and/or LC are located on the vertical CP. Protrusive skeletal mandibular and/or maxillary growth is depicted by UC and/or LC being positioned forward to this vertical CP. Retrusive skeletal mandibular and/or maxillary growth is depicted by UC and/or LC being positioned posterior to this vertical CP. Excessive horizontal mandibular growth is also depicted by the mandibular plane falling below the base of skull instead of tangent to it.

For the purpose of dental evaluation of satisfactory balance and harmony, angularly the long axis of the upper incisor is related to orbitale. Excessive proclination of the upper incisor is depicted by the long axis being positioned posterior to orbitale. Incisors that are too upright are depicted by the long axis being positioned anterior to orbitale. Angulation of the lower incisor is evaluated by its relationship to the symphysis, being best positioned when the long axis approximates the one-third mark of the Ba-Gn plane as it crosses the symphysis, thereby providing good bone support for these teeth. The lower incisors are too proclined if the long axis is positioned too far posteriorly within the symphysis and too upright if it is positioned too far anteriorly within the symphysis. Positionally, the labial surface of the lower incisor should approximate or be positioned slightly forward to the Pt A–Pog (pogonion) plane, depending on subjective soft tissue considerations such as thickness of the lips, desired amount of facial soft tissue convexity, and size of the nose and chin. In the well-balanced face, the incisal edge of the lower incisor should approximate the level of the *Incisal Plane,* a line drawn anteriorly from the Lower Centroid (LC) parallel to the Ba–Pt A plane. The upper incisor should positionally and angularly be properly related to the desired overbite and overjet position of the lower incisor.

Soft tissue (ST) profile balance is best evaluated by utilizing both inner (ST Pog–subnasale) and outer (ST Pog–nasal tip) planes together at the same time. This graphically provides a V-shaped area to view. Lips are generally in balance with the rest of the face when both occupy approximately one-half the space within this area. Visualizing the soft tissue profile in this manner helps relating the soft tissue to the underlying skeletal structures. It also allows for a more objective and subjective evaluation of the nose and chin. For example, if the nose or chin is skeletally in balance but the lips are not, the position and size of the nose and chin need to be evaluated.

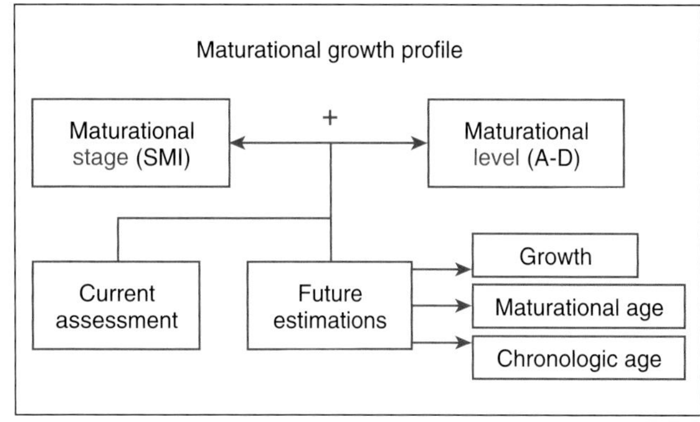

Fig. 3-3 System of Skeletal Maturation Assessment (SMA). *A,* Advanced; *D,* delayed; *SMI,* Skeletal Maturity Indicator.

MATURATIONAL GROWTH PROFILE

Regardless of the treatment mechanics employed, the clinician must responsibly evaluate the maturational profile of the growing patient. Children of the same chronologic age and gender can demonstrate significantly different amounts of growth at varying developmental times. With growth-related problems, there is little justification in formulating a treatment plan that depends exclusively on dental considerations or chronologic age. The clinician cannot ignore the fact that children of the same chronologic age can mature very differently.[10-12]

The *System of Skeletal Maturation Assessment* (SMA) provides the necessary methodology to establish an individualized developmental profile for the patient (Fig. 3-3). This comprehensive system, developed over 30+ years, is easy to learn and provides for both current and future assessments of maxillofacial growth as well as the interrelationships between the patient's maturational and chronologic ages. Information derived from hand-wrist radiographs forms the basis of SMA. Recent interest has focused on evaluating the development of the cervical column, as viewed on lateral cephalometric radiographs, to assess the general stage of maturation. The information derived is diagnostically very limited relative to progressive clinical evaluation and prediction of growth considerations before, during, and after the periods of treatment, including the time of facial skeletal growth cessation.[13,14] The unique SMA approach to the utilization of hand-wrist radiographs thus provides the clinician with individualized patient information that can be directly applied to the timing and nature of treatment.[15]

System of Skeletal Maturation Assessment[16-22]

Identification of a patient's maturational age depends on two mutually important and essential factors: the *stage* of maturation and the *level* of maturation (Fig. 3-3). Other systems judge maturation exclusively on stage of development, as determined by the *Skeletal Maturity Indicator* (SMI) identified on the hand-wrist, cervical, or other radiograph. By not evaluating level of maturation, the clinician is significantly limited in diagnostic and treatment-planning capabilities. The degree by which the individual is advanced, average, or delayed chronologically relative to each SMI represents (1) significantly differing time intervals, (2) differing percentages of total growth completed, (3) differing amounts and rates of incremental growth, and (4) differences in the timing of maxillofacial growth cessation.

Stages of maturation

Development of the hand and wrist follows an orderly progression of skeletal events. The maturational *stage* refers to the highest-ranking SMI found on the hand-wrist radiograph. The *midchildhood* stages (SMIs F-K) of maturation represent a period of low velocity of facial growth (Fig. 3-4).

During *adolescent* development, SMIs 1, 2, and 3 represent a period of accelerating growth rate. SMIs 4 through 7 represent a period of very high growth rate, including the period of peak velocity of development (SMIs 5 and 6). SMIs 8 through 11 represent a period of deceleration in facial growth velocity, resulting in *adulthood,* generally associated with a time of skeletal growth termination.

During the midchildhood to late-childhood period of development, six distinct and progressive ossification events occur that are associated with SMA. These include the appearance and overlapping of the trapezoid and trapezium carpal bones and epiphyseal widening (Fig. 3-5). This *preadolescent* period of development is generally associated with a very low rate of facial growth (see Fig. 3-4).

From the beginning of adolescence to adulthood, the *stage* sequence of developmental events involves 11 main SMIs plus 6 intermediate SMIs. The main adolescent SMIs include completed epiphyseal widening, appearance of the adductor sesamoid of the thumb, bilateral epiphyseal capping, and bilateral epiphyseal-diaphyseal fusion (Fig. 3-6).

The SMI 1-3 period of development is associated with a progressive acceleration of growth rate. As seen in Figure 3-4, the SMI 4-7 period of development is associated with a high growth rate. The SMI 5-6 period is generally associated with the time of peak velocity. The late SMI 8-11 period of development is associated with a progressive deceleration of facial skeletal growth. Adulthood is generally associated with adulthood, a time of skeletal growth termination.

The intermediate SMIs have been selected because of their strong clinical relevance (Fig. 3-7). These transitional stages of maturation include the processes of unilateral epiphyseal capping, midline epiphyseal-diaphyseal fusion of two fingers and midline plus unilateral epiphyseal-diaphyseal fusion, and completed epiphyseal-diaphyseal fusion of the radius. The SMIs are readily identifiable because they are simply identified as transitional bony events that occur between the 11 main adolescent stages.

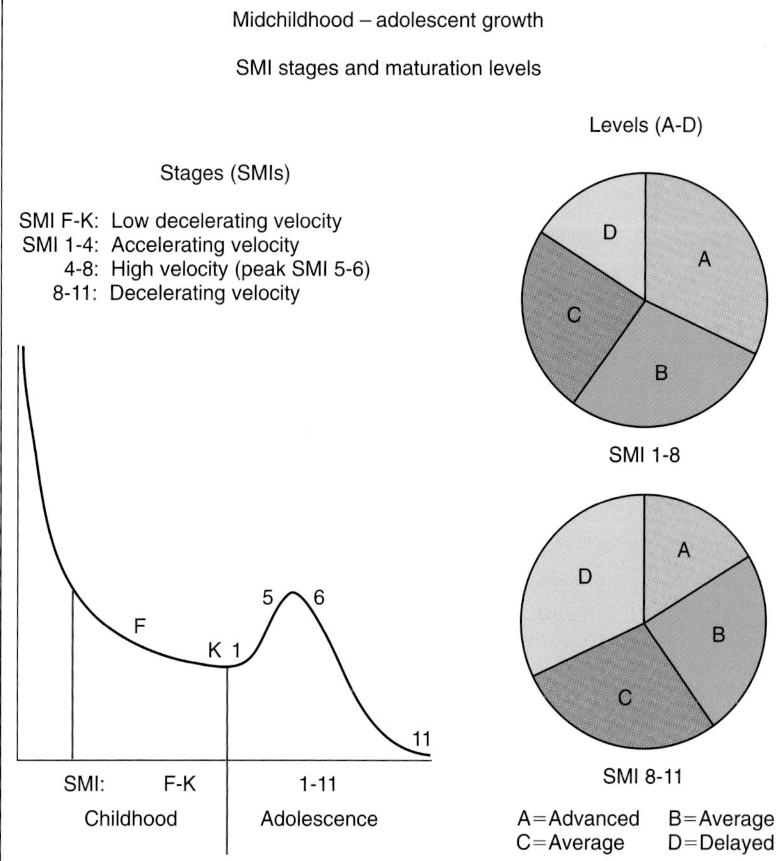

Fig. 3-4 Stages and levels of maturation relative to growth velocity.

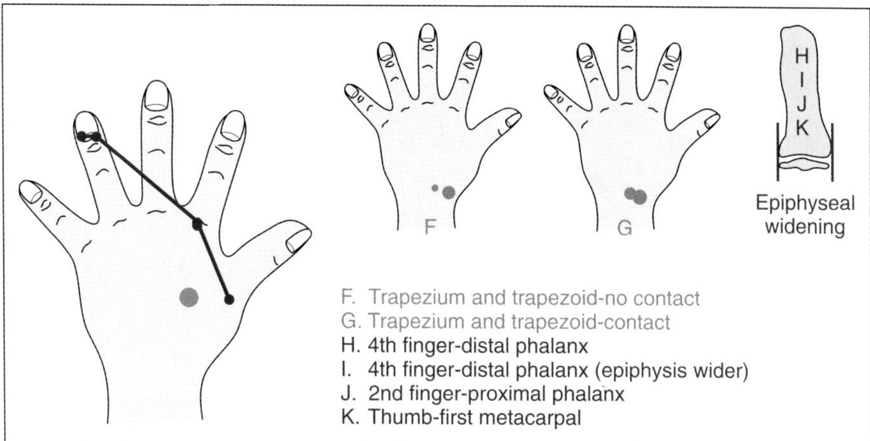

Fig. 3-5 Midchildhood to late-childhood Skeletal Maturity Indicators (SMIs).

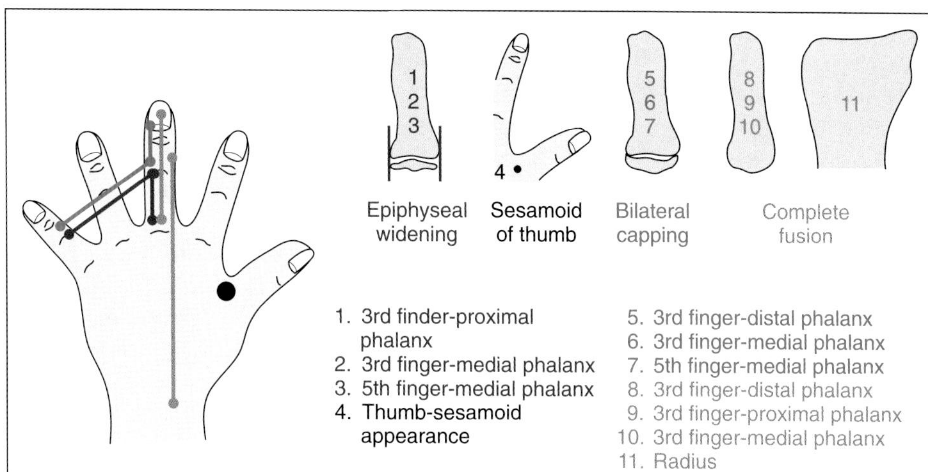

Fig. 3-6 Main adolescent SMIs.

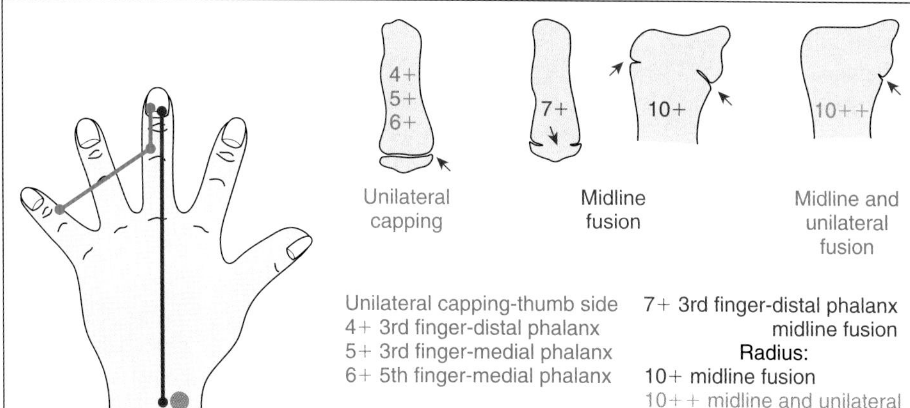

Fig. 3-7 Intermediate adolescent SMIs.

These intermediate SMIs are associated with the periods immediately before, during, and immediately after the time of peak velocity of maxillary and mandibular growth and during the late adolescent period of decelerating growth, when the percentages and the time of total growth completed can be estimated. SMIs 4+, 5+, 6+, and 7+ all occur around the period of very high growth velocity. For many patients, this period of both maxillary and mandibular peak growth rate is a clinically important time when growth modification treatment can be effective. As mentioned previously, chronologic age is not a reliable indicator to determine this developmental timing; changes are occurring rapidly at this time. The late maturational intermediate *stages* 10+ and 10++ are particularly important to identify when craniofacial surgery is planned. Frequently, "delayed (*level* D) maturers" continue to grow during this period, often significantly, and surgical intervention must be delayed. "Advanced (*level* A) maturers" exhibit significantly less growth during this late adolescent period, and therefore surgery can be initiated at an earlier chronologic age.

Levels of maturation

Individuals who demonstrate the same *stage* (SMI) of maturation, as seen on the hand-wrist radiograph, are most likely to demonstrate differing *levels* of maturation; this is a significant clinical factor to consider. For example, as also depicted in Figure 3-4, during most of the developmental process, children of a younger-than-average chronologic age relative to a particular *stage* (SMI) of development are considered "advanced maturers"; they grow more rapidly and quickly than average or delayed individuals up until the time of late adolescence (~SMI 8). These individuals then tend to become developmentally "burnt out" and grow to maturity, but at a slower rate, and demonstrate significantly less incremental skeletal changes and different rates of growth. "Delayed maturers" demonstrate the opposite pattern, demonstrating continued growth over longer periods. With delayed maturers, late adolescence typically lasts longer relative to average or advanced maturers and attempts to "catch up" in terms of the amount of incremental growth. The more advanced or delayed the maturation *level* is from average values, the more evident these varying patterns become.[23-25]

Table 3-1 compares four children (A, B, C, and D) relative to differing *levels* of maturation and their respective chronologic ages and percentages of total mandibular growth completed at SMI *stages* 1, 4, and 11 (adulthood). The chronologically youngest *Patient A* (advanced maturationally) demonstrated the largest percentages of total mandibular growth value. The chronologically oldest *Patient D* (delayed maturationally) demonstrated the smallest percentages of total mandibular growth value. *Patient B* (average but closer to advanced maturationally) and *Patient C* (average but closer to delayed maturationally) demonstrated a progression of this same pattern. The advanced (*level* A) maturer demonstrated the shortest time of adolescent development, and the delayed maturer demonstrated the longest time of adolescent development. Within each maturational *level* subgroup, this same progression of developmental pattern exists, such as when comparing two or more *level* A maturers who have differing chronologic ages.

With factors related to clinical diagnosis and treatment planning, the importance of evaluating both maturational *stage* and maturational *level* together cannot be overemphasized. The clinician must know when, how long, and how much maxillary and mandibular growth will occur in the future for the patient. The time of termination of facial growth varies considerably relative to the maturational *level* but is predictable using SMA.[15]

DIAGNOSIS AND TREATMENT PLANNING

Rational diagnosis and treatment planning for growth-related problems depends on the integration of factors that reveals both the morphological evaluation of facial form and the maturational growth profile of the patient (see Fig. 3-1).

For example, how does the clinician formulate a plan evaluating only the morphological characteristics of the face without knowing how the patient is expected to develop relative to the timing, rates, and amounts of growth during and after treatment? Will growth be terminated during the treatment period, or do significant growth considerations need attention during the retention and postretention periods? Does it make sense to treat similar orthodontic problems the same way if growth considerations demonstrate relevant differences? Does it make sense to judge the nature and timing of treatment strictly on the dentition, when it has been clearly demonstrated that little correlation exists between dental and skeletal development and chronologic age?[26]

In many cases, waiting to initiate treatment for more permanent teeth to erupt excludes treatment that would be more advantageous during the missed-growth periods, such as the need for extraction of teeth. Why does some early treatment work well for one patient and poorly for another?

TABLE 3-1

Examples of Percentages and Amounts of Total Growth Completed Relative to Maturation Levels

	% Total Growth	CA	% Total Growth	CA	% Total Growth	CA	Total Time 1-11
Level	SMI 1		SMI 8		SMI 11		
A	88.71	8.484	97.78	11.251	100	13.074	4.590
B	88.26	9.357	97.19	12.261	100	14.291	4.934
C	87.63	11.302	96.47	14.265	100	17.725	6.426
D	86.83	12.375	95.76	15.267	100	19.442	7.067

CA, Chronologic age; *SMI*, Skeletal Maturity Indicator.

The most important principle always to remember when diagnosing and formulating a treatment plan is that every growing individual demonstrates his or her own unique maturational pattern of development, regardless of chronologic age, gender, facial form, or stage of dentition.

Clinical Examples

To illustrate further the value of this cephalomorphic and biological approach to diagnosis and treatment planning, the following four case examples are presented with select diagnostic and treatment plan options relative to variations in craniofacial form and maturational skeletal development:

Case A

This individual demonstrates a Class II skeletal pattern in which the maxilla and mandible are not harmoniously related to each other (Fig. 3-8). The maxilla (upper face) is positioned too far anteriorly and the mandible (lower face) too far posteriorly, resulting in a convex facial profile. The lower face is deficient in vertical development. All the upper teeth are positioned too far anteriorly, with a resultant excess of anterior overbite and overjet. The upper incisors need to be retracted into a better positional and angular relationship. Because of the deficiency in lower vertical facial development, the lower incisors are positioned too superiorly. The lower incisors need to be uprighted so that they are more satisfactorily supported with bone. Both upper and lower lips are positioned too far anteriorly relative to the nose and chin.

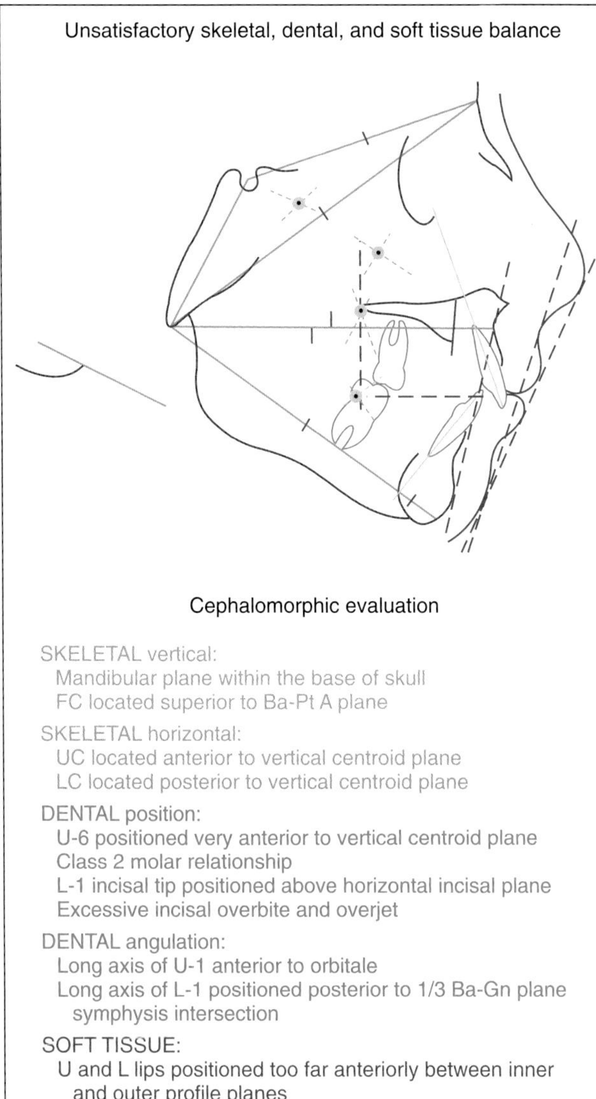

Fig. 3-8 Cephalomorphic evaluation of clinical case A.

As seen in Table 3-2 regarding Case A, to illustrate some of the maxillary and mandibular comparative growth differences between chronologically advanced (*level* A) and delayed (*level* D) patients at four different SMI *stages*, it becomes evident that clinical planning must be modified relative to the patient's specific maturational profile. In these examples the advanced and delayed individuals exhibit approximately a 3- to 6-year difference in chronologic age at the same maturational *stages*, as identified on the hand-wrist radiographs. For example, the 11-year-old advanced maturer would benefit from maxillary headgear treatment at age 9, a high-velocity period of maxillary and mandibular growth (SMI 3), but not at age 11 (SMI 9), a rapidly decelerating–velocity period of growth. The 13-year-old delayed maturer would benefit from maxillary headgear treatment at age 12 (SMI 3) to approximately 15 (SMI 8), a high-velocity period of maxillary and mandibular growth.[18] Extractions may more likely be the treatment of choice in relation to the advanced maturer. The profile is extremely convex in this example. Optimally, treatment should take advantage of more downward and forward mandibular growth and maxillary restriction caused by the headgear effect, whether maxillary headgear, Herbst, or other functional appliance. Because the lower face needs to be developed more vertically, correlating treatment with a high growth rate is important even in cases that demonstrate a vertical growth pattern. Clockwise rotation of the mandible is usually considered to

TABLE 3-2

Case A: Examples of Chronologic Age and Percentages of Total Maxillary and Mandibular Growth Completed Relative to Maturational Stage/Level

	Chronologic Age		Maxilla % Total Growth Completed		Mandible % Total Growth Completed	
SMI	A	D	A	D	A	D
3	8.955	12.790	94.45	91.43	92.53	87.30
6	9.649	14.261	96.53	94.44	93.49	92.52
9	11.305	16.629	99.19	97.47	98.30	96.72
11	13.074	19.442	100	100	100	100

Unsatisfactory skeletal, dental, and soft tissue balance

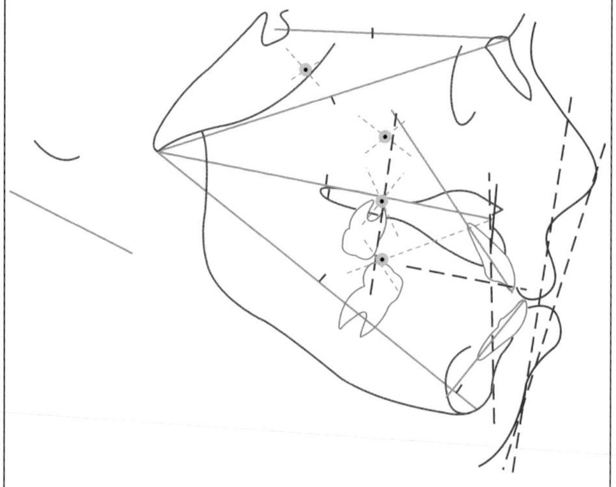

Cephalomorphic evaluation

SKELETAL vertical:
Mandibular plane inferior to base of skull

SKELETAL horizontal:
UC located posterior to vertical centroid plane
LC located anterior to vertical centroid plane

DENTAL position:
U-6 positioned posterior to vertical centroid plane
Class 3 molar relationship
L-1 incisal tip positioned below horizontal incisal plane
Anterior cross-bite, open-bite, negative overbite and overjet
L-1 positioned very anterior to A-pog plane

DENTAL angulation:
Long axis of U-1 very posterior to orbitale
Long axis of L-1 positioned slightly posterior to 1/3 Ba-Gn plane symphysis intersection

SOFT TISSUE:
L-lip positioned anterior to outer profile plane

Fig. 3-9 Cephalomorphic evaluation of clinical case B.

be disadvantageous in a vertical growth pattern, but if properly timed during a high-velocity growth period, it "self-corrects." As also seen in Table 3-2, the advanced maturer continues to demonstrate a higher percentage of total growth completed, which directly translates into more maxillary and mandibular incremental growth at the progressive maturational *stages*.

Case B

This individual demonstrates a Class III skeletal pattern in which the maxilla and mandible are not harmoniously related to each other (Fig. 3-9). The maxilla (upper face) is positioned too far posteriorly and the mandible (lower face) too far anteriorly, resulting in a prognathic mandible, retrusive maxilla, and a comparative soft tissue profile. The lower face demonstrates a horizontal skeletal pattern of growth with some excess in vertical dimension. All the upper teeth are positioned too far posteriorly, with resultant severe negative incisal overjet and associated crossbite relationships. Because of the maxillomandibular skeletal imbalance, the lower incisors are extremely positioned too far anteriorly and inferiorly. In regard to sufficient alveolar bone support, the angulation of the lower incisor is satisfactory at this time. The lower lip is positioned too far anteriorly, resulting in a concave facial profile.

As seen in Table 3-3 regarding Case B, with this example the advanced (*level* A) maturer entered the high-velocity *stage* of skeletal development (SMI 3) at age 9 years, whereas the delayed (*level* D) maturer entered this same period at almost 13 years of age. The advanced maturer completed adolescence at age 13, whereas the delayed maturer reached adulthood after age 19. Because this case requires surgical intervention to establish a more harmonious facial balance, it becomes evident that during late adolescence (SMI 10) the delayed individual demonstrates significantly less total mandibular growth completed than the advanced individual. In this example the advanced maturer became skeletally "burnt out" and exhibited minimal continued maxillary and mandibular growth during this late period compared with the delayed mature individual, who continued to grow skeletally, trying to "catch up." For these reasons, with advanced maturers, surgery often can be initiated at a significantly

TABLE 3-3

Case B: Examples of Chronologic Age and Percentages of Total Maxillary and Mandibular Growth Completed Relative to Maturational Stage/Level

	Chronologic Age		Maxilla % Total Growth Completed		Mandible % Total Growth Completed		S–Pt A		S-Gn	
SMI	A	D	A	D	A	D	A	D	A	D
3	8.955	12.790	94.45	91.43	92.53	87.30	110.0	110.00	123.0	123.0
10	12.260	17.200	99.69	97.53	99.06	97.31	115.76	116.71	131.03	135.31
11	13.074	19.442	100	100	100	100	116.11	119.43	132.19	138.62

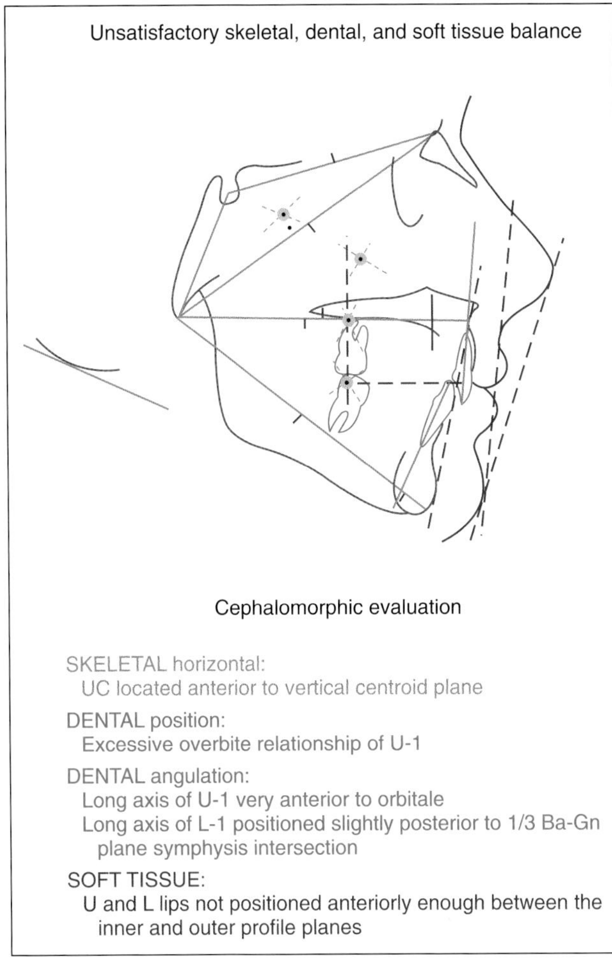

Fig. 3-10 Cephalomorphic evaluation of clinical case C.

earlier chronologic age, even before adulthood is reached. This can provide a much-needed psychological benefit at a relatively young age. For these reasons, intermediate SMI *stages* are used to analyze the projections more definitively.

Case C

This individual demonstrates a Class II skeletal pattern in which the maxilla (upper face) and mandible (lower face) are not harmoniously related to each other (Fig. 3-10). The maxilla is positioned too far anteriorly. The lower face (mandible) is well positioned horizontally and vertically relative to the total face and skull. The molars and lower incisors are generally well positioned, although the location of the lower incisor would be more favorably related to the profile if it was repositioned more labially to the Pt A–Pog plane, resulting in less accentuation of the nose. The upper incisors are positioned too far anteriorly and are in an excessive overbite and overjet relationship. The upper incisors are extremely upright and need to become more procumbent. Even though the maxilla is skeletally positioned too far anteriorly, both upper and lower lips are positioned too retrusively within the two profile planes, indicating that the nose is esthetically too large and prominent.

TABLE 3-4

Case C: Examples of Chronologic Age and Percentages of Total Maxillary and Mandibular Growth Completed Relative to Maturational Stage/Level

	Chronologic Age		Maxilla: % Total Growth Completed		Mandible: % Total Growth Completed	
SMI	A	D	A	D	A	D
2	8.879	12.564	93.85	91.07	91.88	87.24
6	9.649	14.261	96.53	94.44	93.49	92.52
8	11.251	15.267	98.91	97.46	97.78	96.76
11	13.074	19.442	100	100	100	100

As seen in Table 3-4 regarding Case C, the chronologic ages and the percentages of total growth corresponding with the four SMI *stages* demonstrate clearly that basing treatment timing on chronologic age alone is not rational. In the examples shown, peak velocity of facial growth is reached at approximately 9.5 years of age for the advanced maturer (*level* A) and after 14 years of age for the delayed maturer (*level* D). Maxillary headgear or other growth-related treatment would work well with the advanced maturer at SMI 6, but not with the delayed maturer at the same SMI 6 *stage* of development. Such treatment would work well for the delayed maturer at approximately 14 years of age, but not for the advanced maturer, who would have reached adulthood by that age. Growth-related treatment must be maturationally correlated. The percentages of total growth values reflect these significant differences.

Case D

This individual's upper face (maxilla) demonstrates skeletal protrusion (Fig. 3-11). The mandible demonstrates good horizontal balance relative to the total face. A horizontal direction of lower facial growth is evident relative to the mandibular plane's reference to the base of the skull. A balanced vertical skeletal relationship exists between the upper and lower face. The molars are in a moderate Class II relationship. The lower incisors are overerupted into a deep-bite relationship and are also positioned far lingually relative to the skeletal profile. The upper incisors are positioned too far anteriorly, resulting in an extreme overbite and overjet relationship. Because of the incisal pattern, the lower lip is curled and positioned lingually to the upper lip. The relationship between upper and lower lips is unfavorable.

As seen in Table 3-5 regarding Case D, significant growth-related and dental factors contribute to this imbalanced face. If the upper facial skeletal protrusion is to be corrected, growth-related treatment will have to be initiated at approximately chronologic age 10 for the advanced (*level* A) maturer or at approximately age 14 for the delayed (*level* D) matur-

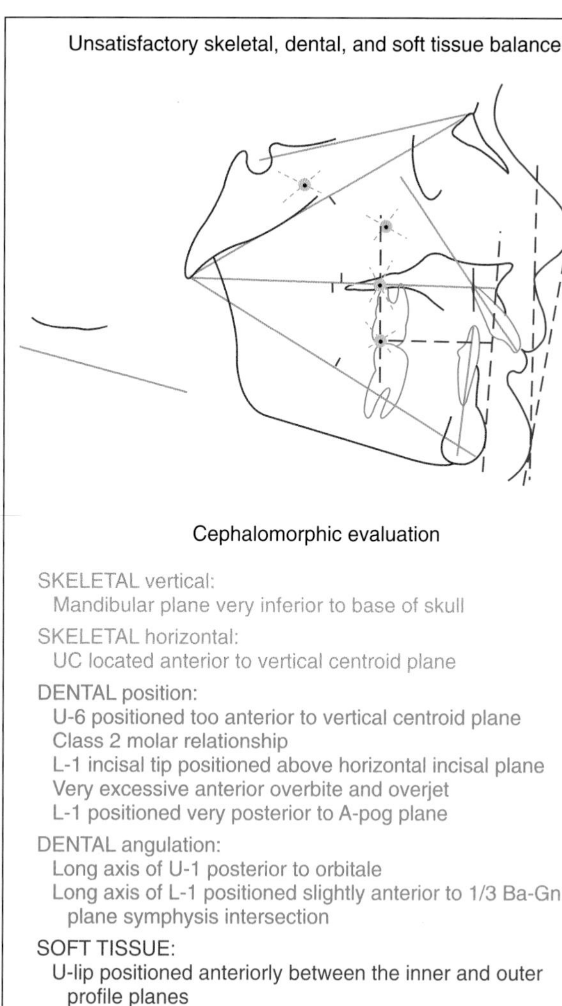

Fig. 3-11 Cephalomorphic evaluation of clinical case D.

ers. Timing treatment maturationally in this manner means it will correlate well with the high-velocity period of facial growth. At age 14 the advanced maturer has already reached adulthood. Initiating treatment that is not correlated with the specific maturational patterns of the patient compromises the result and usually extends the active treatment time. Dentally, the lower incisors need to be depressed and tipped labially. The upper incisors need to be retracted and uprighted. This should improve the soft tissue profile significantly, allowing the upper lip to move posteriorly and the lower lip anteriorly.

MONITORING OF GROWTH AND TREATMENT PROGRESS

When treatment for a particular patient involves significant growth considerations, continued facial development and treatment progress must be carefully monitored. The inherent skeletal patterns exhibited by the patient before treatment most likely will continue until adulthood,[1-3] so it is also often necessary to monitor development up until the time

TABLE 3-5

Case D: Examples of Chronologic Age and Percentages of Total Maxillary and Mandibular Growth Completed Relative to Maturational Stage/Level

	Chronologic Age		Maxilla % Total Growth Completed		Mandible % Total Growth Completed	
SMI	A	D	A	D	A	D
3	10.007	14.414	94.45	91.43	92.53	87.30
5	10.641	15.418	95.98	93.67	92.83	91.74
8	13.093	17.202	98.91	97.46	97.78	95.76
11	14.388	20.096	100	100	100	100

of growth termination. Thus it is often prudent to continue growth modification into the retention phase of treatment.

Superimpositions

To depict the effects of treatment and growth over time, the CentroGraphic Analysis (CGA) provides a rational means of superimposition of radiographic head plates. Downward and forward growth of the jaws and changes within the cranial base caused primarily by growth at the spheno-occipital suture are depicted. Nasion (Na) moves upward and forward; basion (Ba) moves downward and backward.

As shown in Fig. 3-12, two or more serial tracings are superimposed on their respective Facial Centroid Axes (FCAs) and registered on the Cranial Centroid (CC). The *Facial Centroid Axis* (FCA) is defined as a plane formed between the CC and gnathion (Gn). Experience has demonstrated that this method of superimposition is the most satisfactory method for depicting total facial changes relative to growth and treatment results.

CentroPrints

The CentroPrint shows the clinician diagrammatically how treatment is progressing. Figure 3-13 represents a serial CentroPrint of a typical Class II patient exhibiting skeletal maxillary protrusion, a Class II molar relationship, lack of vertical development of the lower face, deep anterior bite, excessive overjet and overbite, and a soft tissue profile that is convex with the lower lip "rolled" under the upper anterior teeth. The patient's maturational age was SMI 1-A at the start of treatment, which represents a period of accelerating velocity of maxillary and mandibular growth. Treatment involved a maxillary headgear, with the outer arms adjusted to increase vertical development of the lower face and to hold the upper molars in place while the mandible grew downward and forward. Treatment also included a utility arch to depress the lower anterior teeth and upright the lower molars to

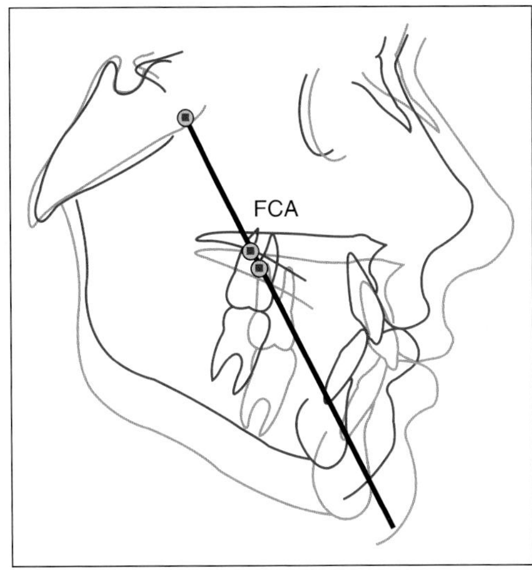

Fig. 3-12 CentroGraphic superimposition on Facial Centroid Axis (FCA).

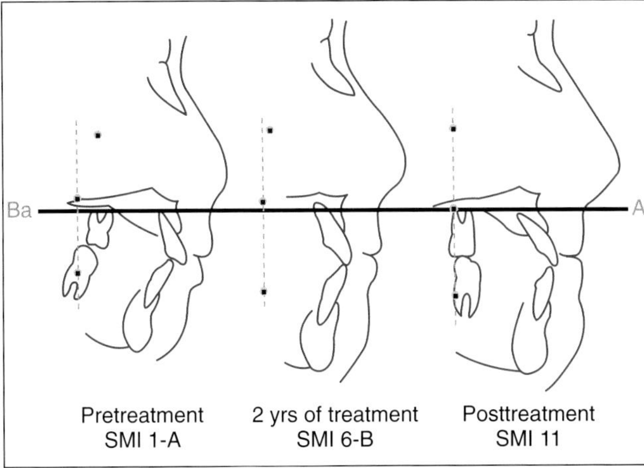

Fig. 3-13 CentroPrint evaluation of serial growth and treatment changes.

increase further the vertical dimension of the lower face. In this case, disadvantageous clockwise rotation of the mandible is transient (not permanent) because of the self-correction associated with the upcoming very-high-velocity period of growth (SMI 4-7). The CentroPrint in Fig. 3-13 demonstrates the following:

- Progressive vertical development of the lower face
- Skeletal influence of the headgear on establishing a more harmonious maxillary-to-mandibular relationship
- Establishment of a Class I molar relationship
- Reduction of excessive dental overbite and overjet
- Positional and angular incisor corrections and improvement of the soft tissue profile

The CentroPrint is a valuable clinical aid for periodically evaluating the progress of orthodontic treatment.

CONCLUSION

Diagnosis and treatment planning require an individualized evaluation of every orthodontic patient. Because every patient demonstrates his or her own unique patterns of morphological and maturational development, the orthodontist is obligated to recognize these variations and to apply developmental factors directly to the timing and type of clinical treatment. Even individuals of the same chronologic and dental age typically demonstrate wide variations in skeletal maturation and facial morphology. For these physiological and clinical reasons, the cephalomorphic CentroGraphic Analysis (CGA) and Skeletal Maturation Assessment (SMA) have been developed and are routinely applied in a coordinated manner to achieve a rational case analysis. Both of these diagnostic techniques have proved to be easy to learn and apply.

References

1. Brodie A: On the growth of the jaws and the eruption of the teeth, *Angle Orthod* 12:109-123, 1942.
2. Nanda RS: The rates of growth of several facial components measured from serial cephalometric roentgenograms, *Am J Orthod* 41:658-673, 1975.
3. Brodie A: Facial patterns, *Angle Orthod* 16:75-87, 1946.
4. Moss ML: The dialectics of craniofacial growth research: it is time for a new synthesis. In McNamara JA, Carlson DS, Ribbens KA, editors: *The effects of surgical intervention on craniofacial growth*, Monograph 12, Craniofacial Growth Series, Ann Arbor, 1982, Center for Human Growth and Development, University of Michigan.
5. Enlow DH: Craniofacial growth mechanisms: normal and disturbed. In McNamara JA, Carlson DS, Ribbens KA, editors: *The effects of surgical intervention on craniofacial growth*, Monograph 12, Craniofacial Growth Series, Ann Arbor, 1982, Center for Human Growth and Development, University of Michigan.
6. Fishman LS: Individualized evaluation of facial form, *Am J Orthod Dentofacial Orthop* 111:510-517, 1997.
7. Keim RG: Achieving facial harmony through orthodontics, *J Cal Dent Soc* 30:825-830, 2002.
8. Dolce C, Schader RE, McGorray SP, Wheeler TT: Centrographic analysis of 1-phase versus 1-phase treatment for Class II malocclusion, *Am J Orthod Dentofacial Orthop* 121:195-200, 2005.
9. Fishman LS: Misinterpretation of centrographic analysis and Class II treatment, *Am J Orthod Dentofacial Orthop* 122:321-322, 2006.
10. Nanda RS, Dandajena T: The role of headgear in growth modification, *Semin Orthod* 12:25-33, 2006.
11. Fishman LS: Chronologic versus skeletal age: an evaluation of craniofacial growth, *Angle Orthod* 49:51-63, 1979.
12. Houston WJ: Relationships between skeletal maturity estimated from hand-wrist radiographs and the timing of the adolescent growth spurt, *Eur J Orthod* 2:81-93, 1980.
13. Grave K, Townsend G: Hand-wrist and cervical vertebral maturation indicators: how can these events be used to time Class II treatments? *Aust Orthod* 19:33-45, 2003.

14. Baccetti T, Franchi L, McNamara JA: An improved version of the cervical vertebral maturation (CVM) method for the assessment of mandibular growth, *Angle Orthod* 72:316-323, 2002.
15. www.GrowthTek.com.
16. Fishman LS: Radiographic evaluation of skeletal maturation, a clinically oriented study based on hand-wrist films, *Angle Orthod* 52: 88-112, 1982.
17. Fishman LS: Maturational patterns and prediction during adolescence, *Angle Orthod* 57:178-193, 1987.
18. Kopecki GR, Fishman LS: Timing of cervical headgear treatment based on skeletal maturation, *Am J Orthod Dentofacial Orthop* 104:162-169, 1993.
19. Flores-Mir C, Nebbe B, Major PW: Use of skeletal maturation based on hand-wrist radiographic analysis as a predictor of facial growth: a systematic review, *Angle Orthod* 74:118-124, 2004.
20. Subtelny JD: Early orthodontic treatment. In Fishman LS, editor: *Maturational development and facial form relative to treatment timing,* Carol Stream, Ill, 2000, Quintessence, pp 265-285.
21. Fishman LS: Readers forum: can cephalometric x-rays of the cervical column be used instead of hand-wrist x-rays to determine a patient's maturational age? *Am J Orthod Dentofacial Orthop* 122:18A-19A, 2002.
22. Revelo B, Fishman LS: Maturational evaluation of ossification of the midpalatal suture, *Am J Orthod Dentofacial Orthop* 105:288-292, 1994.
23. Burstone CI: Process of maturation and growth prediction, *Am J Orthod* 49:907-919, 1963.
24. Fishman LS: Discovering the uniqueness of the individual, *Am J Orthod Dentofacial Orthop* 99:20A-21A, 1991.
25. Silveira AM, Fishman LS, Subtelny JD, Kassebaum DK: Facial growth during adolescence in early, average and late maturers, *Angle Orthod* 62:185-189, 1992.
26. So LL: Skeletal maturation of the hand and wrist and its correlation with dental development, *Aust Orthod J* 15:1-9, 1997.

CHAPTER 4

Occlusal Patterns in Orthodontic Patients: Using the Occlusal Force Measuring System

Yukio Kitafusa

The purpose of orthodontic treatment is to prevent and improve functional malocclusion so that comprehensive and effective masticatory function can be established.[1] The physiological importance of the stomatognathic system is indispensable for normal structure and function. Studies have shown that malocclusion patients have lower masticatory function than patients with normal occlusion,[2,3] resulting in a general decrease in oral function caused by occlusal disharmony, less occlusal force and chewing ability, and other issues. The reasons why subjects with malocclusion have poorer masticatory performance are not completely understood. However, three factors that might influence masticatory performance are (1) the number and area of occlusal contacts, (2) occlusal forces as reflected by maximum bite force, and (3) the amount of lateral excursion during mastication. Masticatory function can be improved by orthodontic treatment, but it is extremely difficult to measure the degree of improvement.

To better evaluate the effectiveness of treatment, the focus of diagnosis should be more on *occlusal force* and *occlusal contacts*. The investigation of occlusal force began with Borelli's mandibular force meter[4] in 1681 and was followed by various other studies. The predominant methods for measuring occlusal force are (1) cantilever,[5] (2) oil pressure, (3) Brinnel hardness,[6] (4) electricity,[7,8] (5) T-scan,[9] and (6) Prescale.[10,11] Dahlberg[12] reported that there are 32 points of occlusal contact area (26 in molar region). Hellman[13] measured the contact areas at centric occlusion and described 138 contact points in an ideal occlusion by classifying (1) the contact condition, (2) the contact with cusp and fissure, (3) the contact with marginal ridge and interdental embrasure, and (4) the contact with marginal ridge and fissure.

A recent shift in the interpretation of occlusal force has resulted from the "T-scan" system and its use with image-analysis technology. The T-scan system is an occlusal measuring device that was created by Maness et al.[14] in 1987. Its primary application is in measuring the differences in electrical resistance, which is representative of occlusal force. However, Patyk et al.[15] reported that the sensor of the T-scan system is thick and tends to dislocate the mandible because of the inherent flexibility in the system. Also, the T-scan system has a narrow measurement range for occlusal force, as well as varying sensitivity at different measurement locations within that range. However, the recent development of the Dental Prescale Occluzer System (Fuji Film, Tokyo, Japan) allows for easy measurements of occlusal contact areas and pressures in occlusion. This system is used widely in Japanese orthodontics. Uchiyama et al.[16] confirmed a high rate of reproduction and reliability in the occlusal contact area measurement taken by this system. Nagai et al.[17] reported that pressure-sensitive sheets are useful in the study of occlusal status of mandibular prognathism. Also, Asano et al.[18] obtained reliable results using the system when examining the change in occlusal force and contact areas during retention.

This chapter addresses the evaluation of occlusal patterns, especially occlusal contact areas and pressures in orthodontic patients, using the Dental Prescale Occluzer System.

DENTAL PRESCALE OCCLUZER SYSTEM

The Dental Prescale Occluzer System consists of pressure-sensitive sheets (Dental Prescale), an analyzing computer (Occluzer), and a data-saving computer (Macintosh Power Book) (Figs. 4-1 and 4-2). The density of color formation on the pressure-sensitive sheets depends on the level of pressure applied. The color formations on the sheets are read by the Occluzer with a color-imaging scanner. The magnitude of occlusal pressure and force is estimated by examining the identified color density and area data.[19]

Prescale Sheet Design

The Dental Prescale incorporates a monosheet design. First, a developer solution is coated over a base layer of polyethylene terephthalate (PET) film. Microcapsules of various dimensions that contain color former are uniformly distributed across this developer layer. Both sides are then vacuum-wrapped in an ultrathin layer of PET film. Special measures are taken throughout the manufacturing process to ensure that each Dental Prescale sheet is completely sterile.

When the Prescale sheet is subjected to pressure, the microcapsules break and release a colorless, clear leuco (white) dye. This dye reacts with the developer layer and turns red. Because the microcapsules can withstand various pressures, depending on their size and thickness, the shade and intensity of the dye will vary with the amount of pressure applied to the Prescale sheet; greater pressure yields deeper color. Large and thin microcapsules break when subjected to relatively low pressure, whereas small and thick microcapsules only break when subjected to greater pressure. The shade of red produced darkens in proportion to the number of capsules that break.[19]

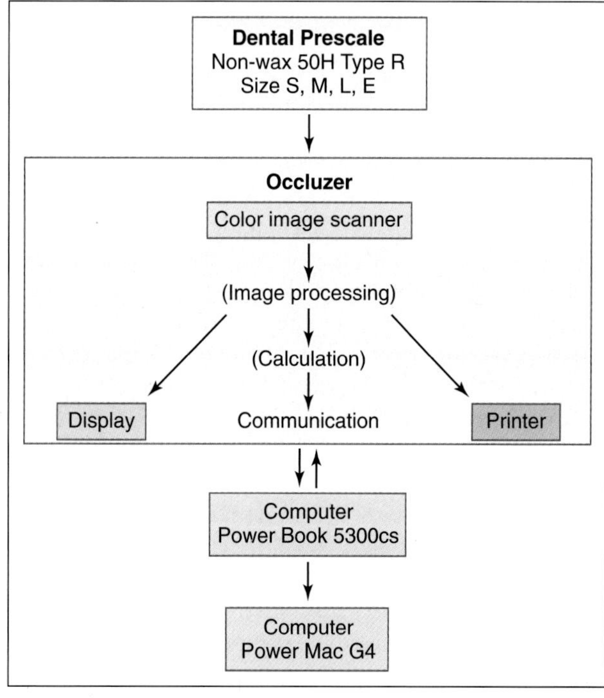

Fig. 4-1 Diagram of Dental Prescale Occluzer System.

Occlusal Force Measuring System

The Occluzer FPD-703 (Fuji Film), an occlusal force measuring system, consists of a scanner, treating board, monitor, thermal printer, and mouse. Measuring begins when the Prescale image is scanned into the computer. The computer then reads the color formation (information provided by Prescale) at 100 dots per inch (dpi) and identifies data with the treating board. The process is completed when the information is expressed in analog data form.

The Dental Prescale 50H Type R (Fuji Film) used in this study is horseshoe shaped so that it fits on the dental arch. There are four sizes available: S, M, L, and E.

In previous studies, modeling compounds,[20] a shellac bite plate,[21,22] and a silicone block[23] were used to mark the occlusal contacts. The Dental Prescale is more precise and convenient than these methods. Type R is more precise and thicker than Type W. Moreover, only the contact area between upper and lower teeth is marked in Type R.

Analysis

Analyzing the results of the Dental Prescale involves the following measurements:

- *Occlusal contact area* ("Area") is the area color-formatted by the Prescale. Low occlusal forces cannot be calculated under the measuring range of the Prescale. The units are given in square millimeters (mm^2).
- *Average occlusal pressure* ("Average" ["Ave"]) is the occlusal force per unit area, expressed in megapascals (MPa).
- *Occlusal force* ("Force"). is calculated by multiplying average occlusal pressure and occlusal contact area. The units are given in newtons (N); 1 N ≅ 0.1 kilogram-force (kgf).

When using the Dental Prescale, the subject sits in the dental chair in a relaxed position. After a "warm-up" that

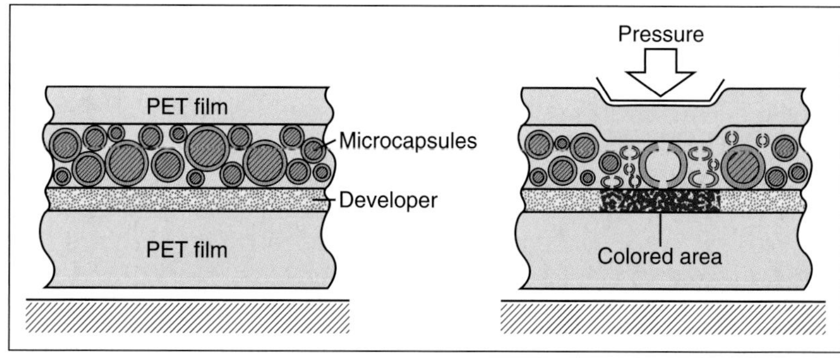

Fig. 4-2 Structure of Dental Prescale pressure-sensitive sheet and mechanism of color formation. *PET,* Polyethylene terephthalate.

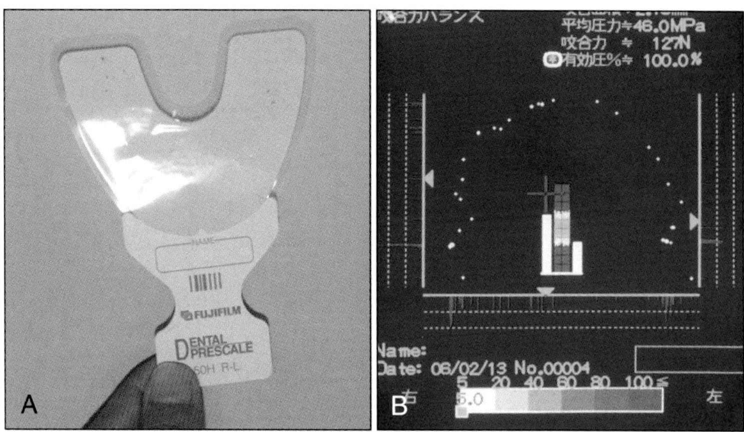

Fig. 4-3 **A,** Dental Prescale pressure-sensitive sheet. **B,** Sample data displayed on analyzing computer.

consists of mild to strong biting two or three times, the patient is directed to bite the Prescale sheet (Fig. 4-3, *A*) only once and hold the bite for 5 seconds. The Prescale sheet is then inserted into the Occluzer to analyze the data (Macintosh Power Book5300cs, Power Mac G4), the occlusal contact areas (mm^2), pressure on each occlusal contact area (MPa), and all the occlusal forces (N) (Fig. 4-3, *B*).

CLINICAL STUDY

Subjects

In this clinical study, subjects with different malocclusions and various facial patterns were selected from incoming patients at the Kitafusa Orthodontic Clinic (Asahi, Chiba, Japan). Subjects with normal occlusion were chosen from office staff and their friends. These subjects had no missing or decayed teeth and had not undergone any orthodontic or prosthodontic treatment. The normal-occlusion subjects displayed a Class I molar relationship, as defined by Angle classification.

Normal-occlusion and malocclusion subjects were distributed as shown in Table 4-1. Subjects with maxillary protrusion were classified into two types: those with greater than 5 mm of overbite ("ov" [over] type), and those with less than 5 mm of overbite ("un" [under] type). Cephalometric analyses were done for all the patients (Table 4-2). Facial angles measured were facial axis (FX), facial depth (FD), mandibular plane (MP), and mandibular arc (MA). Lower facial height (LFH) and total facial height (TFH) were also measured). Facial patterns were classified according to the Ricketts method (Table 4-3) and analyzed cephalometrically (Table 4-4).

Methods

Biting force was recorded for subjects with normal occlusion, subjects with various malocclusions, and subjects representing the seven facial patterns using the pressure-sensitive sheets (Dental Prescale 50H Type R). The data obtained were classified for each group, and statistical analysis was performed using Microsoft Excel 8.0. Data from each group of normal-occlusion and malocclusion subjects and facial pattern subjects were tested by the Stat-View J 5.0. One-way Factorial Analysis of Variance (ANOVA) and Multiple Comparison tests and the Scheffe method were used later to determine significant differences among groups.

TABLE 4-1

Distribution of Normal Occlusion and Malocclusion in Dental Prescale Subjects

Normal/Malocclusion	Number	Average Age
Normal occlusion	10	14.10 ± 4.27
Crowding	21	12.73 ± 7.12
Mandibular protrusion	19	10.96 ± 4.27
Maxillary protrusion (ov)	18	12.79 ± 5.52
Maxillary protrusion (un)	10	14.21 ± 7.63
Lateral crossbite	5	13.20 ± 7.10
Open bite	20	12.51 ± 5.25
TOTAL	103	12.93 ± 7.30

ov, Greater than ("over") 5 mm overbite; *uv*, less than ("under") 5 mm overbite.

Results

The occlusal patterns in subjects with normal occlusion and in those with malocclusions were analyzed. Table 4-5 and Figure 4-4 shows the average value of occlusal contact areas ("Area"), average occlusal pressure on occlusal contacts ("Average"/"Ave"), and all the occlusal force ("Force" = "Ave" × "Area"). The results are as follows:

1. **Normal-occlusion group.** Values of "Area" and "Force" were highest when compared with each malocclusion group. However, "Average" was not significantly higher but rather was similar to the average values.
2. **Mandibular protrusion group.** Despite values of "Average" being the lowest, "Area" was the highest in the

TABLE 4-2

Cephalometric Data of Facial Angles in Dental Prescale Study Subjects: Average ± SD (degrees)

Normal/Malocclusion	FX	FD	MP	LFH	MA	TFH
Normal occlusion	86.52 ± 2.98	84.30 ± 3.43	29.64 ± 3.62	46.44 ± 1.50	31.82 ± 4.81	58.50 ± 2.11
Crowding	84.46 ± 4.25	84.41 ± 3.05	32.39 ± 4.66	48.22 ± 4.17	33.30 ± 4.18	61.14 ± 4.56
Mandibular protrusion	89.24 ± 3.23	87.60 ± 4.27	28.39 ± 5.99	44.67 ± 4.08	33.80 ± 6.96	57.32 ± 4.58
Maxillary protrusion (ov)	83.84 ± 2.54	83.46 ± 2.55	31.43 ± 3.10	46.30 ± 3.32	34.88 ± 2.64	58.72 ± 3.49
Maxillary protrusion (un)	85.34 ± 3.75	85.28 ± 2.20	31.66 ± 4.55	45.03 ± 3.80	31.53 ± 4.98	59.93 ± 4.23
Lateral crossbite	83.12 ± 5.49	85.46 ± 2.74	34.54 ± 4.41	49.68 ± 5.06	29.18 ± 6.63	65.20 ± 4.85
Open bite	83.26 ± 5.55	85.45 ± 3.26	33.70 ± 5.87	51.47 ± 5.88	31.00 ± 4.58	64.09 ± 6.04

SD, Standard deviation; *FX,* facial axis angle; *FD,* facial depth angle; *MP,* mandibular plane angle; *LFH,* lower facial height; *MA,* mandibular arc angle; *TFH,* total facial height.

TABLE 4-3

Distribution of Facial Patterns in Dental Prescale Study Subjects

Pattern	Number	Average Age
Severe dolichofacial	17	13.23 ± 2.77
Dolichofacial (dolicho)	19	12.25 ± 3.70
Mesiofacial, tendency to dolichofacial	17	13.37 ± 8.23
Mesiofacial (mesio)	19	11.38 ± 6.51
Mesiofacial, tendency to brachyfacial	22	11.33 ± 4.74
Brachyfacial (brachy)	13	12.45 ± 6.99
Severe brachyfacial	17	12.44 ± 4.81
TOTAL	124	12.35 ± 5.39

mandibular protrusion group after the normal-occlusion group. "Force" also was highest in this group after the normal-occlusion group.

3. **Crowding group.** "Area" and "Force" showed high values in the crowding malocclusion group similar to the mandibular protrusion group. "Average" was lowest, after the mandibular protrusion group.
4. **Maxillary protrusion group.** In "Area" and "Force" the maxillary protrusion ("un") and maxillary protrusion ("ov") groups had significantly different values. The "un" was near average in all groups and was higher than "ov" in "Area" and "Force." However, the "Average" for "ov" was near average and higher than for "un."
5. **Lateral crossbite group.** "Average" was highest after the normal-occlusion group, and "Area" and "Force" were second lowest in value.
6. **Open-bite group.** "Area" and "Force" were lowest in all subject groups; however, "Average" was highest in all groups.

To summarize the results, force decreased in the following order: normal occlusion, mandibular protrusion, crowding, maxillary protrusion (un), lateral crossbite, maxillary protrusion (ov), and open bite.

Table 4-6 lists the statistical data for the significant differences among normal-occlusion and malocclusion groups.

Within occlusal contact area, normal occlusion vs. open bite, crowding vs. open bite, and mandibular protrusion vs. open bite displayed significant differences. Within average pressure, no significant differences were recognized. Within occlusal force, normal occlusion vs. maxillary protrusion (ov), normal occlusion vs. open bite, crowding vs. open bite, and mandibular protrusion vs. open bite, there were significant differences.

Table 4-7 and Figure 4-5 show the average values of "Area," "Average," and "Force" among the different facial pattern groups, as follows:

1. **Severe dolichofacial** *(dolicho)* **pattern.** "Area" and "Force" were the lowest of all groups. "Average" was slightly higher than the average value.
2. **Dolichofacial pattern** ("dolicho"). This type of pattern showed second lowest on "Area" and "Force". "Average" showed the highest in all groups.
3. **Mesiofacial** *(mesio)* **pattern tendency to dolichofacial.** "Area" and "Force" showed third lowest. "Average" showed almost the same as severe dolichofacial pattern.
4. **Mesiofacial pattern.** "Area", "Average", and "Force" were midway between the high and low positions.
5. **Mesiofacial pattern tendency to brachyfacial** *(brachy).* "Area" and "Force" were the third highest of all groups. "Average" was almost near to average values.
6. **Brachyfacial pattern** ("brachy"). "Area" was almost the same as the severe brachy pattern, but was the highest value of all groups. "Average" was the lowest of all groups, and "Force" was second highest.
7. **Severe brachyfacial pattern.** "Force" was the highest of all groups. "Area" was nearly as high as brachyfacial pattern. "Average" was close to average.

Table 4-8 shows the statistical data of significant differences among facial pattern groups.

Within occlusal contact area

The following facial pattern subjects displayed significant differences within the occlusal contact area ("Area"):

- Severe brachy pattern vs. mesio pattern tendency to dolicho
- Severe brachy pattern vs. dolicho pattern

TABLE 4-4

Cephalometric Data of Facial Patterns in Dental Prescale Subjects: Average ± SD (Degrees)

Pattern	FX	FD	MP	LFH	MA	TFH
Severe dolichofacial	82.64 ± 5.74	84.17 ± 3.03	35.40 ± 5.98	50.60 ± 6.72	30.86 ± 5.47	63.97 ± 7.09
Dolichofacial (dolicho)	84.91 ± 3.70	84.09 ± 2.79	33.11 ± 4.54	48.46 ± 4.31	31.41 ± 4.10	60.69 ± 4.31
Mesio, tendency to dolicho	83.22 ± 4.08	83.74 ± 2.82	34.52 ± 4.25	49.08 ± 3.19	31.57 ± 4.80	62.79 ± 4.74
Mesiofacial (mesio)	83.66 ± 3.22	83.64 ± 2.45	32.88 ± 2.94	47.87 ± 3.93	29.86 ± 4.86	62.64 ± 3.50
Mesio, tendency to brachy	87.45 ± 2.88	87.26 ± 3.74	29.79 ± 2.99	46.20 ± 1.99	32.11 ± 4.30	59.33 ± 2.78
Brachyfacial (brachy)	86.47 ± 2.96	85.58 ± 2.64	29.09 ± 3.13	45.73 ± 3.23	34.37 ± 3.24	58.37 ± 3.11
Severe brachyfacial	90.72 ± 3.30	88.67 ± 3.06	24.95 ± 3.49	41.05 ± 2.33	38.74 ± 3.48	53.73 ± 2.38

SD, Standard deviation; *FX*, facial axis angle; *FD*, facial depth angle; *MP*, mandibular plane angle; *LFH*, lower facial height; *MA*, mandibular arc angle; *TFH*, total facial height.

TABLE 4-5

Occluzer Values of Facial Angles in Dental Prescale Subjects

	Contact Area (mm²)		Pressure (MPa)		Occlusal Force (N)	
Normal/Malocclusion	Average	SD	Average	SD	Average	SD
Normal occlusion	8.48	2.67	51.09	7.71	423.27	113.92
Mandibular protrusion	7.60	3.80	46.13	6.79	348.91	172.02
Crowding	7.49	3.58	46.95	5.39	346.10	154.16
Maxillary protrusion (un)	6.04	3.12	47.22	5.32	281.46	141.22
Lateral crossbite	4.80	1.80	51.12	10.28	245.62	104.22
Maxillary protrusion (ov)	4.70	3.25	50.14	8.80	222.37	146.79
Open bite	3.33	1.36	52.16	6.02	170.92	68.74
AVERAGE	5.64	2.11	50.03	3.12	273.32	94.97

MPa, Megapascals; *N*, newtons (1 N ≅ 0.1 kg-force); *SD*, standard deviation.

- Severe brachy pattern vs. severe dolicho pattern
- Brachy pattern vs. mesio pattern tendency to dolicho
- Brachy pattern vs. dolicho pattern
- Brachy pattern vs. severe dolicho pattern
- Mesio pattern tendency to brachy vs. dolicho pattern
- Mesio pattern tendency to brachy vs. severe dolicho pattern
- Mesio pattern vs. dolicho pattern
- Mesio pattern vs. severe dolicho pattern

Within average pressure

The following facial pattern subjects displayed significant differences within average pressure ("Average"):

- Brachy pattern vs. dolicho pattern
- Mesio pattern tendency to brachy vs. dolicho pattern
- Mesio pattern vs. dolicho pattern

Within occlusal force

The following facial pattern subjects displayed significant differences within occlusal force ("Force"):

- Severe brachy pattern vs. mesio pattern tendency to dolicho
- Severe brachy pattern vs. mesio pattern tendency to dolicho
- Severe brachy pattern vs. dolicho pattern
- Severe brachy pattern vs. severe dolicho pattern
- Brachy pattern vs. mesio pattern tendency to dolicho
- Brachy pattern vs. dolicho pattern
- Brachy pattern vs. severe dolicho pattern
- Mesio pattern tendency to brachy vs. dolicho pattern
- Mesio pattern tendency to brachy vs. severe dolicho pattern
- Mesio pattern vs. dolicho pattern
- Mesio pattern vs. severe dolicho pattern
- Mesio pattern tendency to dolicho vs. severe dolicho pattern

Discussion

Previously, Yurkstas and Manly[24] measured effective occlusal contact area using comparameter and Photovolt reflectometer with wax registration; the average effective occlusal area was 48.4 mm² for subjects with complete dentition. Araki et al.,[25] using the Dental Prescale with five

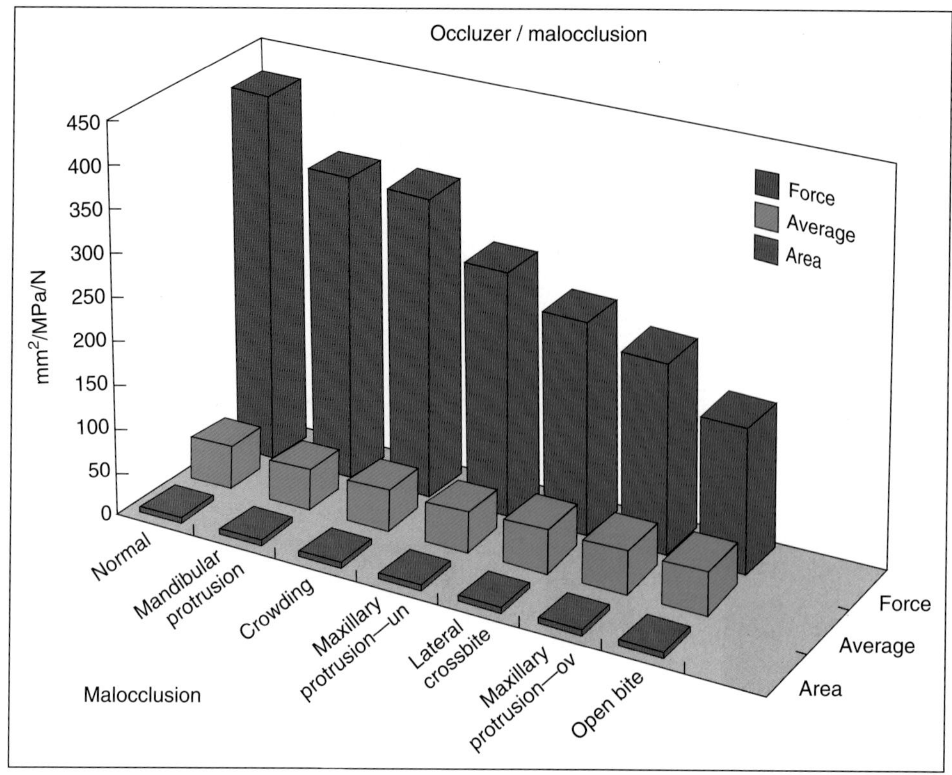

Fig. 4-4 Occluzer values of normal subjects and groups with malocclusion. *un*, Under 5 mm overbite; *ov*, over 5 mm overbite; *MPa*, megapascals; *N*, newtons.

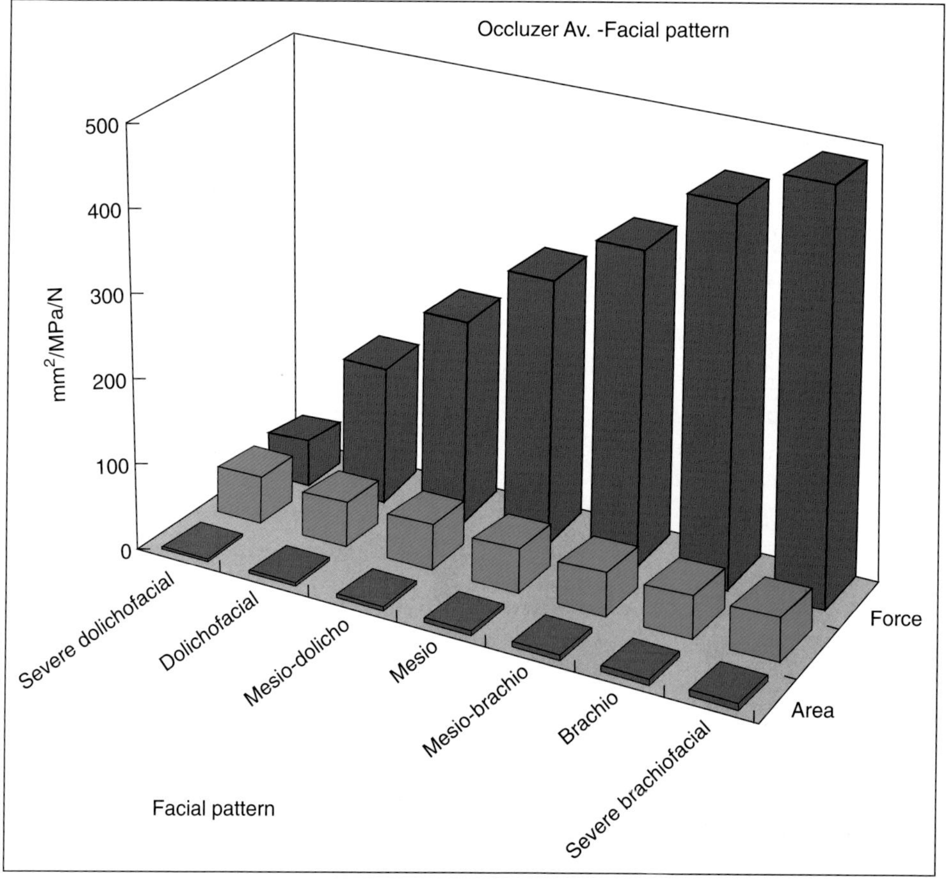

Fig. 4-5 Occluzer values of facial patterns. *MPa*, Megapascals; *N*, newtons.

TABLE 4-6

Results of ANOVA and Scheffe Method for Normal Occlusion and Malocclusion in Dental Prescale Subjects

	Contact Area		Average Pressure	Occlusal Force	
	p		*p*	*p*	
Normal/crowding	0.9944		0.8777	0.9123	
Normal/mandibular protrusion	0.9967		0.7227	0.9159	
Normal/maxillary protrusion (ov)	0.1527		>0.9999	0.0450	*
Normal/maxillary protrusion (un)	0.7239		0.9328	0.4212	
Normal/lateral crossbite	0.5801		>0.9999	0.4921	
Normal/open bite	0.0080	†	>0.9999	0.0024	†
Crowding/mandibular protrusion	>0.9999		>0.9999	>0.9999	
Crowding/maxillary protrusion (ov)	0.2710		0.9152	0.2863	
Crowding/maxillary protrusion (un)	0.9354		>0.9999	0.9371	
Crowding/lateral crossbite	0.8041		0.9610	0.9093	
Crowding/open bite	0.0093	†	0.4643	0.0197	*
Mandibular protrusion/maxillary protrusion (ov)	0.1811		0.7444	0.2123	
Mandibular protrusion/maxillary protrusion (un)	0.8926		0.9998	0.9101	
Mandibular protrusion/lateral crossbite	0.7554		0.9018	0.8896	
Mandibular protrusion/open bite	0.0036	†	0.2264	0.0099	†
Maxillary protrusion (ov)/maxillary protrusion (un)	0.9597		0.9640	0.9633	
Maxillary protrusion (ov)/lateral crossbite	>0.9999		>0.9999	>0.9999	
Maxillary protrusion (ov)/open bite	0.9307		0.9916	0.9708	
Maxillary protrusion (un)/lateral crossbite	0.9963		0.9773	0.9997	
Maxillary protrusion (un)/open bite	0.3942		0.6491	0.5206	
Lateral crossbite/open bite	0.9886		>0.9999	0.9783	

ANOVA, Analysis of variance; *p*, probability.
*Five percent level significance difference.
†One percent level significance difference.

TABLE 4-7

Occluzer Values of Facial Patterns in Dental Prescale Subjects

	Contact Area (mm^2)		Pressure (MPa)		Occlusal Force (N)	
Pattern	**Average**	**SD**	**Average**	**SD**	**Average**	**SD**
Severe dolicho	1.99	1.06	49.26	10.90	34.72	45.70
Dolichofacial	2.92	1.01	56.08	8.25	159.23	50.38
Mesio, tendency to dolicho	4.92	2.03	49.19	5.70	243.29	106.29
Mesiofacial	6.83	2.47	46.28	7.30	314.57	108.65
Mesio, tendency to brachy	7.76	2.71	47.16	7.45	355.91	114.19
Brachyfacial	9.8	5.14	45.58	6.93	423.34	161.74
Severe brachy	9.69	3.69	47.57	5.81	457.28	169.04
AVERAGE	6.27	3.11	48.73	3.52	284.04	149.95

SD, Standard deviation.

normal-occlusion subjects, found that the average "Area" was 12.9 mm^2, "Average" 35.0 MPa, and "Force" 458 N. Kayukawa et al.,[2] also using the Dental Prescale with five normal-occlusion subjects, reported that the average "Area" was 42.8 mm^2, "Average" 7.42 MPa, and "Force" 315.6 N. These data differ from the author's results because of the use of pressure-sensitive sheets. Yurkstas and Manly[24] used Pink Base Plate Wax: Araki et al.[25] and Kayukawa and Kayukawa[2] used 30H Type W.

The range of "sensitive gain" for a 30H sheet is 3 to 13 MPa and for a 50H sheet is 5 to 150 MPa. Ogata et al.[26] reported on the reproducibility of Dental Prescale in which

TABLE 4-8

Results of ANOVA and Scheffe Method for Facial Patterns in Dental Prescale Subjects

	Contact Area		Average Pressure		Occlusal Force	
	p		*p*		*p*	
Severe brachy/brachy	>0.9999		0.9976		0.9946	
Severe brachy/mesio-B	0.5990		>0.9999		0.2747	
Severe brachy/mesio	0.1598		0.9997		0.0343	*
Severe brachy/mesio-D	0.0008	†	0.9990		0.0001	†
Severe brachy/dolicho	<0.0001	†	0.1028		<0.0001	†
Severe brachy/severe dolicho	<0.0001	†	0.9985		<0.0001	†
Brachy/mesio-B	0.5997		0.9991		0.8053	
Brachy/mesio	0.1743		>0.9999		0.2946	
Brachy/mesio-D	0.0013	†	0.9460		0.0058	†
Brachy/dolicho	<0.0001	†	0.0271	*	<0.0001	†
Brachy/severe dolicho	<0.0001	†	0.9334		<0.0001	†
Mesio-B/mesio	0.9789		>0.9999		0.9679	
Mesio-B/mesio-D	0.1353		0.9952		0.1611	
Brachy/dolicho	<0.0001	†	0.0423	*	0.0001	†
Brachy/severe dolicho	<0.0001	†	0.9931		<0.0001	†
Mesio/mesio-D	0.6475		0.9728		0.7385	
Mesio/dolicho	0.0068	†	0.0238	*	0.0099	†
Mesio/severe dolicho	0.0002	†	0.9644		<0.0001	†
Mesio-D/dolicho	0.5882		0.3180		0.5571	
Mesio-D/severe dolicho	0.1359		>0.9999		0.0225	*
Dolicho/severe dolicho	0.9830		0.2960		0.7968	

Mesio-B, Mesiofacial pattern tendency to bradyfacial; *mesio-D,* mesiofacial pattern tendency to dolichofacial.
*Five percent level significance difference.
†One percent level significance difference.

the 30H sheet had a narrow range, not covering the full range. Kumagaya et al.[27] reported that the measuring accuracy of Type W is significantly lower than for Type R. Therefore the author thought that the best way to obtain accurate results was with the 50H Type R pressure-sensitive (Prescale) sheets, which were used in this study.

Occlusal patterns in subjects with normal occlusion and malocclusion

Occlusal patterns of normal-occlusion subjects had highest values in Area and Force. Area (color formation of Prescale) is considered wider in normal occlusion than in malocclusion. As Area in normal occlusion widens, Force becomes stronger, because Force = Average × Area. In malocclusion, Area, Average, and Force decreased in order from mandibular protrusion, crowding, maxillary protrusion ("un"; <5 mm overbite), lateral crossbite, maxillary protrusion ("ov"; >5 mm overbite), and open bite. In Area and Force, some subjects of the mandibular protrusion group and the crowding group were close to the normal-occlusion group data.

Occlusal function is considered to be a closed condition; however, it needs to be studied more using an electromyographic (EMG) device. The open-bite group was lowest in Area and Force, and the poor occlusal function was believed to be related to muscle function, especially digastric muscle function.[13] Also, more advanced systematic studies are needed.

The center of the occlusal force and distribution was confirmed; in the normal-occlusion group, it was in the center bilaterally and near the left and right first molar area anteroposteriorly. In the open-bite group and maxillary-protrusion group, it was confirmed to be positioned more posteriorly. Therefore, to establish occlusal stability in the retention period, the center of occlusal force and distribution in these groups must be changed more anteriorly and must have an improved occlusal pattern.[2]

Occlusal patterns in facial pattern subjects

In general, craniomandibular form is related to oral function.[28] In their study of the relationship between masticatory function and craniomandibular form, Proffit, Fields, and Nixon[3] reported that maximum occlusal force for subjects with a long face was lower than for those with a normal-length face. Park[29] reported that dolichofacial subjects were lower than brachyfacial and mesiofacial subjects in the EMG cycle zone of masticatory muscles.

Muscle action is strong in the brachyfacial pattern but weak in the dolichofacial pattern. The occlusal pattern of the brachyfacial pattern tends to be strong at the occlusal contact area and in occlusal force, whereas the dolichofacial pattern tends to be weak. The results of this study prove this hypothesis.

CONCLUSION

The diagnosis associated with occlusal contacts is the key in evaluating the efficacy of orthodontic treatment. This system provides reliable results and data for measuring occlusal patterns. Application of the Dental Prescale Occluzer System for observing changes in the occlusion of orthodontic patients may help in evaluating the condition of occlusion at the initial examination and during follow-up. The author recommends considering the different facial patterns when applying Dental Prescale for clinical diagnosis in orthodontics.

References

1. Tweed CH: *Clinical orthodontics*, St Louis, 1966, Mosby, pp 33-34.
2. Kayukawa W, Kayukawa H: Occlusal patterns of masticatory patients using measuring system of occlusal pressure, *J Jpn Assoc Adult Orthod* 2:61-68, 1955.
3. Proffit WR, Fields HW, Nixon WL: Occlusal forces in normal and long-face adults, *J Dent Res* 62:566-571, 1983.
4. Kawakami M: Masticatory pressures, *Koku Byogakkai Zasshi* 2:15-20, 1928.
5. Konishi S: Study on occlusal pressure in human normal teeth, various diseases and prosthodontics, *Jpn J Koku* 8:427-458, 1959.
6. Wirz J: Der Kaueffect bei Steggelenkprothestragern, *Schew Mschr Zhanheiik* 74:586-590, 1964.
7. Haga M: A prosthodontic occlusal problem, *Shikwa Gakuho* 67:841-858, 1967.
8. Howell AH, Manly RS: An electronic strain gauge for measuring oral forces, *J Dent Res* 27:705-712, 1948.
9. Tokumura K et al: Study on T-scan system, *Jpn J Prosthod* 33:1037-1043, 1989.
10. Kinoshita S et al: A new measuring method of occlusal contact and occlusal pressure using Prescale, *Jpn J Periodontol* 21:475-484, 1979.
11. Nikawa Y et al: Application of Prescale to dental field, *Shika Hyoron* 448:92-100, 1980.
12. Dahlberg B: The masticatory effect, *Acta Med Scand Suppl*, Lund: Hakan Ohlssons Boktryckeri, 1942.
13. Hellman M: Variations in occlusion, *Dent Cosmos* 63:608-619, 1921.
14. Maness WL, Benjamin M, Podoloff R, et al: Computerized occlusal analysis: a new technology, *Quintessence Int* 18:287-292, 1987.
15. Patyk A, Lotzmann U, Paula JM, et al: Ist das T-scan-system eine diagnostisch relevante methode zur okklusionskontrolle? *ZWR* 98:686-694, 1989.
16. Uchiyama N et al: An evaluating method of occlusal contact areas using measuring system for biting pressure, *J Jpn Orthod Soc* 56:92-99, 1997.
17. Nagai I et al: Use of a pressure-sensitive sheet to evaluate occlusal status in patients with mandibular prognatism, *J Jpn Oral Surg Soc* 46:9-15, 2000.
18. Asano M et al: The change of occlusal force and occlusal contact area during retention, *Nihon Univ Dent J* 70:581-600, 1996.
19. Dental Prescale Occluzer brochure, Fuji Film.
20. Ochiai M: A study on the occluding contacts of dental arch and each tooth the various positions of occlusion, *Nihon Univ Dent J* 38:448-495, 1964.
21. Hiranuma K: A study of occlusal contacts and masticatory effects, *Jpn J Prosthod* 1:17-36, 1957.
22. Inagawa E: A study of occlusal contacts in natural dentition, *Shikwa Gakuho* 70:69-92, 1970.
23. Nakao K: Occlusal facets and contacts in normal dentition (intercuspal position), *Koku Byogakkai Zasshi* 14:1-21, 1970.
24. Yurkstas A, Manly RS: Measurement of occlusal contact area effective in mastication, *Am J Orthod* 35:185-195, 1949.
25. Araki A et al: Consideration for clinical application of new occlusal evaluating system using Dental Prescale/Occluzer, *Dent Outlook* 84:1007-1019, 1994.
26. Ogata T et al: The reproducibility of occlusal contacts in children with Dental Prescale, *Jpn J Pediatr* 32:480-487, 1994.
27. Kumagaya H et al: Occlusal examination with occlusal patterns, *Dent Outlook* 86:233-240, 1995.
28. Enlow EH: *Handbook of facial growth*, Philadelphia, 1971, Saunders, pp 147-185.
29. Park I: A study of the craniomandibular skeletal form and masticatory muscle electromyogram, *Shikwa Gakuho* 91:837-869, 1991.

CHAPTER 5

Three-Dimensional Superimposition for Quantification of Treatment Outcomes

■ *Lucia H.S. Cevidanes, Martin Styner, and William R. Proffit*

Superimposition of serial radiographs on a stable reference structure is necessary to evaluate growth or treatment changes. Three-dimensional (3D) imaging from cone-beam (CB) computed tomography (CT), axial CT, magnetic resonance imaging (MRI), or surface laser scans offers improved diagnostic information and, perhaps more importantly, provides a better way to evaluate the changes resulting from treatment and the consequent skeletal and soft tissue adaptive responses to treatment.[1-8] In two-dimensional (2D) cephalometrics the cranial base is often used for this purpose because it shows minimal changes after neural growth is completed. The 2D cephalometric representations of the 3D craniofacial structures cannot answer many questions regarding treatment-response mechanisms and localized changes resulting from growth.[9,10] In contrast, 3D assessments provide substantial information in this regard, but pose a challenge in the choice of superimposition landmarks and structures. Although 2D landmark location is hampered by identification of hard and soft tissues on x-ray films due to the superimposition of multiple structures, locating 3D landmarks on complex, curving structures is significantly more difficult. As Bookstein[11,12] noted, there are no suitable operational definitions for craniofacial landmarks in the three planes of space: coronal, sagittal, and axial.

In the context of facial changes, superimposition should not rely on landmark identification or on "best-fit" techniques on structures that change with growth and treatment. Maxillomandibular changes need to be assessed relative to stable structures that have not been altered with growth or treatment. To better understand soft and hard tissue facial forms and changes with growth and treatment, as well as to create normative databases and predict changes, registration on the whole surface of the cranial base is the best method. This chapter demonstrates the use of a fully automated, voxelwise, rigid registration at the cranial base and application of 3D superimposition methods to evaluate anatomical structures displaced by growth, surgery, or other treatment.

METHODOLOGY FOR SURFACE REGISTRATION

Image Acquisition

The use of 3D images for treatment planning and follow-up raises concerns regarding radiation dose. Cone-beam CT (CBCT) equipment specialized for maxillofacial imaging now offers a relatively low-dose and convenient way to follow changes in facial morphology in three dimensions. CBCT scans of the cases presented in this chapter were acquired with the NewTom 3G (AFP Imaging, Elmsford, N.Y.), with a 36.3-microsievert (μSv) acquisition dose for a maxillary and mandibular scan. This is a major reduction from 314 μSv for conventional axial CT. There is a decrease in the signal/noise ratio with CBCT, but there is complete visualization of the facial structures, with spatial resolution of 0.36 mm in isotropic voxels. The imaging protocol used a 12-inch field of view to include the entire facial anatomy.

Image Analysis

Analysis of serial CBCT images to evaluate changes over time is done in a sequence of four steps: (1) model construction, (2) image registration, (3) transparency overlay, and (4) quantitative measurement.

Construction of virtual 3D surface models

Longitudinal quantitative assessment of growth and surgical correction requires construction of 3D surface models. The image-analysis tools for this purpose are modifications of open-source, freely available software from the U.S. National Institutes of Health (NIH, Bethesda, Md.).

Segmentation involves outlining the shape of anatomical structures visible in the cross sections of a volumetric data set from CBCT images and is performed with the Insight SNAP tool (Cognitica, Chapel Hill, N.C.).[13] Many standard automatic segmentation methods fail when applied to the complex anatomy of patients with facial deformity. The methods described by Gerig et al.[14] address these technical difficulties and have been adapted by Cevidanes et al.[8] to construct 3D craniofacial models. The 3D virtual models usually are built from a set of about 300 axial cross-sectional slices for each image, with the voxels reformatted for an isotropic of 0.5 × 0.5 × 0.5 mm. This resolution is used because although higher spatial resolution with smaller slice thickness is possible, it increases image file size and requires greater computational power and user interaction time without significantly improving the quality of assessment of changes between time points. After segmentation with the Insight SNAP tool, these files are converted from volumetric data into surface meshes for the 3D shape-analysis procedures.

Image registration

Image registration is a core technology for many imaging tasks. The two obstacles to widespread clinical use of nonrigid (elastic and deformable) registration are computational cost and quantification difficulties as the 3D models are deformed. Nonrigid registration would be required to create a composite of several different jaw shapes to guide the construction of template or standard, normal 3D surface models. To evaluate longitudinal changes, however, rigid registration is acceptable.

Using rigid registration and imagine software,[15] the authors mask anatomical structures displaced with growth or treatment and then perform a fully automated, voxelwise, rigid registration at the cranial base.

For superimposition of CBCT scans of subjects in whom cranial base growth is complete, registration of virtual 3D surface models is done using the whole surface of the cranial base (Fig. 5-1, *A* and *B*). To evaluate within-subject changes with growth and treatment, the anterior cranial fossae and the ethmoid bone surfaces can be used in the registration procedure because the growth of these structures is completed in early infancy. In this way the anterior cranial base of the CBCT images is used as the reference for superimposing different time points (Fig. 5-1, *C* and *D*). Rotational and translational parameters are calculated and then used to register 3D models from before and after treatment on the cranial base (Fig. 5-1, *E* and *F*). After registration, the overlay of the 3D models is assessed using University of North Carolina (UNC) Valmet and MeshValmet software (modifications of NIH Valmet). These software packages allow the visual and quantitative assessment of the location and magnitude of changes over time through graphical overlays and calculation of the euclidean distances between the surfaces of the 3D models at different time points.

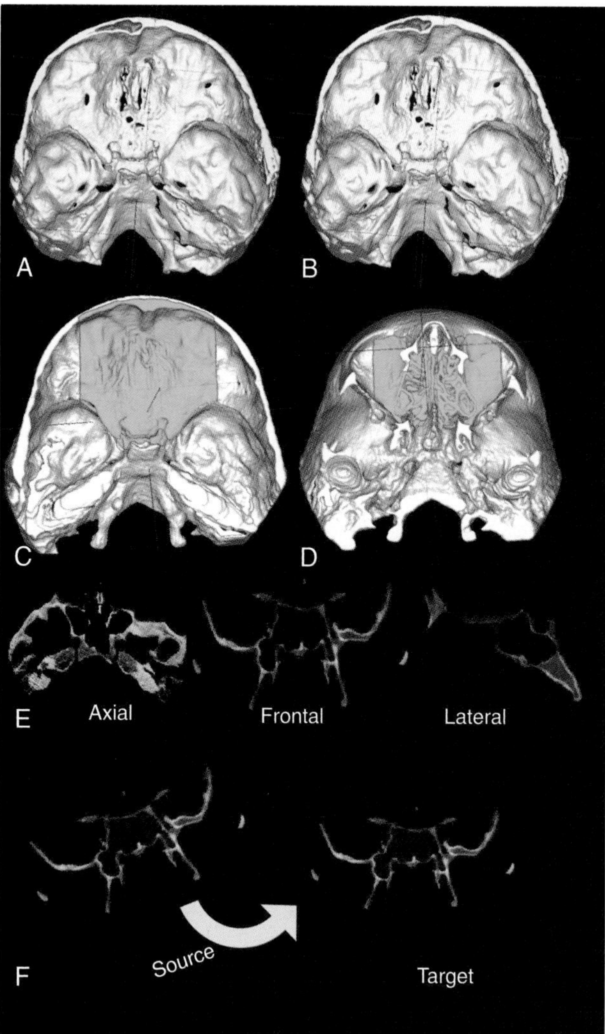

Fig. 5-1 Superimpositions of 3D models of growing children differ from those of adult patients. **A,** Pretreatment image, and **B,** posttreatment image, from superimposition of 3D surface models of a nongrowing subject in whom the whole surface of the cranial base was used for registration of the images. **C,** Superior view, and **D,** inferior view, of 3D surface models after treatment used for assessment of growth and treatment changes. Note that for growing subjects, the anterior cranial fossa surface has been used for registration because this area has completed growth in early infancy, so that the superimpositions describe growth relative to the individual cranial base. **E,** Gray-level–intensity image containing only the cranial fossa for calculation of registration parameters. **F,** Fully automated calculation of rotational and translational parameters between the images.

Transparency overlay

The next step in the analysis involves overlaying the 3D model surfaces that are registered in the same coordinate system with another tool, CMF software (Maurice Müller

Institute, Bern, Switzerland).[16] This tool allows different degrees of transparencies to assess visually the boundaries of the maxillomandibular structures between superimposed models at two different time points. This clearly identifies the location, magnitude, and direction of mandibular displacements and also allows quantification of vertical, transverse, and anteroposterior bone displacements and remodeling that accompany growth and response to treatment.

Quantitative measurements

In evaluation of surgical treatment, precise quantitative measurement is required to assess (1) the placement of bones in the desired position, (2) the position of surgical cuts and fixation screws and plates relative to risk structures, and (3) the location and amount of posttreatment bone remodeling. Landmark-based measurements present errors related to landmark identification. Andresen et al.[17] and Mitteroecker et al.[18] proposed the use of "semilandmarks," or landmarks plus vectors and tangent planes that define their location, but information from the whole curves and surfaces must also be included.

Gerig et al.[14] proposed the use of *color maps* generated from closest-point distances between the surfaces. This method measures closest distances, not corresponding distances between anatomical points on two or more longitudinally obtained images. However, using the MeshValmet and CMF tools allows calculation of thousands of distances in millimeters between surface triangles at two different time points, so that the difference between the two surfaces at any location can be quantified. After combining all 3D models at various time points, specific regions of interest, such as the anterior surface of the maxilla, chin prominence, condyles, and posterior border of the rami, can be selected and analyzed (Fig. 5-2).

The quantitative changes are visualized using color maps, which can be used to indicate inward *(blue)* or outward *(red)*

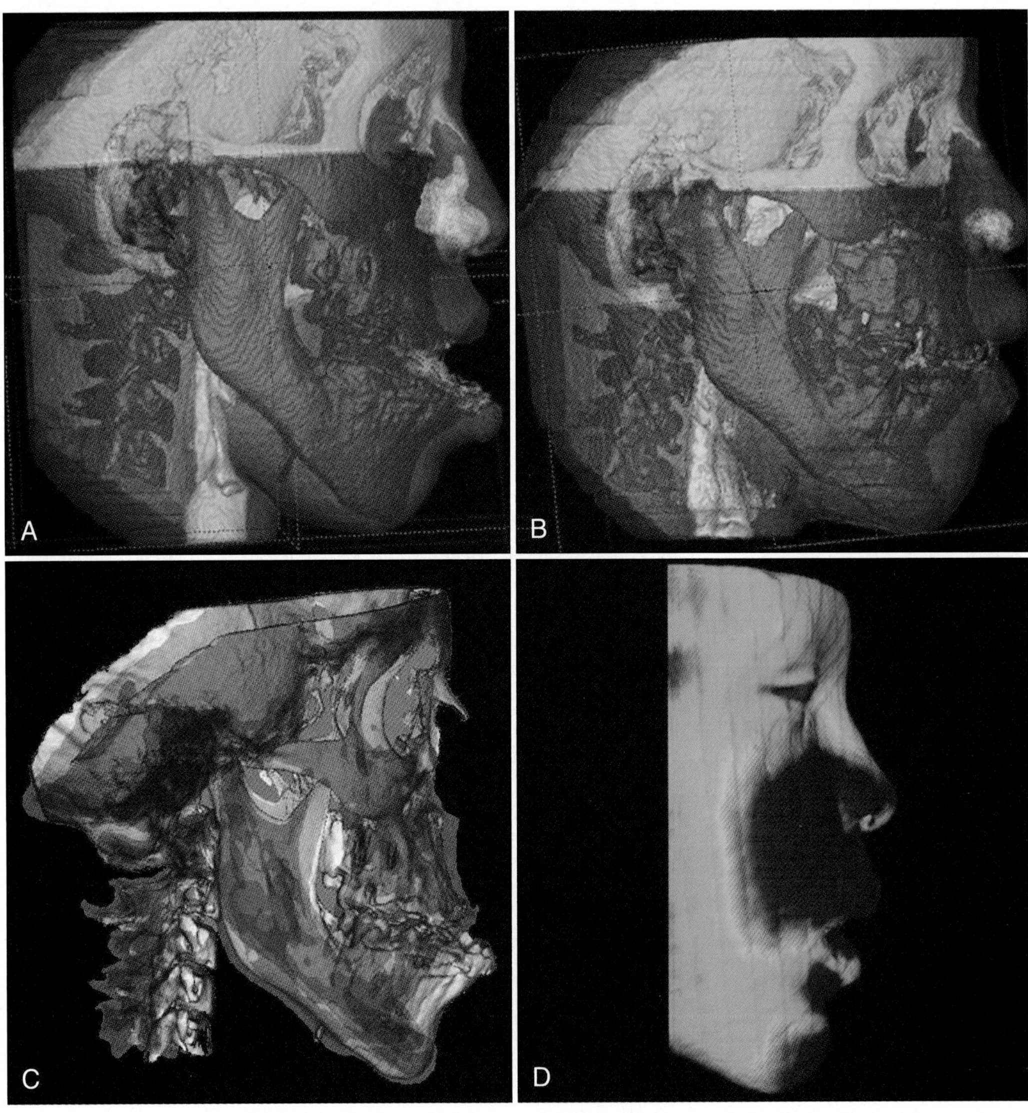

Fig. 5-2 **A,** Pretreatment image, and **B,** 1-year follow-up image, of surgical patient. **C,** Visualization of skeletal changes (in *white* and *red*) superimposed on the cranial base with semitransparency. **D,** Quantification of soft tissue changes for this patient using surface distance color maps.

displacement between overlaid structures. An absence of displacement is indicated by the *green* color code. For example, in mandibular advancement, forward displacement would be shown in a *red* color code in the anterior surface of the chin and in a *blue* color code in the posterior surfaces. A medial displacement of the condyles and rami will display *red* medial surfaces and *blue* lateral surfaces. No postsurgical change would be shown as a green color. This method has been validated and used since 2005.

CLINICAL FINDINGS FROM 3D REGISTRATION ON CRANIAL BASE SURFACE

The authors have used longitudinal CBCT images to evaluate postsurgical changes in the position and contours of the maxilla and mandible (including changes in location and shape of condyles) relative to the registration on the cranial base surface. Longitudinal CBCT scans before surgery, immediately after surgery, at splint removal, and 1 year after surgery allow comparisons of changes between any selected times (Figs. 5-3 and 5-4). Rotation of the mandibular rami results in short-term and long-term changes in the spatial position of the chin that can contribute or diminish the surgical correction (Fig. 5-5). Small, condylar displacements and modest remodeling of condyles (mean surface distances <2 mm) are observed in most patients after both mandibular advancement and two-jaw Class III surgery, but individual cases show significant condylar remodeling with net resorption after mandibular surgery.

When only maxillary surgery is done, the mandibular condyles change position if there is any vertical change (as almost always is the case) by rotating around their long axis. This requires slight remodeling of the condyles, but only small changes are seen after maxillary surgery[19] (Fig. 5-6). When a mandibular ramus osteotomy is done, the condyles must rotate transversely (across the long axis) a few degrees when the condylar and tooth-bearing segments are reconnected. The rotation of the medial pole is *inward* if the mandible is advanced (see Fig. 5-4, *A*) and *outward* if the mandible is set back (see Fig. 5-4, *B*).

Remodeling begins quite soon after the surgery. Changes can be visualized at 6 weeks (and probably earlier), but remodeling continues throughout the first year. For example, 2D measures might indicate increases in mandibular skeletal length and mandibular plane angle 2 years after surgery that negate the outcomes of mandibular surgery. However, 3D image analysis can establish whether the observed 2D changes are actually caused by remodeling on the posterior surfaces of the mandibular condyles, with an accompanying rotation of the mandibular rami unilaterally or bilaterally, or by remodeling at the surgical site. Currently, insufficient evidence exists to indicate whether differently shaped mandibular rami and condyles might dictate different surgical approaches.

CHALLENGES IN CLINICAL APPLICATION AND ROLE OF FUTURE INVESTIGATIONS

Analysis of 3D CBCT images is much more complex than analysis of 2D cephalometric radiographs. Superimposition on landmarks, the usual method for cephalometric analysis, is not satisfactory in analysis of 3D images. The cephalometric landmarks cannot be found consistently as images are rotated away from the midsagittal plane. With the method developed at UNC, a cranial base superimposition focused on the surface contours of the bone overcomes the landmark problem. In essence, instead of three or four landmark points, the superimposition is based on thousands of points.[8] This allows a detailed analysis of surface contour changes in the position of both the maxilla and the

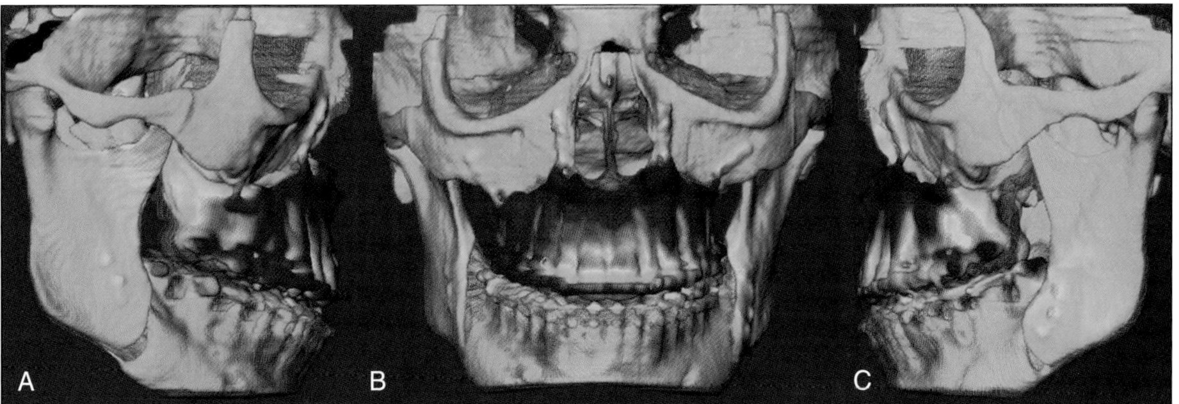

Fig. 5-3 **A** to **C**, Superimposition of presurgery and postsurgery models of nongrowing patient showing surface distances between two models. Surface of cranial base was used for registration. Cranial base color map is green (0 mm surface distance), showing adequate match of before and after models for cranial base structures. Note that maxilla was brought forward, as shown in red. Mandibular setback precisely maintained rami position, sliding mandibular corpus posteriorly, with slight counterclockwise rotation to correct open-bite tendency.

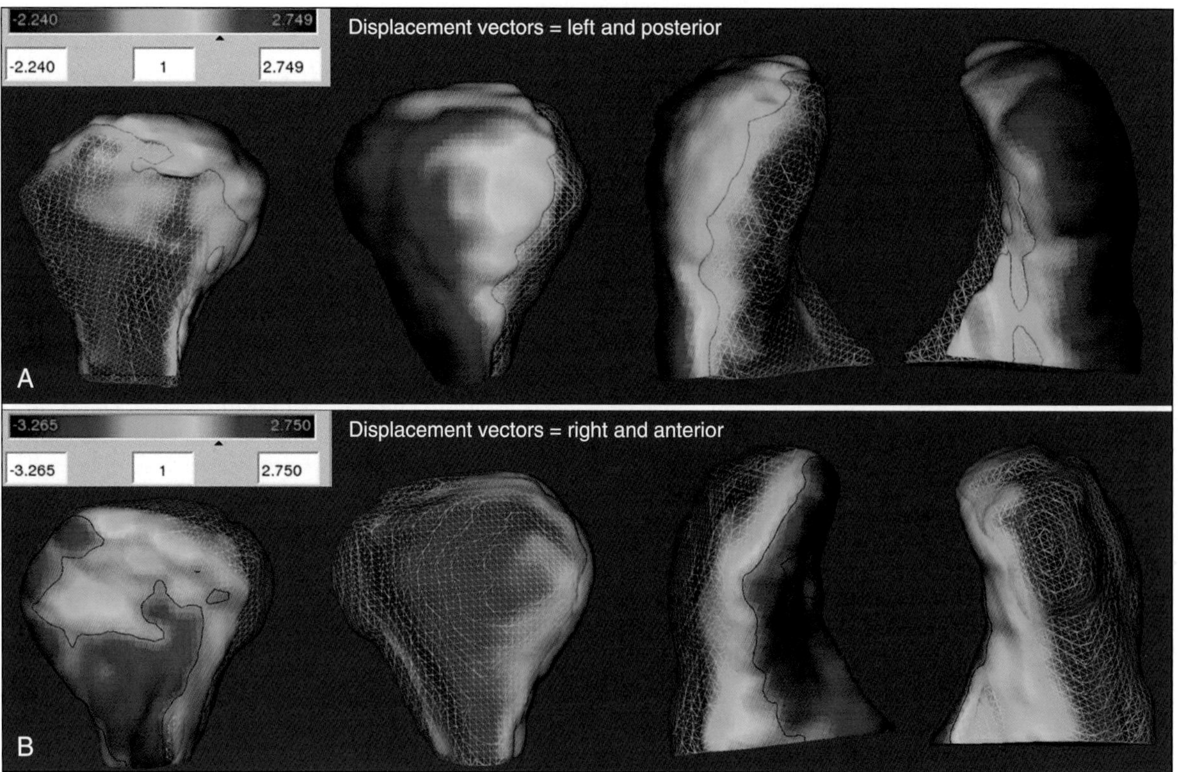

Fig. 5-4 Direction of displacement of a specific anatomical region, in this patient the left mandibular condyle, is clearly identified with the methods described. Color-coded display of displacement showing rotation of the medial pole inward when the mandible was advanced **(A)** and outward if the mandible was set back **(B)**.

mandible from any perspective. Also, a highly detailed analysis of changes in the mandibular condyles can be visualized using color maps, so that all areas in the jaws or condyle that have changed from the previous CT are colored to distinguish both direction and amount of change[9] (see Fig. 5-1).

Currently available commercial software does not allow construction of virtual 3D surface models, but rather displays a 3D rendering that is a projection of the 3D structure of the face for visualization purposes. The implementation of registration tools using "best fit" between the 3D renderings does not allow quantification of local changes with treatment but would allow overall visualization (Figs. 5-7 and 5-8).

The superimposition methods presented in this chapter allow not only visualization, but also precise localization of the skeletal remodeling or adaptation that has occurred in the maxilla or mandible. This approach to 3D image analysis methods has been streamlined and continuously updated with new methods for quantification, with collaboration from the Maurice Müller Institute, the medial image analysis group in the UNC Department of Computer Science, the UNC Neuroimaging Laboratory, and the statistical modeling group in the UNC Biomedical Research Imaging Center.

The recent emphasis on soft tissues as the limiting factor in treatment and on soft tissue relationships in establishing the goals of treatment has produced major changes in diagnosis and treatment planning. This is a paradigm shift away from the previous emphasis on dental occlusion and hard tissue relationships, and cephalometric analysis will play a smaller role and clinical examination of facial proportions a more important role.

Clinical research is beginning to provide data from 3D soft tissue analysis, but the added value of 3D photographs still needs to be assessed in carefully controlled studies. Although the superimposition methodology presented here allows quantification of soft tissue surface changes from any 3D data set (Fig. 5-9), its application to other imaging modalities such as laser scanners and 3D cameras has not yet been assessed.

CONCLUSION

The methodology presented in this chapter has been applied to research in progress. Currently, the superimposition of 3D surface models is still too time-consuming and computing intensive to apply these methods to routine clinical use, but current work has focused on making a simplified analysis available in the near future.

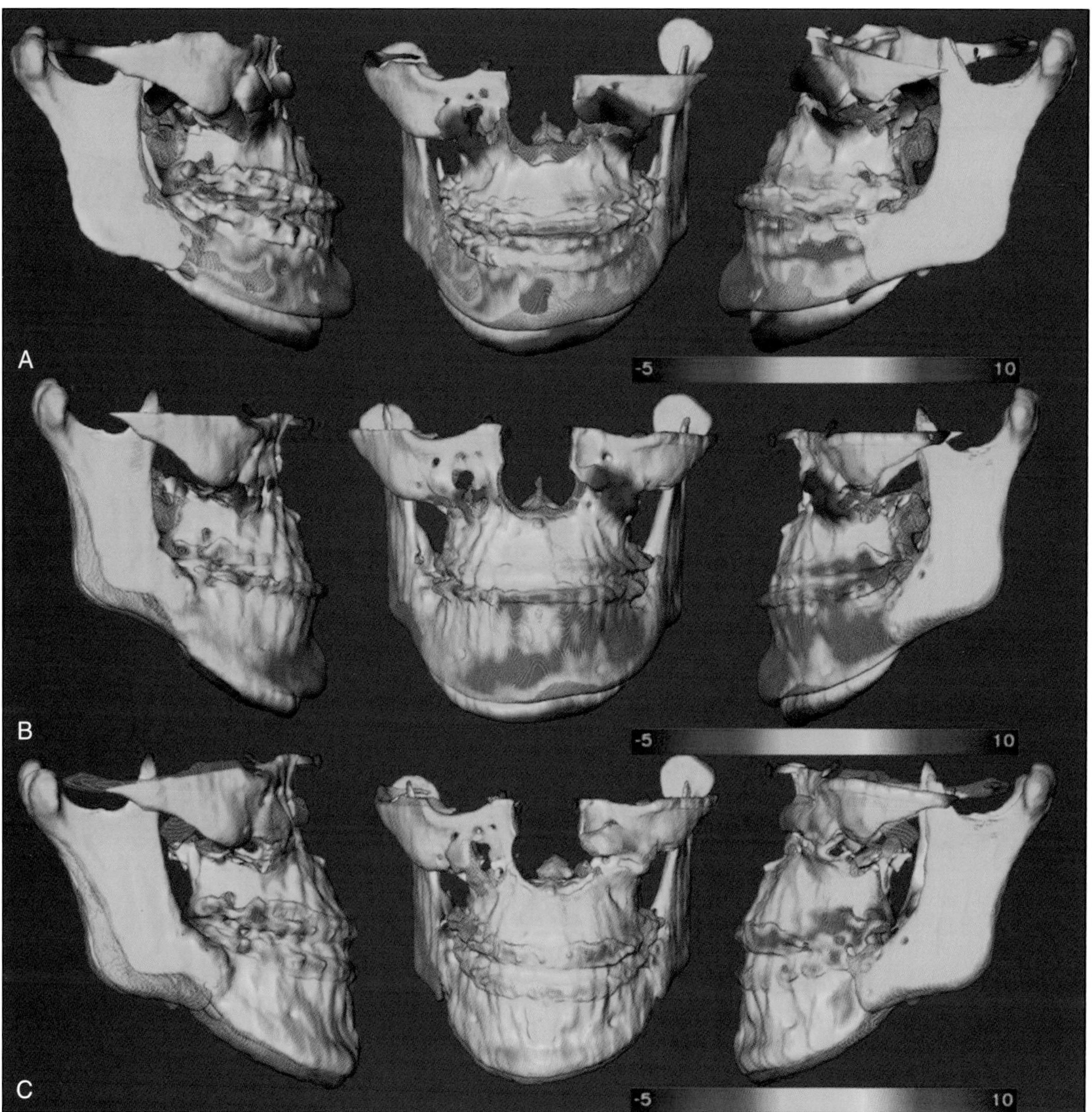

Fig. 5-5 Three-dimensional models before surgery, at surgical splint removal, and 1 year after surgery of patient treated with maxillary advancement and mandibular setback. **A,** Superimposition of presurgery (transparent) and postsurgery (color map) models at splint removal showing surface distances between the two models. Surface of cranial base was used for registration. Note that maxilla was brought forward and downward, as shown in red. Mandibular setback precisely maintained rami position, sliding mandibular corpus posteriorly. **B,** Surface distances between presurgery (transparent) and 1-year postsurgery (color map) models show the maxillary advancement and mandibular setback. **C,** Surface distances between splint removal (transparent) and 1-year postsurgery (color map) models show the mandibular ramus and corpus adaptation after surgery.

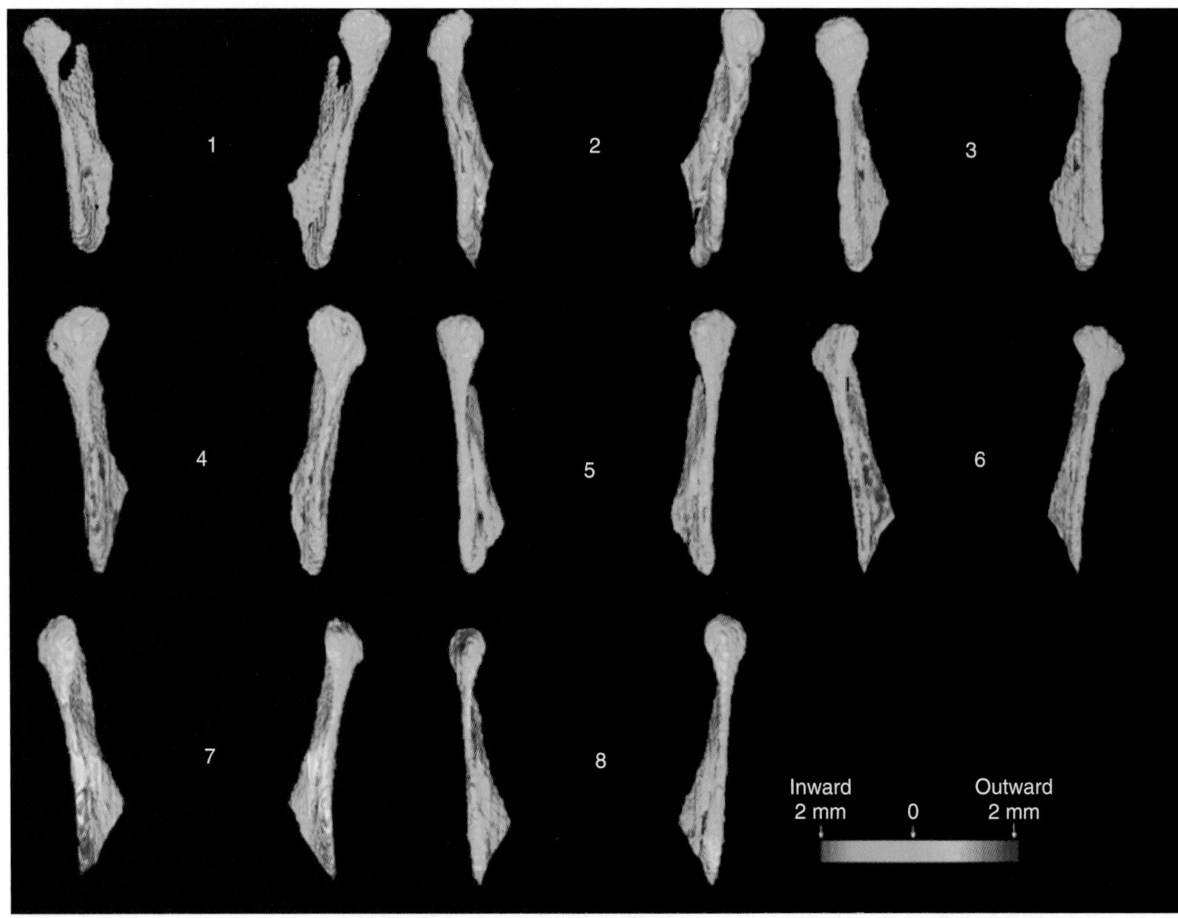

Fig. 5-6 Posterior view of 3D models of mandibular condyle and ramus at 1 week after surgery superimposed with 1-year postsurgery models for eight patients treated with maxillary surgery only. Note that only small changes are seen after maxillary surgery.

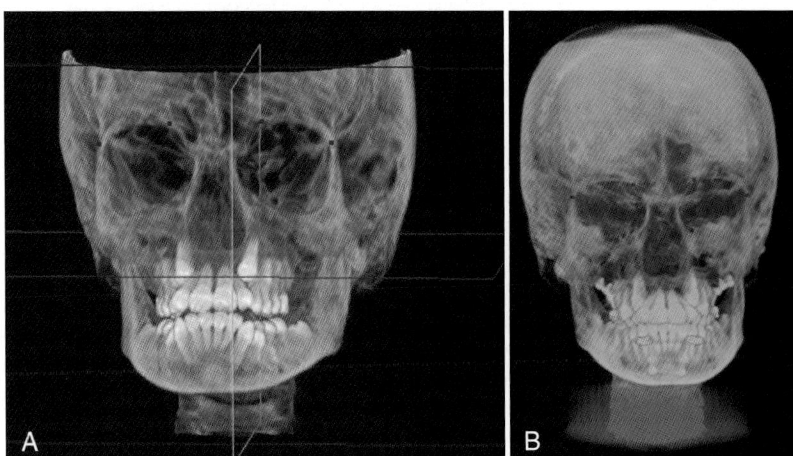

Fig. 5-7 Superimposition with Invivo software 3.1 (Anatomage, San Jose, Calif.). Choice of 3D landmarks on 3D surface renderings to register images **A,** before treatment, and **B,** after treatment.

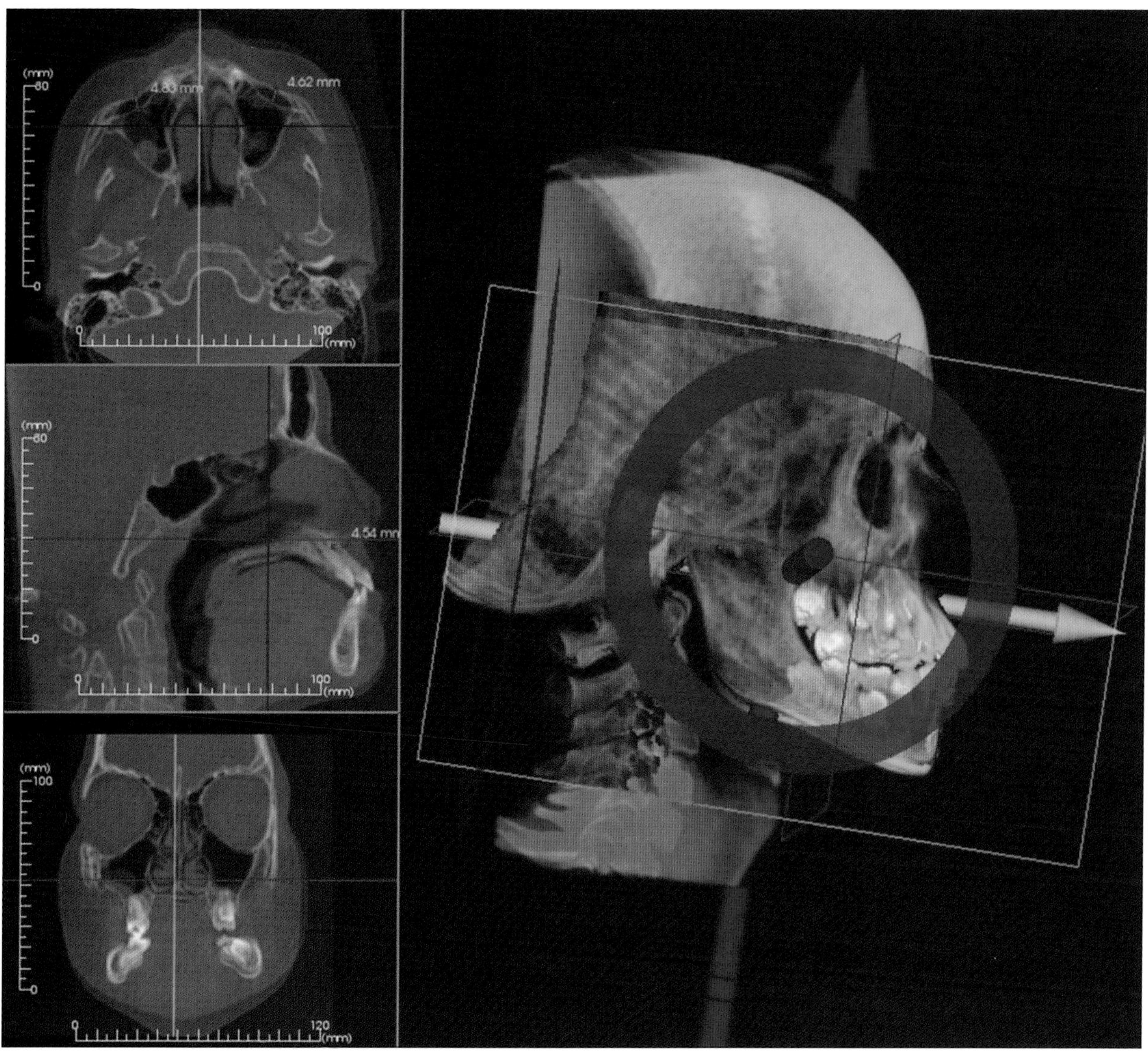

Fig. 5-8 Manual adjustment of *x*, *y*, and *z* axes to superimpose 3D renderings with visualization of maxillary advancement after manual registration on the cranial base. Note that quantification of changes can only be done in 2D cross-sectional slices, and that the registration is not adequate in all three planes, as shown in the anteroposterior cross section.

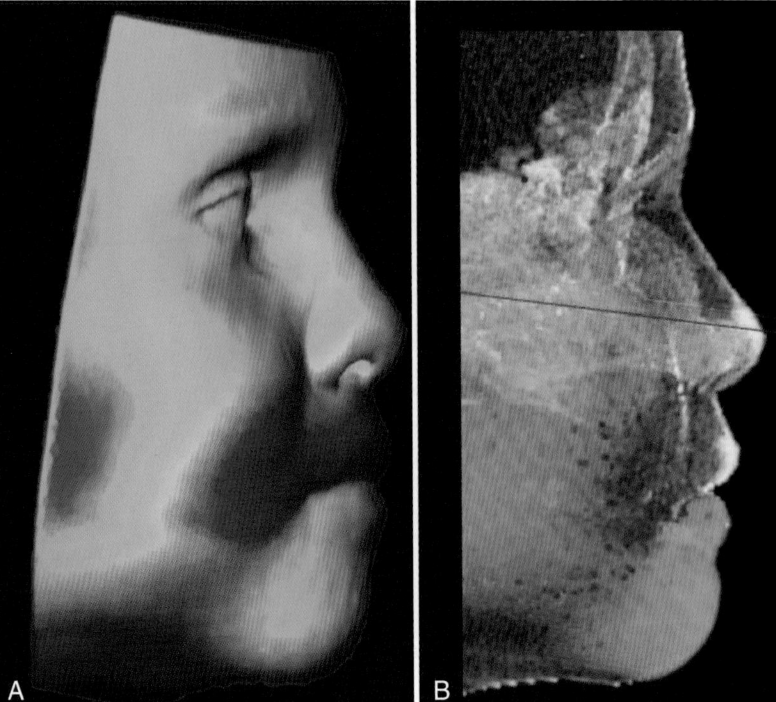

Fig. 5-9 Visualization of soft tissue changes for 3D virtual models registered on the cranial base. **A,** Registration of 3D surface models displayed with CMF software showing color map of thousands of 3D surface distances that describe the soft tissue changes. **B,** Registration of 3D renderings with Invivo software that allows visualization of soft tissue changes with treatment.

References

1. Baumrind S, Moffitt FH, Curry S: The geometry of three-dimensional measurement from paired coplanar x-ray images, *Am J Orthod* 84:313-322, 1983.
2. Cevidanes LHS, Franco AA, Gerig G, et al: Assessment of mandibular growth and response to orthopedic treatment with 3-dimensional magnetic resonance images, *Am J Orthod Dentofacial Orthop* 128:16-26, 2005.
3. Cevidanes LHS, Franco AA, Gerig G, et al: Comparison of relative mandibular growth vectors with high-resolution 3-dimensional imaging, *Am J Orthod Dentofacial Orthop* 127:27-34, 2005.
4. Harrell WE Jr, Hatcher DC, Bolt RL: In search of anatomic truth: 3-dimensional digital modeling and the future, *Am J Orthod Dentofacial Orthop* 122:325-330, 2002.
5. Kau CH, Richmond S, Incrapera A, et al: Three-dimensional surface acquisition systems for the study of facial morphology and their application to maxillofacial surgery, *Int J Med Robot* 3:97-110, 2007 (review).
6. Kau CH, Zhurov A, Richmond S, et al: The 3-dimensional construction of the average 11-year-old child face: a clinical evaluation and application, *J Oral Maxillofac Surg* 64:1086-1092, 2006.
7. Togashi K, Kitaura H, Yonetsu K, et al: Three-dimensional cephalometry using helical computer tomography: measurement error caused by head inclination, *Angle Orthod* 72:513-520, 2002.
8. Cevidanes LHS, Bailey LJ, Tucker GR, et al: Superimposition of 3D cone-beam CT models of orthognathic surgery patients, *Dentomaxillofac Radiol* 34:369-375, 2005.
9. Cevidanes LH, Bailey LJ, Tucker SF, et al: Three-dimensional cone-beam computed tomography for assessment of mandibular changes after orthognathic surgery, *Am J Orthod Dentofacial Orthop* 131:44-50, 2007.
10. Ghafari J, Baumrind S, Efstratiadis SS: Misinterpreting growth and treatment outcome from serial cephalographs, *Clin Orthod Res* 1:102-106, 1998.
11. Bookstein FL, Schafer K, Prossinger H, et al: Comparing frontal cranial profiles in archaic and modern homo by morphometric analysis, *Anat Rec* 257:217-224, 1999.
12. Bookstein FL: *Morphometric tools for landmark data*, Cambridge, Mass, 1991, Cambridge University Press, p 435.
13. Yuskevich PA, Piven J, Hazlett HC, et al: User-guided 3D active contour segmentation of anatomical structures: significantly improved efficiency and reliability, *Neuroimage* 31:1116-1128, 2006.
14. Gerig G, Jomier M, Chakos M: Valmet: a new validation tool for assessing and improving 3D object segmentation, *Med Image Comput/Comput Assist Interv* 2208:516-528, 2001.
15. Rueckert D, Sonoda LI, Denton E, et al: Comparison and evaluation of rigid and nonrigid registration of breast MR images, *Proc SPIE Med Imaging* 3361:78-88, 1999.
16. Chapuis J, Rudolph T, Borgesson B, et al: 3D surgical planning and navigation for CMF surgery, *Proc SPIE Med Imaging* 5367:403-410, 2004.
17. Andresen R, Bookstein FL, Conradsen K, et al: Surface-bounded growth modeling applied to human mandibles, *IEEE Trans Med Imaging* 19:1053-1063, 2000.
18. Mitteroecker P, Gunz P, Bookstein FL: Semilandmarks in three dimensions, *Evol Dev* 7:244-258, 2005.
19. Cevidanes LHS, Styner M, Phillips C, et al: 3D morphometric changes 1 year after jaw surgery biomedical imaging: macro to nano. In *Proceedings of the IEEE International Symposium*, Washington, DC, 2007, pp 1332-1335.

CHAPTER 6

Adhesives and Bonding in Orthodontics

■ *Serdar Üşümez and Nejat Erverdi*

Dentistry in general, and orthodontics in particular, strongly rely on advances in material science. However, these advances do not attract as much attention as the extraction/nonextraction dilemma, the effects of orthodontics on facial esthetics, or the one phase/two phase debate. Indeed, materials often seem less important than these issues. Nonetheless, material development has probably had the greatest single effect on the practice of orthodontics since the introduction of modern orthodontics by Edward H. Angle. The changes in orthodontic clinical practice following the introduction of superelastic wires in the 1980s attest to this effect.[1]

Another important development in orthodontics was the introduction of direct bonding. With the development of reliable and reproducible bonding techniques to enamel surfaces, cemented bands were replaced by bonded brackets on incisor, cuspid, and bicuspid teeth.[2,3] The many advantages of bonded brackets over cemented bands include esthetic improvement, elimination of band seating, and the need for tooth separation as well as elimination of band material thickness, which affected the arch length. Improved oral hygiene through easier access to the interproximal dental areas helps reduce the risk of enamel decalcification. Accessibility to the interproximal area also allows for earlier detection of caries at these sites and their restoration, improved access to interproximal contacts for air-rotor stripping, and elimination of the need for posttreatment space closure. The ability to bond partially erupted and malaligned teeth enable earlier force application during treatment, which was previously not possible with banded attachments.[4-6]

Direct bonding of orthodontic attachments has also increased the acceptability of orthodontic appliances by the public and popularized orthodontic treatment, thus increasing new enrollments each year. Advances in direct bonding have led to new techniques such as lingual orthodontics that could not be used with circumferential bands.

ORTHODONTIC APPLIANCE

At present, direct bonding is the method of choice for attaching orthodontic appliances. However, most bracket bases do not chemically bond to enamel or resin. For most clinical applications, removal or failure of bonded metal brackets occurs at the weaker resin-metal interface.[7-17] The improvement in this macromechanical interface is of critical importance. Bracket base designs include mesh wires, perforations, and undercuts, to provide mechanical interlocking with the resins that have been developed.[18] Some companies also add smaller-scale micromechanical retention, obtained through abrasion, etching, or spray coating, along with retention from the meshes.[1] Many bracket base designs are available for clinical use,[19,20] such as standard mesh base (Ultraminitrim, Dentaurum, Ispringen, Germany), supermesh base (Microarch, GAC International, Bohemia, N.Y.), integral base (Dyna-Lock, 3M Unitek, Monrovia, Calif., and Microloc, GAC International), microetched base (Miniature Twin, 3M Unitek), and laser-structured base (Discovery, Dentaurum) (Fig. 6-1).

Although mesh pad is most often used for retention, improving these other systems has been the goal of many research projects.[21-26] One study found that a new type of laser-structured base retention resulted in double the bond strength produced by foil mesh, without compromising debonding characteristics.[27] The laser-structured Discovery (Dentaurum), integral-based Microloc (GAC International), and microetched-based Miniature Twin (3M Unitek) performed statistically better than the mesh-based brackets with the light-cured composite resin used in another study.[28]

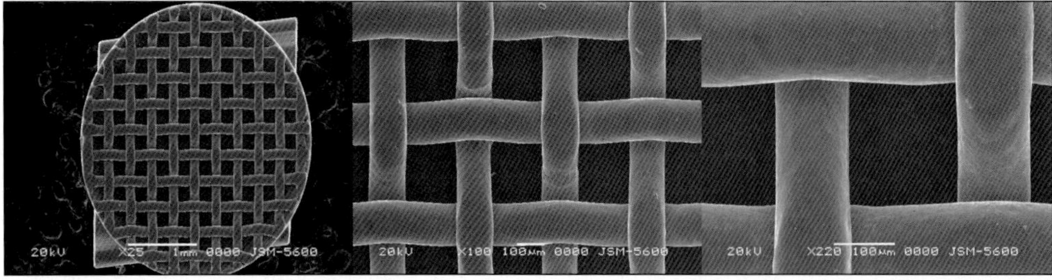

Fig. 6-1 Scanning electron microscopy (SEM) views of a standard mesh-base bracket (Ultraminitrim, Dentaurum, Ispringen Germany). Bracket bases present a retentive base for holding the cured resin. Mesh pad is the system most frequently used for retention.

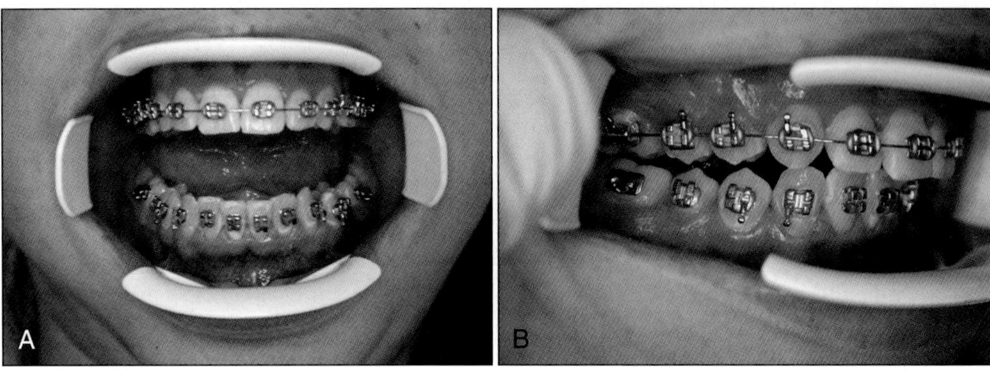

Fig. 6-2 **A,** OptiView (Kerr Hawe) is a flexible lip and cheek retractor that can be easily moved to either side **(B)** when placing premolar brackets for a direct view.

SURFACE PREPARATION AND BRACKET BONDING

Bonding of brackets and other orthodontic attachments is a crucial stage in the treatment process. Minor errors at this stage will be dramatically reflected in the active treatment phase in the form of improper alignment of teeth; premature failure of attachments, which will require time-consuming and costly replacements; and increased susceptibility to demineralization around the attachment. This seemingly "easy" stage should never be underestimated, and care should be taken when bonding each attachment. The principles of "ideal" bonding are not specific to orthodontics and are well addressed by other disciplines of dentistry that use adhesive resins. The basic principles for a successful bonding are (1) cleaning the adhesive surfaces, (2) providing good wetting, (3) ensuring intimate adaptation, (4) making use of every possible bonding force, and (5) providing good curing (polymerization).

Preparation for Bonding

Cleaning

The labial or lingual adhesive surface of teeth should be free of calculus and plaque for efficient bonding. This is most frequently performed by using pumice prophylaxis. However, enamel pumicing before etching has been found of limited value when the tooth surfaces are free from visible plaque precipitation, and pumicing might not be an integral part of the etching process because neither bond strength nor enamel-surface etch pattern is altered by pumicing clean enamel.[29] Despite not being mandatory, pumicing will help the clinician to achieve more optimal results, particularly when bonding posterior teeth, which are sometimes out of reach of efficient brushing activity.[30]

Preparing the working area

Moisture control is crucial during orthodontic bonding because moisture contamination of pretreated enamel can cause failure of the bond or weakening of the shear bond strength. Salivary control and maintenance of a dry working field are essential throughout the bonding procedure, usually accomplished by lip expanders, cheek retractors, saliva ejectors, and cotton rolls. The wire cheek retractor is the most common form of retractor but causes difficulty in bonding the posterior region because it is difficult to swing on either side. Careful bracket placement is important when the wire cheek retractor is used. A useful alternative to wire retractors is the OptiView (Kerr Hawe, Bioggio, Switzerland), which is easily moved to either side when placing premolar brackets (Fig. 6-2). This versatile retractor is also available in "petit" size.

Antisialagogue agents

Antisialagogues are agents that counteract any influence that promotes the flow of saliva. These chemicals may provide quick and excellent saliva flow restriction.[5] However, a recent randomized clinical trial found no statistically significant effect of atropine sulfate premedication on bond failure rates.[31] The advantage of atropine sulfate is questionable and should be avoided.

Enamel Pretreatment

Conventional adhesive systems use three different agents—enamel conditioner, primer solution, and adhesive resin—in the process of bonding orthodontic brackets to enamel. Untouched enamel surface is hydrophobic, and wetting is limited. This makes bonding to intimate enamel surface a challenging procedure. Enamel pretreatment or surface conditioning is necessary to make successful bonds, usually accomplished by etching the surface by various acids.

The most frequently used etchant is 37% orthophosphoric acid. Phosphoric acid is an inorganic substance. Many authors reported changes in surface characteristics, loss of enamel substance, and white, frosty appearance from decalcification and crystal structure deformation with this acid.[32-36]

Bonding to enamel with acid etching has significantly changed and facilitated clinical practice in all fields of dentistry. Characteristics of the enamel surface are altered by acid dissolution, which creates microporosities that result in a micromechanical bond[37] (Fig. 6-3).

The orthophosphoric acid is applied over the enamel surface for 30 seconds after careful isolation of the operative field. The etching time can range from 15 to 60 seconds without compromising the *shear bond strength* (SBS). Etching duration shorter than 15 seconds or longer than 60 seconds has been shown to decrease SBS. At the end of the etching period, the bulk of the etchant is cleaned off the teeth with a cotton roll, and the teeth are rinsed with abundant water spray. A powerful evacuator is crucial for increased efficiency in collecting the etchant-water rinse. The teeth are then thoroughly dried with a moisture-free and oil-free air source to obtain the well-known "frosty" appearance (Fig. 6-4).

Teeth that do not appear frosty should be reetched. Saliva contamination does not require rerinsing, but blood contamination has been shown to decrease SBS, and teeth contaminated with blood should be rerinsed and dried.[5,38,39] A protective liquid polish (e.g., BisCover, Bisco, Inc., Schaumburg, Ill.) may be applied to the etched surface before contamination can occur, to prevent the adverse effect of blood contamination.[38] This product may also be beneficial in difficult bonding areas, such as partially erupted or impacted teeth.

Alternatives to orthophosphoric acid etching

Use of milder acids. Research showed that 10% maleic acid, which is believed to decrease mineral loss alone, may produce similar bond strengths to 37% orthophosphoric acid.[37,40-43] However, the use of maleic acid have never been popularized. Gottlieb, Nelson, and Vogels[44] reported that 95.6% of U.S. orthodontists never used maleic acid, 3.9% used it occasionally, and 0.5% used it routinely.

Laser etching. Laser treatment of dental enamel causes thermally induced changes within the enamel to a depth of 10 to 20 μm, depending on the type of laser and the energy applied to the enamel surface. Laser etching involves a process of continuous vaporization and microexplosions caused by vaporizing the water trapped within the hydroxyapatite matrix (Fig. 6-5). The degree of surface roughening depends on the system used and the wavelength of the laser.[17,45] The results on achieved SBS vary, and in general, lasers currently are unable to produce a standard, reliable etching pattern.[17,46,47]

Sandblasting. Another method of enamel pretreatment is the "air-abrasive technique" (sandblasting).[48-50] However, even the enamel loss resulting from sandblasting at low pressure and short exposure time was found to be smaller than in acid etching. The bond strengths achieved with sandblasting alone were not clinically acceptable.[51-53]

Crystal growth. In 1979, Maijer and Smith[54] reported a method of bonding that involved crystal growth on the enamel surface. This system consists of a polyacrylic acid treatment liquid containing a sulfate component that reacts with the calcium in the enamel surface to form a dense growth of small, needle-shaped crystals. The crystal buildup on the enamel serves as an additional retentive mechanism for the resin that bonds the orthodontic attachment to the teeth. Micromechanical interlocking is created at the enamel surface, and most of the problems associated with conventional acid etching are said to be eliminated.[54,55]

Although debonding and adhesive cleanup were facilitated with this technique, achieved SBS values consistently remained below those of conventional acid etching.[56-59]

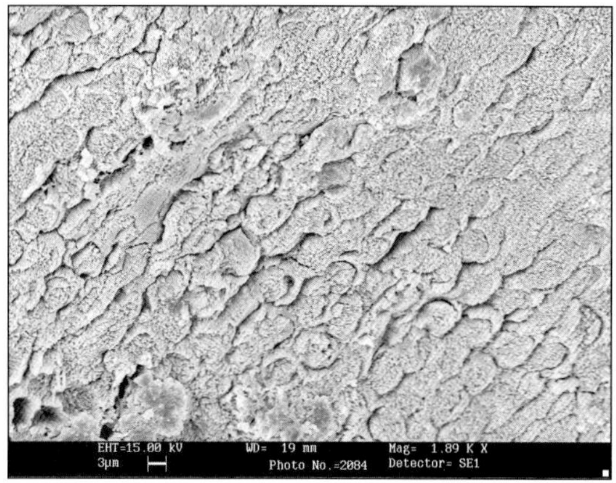

Fig. 6-3 Characteristics of the enamel surface are altered by acid dissolution, which creates microporosities that result in a micromechanical bond. This surface irregularity is clinically observed as the well-known "frosty" appearance.

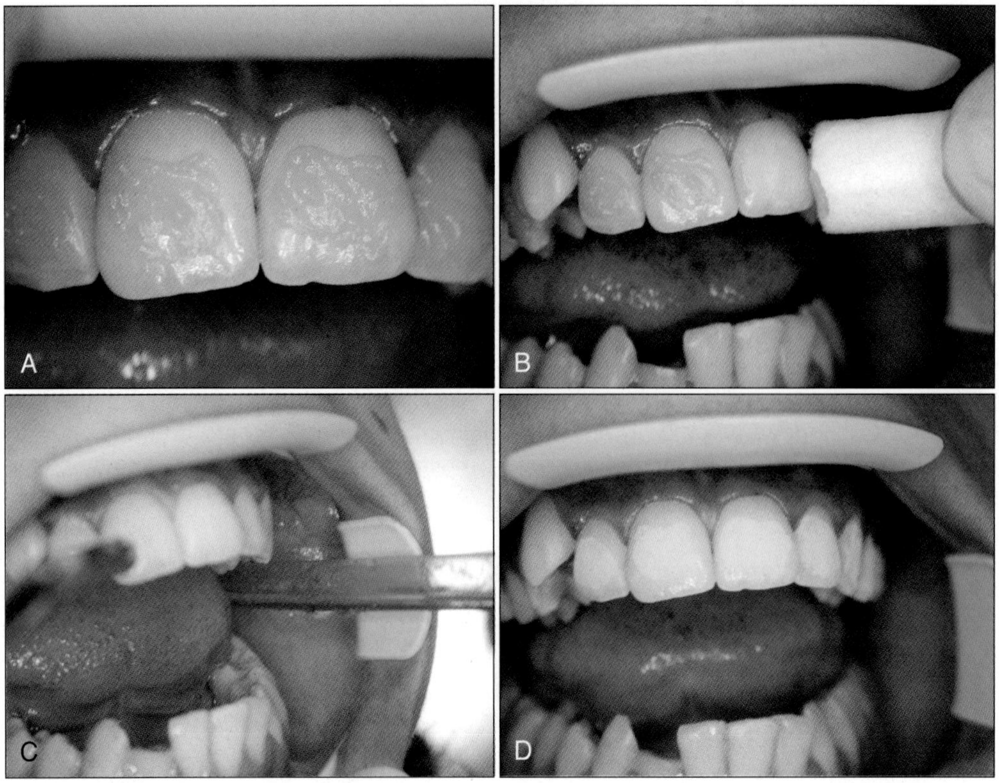

Fig. 6-4 **A,** Phosphoric acid gel is applied over the enamel surface for 30 seconds. **B,** At the end of the etching period, the bulk of the etchant is cleaned off the teeth with a cotton roll, and the teeth are rinsed with abundant water spray. **C,** The teeth are then thoroughly air-dried to obtain the frosty appearance (**D**).

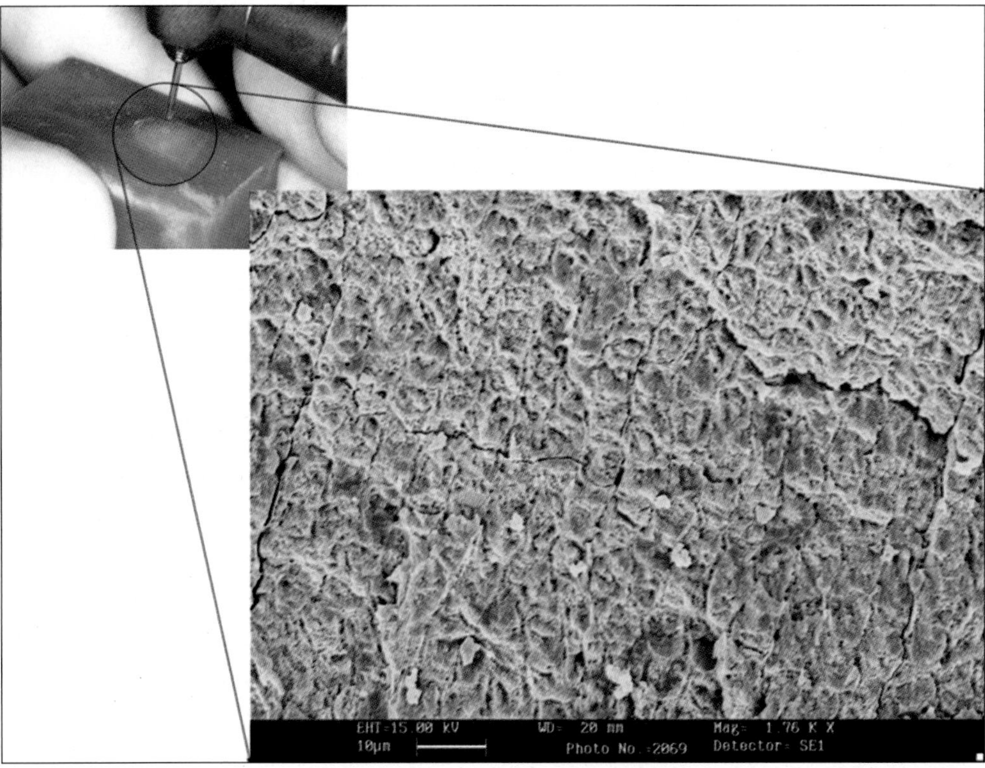

Fig. 6-5 Laser irradiation from a sapphire probe causes thermally induced changes within the enamel to a depth of 10 to 20 μm, depending on the laser and energy applied.

Sealing and Priming

Application of a thin layer of bonding agent (sealant, primer) over the entire etched enamel surface is suggested by all the manufacturers (Fig. 6-6). If excessive, the coating should be thinned by a gentle air burst. A thick layer may cause "drifting" before curing is initiated and may interfere with the precise adaptation of the bracket base.

Separate curing of the bonding agent is not necessary, even when light-cured products are used. The layer may be precured in difficult-to-reach areas where moisture contamination is likely. Reapplication of the sealed layer is not required when saliva contamination occurs, but the area should be air-dried before bracket placement.

Self-etching primers

A unique characteristic of some new bonding systems in operative dentistry is that they combine the *conditioning* and *priming* agents into a single, acidic primer solution for simultaneous use on both enamel and dentin (Fig. 6-7). Combining conditioning and priming into a single treatment step results in improved chair-side efficiency and cost-effectiveness for the clinician and saves time for patients.[60,61]

In a self-etching primer (SEP) the active ingredient is a methacrylated phosphoric acid ester. The phosphoric acid and methacrylate group are combined into a molecule that etches and primes at the same time. The phosphate group dissolves the calcium and removes it from the hydroxyapatite. The removed calcium forms a complex with the phosphate group and is incorporated into the network when the primer polymerizes. Agitating the primer on the tooth surface serves to ensure that fresh primer is transported to the enamel surface. Etching and monomer penetration to the exposed enamel rods are simultaneous. In this manner, the depth of the etch and depth of the primer penetration are identical.

Bonding with an SEP is significantly faster than using conventional acid etching (75.5 vs. 97.7 seconds per bracket),[62,63] and recent studies indicate that SEPs may provide similar SBS values and failure characteristics.[16,62,64] However, it should be noted that pumicing before the use of an SEP is crucial.[30]

Conventional acid etching is still the "gold standard" for bracket bonding, and clinical observations indicate that use of milder self-etching systems increase the bond failure rates.[5]

Types of Adhesives

Composite resins

A large number of dental composite products have appeared in the past 15 years, all having simple, common characteristics. They are all combinations of silane-coated inorganic filler particles with dimethacrylate resin, either bisglycidil methacrylate (BISGMA) or urethane dimethacrylate (UDMA). In some cases, a proportion of a lower-molecular-weight monomer such as triethyleneglycol dimethacrylate (TEGDMA) is introduced to lower the viscosity. The filler particles used are barium silicate glass, quartz, or zirconium silicate, usually combined with 5% to 10% weight of microscopic (0.04-μm) particles of colloidal silica. Modern dental composite materials are thus a blend of glass or ceramic particles dispersed in a photopolymerizable synthetic-organic resin matrix. The polymer materials are blended with the finely divided inorganic material, such as barium aluminosilicate glass or other glass composition, having an effective amount of radiopaque oxide that renders the resultant glass radiopaque to x-rays.[65-67]

Many independent investigations indicate that the filled BISGMA resins have the best physical properties and are the strongest adhesives for metal brackets.[68-70] Reported failure rates for steel mesh–based brackets directly bonded with highly filled diacrylate resins are as low as 1% to 4%.[70]

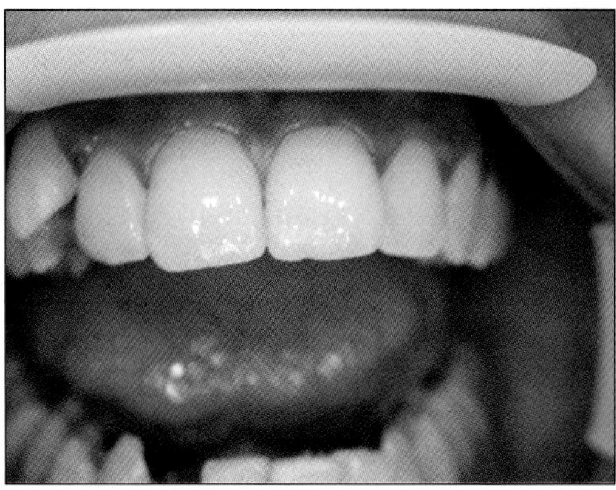

Fig. 6-6 Thin layer of bonding agent is applied over entire etched enamel surface with a microbrush. The coating may be thinned by a gentle air burst for 1 to 2 seconds. A thick layer may cause "drifting" before curing is initiated and may interfere with the precise adaptation of the bracket base.

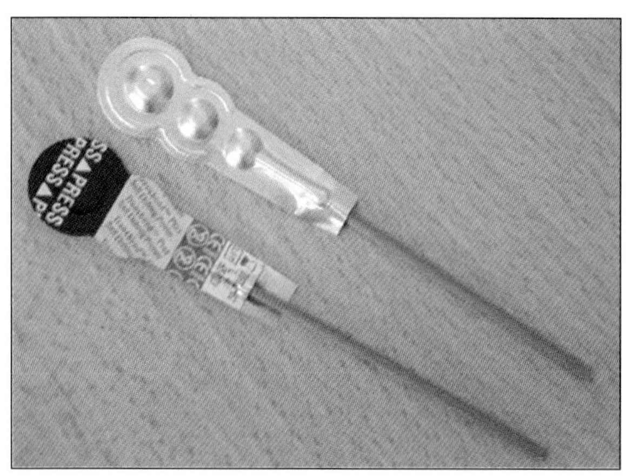

Fig. 6-7 Transbond Plus self-etching primer (3M Unitek).

Glass ionomer cements

Glass ionomer cements have distinctive properties that make them potentially useful in clinical orthodontics. First, they adhere to both enamel and metal.[71] Second, these cements release fluoride and therefore may prevent enamel decalcification.[72] Third, glass ionomer cements can be removed with much less difficulty than composite resin after debonding,[73] because the cement remaining on the tooth surface can be desiccated by simply air drying it,[74] thus rendering it more friable.[75]

Recent research also demonstrated that the use of resin-modified glass ionomer cement (RM-GIC) alone can significantly decrease enamel demineralization compared with composite resin.[76] Although the increased fluoride release from the glass ionomer cements has the potential for lessening decalcification around orthodontic brackets, SBS of the material is relatively low compared with composite adhesive.[77]

It is advisable to limit use of glass ionomer cement to at-risk orthodontic patients to provide preventive actions and potentially remineralize early (subclinical) enamel demineralization.[76]

Cytotoxicity of orthodontic resins

Regardless of polymerization method, in vitro studies have shown that the polymerization reaction that produces the cross-linked polymer matrix from the dimethacrylate resin monomer is never complete; 15% to 50% of the methacrylic group remains unreacted (32.4% and 44.5% for Transbond LR and Lightcure LR orthodontic adhesives, respectively).[67,78-80] Because of the material industry's efforts, the percentage of unbound monomers has been decreased in the past decade, but the problem remains. The quantity of residual monomers is less than a tenth of the remaining methacrylic groups, evaluated as 1.5% to 5%, but sufficient to cause major cytotoxic effects.[67,81]

Monomers identified in orthodontic composites (Transbond XT, Transbond LR, Reliance Light Bond, Reliance FlowTain, Fuji Ortho LC) by liquid chromatography include bisglycidil methacrylate (BISGMA), triethyleneglycol dimethacrylate (TEGDMA), urethane dimethacrylate (UDMA), and 2-hydroxyethyl methacrylate (HEMA) in the 0 to 99.8 µM range.[82] Resins and RM-GIC also release ions such as fluoride, strontium, and aluminum.[67] These unbound free monomers seem to be directly responsible for the cytotoxicity of resin composites on pulp and gingival cells and are implicated in the allergic potential of the material.[80]

Leaching of some ions also seems to be implicated in cell alterations. Depletion of glutathione, production of reactive oxygen species, and a few other molecular mechanisms have been identified as key factors leading to apoptosis and pulp necrosis. In addition, resin monomers stimulate the development of cariogenic bacteria at the interface between the material and the walls of the cavity.[67,83,84]

Currently, it seems inevitable to avoid this resin monomer and ion release. However, some simple and basic precautions may help prevent or decrease the adverse effects of these materials on patients. First, the amount of composite resin used should be kept at a minimum, and any excess resin ("flash") around the orthodontic attachments should be removed before the resin is polymerized. Minimizing the use of adhesive material may be more important when bonding fixed orthodontic retainers because these are left in the oral environment for a long time and are exposed to the cavity, unlike resin beneath the bracket base. Also, the speed of monomer release is maximal in the first 10 to 60 minutes.[82] It might be advisable to have the patients wash their mouth right after the bonding session, or have them spit into a disposable cup for the first 30 minutes when resin is used after topical fluoride applications.

Light Sources in Orthodontics

The introduction of light-cure adhesives not only removed a step in the bonding procedure, but also allowed practitioners to choose when to initiate the adhesive curing cycle after bracket placement. Light-curing resin composites were introduced in the 1970s. In light-cure adhesives, the curing process begins when a photoinitiator is activated. Most dental photoinitiator systems use camphoroquinone as the diketone absorber, with the absorption maximum in the blue region of the visible light spectrum at a wavelength of 470 nanometers (nm).[71,85]

The light-polymerized resins offer the advantage of extended, although not indefinite, working time. This provides the opportunity for assistants to place the brackets, with the orthodontist following up with any final positioning. Light-cured adhesives are particularly useful when a "quick set" is required, such as rebonding one loose bracket or placing an attachment on an impacted canine after surgical uncovering, with the risk for bleeding. Light-cured adhesives are also advantageous when extralong working time is desirable, as when difficult premolar bracket positions need to be checked and rechecked with a mouth mirror before the bracket placement is considered optimal.[5]

The first light-cured resin products were polymerized with ultraviolet light, with later versions cured by visible light, which has a wavelength between 400 and 500 nm. An advantage of using visible light is greater depth of polymerization in shorter periods.[86] Full bonding of upper and lower arches with a conventional tungsten-quartz halogen light source at 40 seconds per bracket may require 15 to 20 minutes.[87-89] The long cure times are inconvenient for the patient, impractical with children, and uncomfortable for the orthodontist and results in lost chair time. A more efficient and faster curing light is needed.[90]

Conventional halogen lights

Currently, the most popular method of delivering blue light is halogen-based light-curing units[91] (e.g., Ortholux XT, 3M Unitek; Fig. 6-8). These provide a light intensity of about 500 mW/cm^2 and a wavelength range of 420 to 500 nm. Halogen bulbs produce light when electrical energy heats a small tungsten filament to high temperatures.[92] Despite their common use in dentistry, halogen bulbs have several disadvantages. The basic principle of light conversion by this tech-

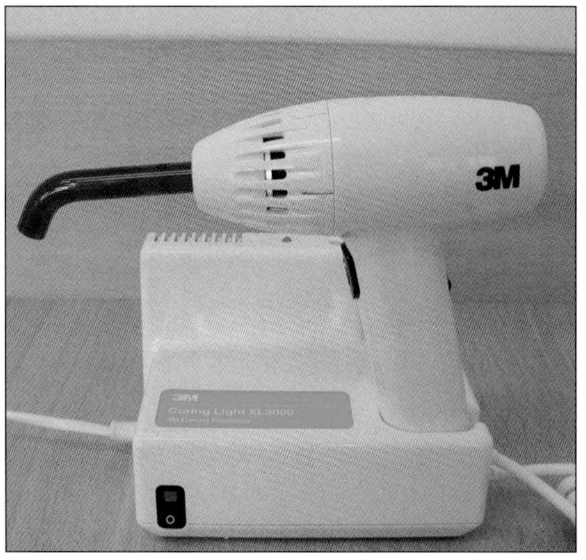

Fig. 6-8 Ortholux XT conventional halogen curing light (3M Unitek).

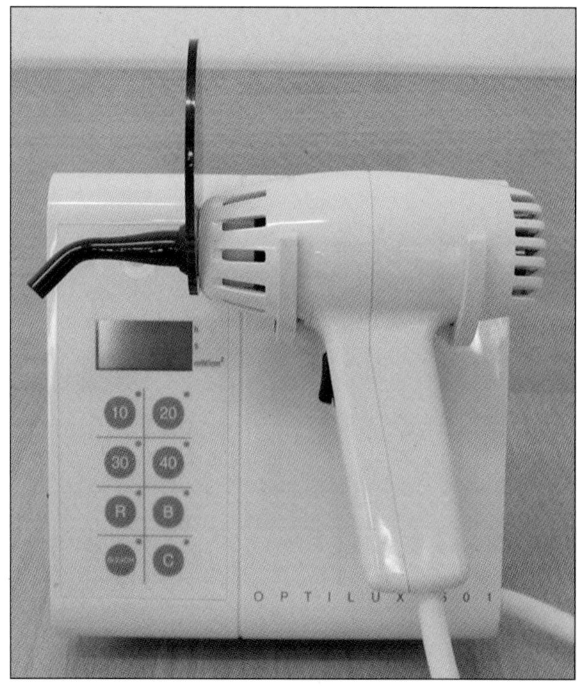

Fig. 6-9 Optilux 501 high intensity halogen curing light (Demetron/Kerr Corp.).

TABLE 6-1

Recommendations for Light Curing Various Adhesives with Different Light Sources

Adhesive	Suggested Time of Light Exposure (seconds) Conventional Halogen Transbond XL	Fast Halogen Optilux 501	Plasma Arc Light Power Pac
Transbond XT (3M Unitek)	40	10	3
Light Bond (Reliance)	40	20	3
Quick Cure (Reliance)	10	6	3
Transbond LR (3M Unitek)	20	10	6
Light Cure Retainer (Reliance)	40	10	15

Data from Üşümez S, Büyükyilmaz T, Karaman AI: *Am J Orthod Dentofacial Orthop* 123(6):641-668, 2003; and Hotz P, McLean JW, Seed I, Wilson AD: *Br Dent J* 142:41-47, 1977.

nique is said to be inefficient because the light power output is less than 1% of the consumed electrical power. Halogens also have a limited effective life of approximately 100 hours because of the degradation of the bulb's components by the high heat generated.[91,93,94] The halogen lights can cure orthodontic composite resins in 20 seconds and light-cured RMGICs in 40 seconds per bracket.[5,95] Table 6-1 provides the authors' recommendations for light curing various adhesives with different light sources.[14,71]

High-intensity halogen lights ("fast halogens")

Halogen lights were followed by "fast halogens" with halogen bulbs of increased light intensity and "turbo tips" to focus the light emitted (e.g., Optilux 501, Demetron/Kerr Corp., Orange, Calif.; Fig. 6-9). These provide a light intensity of 800 to 900 mW/cm^2 and a wavelength range of 400 to 505 nm. Fast halogens can reduce curing time to half that needed with conventional halogen lights.[5,90]

Plasma arc units

Plasma arc lamps have a tungsten anode and a cathode in a quartz tube filled with xenon gas. The gas becomes ionized and forms a plasma that consists of negatively and positively charged particles and that generates an intense white light when an electrical current is passed through the xenon. Plasma arc lights are contained in base units rather than in the "guns" because of the high voltage used and heat generated[5,90] (Fig. 6-10). Plasma arc light sources do not emit distinct frequencies, but rather continuous-frequency bands that are much narrower than those of conventional lights. Consequently, less radiation is filtered with undesired frequencies. Plasma arc lights provide a light intensity of 1200 to 1500 mW/cm^2 and a wavelength range of 380 to 495 nm. Because of the high intensity, manufacturers claim that 1 to 3 seconds of plasma irradiation cures many resin composites to hardness comparable with that achieved after 40 seconds of conventional curing lights.[71,96]

Rapid composite curing with the plasma arc lights clearly is beneficial for the clinician. However, high-intensity plasma arc lights may not be compatible with every orthodontic adhesive.[14,71] The clinician should perform a basic compatibility test before using these light sources with some orthodontic adhesives.

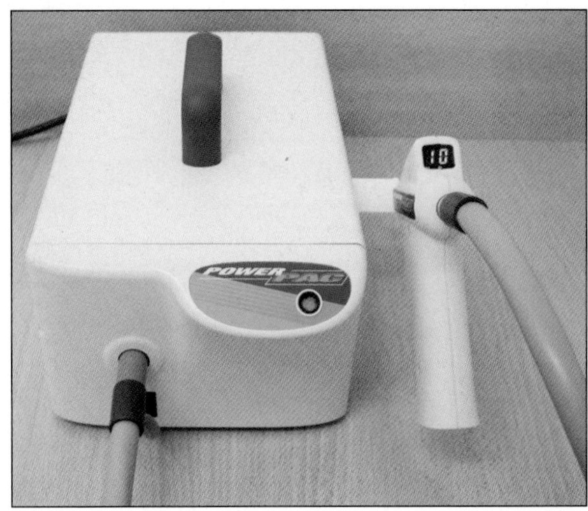

Fig. 6-10 Plasma curing light (PowerPac, American Medical Technologies, Corpus Christi, Tex.). Plasma arc lights are contained in base units, and light energy is delivered to the gun tip with a flexible cord.

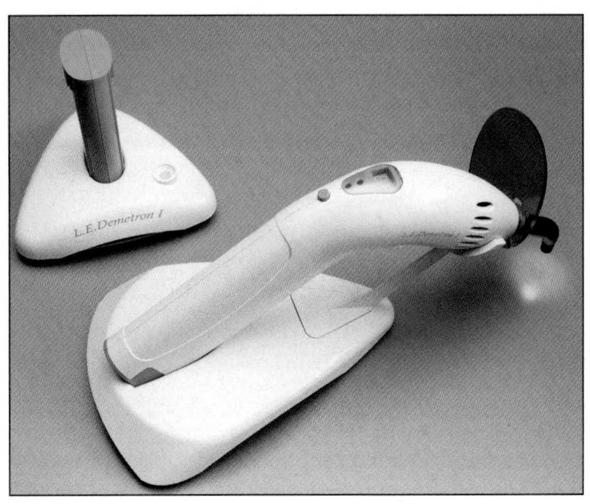

Fig. 6-11 LEDemetron LED curing light (Demetron/Kerr Corp.). (From Boyd LRB: *Dental instruments: a pocket guide,* ed 3, St Louis, 2009, Mosby-Elsevier.)

Another concern with plasma arc lights is the high heat generated.[97,98] Zach and Cohen[99] reported permanent pulp damage in primates when the pulpal temperature rose above 42.5° C. The increase in pulpal temperature in a restorative preparation was found to reach 5.16° C with plasma arc light, versus only 1.86° C with conventional halogen.[100] In orthodontic bonding the untouched enamel and dentin layer may provide additional heat insulation, and thus the use of the plasma arc light for curing orthodontic adhesives for 5 to 10 seconds should be safe in regard to the pulp temperature.[5,101]

Also, studies have shown that plasma arc–generated blue light causes some damage to cells, particularly to DNA, and thus a long curing time exceeding that recommended can cause biological damage to oral tissue.[102,103]

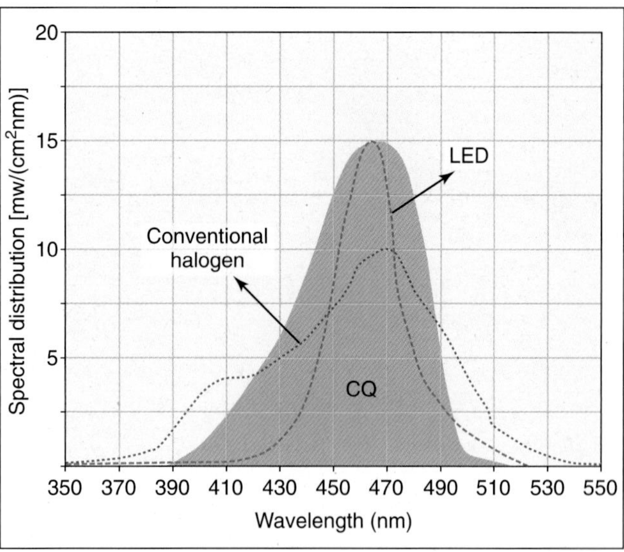

Fig. 6-12 Spectral distribution/wavelength graphic demonstrates that the peak of LED light sources coincide better with the absorption peak of camphoroquinone *(CQ).* This means that a photon emitted by an LED source is more likely to activate a camphoroquinone molecule.

Light-emitting diodes

Mills, Jandt, and Ashworth[91] proposed solid-state light-emitting diode (LED) technology for the polymerization of light-activated dental materials to overcome the disadvantages of halogen visible-light curing units (Fig. 6-11). LEDs use junctions of "doped" semiconductors to generate light instead of the hot filaments used in halogen bulbs.[104] LEDs have a lifetime of over 10,000 hours and undergo little degradation of output over this time.[105] LEDs do not require filters to produce blue light, are resistant to shock and vibration, and take little power to operate.[91] Earlier LED designs provided unsatisfactory with metal brackets, possibly because of their low power output.[13]

Current LED light sources combine high power output (~1000 mW/cm^2) with a very narrow wavelength range of about 465 nm, which matches well with the absorption peak of camphoroquinone (Fig. 6-12). These light sources are currently replacing the conventional halogens in all dental fields.

Safe operation of curing lights

The normal spectral output from a visible-light curing (VLC) unit extends into both ultraviolet (UV) and infrared (IR) ranges. This spectral region is often referred to as the *retinal hazard region.* Inexpensive bandpass filters incorporated into the VLC unit eliminate unnecessary light energy, although extraneous visible light still reaches the operator's eye during the curing process (Fig. 6-13).

This light energy is dangerous because the cornea, lens, and vitreous fluid of the eye are transparent to these wavelengths, and the light energy is absorbed in the retina. Damage to the retina is possible through thermal or photo-

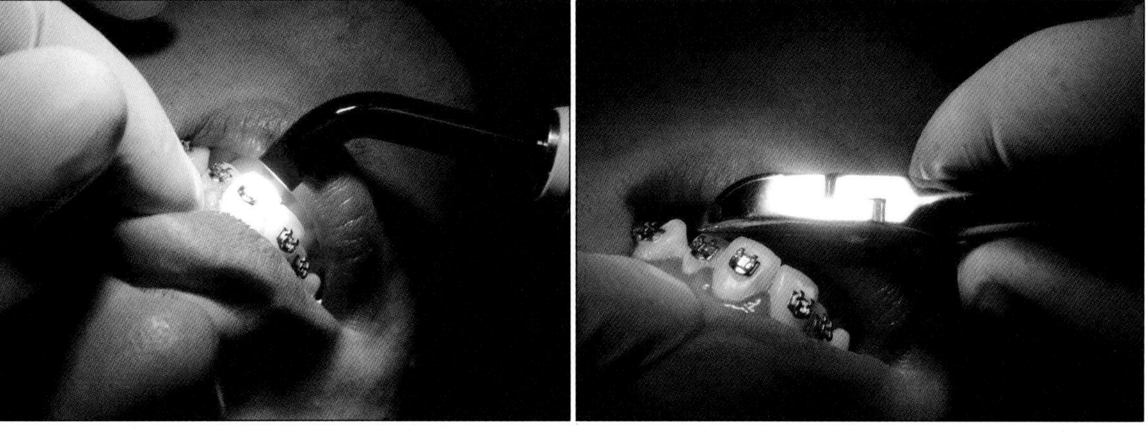

Fig. 6-13 Normal spectral output from a visible-light curing unit extends into both ultraviolet and infrared ranges (retinal hazard region).

chemical processes. Photochemical damage to photoreceptor cells of the retina can degrade overall light or color sensitivity, and the IR wavelengths may cause cataract formation in the lens[106] (Fig. 6-14).

What makes UVA and blue light hazardous? Research shows that when blue light strikes the retina, the light waves inhibit the formation of the chemical cytochrome-*c* oxidase. This chemical is an important part of retinal cells because it transports oxygen to photoreceptor and other retinal cells. Without cytochrome-*c* oxidase, the cells become deprived of oxygen and eventually die. When enough cells die, retinal degeneration occurs.[107-110]

Similar research demonstrated that the retinal damage done was a feature of the *wavelength,* not the duration or frequency, of exposure. This means that even a short exposure to blue light can cause retinal damage without adequate protection. Often the lesions from UVA and blue light are scattered on the retina. Only when enough of them appear and coalesce does a vision loss become noticeable. This is why vision loss is not immediate, but often takes many years to manifest.[107-110]

On average, orthodontists bond up to 20 attachments per day. With an acceptable curing time of 20 seconds per tooth, they spend 28 hours per year holding the light gun, even longer than their restorative colleagues.

Individuals with a history of retinal disease should seek advice from their ophthalmologist before operating the unit. This group of individuals must take extreme care and comply with all safety precautions, including the use of suitable light-filtering safety goggles.[102,103,111,112]

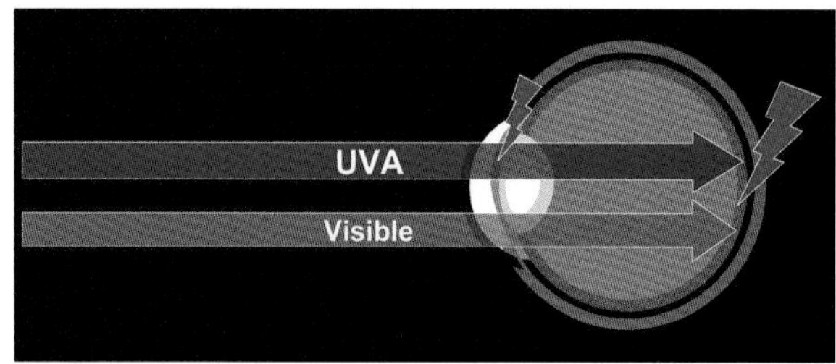

Fig. 6-14 Overexposure to light energy is dangerous because the cornea, lens, and vitreous fluid of the eye are transparent to these wavelengths, and the light energy is absorbed in the retina. *UVA,* Ultraviolet light type A.

Direct Bonding

Premedication

Initial activation of the orthodontic attachments may cause significant discomfort to the patient. Recent research revealed that patients premedicated with 550 mg of naproxen sodium 1 hour before archwire placement had significantly lower levels of pain at 2 hours, 6 hours, and later that night after adjustment than patients taking placebo.[113] Analgesic premedication may be considered before proceeding to the bonding stage.

Bonding procedure

A successful bracket bonding procedure[5,9,70] consists of the following steps. First, the bracket is gripped with reverse-action tweezers, and the adhesive is applied to the bracket base. It is important that the adhesive be evenly distributed on the bracket base without leaving a gap between the adhesive (Fig. 6-15). Presence of such a gap may act as the weakest link in the chain and lead to premature failure of the attachment. The bracket is then placed on the tooth immediately.

A scaler or a round probe is used to position the bracket on the tooth surface in occlusogingival, mesiodistal directions and in correct angulation. Direct visualization is limited in the posterior area because of tissue stretching from cheek retractors. Correct positioning of posterior teeth requires effort and checking from the occlusal surface with a mirror (Fig. 6-16). Alternatively, these teeth may be bonded separately, or a more flexible type of cheek retractor may be used

Fig. 6-15 Direct-bonding procedure. The bracket is gripped with reverse action tweezers and the adhesive is applied to the bracket base. It is important that the adhesive is evenly distributed on the bracket base without leaving any gap between the adhesive. This can be achieved with a small dental instrument.

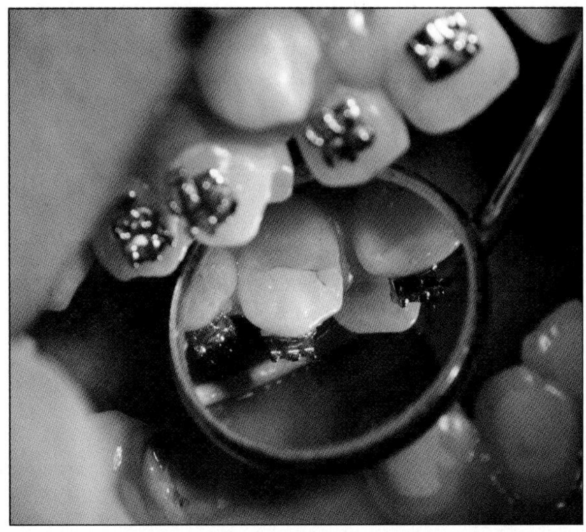

Fig. 6-16 Direct-bonding procedure. Direct visualization is limited in the posterior area due to tissue stretching as a result of cheek retractors. Correct positioning of posterior teeth should be checked from the occlusal surface with a mirror.

for direct visualization. The placement of orthodontic brackets is guided either by localizing the center of the clinical crown or by measuring the distance from the incisal edge. It is suggested that bracket bonding guided by measuring the distance from incisal edge may result in improved placement for anterior teeth. Archwire bending or bracket repositioning is still necessary to compensate for the inaccuracies with both techniques.[114]

The attachment is then pressed onto the enamel surface with the scaler or the probe. The fitting of the bracket base to the contour of the tooth is important. Improper fitting of the base leads to unwanted tooth movement, usually in the form of rotation.

It is important to avoid placing the brackets too far gingival, unless dictated by the opposing teeth, as is sometimes the case in the lower arch. This leads to incomplete expression of the torque value built into the bracket and improper hygiene conditions. The brackets may come into contact with the gingival margin, particularly after intrusive tooth movement, because the gingival margin and the mucogingival junction move in the same direction as the teeth by only 79% and 62%, respectively. A statistically significant decrease of the clinical crown length has also been observed after intrusion.[115]

Any excess material expressed around the bracket is removed with a scaler before the material sets or the light polymerizes it. The suggested light-curing times can be monitored according to Table 6-1. Removal of the "flash" around the margins is important to maintain proper oral hygiene throughout the treatment. Some manufacturers add a coloring agent to assist in the visualization of the excess adhesive (APC Plus, 3M Unitek), although recent research reveals that this method does not reduce the amount of excessive adhesive around orthodontic brackets.[116]

After completion of bracketing, the position of each bracket should be checked carefully. Any attachment that is not in proper position should be removed and rebonded immediately. Rebondings postponed to later appointments will take much longer to perform and may lead to compromised results. Motivational oral hygiene and brushing instructions should follow.[117] The use of additional postoperative doses of analgesics may be recommended to control orthodontic pain completely.[118]

Bonding to artificial tooth surfaces

With increased popularity of orthodontic treatment and advances in the esthetic appearance of attachments, more adults are visiting orthodontic clinics. Bracketing of these patients may frequently require bonding to crown-and-bridge restorations fabricated from porcelain and precious metals in addition to amalgam restorations.[5,118-120] This section summarizes current techniques with emphasis on the protection for surrounding periodontal structures. Bonding to an artificial surface requires the use of microetching of these surfaces using 50-μm white or 90-μm aluminum oxide particles at about 7 kg/cm^2 pressure.

Ceramic crowns. The ceramic restorations should be bonded separately under carefully isolated conditions. A barrier gel such as Kool-Dam (Pulpdent Corp., Watertown, Mass.) is suggested whenever a risk exists that the hydrofluoric acid etching gel may flow into contact with the gingiva or soft tissues. The bonding procedure is as follows[5]:

1. Sandblast an area slightly larger than the base of the orthodontic attachment with 50-μm aluminum oxide for 3 seconds.
2. Etch the porcelain with 9.6% hydrofluoric acid gel for 2 minutes.
3. Remove the bulk of the gel with cotton roll, and then rinse using high-power suction.
4. Immediately dry with air, and bond the bracket as usual.

Amalgam. The procedure for bonding to amalgam depends on the size of the amalgam restoration and incorporation of the enamel area. For small amalgam restorations with surrounding sound enamel, the following technique has been suggested[5,119,120]:

1. Sandblast the amalgam alloy with 50-µm aluminum oxide for 3 seconds.
2. Condition the surrounding enamel with 37% phosphoric acid for 15 seconds.
3. Apply sealant, and bond as usual with composite resin.

For large amalgam restoration with minimal enamel inclusion or for amalgam only[5]

1. Sandblast the amalgam filling with 50-µm aluminum oxide for 3 seconds.
2. Apply a uniform coat of metal primer (e.g., Reliance Metal Primer, Reliance Orthodontic Products, Itasca, Ill.) and wait for 30 seconds.
3. Apply sealant, and bond with composite resin.

Gold. In vitro studies report high bond strengths with gold. New technologies include sandblasting, electrolytic tin plating or plating with gallium-tin solution, and use of different types of intermediate primers, as well as new adhesives that bond chemically to precious metals (Superbond C&B, Panavia Ex and Panavia 21; Kuraray America, New York, N.Y.). Clinical results are, however, far from satisfactory when bonding to gold crowns.[5,119,120]

Composite. Bonding to old composite restorations does not usually present a clinical problem provided that the previous surface is removed with a rotary instrument and the old composite thoroughly dried.[5,121,122]

Indirect Bonding

Indirect bonding was first introduced in detail as a concept in 1972 by Silverman and Cohen.[123] There are many proposed advantages associated with indirect bonding,[124,125] and it has even been proposed as the mandatory mode of placement, especially in lingual cases.[126] Clinical and laboratory studies failed to support this advantage of indirect bonding in labial cases, however, with only a small gain in the accuracy of bracket height.[127-129]

Many advocates believe that reduced chair time and delegation of the procedure to assistant staff make indirect bonding cost-effective.[130] Hodge et al.[127] found significant cost savings when using indirect bonding versus direct bonding in a hospital dental clinic. In addition to cost-effectiveness, additional benefits include enhanced patient comfort, elimination of the need for separators and bands, easier ability to rebond brackets and build in overcorrections, better in/out and vertical control, and improved oral hygiene because of generally smaller attachments.[131,132] Other benefits are optimal use of staff, reduced inventory and associated costs, fewer appointments for appliance placement and removal, and overall healthier ergonomics.[129]

In vitro bond-strength studies demonstrate comparable SBS values between the direct and indirect methods.[122,133-136] Bond failure rates reported for in vivo investigations also generally fall within clinically acceptable ranges of 1.4% to 6.5%.[137-142]

Several techniques for indirect bonding are available. The brackets are temporarily bonded to the teeth on the stone models with composite resin, transferred to the mouth with some type of tray into which the brackets become incorporated into the tray, and then bonded all at once using an intermediate sealant.[5,131,143]

Rebonding Loose Brackets

Accidental dislodgement of an orthodontic bracket caused by occlusal trauma, or intentional removal of a bracket to reposition, is common in orthodontic practice.[144] Before rebonding an orthodontic attachment, the orthodontist should consider reconditioning of the enamel surfaces, the use of new or the original brackets, and the recycling and bonding system to be used. In general, SBS of a rebonded bracket has been reported to be comparable to that of the original.[144,145]

The removed bracket should first be inspected for deformation of the slot that may have occurred during breakage. Brackets that seem to be deformed should be replaced with a new bracket. Before proceeding with rebonding, any composite remaining on the tooth surface is removed with a tungsten-carbide bur. The adhesive remaining on the loose bracket is also removed with the bur, until all visible bonding material is removed from the base, with treatment by sandblasting as an option.[144,145] The tooth then is etched with phosphoric acid gel for 30 seconds. A longer etch is advisable. In contrast to initial bonding, the enamel surface may not appear uniform because some areas may retain composite. After priming, the bracket is rebonded. The bond strength for sandblasted rebonded brackets is comparable to the SBS (and subsequent success rate) for new brackets.[144-146]

DEBONDING

Unlike other restorative practices in dentistry, the adhesive system set up at the start of orthodontic treatment is dismantled, and the brackets are removed after completion of the therapy. The debonding phase is as important as the bonding phase and should not be underestimated; doing so may result in significant damage to the enamel surface and unnecessary elongation of the chair time to restore the surface to its original gloss.

Debonding sessions are best scheduled on a certain day of the week or month so that both clinician and staff are concentrated to provide the best debonding service to the patient. Whether metal or ceramic, the brackets should be removed individually after removal of the archwires to avoid force transfer from tooth to tooth, which may increase the risk of enamel crack formation.

Bracket Removal

Steel brackets

A peeling-type force technique was recommended by Zachrisson and Büyükyilmaz[5] to break the adhesive bond without deforming the bracket, to allow recycling. The peeling force is said to create peripheral stress concentrations that cause bonded metal brackets to fail at low force values.[147] This type of removal is advantageous because a break is likely to occur in the adhesive-bracket interface, leaving adhesive remnants on the enamel.[5]

Ceramic brackets

Debonding of ceramic brackets is more likely to cause enamel fracture because ceramic brackets adhere more strongly to the enamel surface and will not flex when squeezed with debonding pliers.[148,149] The risk is lower with ceramic brackets using mechanical retention than those using chemical retention.[148,150-152] The bracket should be lifted off with peripheral force application, as with steel brackets, for easier and safer removal.

One study showed that new designs with a ball reduction band (e.g., Inspire Ice bracket, Ormco Corp., Orange, Calif.) and the vertical debonding slot (e.g., Clarity bracket, 3M Unitek) significantly reduced the risk of ceramic bracket fracture during debonding[21] (Fig. 6-17). The force required to debond the Inspire Ice bracket was significantly lower than that of the Inspire bracket.[153]

Because of the high heat generated, grinding of ceramic brackets with a low-speed handpiece with no water coolant may cause permanent damage or necrosis of dental pulp. Water cooling of the grinding sites is necessary.[154]

Other efforts to facilitate removal of ceramic brackets include thermal debonding[150,155-158] and the use of lasers,[159-161] which are based on heating and softening of the composite resin. Another recent challenge is the modification of the methylmethacrylate resin to initiate self-removal when activated.[162,163] These applications may be less traumatic with less risk of enamel damage, but are still at an introductory stage, with definitive results not yet reported.

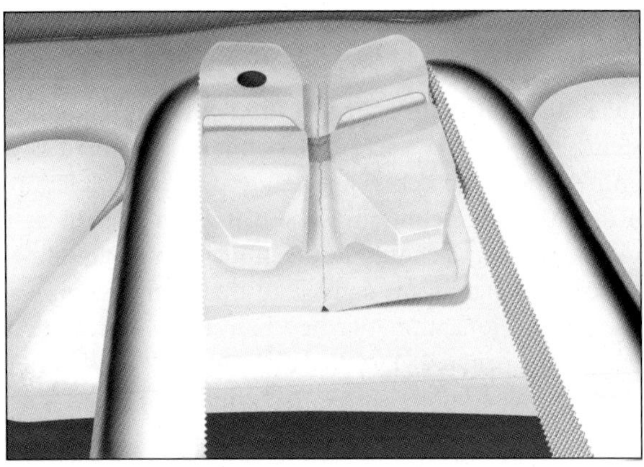

Fig. 6-17 The vertical debonding slot in the Clarity bracket significantly reduces the risk of ceramic bracket fracture during debonding. The two halves of the bracket collapse when the wings are squeezed. (Courtesy 3M Unitek, Monrovia, Calif.)

Residual Adhesive Cleaning

With improvements in the physical and mechanical properties of resin adhesive systems, cleanup of resin remnants after orthodontic bracket debonding has become a clinical problem. The removal of adhesive remnants from tooth surfaces is a final procedure to restore the surface as closely as possible to its pretreatment gloss without inducing iatrogenic damage.[164] If remnants are not completely removed, tooth surfaces are likely to discolor and entrap plaque with time.[165] Many investigators have introduced various resin-remnant removal techniques. Despite the introduction of new methods (e.g., Nd:YAG laser) to remove residues of bonding resin selectively,[166,167] the most common removal techniques use a low-speed handpiece with a tungsten-carbide bur and a high-speed handpiece with a diamond bur.[168-170] The preferred method uses a low-speed handpiece with a round, tungsten-carbide bur.[171,172]

The bulk of the remaining adhesive may be removed with diamond or tungsten-carbide burs attached to a high-speed handpiece. Because of considerable scratching, however, these should not be used closer to the enamel surface.[5,164,165,171,173] When approaching the enamel, a tungsten-carbide bur attached to a low-speed hand piece operating at 30,000 rpm should be used.[5] For this purpose, the bur is moved in one direction as the resin layers are removed.[164] Water cooling is avoided at this stage to improve the contrast between the adhesive and the enamel surface.[5]

Any recontouring considered necessary should be completed at this stage before proceeding to polishing.

Operator Safety During Debonding

Another important but often ignored issue is the inhalation of aerosols produced during the removal of fixed orthodontic appliances. Recent research shows that aerosol particulates produced during enamel cleanup might be inhaled regardless of handpiece speed or the presence or absence of water coolant. This aerosol may contain calcium, phosphorus, silica, aluminum, iron, and lanthanum.[174] Blood, hepatitis B surface antigen (HBsAg) and hepatitis B virus (HBV) DNA were also detected in excess fluid samples of the two hepatitis B carriers.[175] Although the particles most likely are deposited in the conducting airways and terminal bronchi, some might be deposited in the terminal alveoli of the lungs and cleared only after weeks or months.[174]

Studies indicate that orthodontists are exposed to high levels of aerosol generation and contamination during the debonding procedure, and that preprocedural chlorhexidine gluconate mouthrinse appears to be ineffective in decreasing exposure to infectious agents. Barrier equipment should be used to prevent aerosol contamination.[174,176]

Detailing and Polishing

After completion of adhesive removal, the enamel surface may be further polished using various soft disks, cups, and pastes.[164,177] Some authors view this stage as "optional," considering the normal wear of enamel.[5]

PREVENTION AND TREATMENT OF WHITE SPOTS DURING FIXED-APPLIANCE THERAPY AND AFTER DEBONDING

Preventive Measures

White-spot lesion (WSL) demineralization is a significant problem during orthodontic treatment. The primary measure to prevent WSLs is maintenance of maximum oral hygiene with effective brushing and cleaning of the entire dentition throughout orthodontic treatment. Special attention should be given to oral hygiene instruction and monitoring at the patient's initial visit and bonding session and throughout treatment when necessary. Parents should also be informed about the outcomes of failure to brush properly. One cross-sectional study found that 50% of individuals undergoing treatment with braces had a nondevelopmental WSL compared with 25% of controls.[178] Another study found that, even 5 years after treatment, orthodontic patients had a significantly higher incidence of WSLs than a control group of patients who had not had orthodontic treatment.[179] This obvious degree of iatrogenic damage suggests the need for preventive programs using fluoride during fixed-appliance orthodontic treatment.[5,180]

Methods to deliver fluoride to teeth during orthodontic treatment (in addition to fluoridated toothpaste) include the following[180]:

1. Topical fluorides (e.g., mouthrinse, gel, varnish, toothpaste, "tooth mousse")
2. Fluoride-releasing materials (e.g., bonding materials, elastics)

Daily rinsing with dilute (0.05%) sodium fluoride solution throughout treatment and retention, plus regular use of a fluoride dentifrice, is recommended as a routine procedure for all orthodontic patients.[117] Evidence shows that a daily sodium fluoride mouthrinse reduces the severity of enamel decay surrounding a fixed bracket.[180-188] For the self-administration methods of applying fluoride (e.g., fluoride toothpastes and mouthrinses) to be effective, the patient's cooperation is essential.[178,189,190] Compliance rates as low as 13% have been reported for patients asked to decrease their caries risk with a daily fluoride mouthrinse.[191,192]

Professional means of fluoride application have included fluoride-releasing bonding agents, fluoridated elastomeric ligature ties, fluoride varnish, and 10% casein phosphopeptide–amorphous calcium phosphate (CPP-ACP; GC Tooth Mousse, GC America, Alsip, Ill.)[83,187,193-199] (Fig. 6-18). Professional application of 1% chlorhexidine collagen gel is also suggested to control *Streptococcus mutans* level in orthodontic patients with high caries risk.[200] The use of a polymeric

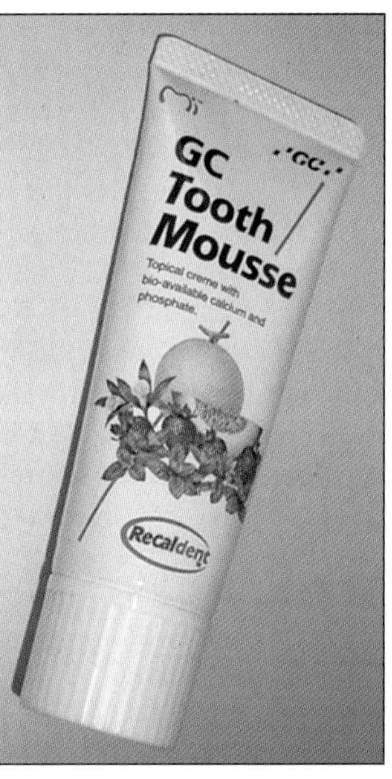

Fig. 6-18 GC Tooth Mousse (GC America) is a water-based, sugar-free cream containing Recaldent CPP-ACP (casein phosphopeptide–amorphous calcium phosphate). When CPP-ACP is applied to the tooth surfaces, it binds to biofilms, plaque, bacteria, hydroxyapatite, and surrounding soft tissue, localizing bioavailable calcium and phosphate.

coating on the tooth surface around the brackets showed almost no demineralization-inhibiting effect.[182]

Fluoridated elastomeric modules were considered to be an ideal solution to supplement fluoride around orthodontic brackets because they do not interfere with routine clinical practice and could ensure a "fresh" delivery of fluoride at each visit.[197,199] Unfortunately, because of their poor mechanical performance and swelling as a result of water absorption, fluoridated elastomers have not provided an acceptable solution to the problem.[192]

The use of glass ionomer cements for bracket bonding also reduces the prevalence and severity of white spots, but the evidence is weak compared with use of composite resins.[181-188,192] Although the increased fluoride release from glass ionomers has the potential for decreasing decalcification around orthodontic brackets, the SBS of some glass ionomer cement material is relatively low.[84] If glass ionomer cement is used in a high-risk patient, Fuji Ortho LC (GC America) and Fuji Ortho Band Paste Pak (GC America) may be considered the material of choice because these adhesives reportedly release more fluoride than other commercially available products.[201]

Patients who undergo orthodontic therapy have changes in their oral environment, such as a low pH, increased retentive sites for *S. mutans*, and increased retention of food particles, which may lead to increased proportions and absolute numbers of salivary *S. mutans*.[202-207] These changes may be partly responsible for the post–orthodontic treatment decalcification in certain cases.[178,208] Øgaard et al.[209] indicated that a high prevalence of caries may be caused by the high cariogenic environment in the plaque around orthodontic appliances. Proper oral hygiene is more difficult to maintain, and pH levels lower than 4.5 have been measured in the plaque around the brackets and the bands during orthodontic treatment.[209] At such a low pH, the remineralization phase is hampered, and more fluoride will not necessarily provide a better cariostatic effect.[210] Therefore, Øgaard and Rølla[210] suggested that fluoride agents could be further improved by the addition of antibacterial agents. Accordingly, the application of Cervitec varnish induced a significant reduction of *S. mutans* in saliva over 1 month[211] and a reduction in the proportion of *S. mutans* in the plaque adjacent to brackets, without adversely affecting SBS.[212] No clinical differences were found in the incidence of incipient enamel demineralization around the bracket bases. The differences decreased over time, becoming statistically insignificant during the third month.[213]

Another, newer method of fighting decalcification is the use of probiotic nutritional products or functional foods. A *probiotic* is a live microbial food supplement that beneficially affects the host by improving intestinal microbial balance. These "beneficial" microorganisms can inhabit a biofilm and protect oral tissue from disease. One mechanism by which these biofilms keep out pathogens is to occupy a space that pathogens might otherwise occupy.[214] An in vitro study suggests that *Lactobacillus rhamnosus* strain GG can inhibit the colonization of streptococcal caries pathogens, thus reducing the incidence of caries in children.[215] A recent double-blind randomized study showed that daily consumption of *Bifidobacterium* DN-173 010 containing 200 g of fruit-flavored yogurt was able to decrease salivary *S. mutans* levels significantly.[216]

Treatment After Bracket Removal

When WSLs are seen at debonding, the orthodontist should allow 2 to 3 months of good oral hygiene without fluoride supplementation. More fluoride applied at this early stage is believed to precipitate calcium phosphate onto the enamel surface and block the surface pores, which limits remineralization to the superficial part of the lesion, and the optical appearance of the white spot is not reduced.[5,217]

When the remineralizing capacity of the oral fluids is exhausted and WSLs are established, microabrasion as described by Gelgör and Büyükyilmaz[218] is an effective way to remove superficial enamel opacities. This technique can eliminate enamel stains with minimal enamel loss. An abrasive gel (18% hydrochloric acid, fine-powdered pumice, and glycerin) is applied by electric toothbrush for 3 to 5 minutes. Monthly repetition of the procedure for 2 or 3 months may be necessary, depending on the severity of the lesions, until the stains gradually disappear.[218]

BONDING FIXED LINGUAL RETAINERS

Many appliance types have been used for the retention of posttreatment tooth position. The first appliances were based on banded fixed appliances,[219] followed by removable retainers.[220] Most recently, bonded fixed retainers have been introduced, consisting of a length of orthodontic wire bonded to the teeth with acid-etched retained composite.[221]

Early bonded fixed retainers were made with plain, round or rectangular orthodontic wires,[222-226] but Zachrisson[221] proposed using multistrand wire. Årtun and Zachrisson[227] first described the clinical technique for use of a multistrand-wire, canine-to-canine, bonded fixed retainer. In this retainer the wire was bonded to the canine teeth only. In 1983, Zachrisson[228] reported the use of multistrand wire in a bonded fixed retainer in which the wire was bonded to all the teeth in the labial segment.[229]

These appliances are shown to perform successfully, and long-term retention of mandibular incisor alignment is acceptable with fixed retainers even after 20 years in most patients.[230,231] Some patients needing re-treatment despite successful retention of fixed lingual retainers has also been reported.[232]

Another issue with the use of fixed lingual retainers is periodontal health. Some consider the retainers compatible with periodontal health even over the long term,[233] whereas others question the appropriateness of lingual fixed retainers as a standard retention plan for all patients, regardless of their attitude toward dental hygiene.[234] Consequently, selection of retention protocol and fixed retainer type may be based on case-specific parameters such as dental and gingival anatomy and oral hygiene status. Regardless of selection, the patient should be given detailed hygiene instruction for healthy preservation of the fixed lingual retainer.

Adhesives Used for Lingual Retainer Bonding

Highly filled resins

Bonded fixed retainers are attached to the teeth with composite. Adhesives used with lingual retainers remain exposed to the oral cavity, so they require certain physical properties and proper management before the curing process. Composites described for this technique include both restorative and orthodontic bonding materials. Thinning of the composite was previously advised to obtain the best handling characteristics, but some difficulty in application remained. Later, several companies developed adhesives for lingual retainer bonding, claiming ease of application and optimal handling characteristics, to allow the clinician to shape and finish the adhesive around the lingual retainer wire for maximum patient comfort. These highly filled, light-cured resin pastes are also said to be a better choice when longevity and durability are required.[5,14] Light-activated composites may have these properties.

Studies have tested the surface hardness[14] and conversion rate[71] of different lingual retainer adhesives. Transbond LR (3M Unitek) yielded significantly higher surface hardness than Concise (3M Unitek) and Light Cure Retainer (Reliance Orthodontic Products), with Concise significantly harder than Light Cure Retainer. Dilution of Concise resin decreased the in vitro surface hardness, which in turn may decrease its clinical abrasion resistance and longevity.[5,14,71]

Regarding suggested curing times with various light sources, according to a monomer conversion study, a similar or higher degree of conversion than the control values could be achieved in 10 to 15 seconds by fast-halogen curing, in 20 seconds by LED curing, and in as low as 6 to 9 seconds by plasma arc curing.[71] High-intensity curing lights have been shown to cause significantly higher microleakage at the wire-adhesive interface, which in turn may decrease the clinical service time of the fixed lingual retainer.[235]

Flowable resins

Flowable resin composites have been made with a variety of formulas and viscosities for different uses.[236-241] Recently, use of flowable composites originally created for restorative dentistry (by increasing resin content of traditional microfilled composites) have been suggested for bonding lingual retainers.[242-244] These composites have advantages over other adhesives because (1) no mixing is required, (2) needle tips on the application syringes allow direct and precise composite placement, (3) the composite is not sticky and flows toward the bulk of the material rather than away from it, (4) no trimming or polishing is required, and (5) chair time is reduced.[242]

Previous reports demonstrated that flowable composites have lower SBS values when used for bonding metallic orthodontic brackets.[245] This leads to the question of whether they can serve as well when used for lingual retainer bonding. A recent study of the authors demonstrated that flowable composites provide SBS and wire pull-out values comparable to a standard orthodontic resin and can be used as an alternative for direct bonding of lingual retainers.[246]

Higher microleakage scores at the wire-adhesive interface and uncertain wear resistance make the use of flowable composites questionable.[247] These resins are best avoided in lingual retainer bonding until long-term clinical studies prove their dependability.

Clinical Procedures

Bonding 3-3 retainer bar (Fig. 6-19)

1. Bend the retainer wire from a plain, round, stainless steel or gold-coated wire of .030- to .032-inch diameter, precisely contacting the lingual surface of all mandibular incisors.
2. Sandblast both ends with 50-μm aluminum oxide powder for about 5 seconds using the Microetcher.
3. Apply prophylactic pumice to the lingual surfaces of both canines.
4. Check the position of the wire in the mouth, and fix with two steel ligatures around the bracket wings of the incisors when satisfactory.
5. Isolate the working area.
6. Etch the lingual surfaces of the canines with phosphoric acid gel for 30 seconds with the retainer wire in place. Rinse and dry.
7. Apply a thin coat of primer on the sandblasted ends of the retainer wire and on the etched enamel.
8. Apply the lingual retainer adhesive of choice to the right and left canines. Shape the resin bulk with microbrush strokes from the gingival margin to the incisal edge. Avoid creating any contour that may trap plaque.
9. Light-cure the composite resin according to instructions for the light source used.
10. Trim the gingival margin and contour the bulk, with a tungsten-carbide bur if necessary.
11. Instruct the patient in proper oral hygiene and use of dental floss or Superfloss (Oral-B, Boston, Mass.) beneath the retainer wire and along the mesial contact areas of both canines. Instruct patients to floss once daily to prevent accumulation of calculus and plaque.

Bonding 3-3 retainer wire (Fig. 6-20)

1. Bend the retainer wire from .0215-inch Penta-One steel wire, precisely contacting the lingual surface of all mandibular incisors.
2. Apply prophylactic pumice to the surfaces to be bonded, and etch with phosphoric acid gel for 30 seconds.
3. Stabilize the retainer wire in place before bonding, using two steel ligatures.[248]
4. Isolate the working area.
5. Apply the lingual retainer adhesive of choice to each tooth. Shape the resin bulk with microbrush strokes from the gingival margin to the incisal edge. Provide sufficient thickness of resin on the wire to resist wear. Avoid creating any contour that may trap plaque.
6. Light-cure the composite resin according to instructions for the light source used.
7. Trim the gingival margin and contour the bulk, with a tungsten-carbide bur if necessary.
8. Instruct the patient in proper oral hygiene and use of dental floss or Superfloss (Oral-B) beneath the retainer wire and along the mesial contact areas of both canines. Instruct patients to floss once daily to prevent accumulation of calculus and plaque.

CONCLUSION

The introduction of adhesive resins and direct bonding opened a new era in the practice of orthodontics. Every orthodontic resident and clinician should acknowledge the importance of adhesives and material science on their profession, and these issues should be an integral part of training programs. The modern orthodontist should have a thorough understanding of available materials to choose the best product available for a particular patient's needs and to achieve the best outcome. Composite resins and light-curing units are an important part of the orthodontist's armamentarium because of direct bonding and advances in the material science. As with any material, composite resins and bonding have particular pros and cons. Questions remain about the biological aspects of free monomers leaching from composite resins and the adverse effects of blue curing lights on operators' vision. These materials and devices should be handled with optimum care and precautions, keeping the safety of patients as the main priority.

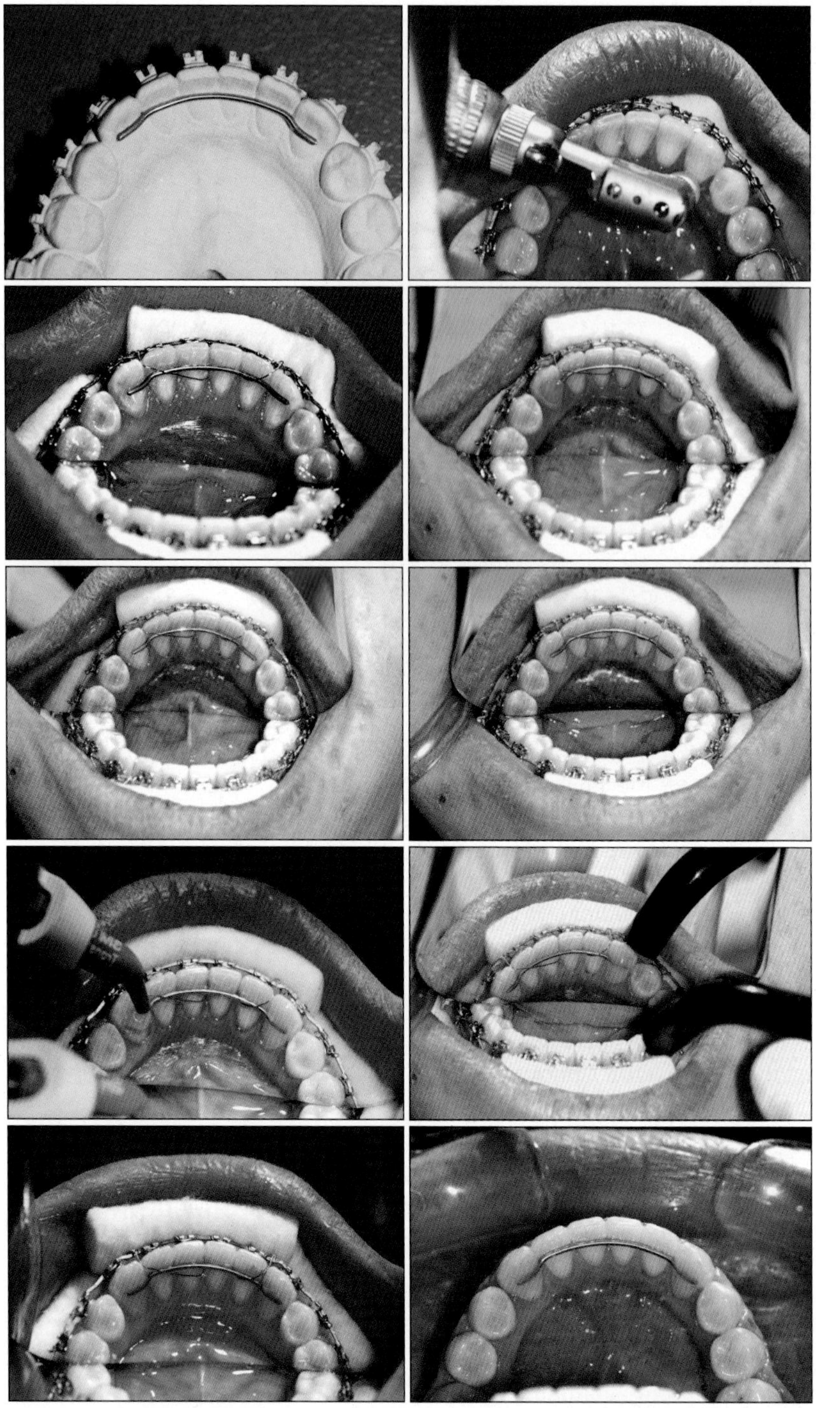

Fig. 6-19 Fabrication of 3-3 retainer bar. The wire is adapted carefully and checked in place before the lingual surfaces are pumiced. The wire is fixed temporarily using steel ligatures, and the canines are etched. The two ends of the bar are bonded using light-cured composite with adequate thickness, and trimmed if necessary.

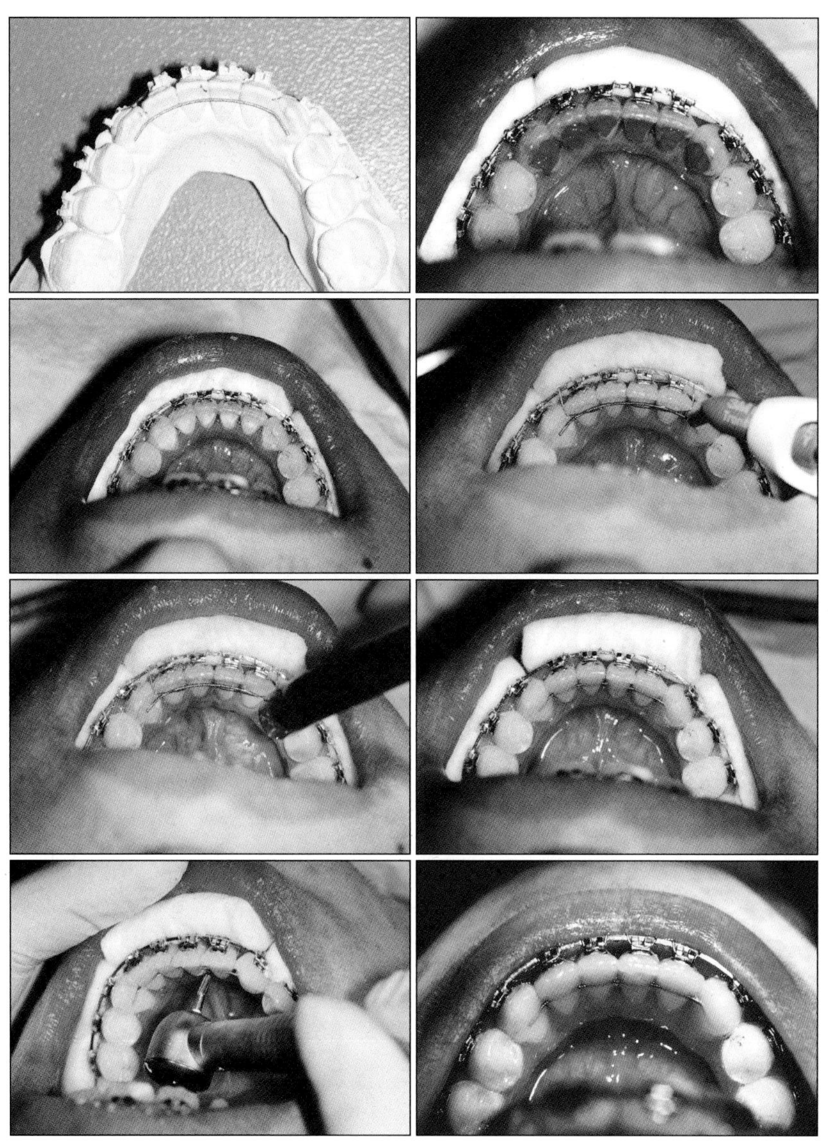

Fig. 6-20 Fabrication of 3-3 flexible wire retainer. Similar to 3-3 bar fabrication (see Fig. 6-19) except that the teeth are etched without the retainer in place.

References

1. Jenkins TS: Adhesives in orthodontics: are we pushing the envelope in the right direction? *Semin Orthod* 11:76-85, 2005.
2. Buonocore MG: *The use of adhesives in dentistry*, Springfield, Ill, 1975, Charles C Thomas.
3. Buonocore M: A simple method of increasing the adhesion of acrylic filling materials to enamel surface, *J Dent Res* 34:849, 1955.
4. Reynolds IR: A review of direct orthodontic bonding, *Br J Orthod* 6:171-178, 1979.
5. Zachrisson BU, Büyükyilmaz T: Bonding in orthodontics. In Graber TM, Vanarsdall RL, Vig KW, editors: *Orthodontics: current principles and techniques,* St Louis, 2005, Elsevier Health Sciences, pp 579-659.
6. Howells D, Jones P: In vitro evaluation of a cyanoacrylate bonding agent, *Br J Orthod* 16:75-78, 1989.
7. Willems G, Carels CEL, Verbeke G: In vitro peel/shear bond evaluation of orthodontic bracket base design, *J Dent* 25:271-278, 1997.
8. Willems G, Carels CEL, Verbeke G: In vitro peel/shear bond strength of orthodontic adhesive, *J Dent* 25:263-270, 1997.
9. Zachrisson BU: Post-treatment evaluation of direct bonding in orthodontics, *Am J Orthod* 75:173-189, 1977.
10. Tavas MA, Watts DC: An in vitro study, *Br J Orthod* 6:207-208, 1979.
11. Greenlaw R, Way DC, Galil KA: An in vitro evaluation of a visible light-cured resin as an alternative to conventional resin bonding systems, *Am J Orthod Dentofacial Orthop* 96:214-220, 1989.
12. Millett DT, Gordon PH: A 5-year clinical review of bond failures with a no-mix adhesive, *Eur J Orthod* 16:203-211, 1994.
13. Üşümez S, Büyükyilmaz T, Karaman AI: Effect of light-emitting diode on bond strength of orthodontic brackets, *Angle Orthod* 74:259-263, 2004.
14. Üşümez S, Büyükyilmaz T, Karaman AI: Effects of fast halogen and plasma arc curing lights on the surface hardness of orthodontic adhesives for lingual retainers, *Am J Orthod Dentofacial Orthop* 123:641-668, 2003.

15. Uysal T, Basciftci FA, Üşümez S, et al: Can previously bleached teeth be bonded safely? *Am J Orthod Dentofacial Orthop* 123:628-632, 2003.
16. Büyükyilmaz T, Üşümez S, Karaman AI: Effect of self-etching primers on bond strength: are they reliable? *Angle Orthod* 73:64-70, 2003.
17. Üşümez S, Orhan M, Üşümez A: Laser etching of enamel for direct bonding with an Er,Cr:YSGG hydrokinetic laser system, *Am J Orthod Dentofacial Orthop* 122:649-656, 2002.
18. Reynolds IR, von Fraunhofer JA: Direct bonding of orthodontic attachments to teeth: the relation of adhesive bond strength to gauze mesh size, *Br J Orthod* 3:91-95, 1976.
19. Maijer R, Smith DC: Variables influencing the bond strength of metal orthodontic bracket bases, *Am J Orthod* 79:20-34, 1981.
20. Sharma-Sayal SK, Rossouw PE, Kulkarni GV, Titley KC: The influence of orthodontic bracket base design on shear bond strength, *Am J Orthod Dentofacial Orthop* 124:74-82, 2003.
21. Bishara SE, Olsen M, VonWald L: Comparisons of shear bond strength of precoated and uncoated brackets, *Am J Orthod Dentofacial Orthop* 112:617-621, 1997.
22. Ødegaard J, Segener D: Shear bond strength of metal brackets compared with a new ceramic bracket, *Am J Orthod Dentofacial Orthop* 94:201-206, 1988.
23. Millett D, McCabe JF, Gordon PH: The role of sandblasting on the retention of metallic brackets applied with glass ionomer cement, *Br J Orthod* 20:117-122, 1993.
24. Regan D, LeMasney B, Van-Noort R: The tensile bond strength of new and rebonded stainless steel orthodontic brackets, *Eur J Orthod* 15:125-135, 1993.
25. Wang WN, Meng CL, Tarng TH: Bond strength: a comparison between chemical coated and mechanical interlock bases of ceramic and metal brackets, *Am J Orthod Dentofacial Orthop* 11:374-381, 1997.
26. MacColl GA, Rossouw PE, Titley KC, Yamin C: The relationship between bond strength and orthodontic bracket base surface area with conventional and microetched foil-mesh bases, *Am J Orthod Dentofacial Orthop* 113:276-281, 1998.
27. Sernetz F, Binder F: Improvement of bond strength of orthodontic titanium brackets and tubes by laser structuring. In *Proceedings of the 5th International Conference on Joining Ceramics, Glass and Metal*, Jena, Germany; *DVS Berichte Band* 184:82-85, 1997.
28. Basciftci FA, Üşümez S, Malkoc S, Orhan M: Effect of orthodontic bracket base structure on shear bond strength, *Turk J Orthod* 19, 2006.
29. Ireland AJ, Sherriff M: The effect of pumicing on the in vivo use of a resin modified glass poly (alkenoate) cement and a conventional no-mix composite for bonding orthodontic brackets, *J Orthod* 29:217-220, 2002.
30. Burgess AM, Sherriff M, Ireland AJ: Self-etching primers: is prophylactic pumicing necessary? A randomized clinical trial, *Angle Orthod* 76:114-118, 2006.
31. Ponduri S, Turnbull N, Birnie D, et al: Does atropine sulphate improve orthodontic bond survival? A randomized clinical trial, *Am J Orthod Dentofacial Orthop* 132:663-670, 2007.
32. Kochavi D, Gedalia I, Anaise J: Effect of conditioning with fluoride and phosphoric acid on enamel surfaces as evaluated by scanning electron microscopy and fluoride incorporation, *J Dent Res* 54:304-309, 1975.
33. Fitzpatrick DA, Way DC: The effects of wear, acid etching and band removal on human enamel, *Am J Orthod* 72:671-681, 1977.
34. Brown CRL, Way DC: Enamel loss during orthodontic bonding and subsequent loss during removal of filled and unfilled adhesives, *Am J Orthod* 74:663-671, 1978.
35. Lehman R, Davidson CL, Duijster PPE: In vitro studies on susceptibility of enamel to caries attack after orthodontic bonding procedures, *Am J Orthod Dentofacial Orthop* 80:61-72, 1981.
36. Shey Z, Brandt S: Enamel loss due to acid treatment for bonding, *J Clin Orthod* 16:338-340, 1982.
37. Bas-Kalkan A, Orhan M, Üşümez S: The effect of enamel etching with different acids on the bond strength of metallic brackets, *Turk J Orthod* 20, 2007.
38. Sayinsu K, Isik F, Sezen S, Aydemir B: Effect of blood and saliva contamination on bond strength of brackets bonded with a protective liquid polish and a light-cured adhesive, *Am J Orthod Dentofacial Orthop* 131:391-394, 2007.
39. Faltermeier A, Behr M, Rosentritt M, et al: An in vitro comparative assessment of different enamel contaminants during bracket bonding, *Eur J Orthod* 29:559-563, 2007.
40. Olsen ME, Bishara SE, Damon P, Jakobsen JR: Evaluation of Scotchbond multipurpose and maleic acid as alternative methods of bonding orthodontic brackets, *Am J Orthod Dentofacial Orthop* 111:498-501, 1997.
41. Hermsen RJ, Vrijhoef MMA: Loss of enamel due to etching with phosphoric or maleic acid, *Dent Mater* 9:332-336, 1993.
42. Baratieri LN, Monteiro S: Influence of acid type (phosphoric or maleic) on the retention of pit and fissure sealant: an in vivo study, *Quintessence Int* 25:749-755, 1994.
43. Goes MF, Sinhoreti MAC, Consani S, Silva MAP: Morphological effect of the type, concentration and etching time of acid solution on enamel and dentin surface, *Braz Dent J* 9:3-10, 1998.
44. Gottlieb EL, Nelson AH, Vogels DS: 1996 JCO Study of orthodontic diagnosis and treatment procedures. Part 1. Results and trends, *J Clin Orthod* 30:615-630, 1996.
45. Von Fraunhofer JA, Allen DJ, Orbell GM: Laser etching of enamel for direct bonding, *Angle Orthod* 63:73-76, 1993.
46. Basaran G, Ozer T, Berk N, Hamamci O: Etching enamel for orthodontics with an erbium, chromium:yttrium-scandium-gallium-garnet laser system, *Angle Orthod* 77:117-123, 2007.
47. Berk N, Başaran G, Ozer T: Comparison of sandblasting, laser irradiation, and conventional acid etching for orthodontic bonding of molar tubes, *Eur J Orthod* 30:183-189, 2008. Epub Feb 8, 2008.
48. Canay Ş, Kocadereli İ, Akça E: The effect of enamel air abrasion on the retention of bonded metallic orthodontic brackets, *Am J Orthod Dentofacial Orthop* 117:15-19, 2000.
49. Katora ME, Jubach T, Polimus MM: Air-abrasive etching of the enamel surface, *Quintessence Int* 9:967-968, 1981.
50. Goldstein RE, Parkins FM: Using air-abrasive technology to diagnose and restore pit and fissure caries, *J Am Dent Assoc* 126:761-766, 1995.
51. Hogervorst WW, Feilzer AJ, Prahl-Andersen B: The air-abrasion technique versus the conventional acid-etching technique: a quantification of surface enamel loss and a comparison of shear bond strength, *Am J Orthod Dentofacial Orthop* 117:20-26, 2000.

52. Olsen ME, Bishara SE, Damon P, Jakobsen JR: Comparison of shear bond strength and surface structure between conventional acid etching and air-abrasion of human enamel, *Am J Orthod Dentofacial Orthop* 112:502-503, 1997.
53. Reisner KR, Levitt HL, Mante F: Enamel preparation between the use of a sandblaster and current techniques, *Am J Orthod Dentofacial Orthop* 111:366-373, 1997.
54. Maijer R, Smith DC: A new surface treatment for bonding, *J Biomed Mater Res* 13:975-985, 1979.
55. Maijer R, Smith DC: Crystal growth on the outer enamel surface: an alternative to acid etching, *Am J Orthod* 89:183-193, 1986.
56. Artun J, Bergland S: Clinical trials with crystal growth conditioning as an alternative to acid-etch enamel pretreatment, *Am J Orthod* 85:333-340, 1984.
57. Jones ML, Pizarro KA: A comparative study of the shear bond strengths of four different crystal growth solutions, *Br J Orthod* 21:133-137, 1994.
58. Knox J, Jones ML: Crystal bonding: an adhesive system with a future? *Br J Orthod* 22:309-317, 1995.
59. Jones SP, Gledhill JR, Davies EH: The crystal growth technique: a laboratory evaluation of bond strengths, *Eur J Orthod* 21:89-93, 1999.
60. Chigira H, Koike T, Hasegawa T, et al: Effect of the self etching dentin primers on the bonding efficacy of dentine adhesive, *Dent Mater* 8:86-92, 1989.
61. Nishida K, Yamauchi J, Wada T, Hosoda H: Development of a new bonding system, *J Dent Res* 72:137, 1993 (abstract).
62. Banks P, Thiruvenkatachari B: Long-term clinical evaluation of bracket failure with a self-etching primer: a randomized controlled trial, *J Orthod* 34:243-251, 2007.
63. Elekdag-Turk S, Isci D, Turk T, Cakmak F: Six-month bracket failure rate: evaluation of a self-etching primer, *Eur J Orthod* 30:211-216, 2008. Epub Jan 23, 2008.
64. Turk T, Elekdag-Turk S, Isci D: Effects of self-etching primer on shear bond strength of orthodontic brackets at different debond times, *Angle Orthod* 77:108-112, 2007.
65. Jones DW: Dental composite biomaterials, *J Can Dent Assoc* 64:732-734, 1998.
66. Tabrizi S, Üşümez S: A comparative evaluation of flowable composites for lingual retainer bonding in orthodontics, Marmara University Health Sciences Institute, 2007 (submitted MS dissertation).
67. Goldberg M: In vitro and in vivo studies on the toxicity of dental resin components: a review, *Clin Oral Invest* 12:1-8, 2008.
68. Buzitta VAJ, Hallgren SE, Powers JM: Bond strength of orthodontic direct-bonding cement-bracket systems as studied in vitro, *Am J Orthod* 81:87-92, 1982.
69. Jost-Brinkman PG, Schiffer A, Miethke RR: The effect of adhesive layer thickness on bond strength, *J Clin Orthod* 26:718-720, 1992.
70. Zachrisson BU, Brobakken BO: Clinical comparison of direct versus indirect bonding with different bracket types and adhesives, *Am J Orthod* 74:62-78, 1978.
71. Hotz P, McLean JW, Seed I, Wilson AD: The bonding of glass ionomer cements to metal and tooth substrates, *Br Dent J* 142:41-47, 1977.
72. Hallgren A, Oliveby A, Twetman S: L(+)-lactic acid production in plaque from orthodontic appliances retained with glass ionomer cement, *Br J Orthod* 21:23-26, 1994.
73. Norevall LI, Marcusson A, Persson MA: Clinical evaluation of glass ionomer cement for bonding, *Eur J Orthod* 17:449, 1995 (abstract).
74. White LW: Glass ionomer cement, *J Clin Orthod* 20:387-391, 1986.
75. Millett DT, McCabe JF: Orthodontic bonding with glass ionomer cement: a review, *Eur J Orthod* 18:385-399, 1996.
76. Sudjalim TR, Woods MG, Manton DJ, Reynolds EC: Prevention of demineralization around orthodontic brackets in vitro, *Am J Orthod Dentofacial Orthop* 131:705.e1-e9, 2007.
77. Bishara SE, Soliman M, Laffoon JF, Warren J: Shear bond strength of a new high fluoride release glass ionomer adhesive, *Angle Orthod* 78:125-128, 2008.
78. Üşümez S, Büyükyilmaz T, Karaman AI, Gündüz B: Degree of conversion of two lingual retainer adhesives cured with different light sources, *Eur J Orthod* 27:173-179, 2005.
79. Ozturk N, Üşümez A, Üşümez S, Ozturk B: Degree of conversion and surface hardness of resin cement cured with different curing units, *Quintessence Int* 36:771-777, 2005.
80. Ferracane JL: Elution of leachable components from composites, *J Oral Rehabil* 21:441-452, 1994.
81. Stanislawski L, Daniau X, Lauti A, Goldberg M: Factors responsible for pulp cell cytotoxicity induced by resin-modified glass ionomer cements, *J Biomed Mater Res* 48:277-288, 1999.
82. Agha MO, Üşümez S: Evaluation of leaching of three different orthodontic bonding resins, Marmara University Health Sciences Institute, 2007 (submitted MS dissertation).
83. Lefeuvre M, Amjaad W, Goldberg M, Stanislawski L: TEGDMA induces mitochondrial damage and oxidative stress in human gingival fibroblasts, *Biomaterials* 26:5130-5137, 2005.
84. Noda M, Wataha JC, Kaga M, et al: Components of dentinal adhesives modulate heat shock protein 72 expression in heat-stressed THP-1 human monocytes at sublethal concentrations, *J Dent Res* 81:265-269, 2002.
85. Althoff O, Hartung M: Advances in light curing, *Am J Dent* 13:77D-81D, 2000.
86. Tirtha R, Fan LP, Dennison JB, Powers JM: In vitro depth of cure of photo-activated composites, *J Dent Res* 61:1184, 1982.
87. Oesterle LJ, Messersmith ML, Devine SM, Ness CF: Light and setting times of visible-light-cured orthodontic adhesives, *J Clin Orthod* 29:31-36, 1995.
88. Weinberger SJ, McConnell RJ, Wright GZ: Bond strengths of two ceramic brackets using argon laser, light, and chemically cured resin systems, *Angle Orthod* 67:173-178, 1997.
89. Kurchak M, DeSantos B, Powers J, Turner D: Argon laser for light-cured adhesives, *J Clin Orthod* 31:371-374, 1997.
90. Büyükyılmaz T, Üşümez S: Die Oberflächenhärte von Kunststoffen für die Befestigung von lingualen Drahtretainern im Laborversuch und im klinischen Einsatz, *Inform Orthod Kieferorthop* 3:205-212, 2003.
91. Mills RW, Jandt KD, Ashworth SH: Dental composite depth of cure with halogen and blue light-emitting diode technology, *Br Dent J* 186:388-391, 1999.
92. Dunn WJ, Taloumis LJ: Polymerization of orthodontic resin cement with light-emitting diode curing units, *Am J Orthod Dentofacial Orthop* 122:236-241, 2002.

93. Jandt KD, Mills RW, Blackwell GB, Ashworth SH: Depth of cure and compressive strength of dental composites cured with blue light-emitting diodes (LEDs), *Dent Mater J* 16:41-47, 2000.
94. Stahl F, Ashworth SH, Jandt KD, Mills RW: Light-emitting diode (LED) polymerization of dental composites: flexural properties and polymerization potential, *Biomaterials* 21:1379-1385, 2000.
95. Sfondrini MF, Cacciafesta V, Pistorio A, et al: Effects of conventional and high-intensity light curing on enamel shear bond strength of composite resin and resin-modified glass ionomer, *Am J Orthod Dentofacial Orthop* 119:30-35, 2001.
96. Hofmann N, Hugo B, Schubert K, Klaiber B: Comparison between a plasma arc light source and conventional halogen curing units regarding flexural strength, modulus, and hardness of photoactivated resin composites, *J Clin Oral Invest* 4:140-147, 2000.
97. Miyazaki M, Hattori T, Ichiishi Y, et al: Evaluation of curing units used in private dental offices, *Oper Dent* 23:50-54, 1998.
98. Pilo R, Oelgiesser D, Cardash HS: A survey of output intensity and potential for depth of cure among light-curing units in clinical use, *J Dent* 27:235-241, 1999.
99. Zach L, Cohen G: Pulp response to externally applied heat, *Oral Surg Oral Med Oral Pathol* 19:515-530, 1965.
100. Ozturk B, Üşümez A, Üşümez S, et al: Temperature rise during adhesive and resin composite polymerization with various light curing sources, *Oper Dent* 29:325-332, 2004.
101. Oesterle LJ, Newman SM, Shellhart WC: Rapid curing of composite with a xenon plasma arc light, *Am J Orthod Dentofacial Orthop* 119:610-616, 2001.
102. Hwang IY, Son YO, Kim JH, et al: Plasma-arc generated light inhibits proliferation and induces apoptosis of human gingival fibroblasts in a dose-dependent manner, *Dent Mater* 24:1-36, 1042, 2008. Epub Dec 31, 2007.
103. Taoufik K, Mavrogonatou E, Eliades T, et al: Effect of blue light on the proliferation of human gingival fibroblasts, *Dent Mater* 24:895-900, 2008. Epub March 4, 2008.
104. Nakamura S, Mukai T, Senoh M: Candela-class high brightness InGaN/AlGaN double heterostructure blue-light-emitting diodes, *Appl Physics Lett* 64:1687-1689, 1994.
105. Haitz RH, Craford MG, Wiessman RH: Handbook of optics, vol 2, New York, 1995, McGraw-Hill, pp 12.1-12.9.
106. http://www.microscopyu.com/articles/fluorescence/lasersafety.html. Accessed Feb 12, 2008.
107. Chen E: Inhibition of cytochrome oxidase and blue-light damage in rat retina, *Graefes Arch Clin Exp Ophthalmol* 231:416-423, 1993.
108. Chen E: Inhibition of enzymes by short-wave optical radiation and its effect on the retina, *Acta Ophthalmol Suppl* 208:1-50, 1993.
109. Chen E, Söderberg PG, Lindström B: Cytochrome oxidase activity in rat retina after exposure to 404 nm blue light, *Curr Eye Res* 11:825-831, 1992.
110. Ham WT Jr: Ocular hazards of light sources: review of current knowledge, *J Occup Med* 25:101-103, 1983.
111. Üşümez S, Goyenc Y, Gunduz K, Uysal T: Are bluc curing lights safe for orthodontists? *Eur J Orthod* 28:e177-e178, 2006.
112. Bruzell Roll EM, Jacobsen N, Hensten-Pettersen A: Health hazards associated with curing light in the dental clinic, *Clin Oral Invest* 8:113-117, 2004.
113. Polat O, Karaman AI, Durmus E: Effects of preoperative ibuprofen and naproxen sodium on orthodontic pain, *Angle Orthod* 75:791-796, 2005.
114. Armstrong D, Shen G, Petocz P, Darendeliler MA: A comparison of accuracy in bracket positioning between two techniques: localizing the centre of the clinical crown and measuring the distance from the incisal edge, *Eur J Orthod* 29:430-436, 2007.
115. Erkan M, Pikdoken L, Üşümez S: Gingival response to mandibular incisor intrusion, *Am J Orthod Dentofacial Orthop* 132:143.e9-e13, 2007.
116. Armstrong D, Shen G, Petocz P, Darendeliler MA: Excess adhesive flash upon bracket placement: a typodont study comparing APC PLUS and Transbond XT, *Angle Orthod* 77:1101-1108, 2007.
117. Zachrisson BU: Fluoride application procedures in orthodontic practice: current concepts, *Angle Orthod* 44:72-81, 1975.
118. Zachrisson BU: Orthodontic bonding to artificial tooth surfaces: clinical versus laboratory findings, *Am J Orthod Dentofacial Orthop* 117:592-594, 2000.
119. Zachrisson BU, Büyükyilmaz T: Recent advances in bonding to gold, amalgam, and porcelain, *J Clin Orthod* 27:661, 1993.
120. Zachrisson BU, Büyükyilmaz T, Zachrisson YØ: Improving orthodontic bonding to silver amalgam, *Angle Orthod* 65:35, 1995.
121. Jost-Brinkmann PG, Can S, Drost C: In vitro study of the adhesive strengths of brackets on metals, ceramic and composite. 2. Bonding to porcelain and composite resin, *J Orofac Orthop (Fortschr Kieferorthop)* 57:132-141, 1996.
122. Klocke A, Shi J, Kahl-Nieke B, Ulrich B: Bond strength with custom base indirect bonding technique, *Angle Orthod* 73:176-180, 2003.
123. Silverman E, Cohen M: A universal direct bonding system for both metal and plastic brackets, *Am J Orthod* 62:236-244, 1972.
124. Brandt S: JCO interviews Dr Elliott Silverman, Dr Morton Cohen, and Dr AJ Gwinnett on bonding, *J Clin Orthod* 4:236-251, 1979.
125. Rossouw PE, Bruwer HC, Stander IA: The rationale behind a viable alternative to direct bonding of orthodontic attachments: indirect bonding, *Ont Dent* 5:19-25, 1999.
126. Scholz RP, Schwarz ML: Lingual orthodontics: a status report. Part 3. Indirect bonding: laboratory and clinical procedures, *J Clin Orthod* 12:812-820, 1982.
127. Hodge TM, Dhopatkar AA, Rock WP, Spary DJ: The Burton approach to indirect bonding, *J Orthod* 28:267-270, 2001.
128. Koo BC, Chung C, Vanarsdall RL: Comparison of the accuracy of bracket placement between direct and indirect bonding techniques, *Am J Orthod Dentofacial Orthop* 3:346-351, 1999.
129. Kalange JT, Thomas RG: Indirect bonding: a comprehensive review of the literature, *Semin Orthod* 13:3-10, 2007.
130. Sheridan JJ: The readers' corner, *J Clin Orthod* 10:543-546, 2004.
131. Thomas RG: Indirect bonding: simplicity in action, *J Clin Orthod* 13:93-104, 1979.
132. Kalange JT: Indirect bonding: a comprehensive review of the advantages, *World J Orthod* 4:301-307, 2004.
133. Hocevar RA, Vincent HF: Indirect versus direct bonding: bond strength and failure location. *Am J Orthod Dentofacial Orthop* 5:367-371, 1988.

134. Milne JW, Andreasen GF, Jakobsen MA: Bond strength comparison: a simplified indirect technique versus direct placement of brackets, *Am J Orthod Dentofacial Orthop* 96:8-15, 1989.
135. Yi GK, Dunn WJ, Taloumis LJ: Shear bond strength comparison between direct and indirect bonded orthodontic brackets, *Am J Orthod Dentofacial Orthop* 5:577-581, 2003.
136. Deahl ST, Salome N, Hatch JP, Rugh JD: Practice-based comparison of direct and indirect bonding, *Am J Orthod Dentofacial Orthop* 132:738-742, 2007.
137. Thompson MA, Drummond JL, BeGole EA: Bond strength analysis of custom base variables in indirect bonding techniques, *Am J Orthod Dentofacial Orthop* 133:9.e15-e20, 2008.
138. Cooper RB, Sorenson NA: Indirect bonding with adhesive precoated brackets, *J Clin Orthod* 27:164-166, 1993.
139. Read MJF, O'Brien KD: A clinical trial of an indirect bonding technique with a visible light-cured adhesive, *Am J Orthod Dentofacial Orthop* 98:259-262, 1990.
140. Aguirre MJ, King GJ, Waldron JM: Assessment of bracket placement and bond strength when comparing direct bonding to indirect bonding techniques, *Am J Orthod* 82:269-276, 1982.
141. Krug AY, Conley RS: Shear bond strengths using an indirect technique with different light sources, *J Clin Orthod* 8:485-487, 2005.
142. Scholz RP: Indirect bonding revisited, *J Clin Orthod* 8:529-536, 1983.
143. Sondhi A: Efficient and effective indirect bonding, *Am J Orthod Dentofacial Orthop* 115:352-359, 1999.
144. Mui B, Rossouw PE, Kulkarni GV: Optimization of a procedure for rebonding dislodged orthodontic brackets, *Angle Orthod* 69:276-281, 1999.
145. Tavares SW, Consani S, Nouer DF, et al: Shear bond strength of new and recycled brackets to enamel, *Braz Dent J* 17:44-48, 2006.
146. Sonis AL: Air abrasion of failed bonded metal brackets: a study of shear bond strength and surface characteristics as determined by scanning electron microscopy, *Am J Orthod Dentofacial Orthop* 110:96-98, 1996.
147. Øilo G: Bond strength testing: what does it mean? *Int Dent J* 43:492-498, 1993.
148. Redd TB, Shivapuja PK: Debonding ceramic brackets: effects on enamel, *J Clin Orthod* 25:475-481, 1991.
149. Årtun J: A post-treatment evaluation of multibonded ceramic brackets in orthodontics, *Eur J Orthod* 19:219-228, 1997.
150. Bishara SE, Fehr DE: Ceramic brackets: something old, something new: review, *Semin Orthod* 3:178-188, 1997.
151. Viazis AD, Cavanaugh G, Bevis RR: Bond strength of ceramic brackets under shear stress: an in vitro report, *Am J Orthod Dentofacial Orthop* 98:214-221, 1990.
152. Winchester LJ: Bond strength of five different ceramic brackets: an in vitro study, *Eur J Orthod* 92:293-305, 1991.
153. Chen HY, Su MZ, Chang HF, et al: Effects of different debonding techniques on the debonding forces and failure modes of ceramic brackets in simulated clinical set-ups, *Am J Orthod Dentofacial Orthop* 132:680-686, 2007.
154. Vukovich ME, Wood DP, Daley TD: Heat generated by grinding during removal of ceramic brackets, *Am J Orthod Dentofacial Orthop* 99:505-512, 1991.
155. Crooks M, Hood J, Harkness M: Thermal debonding of ceramic brackets: an in vitro study, *Am J Orthod Dentofacial Orthop* 111:163-172, 1997.
156. Jost-Brinkman PG, Stein H, Miethke RR, et al: Histologic investigation of the human pulp after thermodebonding of metal and ceramic brackets, *Am J Orthod Dentofacial Orthop* 102:410-417, 1992.
157. Rueggeberg FA, Lockwood P: Thermal debracketing of orthodontic resins, *Am J Orthod Dentofacial Orthop* 98:56-65, 1990.
158. Stratmann U, Schaarschmidt K, Wegener H, et al: The extent of enamel surface fractures: a quantitative comparison of thermally debonded ceramic and mechanically debonded metal brackets by energy dispersive micro- and image-analysis, *Eur J Orthod* 18:655-662, 1996.
159. Ma T, Marangoni RD, Flint W: In vitro comparison of debonding force and intrapulpal temperature changes during ceramic orthodontic bracket removal using a carbon dioxide laser, *Am J Orthod Dentofacial Orthop* 111:203-210, 1997.
160. Rickabaugh JL, Marangoni RD, McCaffrey KK: Ceramic bracket debonding with the carbon dioxide laser, *Am J Orthod Dentofacial Orthop* 110:388-393, 1996.
161. Tocchio RM, Williams PT, Mayer FJ, et al: Laser debonding of ceramic orthodontic brackets, *Am J Orthod Dentofacial Orthop* 103:155-162, 1993.
162. Kawabata R, Hayakawa T, Kasai K: Modification of 4-META/MMA-TBB resin for safe debonding of orthodontic brackets: influence of the addition of degradable additives or fluoride compound, *Dent Mater J* 25:524-532, 2006.
163. Tsuruoka T, Namura Y, Shimizu N: Development of an easy-debonding orthodontic adhesive using thermal heating, *Dent Mater J* 26:78-83, 2007.
164. Campbell PM: Enamel surfaces after orthodontic bracket debonding, *Angle Orthod* 65:103-110, 1995.
165. Hong YH, Lew KKK: Quantitative and qualitative assessment of enamel surface following five composite removal methods after bracket debonding, *Eur J Orthod* 17:121-128, 1995.
166. Thomas BW, Hook CR, Draughn RA: Laser-aided degradation of composite resin, *Angle Orthod* 66:281-286, 1996.
167. Alexander R, Xie J, Fried D: Selective removal of residual composite from dental enamel surfaces using the third harmonic of a Q-switched Nd:YAG laser, *Lasers Surg Med* 30:240-245, 2002.
168. Krell KV, Courey JM, Bishara SE: Orthodontic bracket removal using conventional and ultrasonic debonding techniques: enamel loss and time requirements, *Am J Orthod Dentofacial Orthop* 103:258-266, 1993.
169. Oliver RG, Griffiths J: Different techniques of residual composite removal following debonding: time taken and surface enamel appearance, *Br J Orthod* 19:131-137, 1992.
170. Retief DH, Denys FR: Finishing of enamel surfaces after debonding of orthodontic attachments, *Am J Orthod* 49:1-10, 1979.
171. Zachrisson BU, Årtun J: Enamel surface appearance after various debonding techniques, *Am J Orthod* 75:121-137, 1979.
172. Kim SS, Park WK, Son WS, et al: Enamel surface evaluation after removal of orthodontic composite remnants by intraoral sandblasting: a 3-dimensional surface profilometry study, *Am J Orthod Dentofacial Orthop* 132:71-76, 2007.
173. Gwinnett AJ, Gorelick L: Microscopic evaluation of enamel after debonding, *Am J Orthod* 71:651-655, 1977.
174. Day CJ, Price R, Sandy JR, Ireland AJ: Inhalation of aerosols produced during the removal of fixed orthodontic appliances: a comparison of 4 enamel cleanup methods, *Am J Orthod Dentofacial Orthop* 133:11-17, 2008.

175. Toroglu MS, Bayramoglu O, Yarkin F, Tuli A: Possibility of blood and hepatitis B contamination through aerosols generated during debonding procedures, *Angle Orthod* 73:571-578, 2003.
176. Toroglu MS, Haytaç MC, Köksal F: Evaluation of aerosol contamination during debonding procedures, *Angle Orthod* 71:299-306, 2001.
177. Osorio R, Toledano M, García-Godoy F: Enamel surface morphology after bracket debonding, *ASDC J Dent Child* 65:313-317, 354, 1998.
178. Gorelick L, Geiger AM, Gwinnett AJ: Incidence of white spot formation after bonding and banding, *Am J Orthod* 81:93-98, 1982.
179. Øgaard B: Prevalence of white spot lesions in 19-year-olds: a study on untreated and orthodontically treated persons 5 years after treatment, *Am J Orthod Dentofacial Orthop* 96:423-427, 1989.
180. Benson PE, Shah AA, Millett DT, et al: Fluorides, orthodontics and demineralization: a systematic review, *J Orthod* 32:102-114, 2005.
181. Benson PE, Parkin N, Millett DT, et al: Fluorides for the prevention of white spots on teeth during fixed brace treatment, *Cochrane Database Syst Rev* 3:CD003809, 2004.
182. Derks A, Katsaros C, Frencken JE, et al: Caries-inhibiting effect of preventive measures during orthodontic treatment with fixed appliances: a systematic review, *Caries Res* 38:413-420, 2004.
183. Twetman S, McWilliam JS, Hallgren A, Oliveby A: Cariostatic effect of glass ionomer retained orthodontic appliances: an in vivo study, *Swed Dent J* 21:169-175, 1997.
184. Marcusson A, Norevall LI, Persson M: White spot reduction when using glass ionomer cement for bonding in orthodontics: a longitudinal and comparative study, *Eur J Orthod* 19: 233-242, 1997.
185. Chung CK, Millett DT, Creanor SL, et al: Fluoride release and cariostatic ability of a compomer and a resin-modified glass ionomer cement used for orthodontic bonding, *J Dent* 26:533-538, 1998.
186. Gorton J, Featherstone JD: In vivo inhibition of demineralization around orthodontic brackets, *Am J Orthod Dentofacial Orthop* 123:10-14, 2003.
187. Pascotto RC, Navarro MF, Capelozza Filho L, Cury JA: In vivo effect of a resin-modified glass ionomer cement on enamel demineralization around orthodontic brackets, *Am J Orthod Dentofacial Orthop* 125:36-41, 2004.
188. Czochrowska E, Øgaard B, Duschner H, et al: Cariostatic effect of a light-cured, resin-reinforced glass ionomer for bonding orthodontic brackets in vivo: a combined study using microradiography and confocal laser scanning microscopy, *J Orofac Orthop* 59:265-273, 1998.
189. Geiger AM, Gorelick L, Gwinnett AJ, Griswold PG: The effect of a fluoride program on white spot formation during orthodontic treatment, *Am J Orthod Dentofacial Orthop* 93:29-37, 1988.
190. Jordan C: Prevention of white spot enamel formation during orthodontic treatment, *Gen Dent* 46:498-502, 1998.
191. Geiger A, Gorelick L, Gwinnett AJ, Benson BJ: Reducing white spot lesions in orthodontic populations with fluoride rinsing, *Am J Orthod Dentofacial Orthop* 101:403-407, 1992.
192. Li S, Hobson RS, Bai Y, et al: A method for producing controlled fluoride release from an orthodontic bracket, *Eur J Orthod* 29:550-554, 2007.
193. Sonis AL, Snell W: An evaluation of a fluoride-releasing visible light-activated bonding system for orthodontic bracket placement, *Am J Orthod Dentofacial Orthop* 95:306-311, 1989.
194. Øgaard B, Rezk-Lega F, Ruben J, Arends J: Cariostatic effect of fluoride release from a visible light-curing adhesive for bonding of orthodontic brackets, *Am J Orthod Dentofacial Orthop* 101:303-307, 1992.
195. Frazier MC, Southard TC, Doster PM: Prevention of enamel demineralization during orthodontic treatment: an in vitro study using pit and fissure sealants, *Am J Orthod Dentofacial Orthop* 110:459-465, 1996.
196. Todd MA, Staley RN, Kanellis MJ, et al: Effect of a fluoride varnish on demineralization adjacent to orthodontic treatment, *Am J Orthod Dentofacial Orthop* 116:159-167, 1999.
197. Wiltshire WA: In vitro and in vivo fluoride release from orthodontic elastomeric ligature ties, *Am J Orthod Dentofacial Orthop* 115:288-292, 1999.
198. Gillgrass TJ, Creanor SL, Foye RH, Millett DT: Varnish or polymeric coating for the prevention of demineralization? An ex vivo study, *J Orthod* 28:291-295, 2001.
199. Mattick CR, Mitchell L, Chadwick SM, Wright J: Fluoride-releasing elastomeric modules reduce decalcification: a randomized controlled trial, *J Orthod* 28:217-219, 2001.
200. Alves PV, Alviano WS, Bolognese AM, Nojima LI: Treatment protocol to control *Streptococcus mutans* level in an orthodontic patient with high caries risk, *Am J Orthod Dentofacial Orthop* 133:91-94, 2008.
201. Cacciafesta V, Sfondrini MF, Tagliani P, Klersy C: In vitro fluoride release rates from 9 orthodontic bonding adhesives, *Am J Orthod Dentofacial Orthop* 132:656-662, 2007.
202. Balenseifen JW, Madonia JV: Study of dental plaque in orthodontic patients, *J Dent Res* 49:320-324, 1970.
203. Chatterjee R, Kleinberg I: Effect of orthodontic band placement on the chemical composition of human incisor tooth plaque, *Arch Oral Biol* 24:97-100, 1979.
204. Corbett JA, Brown LR, Keene HJ, Horton IM: Comparison of *Streptococcus mutans* concentrations in non-banded and banded orthodontic patients, *J Dent Res* 60:1936-1942, 1981.
205. Mattingly JA, Sauer GJ, Yancey JM, Arnold RR: Enhancement of *Streptococcus mutans* colonization by direct bonded orthodontic appliances, *J Dent Res* 62:1209-1211, 1983.
206. Scheie AA, Arnesberg P, Krogstad O: Effects of orthodontic treatment on prevalence of *Streptococcus mutans* in plaque and saliva, *Scand J Dent Res* 92:211-217, 1984.
207. Vierrou AM, Manwell MA, Zameck RL, et al: Control of *Streptococcus mutans* with topical fluorides in patients undergoing orthodontic treatment, *J Am Dent Assoc* 113:644-646, 1986.
208. Stratemann MW, Shannon IL: Control of decalcification in orthodontic patients by daily self-administered application of a water-free 0.4% SnF2 gel, *Am J Orthod* 66:273-279, 1974.
209. Øgaard B, Larsson E, Henriksson T, et al: Effects of combined application of antimicrobial and fluoride varnishes in orthodontic patients, *Am J Orthod Dentofacial Orthop* 120:28-35, 2001.
210. Øgaard B, Rølla G: Cariological aspects of treatment with fixed orthodontic appliances. Part II. New concept on cariostatic mechanism of topical fluoride, *Kieferorthop Mitterlung* 6:45-51, 1993.

211. Eronat C, Alpöz AR: Effect of Cervitec varnish on the salivary *Streptococcus mutans* levels in the patients with fixed orthodontic appliances, *J Dent Res* 73(suppl), 1994 (abstract 425).
212. Karaman AI, Uysal T: Effectiveness of a hydrophilic primer when different antimicrobial agents are mixed, *Angle Orthod* 74:414-419, 2004.
213. Twetman S, Hallgren A, Petersson LG: Effect of antibacterial varnish on mutans streptococci in plaque from enamel adjacent to orthodontic appliances, *Caries Res* 29:188-191, 1995.
214. Caglar E, Sandalli N: Probiotics and their effect on dental health, *Turk J Orthod* 18:287-292, 2005.
215. Meurman JH, Antila H, Korhonen A, Salminen S: Effect of *Lactobacillus rhamnosus* strain GG (ATCC 53103) on the growth of *Streptococcus sobrinus* in vitro, *Eur J Oral Sci* 103:253-258, 1995.
216. Germeç D, Çağlar E, Kavaloğlu-Çıldir Ş, et al: Effect of probiotics on mutans streptococci and lactobacilli levels of orthodontic patients. Presented at 10th Symposium of Turkish Orthodontic Society, Ankara, 2007, p 51.
217. Øgaard B, Rølla G, Arends J, et al: Orthodontic appliances and enamel demineralization. 2. Prevention and treatment of lesions, *Am J Orthod Dentofacial Orthop* 94:123-128, 1988.
218. Gelgör IE, Büyükyilmaz T: A practical approach to white spot lesion removal, *World J Orthod* 4:152-156, 2003.
219. Angle EA: Treatment of malocclusion of the teeth, ed 7, Philadelphia, 1907, SS White Manufacturing. In Blake M, Bibby K: Retention and stability: a review of the literature, *Am J Orthod Dentofacial Orthop* 114:299-306, 1998.
220. Hawley CA: A removable retainer, *Int J Orthod* 2:291-298, 1919. In Bearn DR: Bonded orthodontic retainers: a review, *Am J Orthod Dentofacial Orthop* 108:207-213, 1995.
221. Zachrisson BU: Clinical experience with direct-bonded orthodontic retainers, *Am J Orthod* 71:440-448, 1977.
222. Knierim RW: Invisible lower cuspid to cuspid retainer, *Angle Orthod* 43:218-219, 1973.
223. Rubenstein BM: A direct bond maxillary retainer, *J Clin Orthod* 10:43, 1976.
224. Carter RN: Simplified direct-bonded retainer, *J Clin Orthod* 12:221, 1978.
225. Lubit EC: The bonded lingual retainer, *J Clin Orthod* 13:311-313, 1979.
226. Lee RT: The lower incisor bonded retainer in clinical practice: a three year study, *Br J Orthod* 8:15-18, 1981.
227. Årtun J, Zachrisson BU: Improving the handling properties of a composite resin for direct bonding, *Am J Orthod* 81:269-276, 1982.
228. Zachrisson BU: The bonded lingual retainer and multiple spacing of anterior teeth, *J Clin Orthod* 17:838-844, 1983.
229. Bearn DR: Bonded orthodontic retainers: a review, *Am J Orthod Dentofacial Orthop* 108:207-213, 1995.
230. Dahl EH, Zachrisson BU: Long-term experience with direct-bonded lingual retainer, *J Clin Orthod* 25:619-632, 1991.
231. Booth FA, Edelman JM, Proffit WR: Twenty-year follow-up of patients with permanently bonded mandibular canine-to-canine retainers, *Am J Orthod Dentofacial Orthop* 133:70-76, 2008.
232. Katsaros C, Livas C, Renkema AM: Unexpected complications of bonded mandibular lingual retainers, *Am J Orthod Dentofacial Orthop* 132:838-841, 2007.
233. Pandis N, Vlahopoulos K, Madianos P, Eliades T: Long-term periodontal status of patients with mandibular lingual fixed retention, *Eur J Orthod* 29:471-476, 2007.
234. Zachrisson BU: Third-generation mandibular bonded lingual 3-3 retainer, *J Clin Orthod* 29:39-48, 1995.
235. Baysal A, Uysal T, Ulker M, Üşümez S: Effects of high-intensity curing lights on microleakage under bonded lingual retainers, *Angle Orthod* 78:1084-1088, 2008.
236. Attar N, Tam LE, McComb D: Flow, strength, stiffness and radiopacity of flowable resin composites, *J Can Dent Assoc* 69:516-521, 2003.
237. Bayne SC, Thompson JY, Swift EJ Jr, et al: A characterization of first-generation flowable composites, *J Am Dent Assoc* 129:567-577, 1998.
238. Behle C: Flowable composites: properties and applications, *Pract Periodont Aesthet Dent* 10:347-350, 1998.
239. Bonilla ED, Yashar M, Caputo AA: Fracture toughness: nine flowable resin composites, *J Prosthet Dent* 89:261-267, 2003.
240. Labela R, Lambrechts P, Van Meerbeek B, Vanherle G: Polymerization shrinkage and elasticity of flowable composites and filled adhesives, *Dent Mater* 15:128-137, 1999.
241. Moon PC, Tabassian MS, Culbreath TE: Flow characteristics and film thickness of flowable resin composites, *Oper Dent* 27:248-253, 2002.
242. Elaut J, Asscherickx K, Vande Vannet B, Wehrbein H: Flowable composites for bonding lingual retainers, *J Clin Orthod* 36:597-598, 2002.
243. Geserick M, Wichelhaus A: A color-reactivated flowable composite for bonding lingual retainers, *J Clin Orthod* 38:165-166, 2004.
244. Geserick M, Ball J, Wichelhaus A: Bonding fiber-reinforced lingual retainers with color-reactivating flowable composite, *J Clin Orthod* 38:560-562, 2004.
245. Uysal T, Sari Z, Demir A: Are the flowable composites suitable for orthodontic bracket bonding? *Angle Orthod* 74:697-702, 2003.
246. Tabrizi S, Salamis E, Üşümez S: Flowable composites for bonding orthodontic retainers, *Angle Orthod,* 2008 (in press).
247. Uysal T, Ulker M, Baysal A, Üşümez S: Different lingual retainer composites and the microleakage between enamel-composite and wire-composite interfaces, *Angle Orthod* 78:941-946, 2008.
248. Al-Emran S, Barakati R: A method for stabilizing a lingual fixed retainer in place prior to bonding, *J Contemp Dent Pract* 8:108-113, 2007.

CHAPTER 7

The Impact of Bracket Selection and Bracket Placement on Expressed Tooth Movement and Finishing Details

Anoop Sondhi

In the management of a patient's orthodontic treatment, the devil is frequently in the details. In completing a patient's orthodontic treatment, barring any significant complications imposed by skeletal discrepancies, missing teeth, or other conditions, a clinician may spend as much time completing the details as in making the major corrections related to crowding and space closure. Frequently, patients start to become impatient with the process, particularly if the remaining treatment involves second-order and third-order changes in the posterior dentition, which they usually cannot see.

Although necessary adjustments to address these details may not become evident until a certain stage in treatment, many of these details can be foreseen in the original diagnosis and treatment plan, as well as during bracket selection and placement. Although many authors have written extensively on the finishing details in orthodontic treatment, adequate attention has not been given to the potential impact of proper bracket selection and placement on these details.

OBJECTIVE VERSUS SUBJECTIVE ASSESSMENT

Only some of the finishing details discussed here involve variables that are *quantifiable* and therefore can be measured objectively. For example, the desirable overbite at the end of treatment could be identified as either 2 or 3 mm, with reasons cited for either preference. At the end of treatment, it would also be possible to measure (quantify) this variable. Also at the end of treatment, there should be no open spaces in the dental arches, unless the space is specifically targeted for subsequent buildup of a tooth with a restoration; the presence or absence of spaces can be quantified.

A number of other variables involve a high degree of subjectivity, partly because of the personal preferences of patients and clinicians and partly because of the difficulty in quantifying them because of the difficulty in obtaining objective measurements. For example, the degree of mesiodistal tip on the maxillary anterior teeth can be varied to a certain degree, with some differences in the esthetic outcome. Indeed, a range of possible axial inclinations for the maxillary anterior teeth would result in an esthetic appearance that could be pleasing to the patient or the clinician, without significant impact on stability or the patient's long-term dental health and function. Similarly, clinicians may have differing viewpoints on the desirable axial inclinations of the posterior teeth in the transverse plane of space. Most patients are unlikely to give this much thought, but the functional outcome for the patient would clearly be different. Now add, for example, the difficulty in measuring the actual buccolingual inclination of a molar, let alone the difficulty in achieving a consensus on a reference plane to make such measurements.

The point is simple: certain factors in the finishing of an orthodontic case will affect primarily the esthetics of the finished result, other variables will influence primarily the patient's long-term dental health and function, and yet another set of variables will affect both. Some factors are quantifiable and therefore measurable. Other clinical details are more subjective, and either difficult or impossible to quantify. Further, a significant range of orthodontic opinions exists regarding both the appearance and the function of the treatment result, as evidenced by differing opinions between a practitioner of the "Tweed" philosophy and another practitioner of the "Bioprogressive" school of thought. The anterior torque values vary significantly between these two practitioners, with an identifiable difference in the esthetics and the function of the treatment results.

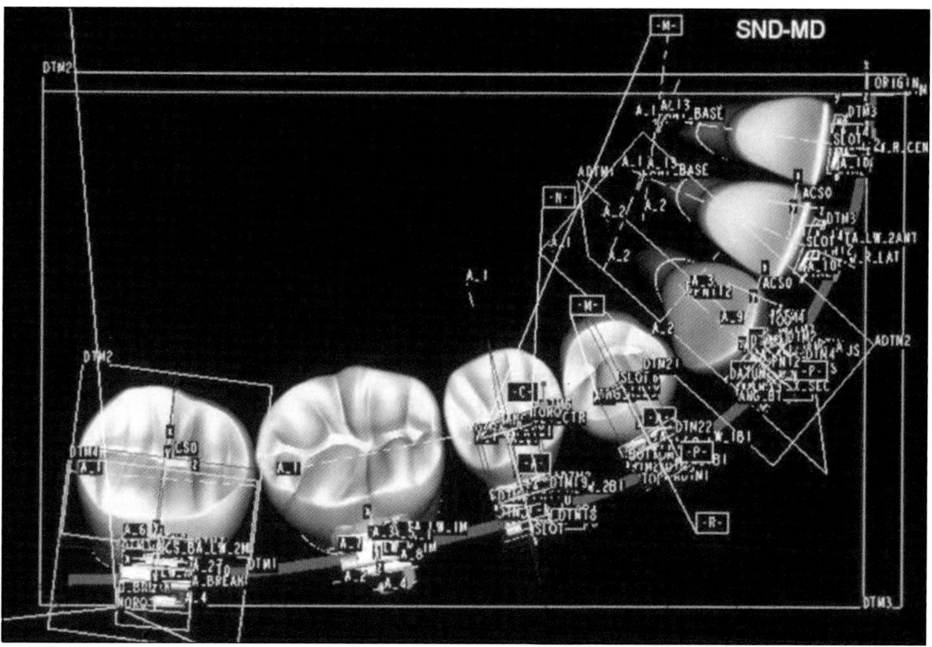

Fig. 7-1 Digitally constructed mandibular dentition, with some of the multiple measurements documenting appliance placement.

Andrews[1] was among the first to present a structured assessment of the treatment result. His definition of the "six keys to normal occlusion" constituted the first real effort to tabulate specific variables that could be measured in the finished orthodontic result. Indeed, this was the foundation of the then-nascent process of developing pretorqued and preangulated appliances. Before that time, torque, tip, and offsets were not "measured," only visually assessed.

THREE-DIMENSIONAL GRAPHIC ANALYSIS

Many pretorqued and preangulated appliance systems are currently available to the orthodontic practitioner. These prescriptions are based on a foundation of clinical principles, as well as the personal and philosophical preferences of the individual clinician. However, objective documentation on the efficacy of these various prescriptions has been lacking in the literature, and most of the evidence presented appears to be anecdotal. Further, a clinician wanting to test a specific prescription must treat a sample of patients over a minimum of 2 to 3 years, to appreciate the clinical details—a cumbersome approach.

Therefore the author's goal was to construct a virtual dentition (Fig. 7-1), progress to the development of a virtual occlusion, and then test the efficacy of the appliance design on the virtual dentition before applying it to the patient. This also allowed objective comparison of the effects of different torques, angulations, and prescriptions.

The purpose of this process was straightforward. Instead of extrapolating treatment results influenced by patient compliance, variations in morphology, and other uncontrollable factors, the impact of appliance designs would be evaluated by creating a standardized virtual dentition free of these influences. Standardized virtual appliances were then applied to this dentition to study the outcome of specific bracket placement, torque, and tip application, varying one factor at a time. For example, with the rest of the dentition and the appliance kept as a constant, a single tooth was identified for variation of the selected torque in the bracket (Fig. 7-2), allowing measurement of the impact of the changed variable on the tooth's finished position. Conversely, to study the impact of a specific orthodontic prescription on the entire dental arch, the dentition could be kept as a standard, and the entire appliance system changed; thus the impact on the combined axial inclinations in all three planes of space could be studied by rotating the model in each plane.

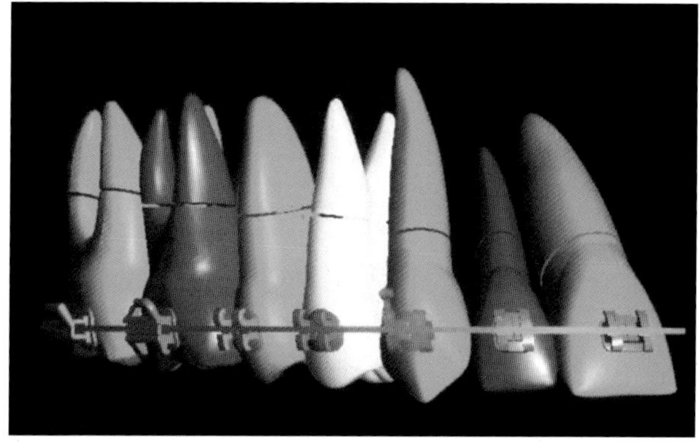

Fig. 7-2 Anterolateral view of a maxillary dental arch, with the maxillary right first premolar isolated to evaluate and modify its axial inclination.

Opinions still differ on assessment of occlusal function and the functional aspects of the occlusion. However, it is widely accepted that "balancing interferences" are undesirable during lateral movements, for both periodontal reasons and concerns about the impact on temporomandibular function. Some authors have identified the impact of occlusal dysfunction associated with a significant lateral shift of the mandible.[2] These functional aspects of occlusal function are usually viewed as "quantifiable," but are not always easy to measure.

SELECTION OF BRACKETS AND TUBES

Although clinicians generally accept that the choice of brackets and bracket systems influences the treatment outcome, the impact of bracket choice and placement on specific finishing details has been inadequately addressed. This point can be illustrated by studying a simple finishing detail that frequently requires significant treatment time and can occasionally vex the clinician.

It became increasingly apparent over the past 20 years that the mandibular second molars ought to be aligned properly within the dental arches at the completion of orthodontic treatment. Although patients would neither recognize nor be concerned about the alignment of the second molars, clinicians are certainly aware of the long-term periodontal and dental health consequences of poorly positioned and poorly inclined mandibular second molars.

Consider, then, that the clinician has a choice of molar tubes from which to select the specific appliance to use on patients. Some clinicians might promote placement of a mandibular first molar tube with a distal offset, providing a mesial-out rotation on the molar and presumably improving the alignment of the dental arch. This harkens back to the days when molar offsets routinely had to be placed in archwires because non-preadjusted appliances did not account for variations in morphology.

However, if we use a mandibular first molar tube with a distal offset and then study the impact on the contact point between the first and second molars, it becomes quickly apparent (Fig. 7-3, *A* and *B*) that an undesirable distolingual rotation of mandibular first molar will be expressed. Clinically, this generally requires compensation by putting an offset in the archwire (Fig. 7-3, *C*). The net result is that

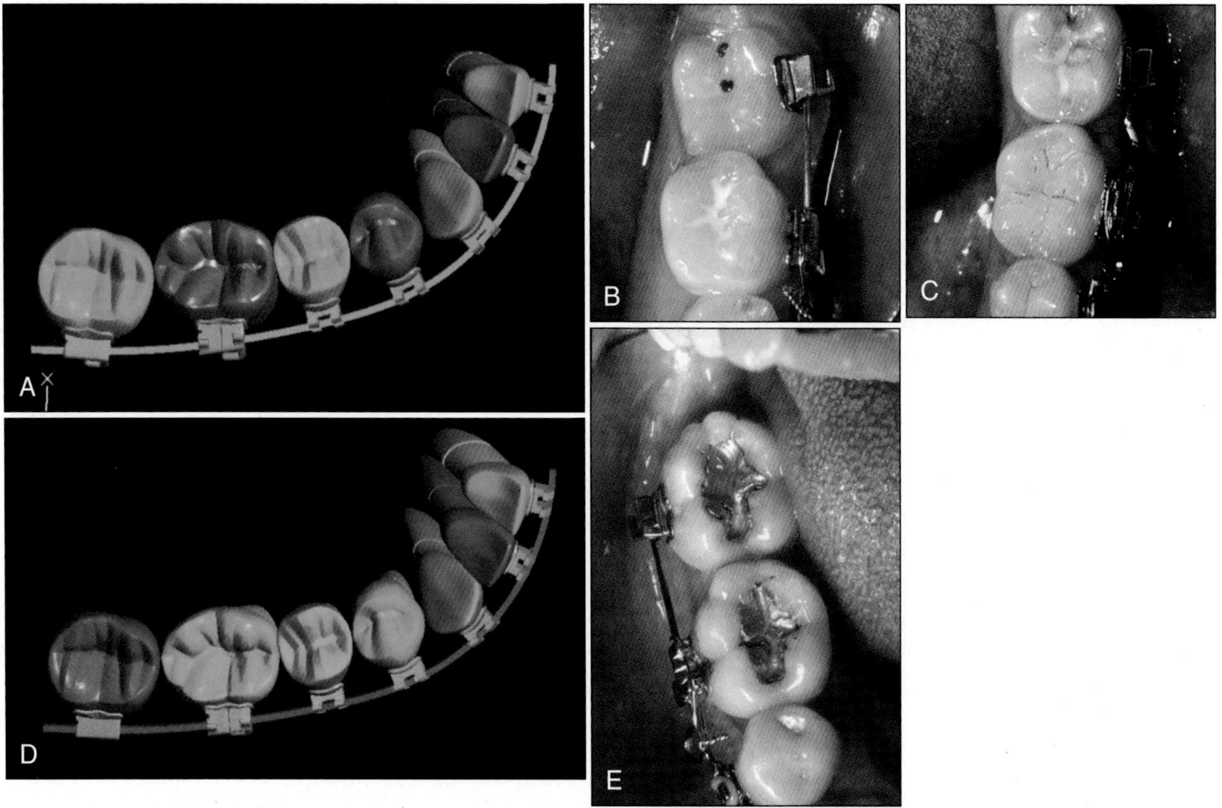

Fig. 7-3 **A,** Effect of distal offset on first molar tube in the mandibular arch. Note the resulting distolingual rotation of the first molar and resulting break in the contact point. **B,** Clinical example of the movement depicted graphically in Fig. 7-2. **C,** Archwire adjustment to offset the distolingual rotation imposed by selecting a tube with a distal offset. **D,** Contact point between mandibular first and second molars if a first molar tube without a distal offset is used. **E,** Clinical illustration of the contact relationship between mandibular first and second molars, achieved by using a molar tube without a distal offset.

the archwire adjustment became necessary to undo the movement expressed by the offset built into the tubes. This would therefore argue for a molar tube that does not have a distal offset (Fig. 7-3, *D* and *E*), because this seems to deliver the desirable outcome in establishing a proper contact relationship between the mandibular first and second molars.

Many such variables need to be considered in the management of orthodontic treatment; this simply illustrates how the choice of molar tubes would influence the finished treatment result and subsequent archwire adjustments.

The decision regarding the effects of tube selection on the rotation of the mandibular first molars must recognize that the morphology of the buccal surface of the mandibular first molar dictates that the mesiodistal position of the tube (or bracket) will influence the tube's final position. However, the ability to affect the mesiodistal position of the tube is limited, even more so with bands, because most practitioners now use preformed bands with prewelded brackets and tubes. Preformed bands greatly inhibit the ability to change the molar's mesiodistal position. Direct bonding might result in slightly greater flexibility, although the preformed shape of the bracket base generally limits the available modification (Fig. 7-4). With indirect bonding, particularly if a custom resin base is created, slightly more flexibility is available to the clinician.

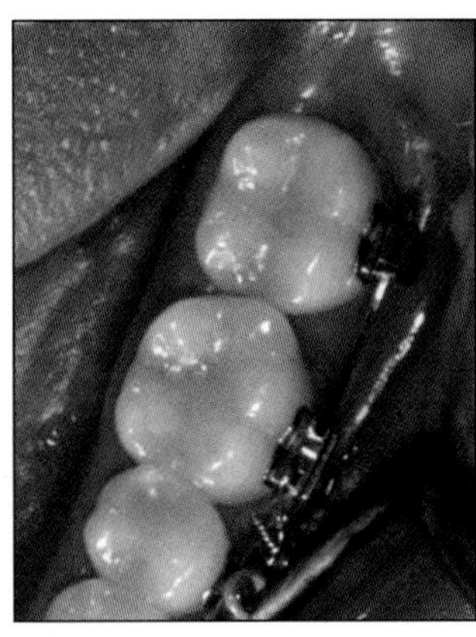

Fig. 7-4 The close adaptation of a molar bonding pad significantly limits the ability to vary the mesiodistal position of the tube with direct bonding. A slight increase in flexibility can be obtained with indirect bonding because a custom resin base is formed.

BRACKET SELECTION AND EFFECT ON THIRD-ORDER MOVEMENTS

Since the advent of pretorqued and preangulated brackets, orthodontists have had a wide choice of torques and angulations. Many pretorqued and preangulated appliance systems are available, and each prescription is based on a foundation of clinical principles, as well as the philosophical preferences of the clinician. Considerable variation exists in the prescribed torques and angulations of the Hilgers and Alexander prescriptions, for example, and further differences in mechanics are introduced by using the .018 slot or the .022 slot. One practitioner treating a patient population may use an Alexander prescription, with +14 degrees of torque on the maxillary central incisors, +7 degrees of torque on the lateral incisors, and −3 degrees of torque on the canines. Another practitioner treating a similar patient population may use the Hilgers prescription, with +22 degrees of central incisor torque, +14 degrees of lateral incisor torque, and +7 degrees of canine torque. These differences are substantial, but the differences become applicable only when full-size archwires are used, a relatively uncommon event. Further, the choice of prescriptions may be governed by the practitioner's philosophy on occlusal function and its potential impact on temporomandibular disorders.[3]

However, virtually all existing treatment methodologies recommend that the torque on the maxillary first and second molars be identical. This is somewhat surprising, given the difference in morphology between these two teeth, and the increasing gradient toward the occlusal surface when viewing the buccal surface of the upper second molars. Consequently, as shown in Figure 7-5, *A*, placing the same degree of torque in the tube on the maxillary second molar as placed on the maxillary first molar will result in a lesser degree of torque expressed on the second molar. The undesirable consequence of this would be a relatively low position of the lingual cusps, thereby creating possible balancing interferences, and perhaps resulting in inadequate settling of the posterior occlusion. The author believes that the torque should be greater for the average second molar than the first molar, because most second molars erupt with a buccal crown inclination and consequent lingual root torque.

To study the degree of torque required in the molar tube to achieve an adequate buccal root torque, the author studied the problem with the three-dimensional (3D) graphic analysis described earlier. Figure 7-5, *A*, shows an occlusal view of the maxillary arch with an appliance system that has 10 degrees of torque on the maxillary first molar and 10 degrees of torque on the maxillary second molar. Figure 7-5, *B*, is a buccal view of the same dental arch with the second molar tube designed to express 10 degrees of lingual crown torque. It is evident that the second molar is not torqued adequately, with the consequent and undesirable extension of lingual cusps into the occlusal plane. Figure 7-5, *C* and *D*, are occlusal views showing the difference when the torque is increased from 10 degrees to 17 degrees on the second molar. Since a full-sized finishing archwire will not be used, the amount of torque on the second molar tube was established at 19 degrees. The author concluded that the differential in torque between the maxillary first and second molars is probably more accurately reflected with a 5-degree differential, and therefore the torque on the first molars has been increased to 14 degrees. Recently, McLaughlin, Bennett, and Trevisi[4] also recommended that the torque on the maxillary second molar be 5 degrees higher than the first molar's torque.

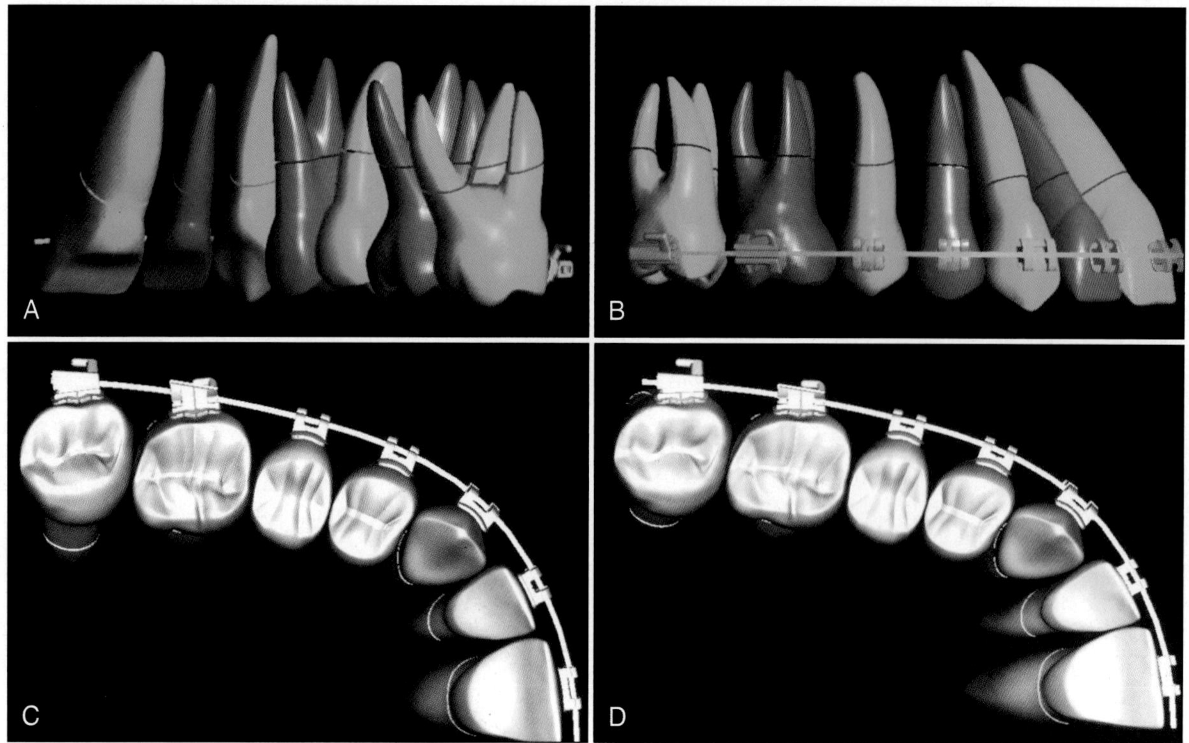

Fig. 7-5 **A,** Difference in expressed lingual crown torque between maxillary first and second molars, when a tube with 10 degrees of lingual crown torque is used on both teeth. The occlusal view of the maxillary arch shows a molar tube that delivers 10 degrees of lingual crown torque on the maxillary first molar and the maxillary second molar. The inadequate lingual crown torque on the maxillary second molar is evident. **B,** Lateral view of the same dental arch with a second molar tube that delivers 10 degrees of lingual crown torque. **C,** Occlusal view of a maxillary arch, demonstrating improved torque in the maxillary second molar. **D,** Lateral view of a maxillary arch, demonstrating balancing interferences from the lingual cusps of the maxillary second molar.

IMPACT OF VERTICAL PLACEMENT ON EXPRESSED TORQUE

In assessing the impact of appliance choice, it is important to remember that it is not the torque in the bracket that counts, but rather the *expressed* torque on the tooth. After all, *teeth* are being positioned, not brackets. Further, the clinician should remember that, with the new higher-resiliency archwires, force diminishes as an activation reaches its final stages. This diminution in force may be significant enough to consider whether 17 degrees of torque in a bracket will be more fully expressed with a steel archwire than a heat-activated Nitinol archwire. This subject has not been adequately investigated.

It is important to discern the differences introduced by vertical changes in bracket position on the expressed torque in different teeth. In drawing a distinction between two teeth, the maxillary canine and the maxillary central incisor, it becomes immediately apparent that the degree of convexity of the labial surface has a profound impact on this variable.

The maxillary central incisor has a labial surface with a mild degree of convexity (Fig. 7-6, *A*). Therefore, when the bracket level is changed (Fig. 7-6, *B* and *C*), the tooth will change in its vertical position relative to the archwire, but only a slight change will occur in the expressed torque. In contrast to the central incisors, when similar changes in the vertical position of the bracket are made on the maxillary canine (Fig. 7-6, *D*), the tooth does not merely change its vertical orientation to the archwire. A rather profound impact on the expressed torque is immediately apparent (Fig. 7-6, *E* and *F*) because of the effect of the convexity on the labial surface of this tooth. This is precisely why it is advisable to select specific torque values for the maxillary incisors and maxillary canines differently; the vertical placement of the bracket can be modified for deep overbites and open bites without introducing a significant compromise in the expressed torque desired by the clinician. As a result, the choice of torque in the bracket is only significant when it is identified in conjunction with specific vertical placement of the bracket on the tooth.

Figure 7-7, *A*, is an anterior view of the maxillary dental arch, with bracket positions selected by the author. Note the vertical position of the maxillary canine and the root angulation in the labiolingual plane. In Fig. 7-7, *B*, the vertical position of the canine bracket has been changed by 1 mm, while keeping other variables in the dental arch and the appliance configuration as a constant. It is evident not only that the canine has extruded, but also that a noticeable change exists in the labiolingual inclination of that tooth. In Fig. 7-7, *C*, the vertical position of the canine bracket has been modified by 2 mm, and it quickly becomes apparent that the tooth not only extrudes, but also shows a rather significant change in the labiolingual inclination. Figure 7-7, *D*, is an occlusal view with the original bracket placement, and Figure 7-7, *E*, is an occlusal view with the bracket having been moved gingivally by 2 mm. The impact of the change in axial inclination, without changing the torque in the bracket or archwire, is noticeable. Figure 7-7, *F*, is a representation of the clinical difficulty this will present, effectively precluding the ability to establish contact between the maxillary and mandibular incisors. This sometimes frustrates clinicians, who are unable to understand why the occlusion will not "settle."

To understand the impact of this information on the day-to-day management of orthodontic patients, one must appreciate that a 2-mm differential between the selected and actual vertical positions of a bracket occurs more often than realized. For example, if a bracket will be placed at a height of 4.5 mm from the cusp tip, and the patient had sufficient bruxism to flatten the cusp tip by 2 mm, the habit of placing the bracket at 4.5 mm will create interference from the canine in the occlusion. Cusp tip wear of 2 mm on the canine is not unusual, and the impact of this information must be carefully evaluated in establishing the finishing details during treatment. An effort to overcome this by deliberate overtorquing, or "stepping out" of the tooth, is unlikely to create a favorable result. In these patients the clinician should consider reshaping the lingual surface of the maxillary canine.

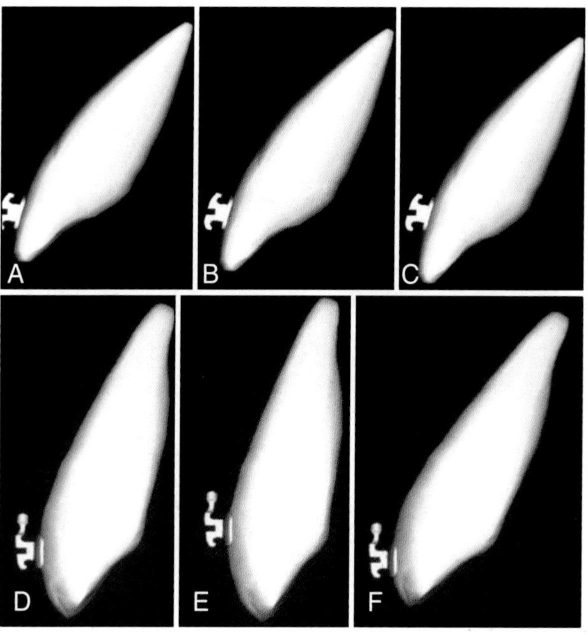

Fig. 7-6 Torque variation by bracket placement. **A** to **C,** Varying vertical positions of the bracket on a maxillary central incisor, with subsequent change in the vertical position of the tooth relative to the archwire. Note that the change in lingual root torque is minimal. **D** to **F,** In contrast, a change in the vertical position of the bracket on the canine results in a fairly profound change in the expressed lingual crown torque.

IMPACT OF TOOTH'S STARTING POSITION ON THE FINISHED RESULT

One of the least understood aspects of treatment with preadjusted appliances is the assumption that a fixed degree of second-order and third-order adjustments built into the bracket will be expressed uniformly in orthodontic treatment. If a bracket has 17 degrees of torque, for example, it is assumed that that torque will result in a uniform outcome, regardless of the starting position of the tooth. This is tenable only if one assumes that the treatment will be completed with a full-sized archwire, that is, a .022 × .028–inch archwire in a .022 × .028–inch slot, or .018 × .025–inch archwire in .018 × .025–inch slot. This is rarely the case. Most practitioners using the .022 × .028–inch slot have indicated that the finishing wires are rarely larger than .021 × .025 inch, and .019 × .025–inch wires are frequently used. The overwhelming majority of clinicians who use the .018 × .025–inch slot use a .016 × .022–inch finishing archwire.

Figure 7-8 provides a diagrammatic representation of the impact of pretreatment tooth position on treatment outcomes. The pronounced lingual inclination of the maxillary incisor crown is intended to reflect the starting position in a significant Class II, Division 2 malocclusion (Fig. 7-8, *A*). Figure 7-8, *B*, demonstrates the finished position of this tooth if a .016 × .022–inch archwire is used in a .018 × .025–inch slot. Figure 7-8, *C* and *D*, demonstrate the starting and finished position of the same tooth if a .018 × .025–inch archwire is used, and it is clear that more lingual root torque will be expressed. Figure 7-8, *E* and *F*, show the effect, using the same bracket and a .016 × .022 archwire, in a labially inclined incisor, such as that seen in a Class II, Division 1 malocclusion. As evident in Fig. 7-8, *G* and *H*, the finished position will be the same if a .018 × .025–inch archwire is used. However, the finished position will be slightly different if a .016 × .022–inch archwire is used, because the archwire will not engage in the third order until the tooth has been retracted to a certain degree. This would support using a higher-torqued central incisor bracket, versus a central incisor bracket with low lingual root torque. It is important to remember that the higher torque on the maxillary anterior teeth is also desirable to preclude the adverse effects of an anterior interference in the occlusion.[3] A bracket with 12 degrees of torque, for example, is not likely to have adequate

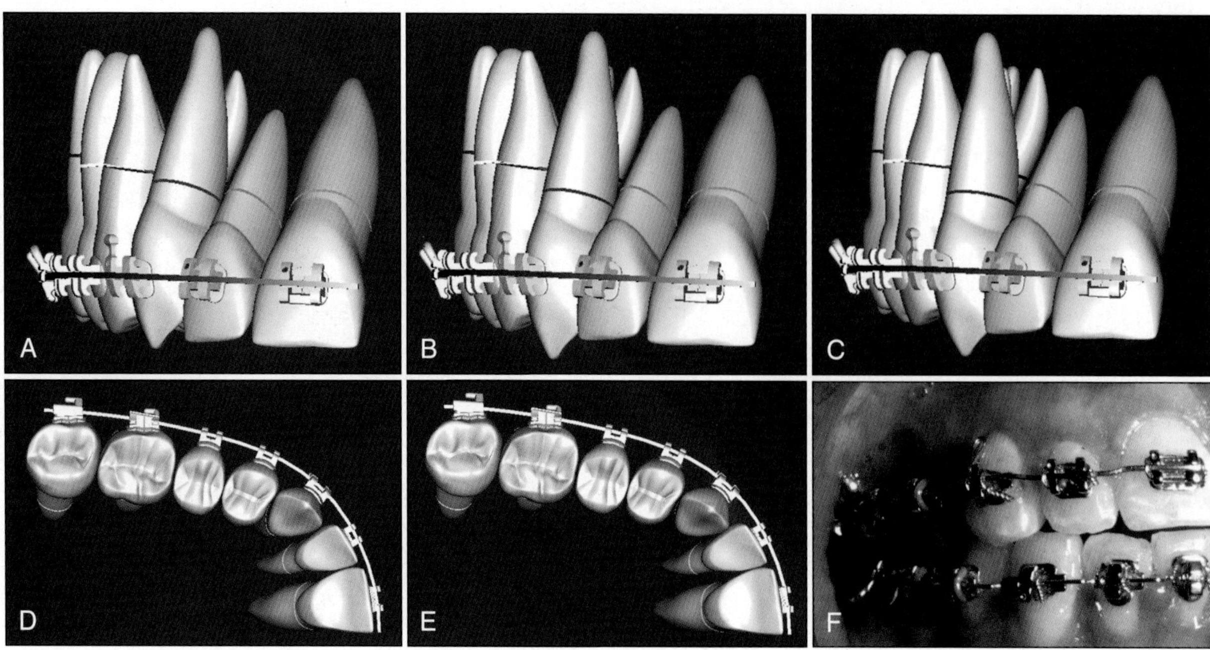

Fig. 7-7 **A,** Anterior view of maxillary dental arch, demonstrating vertical position and axial inclination of the canine, with preferred bracket position selected by the author. **B,** Effect of changing bracket position by 1 mm. Note that the tooth has extruded, and that a noticeable labial root torque has been realized. **C,** Anterior view of the same dental arch, with the bracket repositioned 2 mm gingivally. Note that the tooth does not merely extrude, but also displays a significant increase in labial root torque. **D,** Occlusal view of maxillary dental arch, with the canine bracket positioned at the same vertical level as in *A*. **E,** Occlusal view of the same dental arch, with the bracket repositioned gingivally by 2 mm. Note the degree of lingual crown torque introduced as a result of the vertical change, with a consequent interference of the canine into the occlusion. **F,** Clinical example of a canine with moderate cusp tip wear, and the resulting interference in the occlusion. Note the compensating labial crown torque that has been placed on the tooth. Reshaping of the canine is recommended to establish an occlusion, in addition to preventing excessive crown torque on the tooth.

activation to permit an adequate result for the average Class II, Division 2 case.

These types of factors must be taken into account in the choice of brackets and bracket systems when planning the treatment of patients (because of the profound impact of these variables on the finishing details in the treatment result).[5]

VARIABLE PRESCRIPTION MODULES AND SELF-LIGATION

With the advent and seemingly inexorable growth of self-ligation in clinical practice, it is important for the clinician to appreciate the implications of bracket selection and bracket placement in expressing first-, second-, and third-order movements with a self-ligating appliance. Given the absence of ligation, it is evident that inserting an archwire with added torque into a self-ligating bracket presents an additional challenge, which will vary between the "active" and "passive" bracket systems.

Given the desirability of reducing the additional clinical burden imposed by inserting archwires with significant torque activation, selecting precisely constructed prescriptions would seem valuable in the management of a patient's treatment. Significant variation exists among patient populations, and generalizations are not advisable. Clearly, however, the many "prescriptions" developed and promoted over the years must be challenged in the light of current understanding and technology.

For example, alignment of the maxillary incisors presents in two classic versions for most Class II, Division 2 malocclusions. The first type generally has retroclined maxillary central incisors and proclined maxillary lateral incisors (Fig. 7-9, *A*), whereas the second type presents with significant lingual inclination of all four maxillary incisors (Fig. 7-9, *B*). In the second type, brackets with relatively high torque values may be placed to provide lingual root torque to all four incisors (Fig. 7-9, *C*). However, if the same lateral incisor bracket were used on the first type, with labially proclined maxillary lateral incisors (Fig. 7-9, *A*), the expressed torque would obviously be higher because of the different starting position of the tooth, with an undesirable result (Fig. 7-9, *D*).

Given the vast difference in the starting positions of the lateral incisors in these two presentations, it is appropriate to question whether the same lateral incisor bracket should be used in both cases, simply because that is the value a particular clinician selected in the original development of a prescription. With reference to the previous information regarding the impact that the starting position the tooth will have on expressed torque, it would behoove a thoughtful clinician to recognize that brackets with different tips and torques should be used on these two different lateral incisors.

The author believes that the first step in accepting the concept of *variable prescription modules,* used to refine the effectiveness and efficiency of preadjusted orthodontic appliances, is to recognize and accept the extremes that the clinician is likely to encounter in clinical practice. Over the years, clinical problems have been classified into different categories, such as dolichocephalic, brachycephalic, and mesocephalic. Other processes for classification take into account Angle's classification, in conjunction with other transverse and vertical categories of discrepancy. Regardless of classification in the decision-making process, most clinicians differentiate patients into those who would require higher levels of torque versus those who require lower levels of torque in the expression of third-order movements, with a spectrum of finished positions between these extremes.

Therefore the author's work with digital graphics has been expanded to recognize the variable prescriptions that would be necessary in implementing a high-torque appliance, as in management of Class II, Division 2 malocclusions, and a low-torque appliance, as in management of Class II, Division 1 malocclusions. Figure 7-10 shows the extremes for these prescriptions; *A* demonstrates the expression of a high-torque prescription, *B* a medium-torque prescription, and *C* a low-torque prescription. To recognize the extremes on either side of the spectrum, the graphic analysis assumes the placement of a full-sized archwire. As previously noted, this is an extremely rare event in clinical practice and virtually nonexistent in treatment with self-ligating appliances. Therefore the clinician should define the appliance of choice for a given case and vary the prescriptions as necessary.

The logical extension of variable prescription modules is the incorporation of what may be described as a "range" of brackets with differing tips and torques. For example, in the Class II, Division 2 patient with four retroclined maxillary incisors, the clinician may choose high-torque brackets for all four incisors. However, for the Class II, Division 2 malocclusion with labially inclined maxillary lateral incisors, the

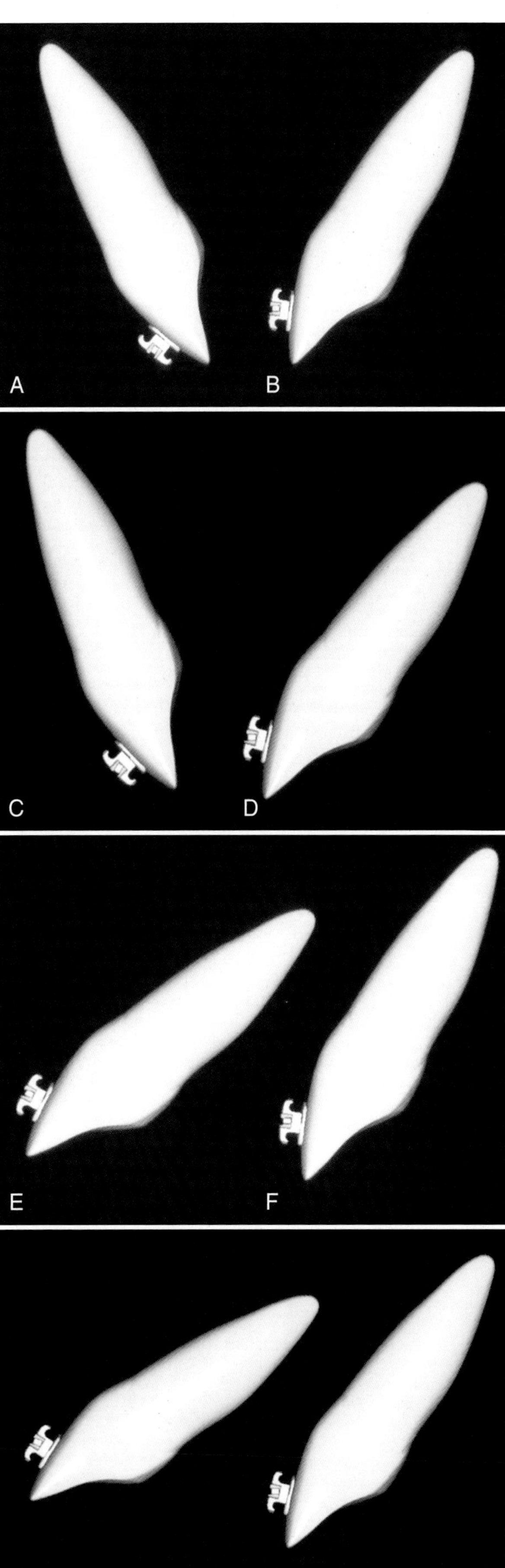

Fig. 7-8 **A,** Lingually inclined maxillary incisor, as seen in Class II, Division 2 malocclusion. **B,** Finished position of tooth in *A,* with .016 × .022–inch *(16 × 22)* archwire in a .018 × .025–inch slot. **C** and **D,** Starting and finished positions of the same tooth with .018 × .025–inch *(18 × 25)* archwire in .018 × .025–inch slot. **E** and **F,** Labially inclined incisor using the same bracket and a .016 × .022–inch archwire. Since the archwire will not block the initial lingual tipping during a retraction, the complete 22 degrees of torque will not be expressed. **G** and **H,** Difference in the finished position of the tooth if an .018 × .025–inch archwire is used.

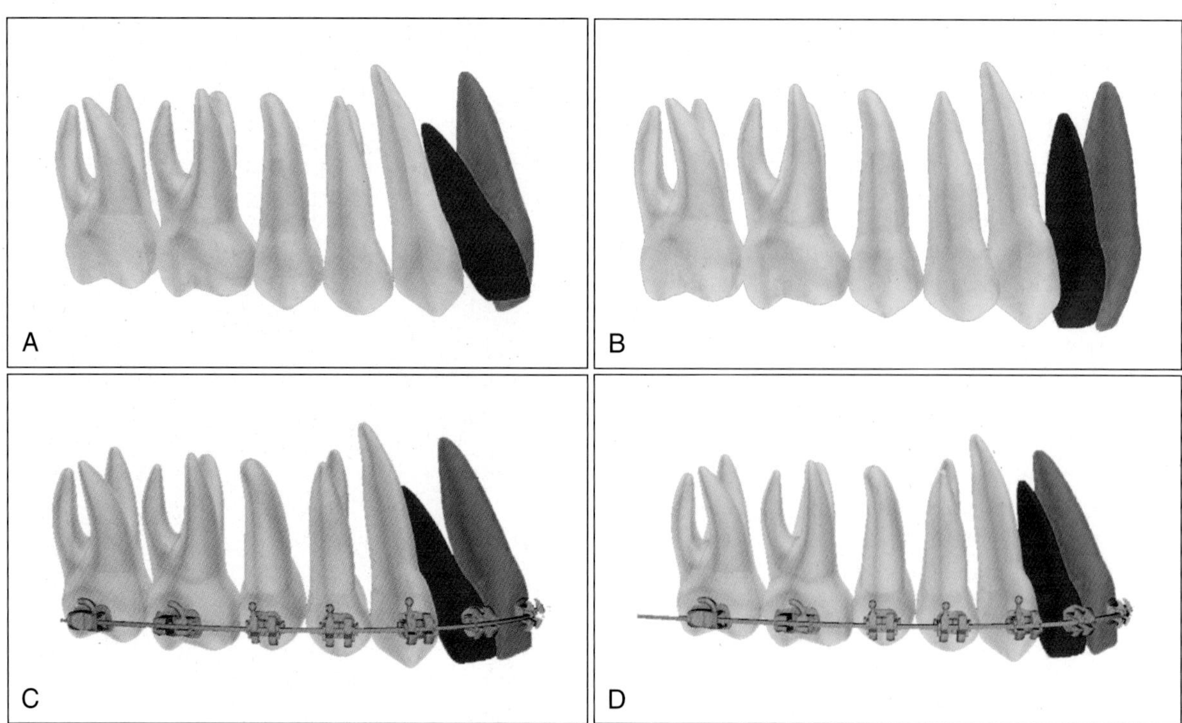

Fig. 7-9 **A,** Classic appearance of Class II, Division 2 malocclusion, with retroclined maxillary central incisors and proclined maxillary lateral incisors. **B,** Another type of Class II, Division 2 malocclusion, with lingual inclination of all four maxillary incisors. **C,** Corrected Class II, Division 2 malocclusion of the type shown in Fig. 7-8, *G* and *H*. This diagram illustrates the SmartClip self-ligating appliance, with pretorqued brackets. **D,** Finished treatment result with the same pretorqued lateral incisor bracket, used on the malocclusion depicted in Fig. 7-8, *G* and *H*. Excessive lingual root torque is depicted.

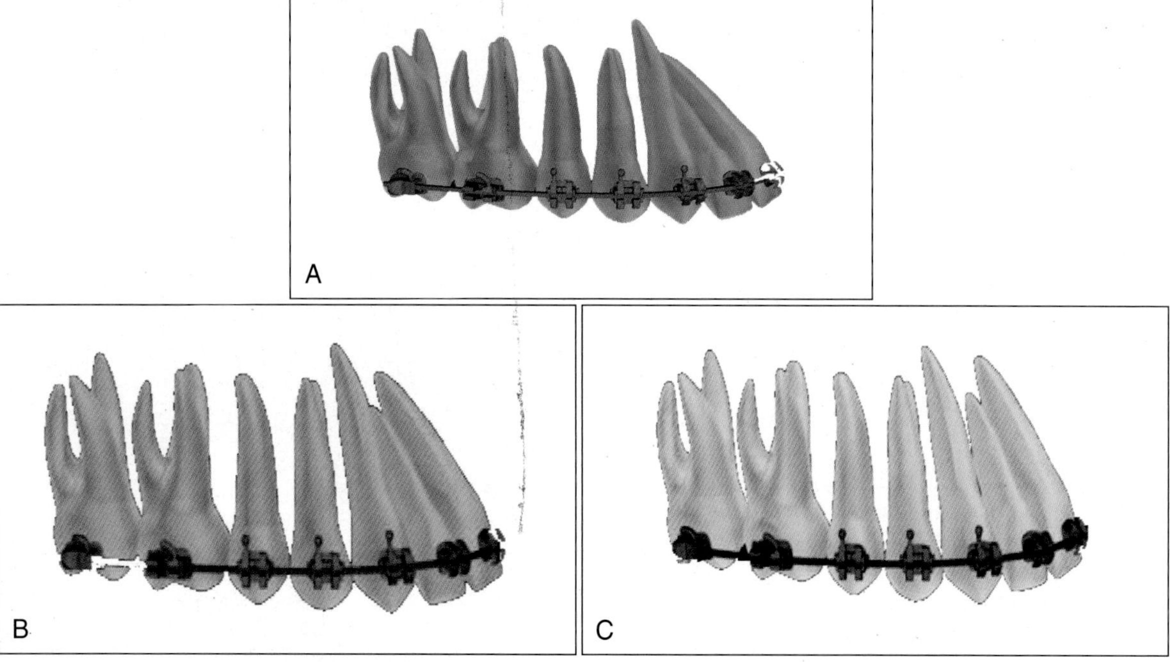

Fig. 7-10 Graphic representations of tooth movement with SmartClip self-ligating appliance. **A,** Expressed tooth movement with high-torque appliance, assuming full-sized finishing archwire. **B,** Expressed tooth positions with medium-torque prescription. **C,** Expressed tooth movement with low-torque prescription.

clinician may choose to combine a high-torque central incisor bracket with a lower-torque lateral incisor bracket. This is consistent with the varying expression of torque in the absence of full-sized archwires. For this reason a "range" of variable prescriptions are described and available to the clinician, to be customized in managing a specific case to maximum advantage. As previously mentioned, with the undesirability of inserting torqued archwires into self-ligating bracket slots, this will further decrease the need to make significant adjustments to finishing archwires in detailing a case.

CONCLUSION

Many different variables in all three planes of space have an impact on the finished orthodontic treatment result, and the impact will depend on the specifics of a clinical problem. A three-dimensional graphic analysis can influence finishing details and choice of brackets, bracket systems, and specific orthodontic prescriptions. The choice of a prescription is not the only decision determining the clinical outcome; significant differences are further introduced by variations in mesiodistal and vertical positioning of the brackets. Clinicians should therefore recognize the need for analyzing bracket placement and choice of prescription together. A prescription offered without specific guidelines on bracket placement has limited value, as do guidelines for specific bracket placement without an understanding of the implied effect on expressed first-, second-, and third-order movements.

Although a "work in progress," the author believes that the virtual and variable approach described here will continue to gain acceptance within the orthodontic profession, with an overall enhancement in the level of effectiveness and efficiency in the management of orthodontic patients.

REFERENCES

1. Andrews L: Six keys to normal occlusion, *Am J Orthod* 62:296-309, 1972.
2. McNamara JA, Seligman DA, Okeson JP: The relationship of occlusal factors and orthodontic treatment to temporomandibular disorders. In *Temporomandibular disorders and related pain conditions. Progress in pain research and management*, vol 4, Seattle, 1995, IASP Press.
3. Sondhi A: Anterior interferences: their impact on anterior inclination and orthodontic finishing procedures, *Semin Orthod* 9:204-215, 2003.
4. McLaughlin RP, Bennett JC, Trevisi HJ: *Systemized orthodontic treatment mechanics,* St Louis, 2001, Mosby.
5. Sondhi A: The implications of bracket selection and bracket placement on finishing details, *Semin Orthod* 9:155-164, 2003.

CHAPTER 8

Quality Orthodontics: Challenging Popular Trends

Björn U. Zachrisson

The new and popular trends in orthodontics, as advocated by orthodontic companies, appliance inventors, and self-proclaimed experts, seem to have reduced clinical orthodontics to the use of self-ligating brackets, high-tech archwires with no need for wire bending, and permanent retention with bonded retainers.[1]

Several influential lecturers on the international circuit demonstrate a purely mechanistic approach to orthodontic treatment and largely disregard the aspects of diagnosis, treatment planning, and treatment objectives. Even in cases with marked crowding, proclined lower incisors, or the six mandibular anterior teeth well above the functional occlusal plane, these "experts" bond orthodontic attachments to all teeth and take a nonextraction treatment approach. Superelastic, round or rectangular archwires without bends are used to level and align the dental arches. By necessity, this leads to lateral expansion of the mandibular canines and premolars and further lower incisor proclination, as evidenced by the cephalometric films and tracings of these individuals. After debonding, the recommendation is that teeth be permanently retained with fixed retainers bonded from first premolar to first premolar.

The purpose of this chapter is to emphasize the long-term follow-up clinical research and experience-based information on proper orthodontic treatment that benefits the patients and ensures optimal treatment and stable results. It addresses the following needs:

- For evidence-based treatment planning
- For archwire bending
- To intrude mandibular rather than maxillary incisors
- To use transpalatal arches as supplements to labial archwires
- For differentiated long-term rather than permanent retention

NEED FOR EVIDENCE-BASED TREATMENT PLANNING

Teeth are positioned exactly in the oral cavity for a reason. Even in a malocclusion, there is equilibrium between forces from the inside and from the outside of the dentition.[2-4] If the orthodontist's purpose is to change tooth positions significantly, the clinical problem is to estimate the amount of change that will remain stable over time.

Malocclusion of the teeth is caused by an interplay between inborn genetic factors and external environmental factors. Edward Angle believed that the environment could be modified by orthodontic treatment, that orthodontic treatment regenerated new bone, and that it would be possible to produce stable ideal occlusions without tooth extractions. However, we know now that bone yields to functional forces, and that premolar extractions are required in some cases.[4] The percentage of extraction cases reflects a judgment as to the importance of how much the equilibrium of environmental forces around the dentition can be modified permanently. There is ample evidence in the literature that expansion in the lower arch, particularly in the canine region, is unstable, with little or no evidence to the contrary.[4,5] Transverse expansion across the canines is almost never maintained, probably because of lip pressures at the corners of the mouth.[4] It is important, therefore, to avoid an increase in the normal mandibular intercanine width (25-26 mm) during orthodontic treatment.[6-11] Some excellent clinical long-term studies have demonstrated that not only the mandibular intercanine distance, but also the patient's pretreatment mandibular arch form, should constitute a guide to arch shape.[11-13]

The lower incisor position in space is also controlled by a balance of muscle forces, which may lie within a narrow zone of stability.[2,3] Moving lower incisors forward more than

2 mm is problematic for stability, probably because lip pressure seems to increase sharply at that point.[4] Further research is needed before evidence-based clinical guidelines on lower incisor proclinations can be established.

NEED FOR ARCHWIRE BENDING

Individualized archwire bends should be used to secure early and full correction of all rotations in the original malocclusion. The main reason is that even slightly broken contacts (Fig. 8-1, *A*) in both untreated cases and treated cases are the predictable starting points for relapse and later increased crowding.[14]

Slight undercorrection of previously rotated teeth is not easy to detect clinically. The size of the archwire bends necessary to produce full-rotation correction is often remarkably large (Fig. 8-1, *B*). This results from the slack between the archwire slot and the wire. Fine details must be checked toward the end of treatment by careful comparison with the pretreatment plaster models. In the maxilla, a mouth mirror is necessary to check the incisor region.[14] If these steps are not taken, an undercorrected case may look good or even excellent on clinical examination in the orthodontist's chair.

Small, meticulous archwire bends will also help ensure that the distal contact areas of the mandibular lateral incisors are placed slightly labial to the mesial contact points of the mandibular canines, and that the teeth are retained in these positions (Fig. 8-1, *C*). This is particularly important when the distal aspects of one or both lateral incisors are lingually displaced at the start of treatment. The mandibular anterior region is the most common area for increased crowding and relapse after treatment. Moderate crowding can be masked if the four incisors are positioned as a block outside the mesial contacts of the mandibular canines.[15]

Careful archwire bends are also necessary to provide the desired and symmetrical axial inclinations (crown torque) of the maxillary and mandibular canines and premolars before appliance removal, to provide a full and radiant smile[16] (Fig. 8-2). No straight-wire approach or "fully programmed preadjusted appliance" used by an orthodontist without wire bending can place every tooth in correct position in all three planes of space.[5]

NEED TO INTRUDE MANDIBULAR RATHER THAN MAXILLARY INCISORS

Analogous with recent concepts of treatment planning in general and esthetic dentistry,[17,18] the mechanical intrusion of maxillary incisors in orthodontics should be made with the utmost care to avoid "hiding" these teeth behind the upper lip. In most deep-bite cases, intrusion of the mandibular teeth should be done.

Maxillary Intrusion Arch Versus Bite Plate

Lindauer, Lewis, and Shroff[19] recently made a comparative clinical and cephalometric analysis of the effects of two common procedures to reduce deep overbite in 40 patients: maxillary incisor intrusion using an intrusion arch and posterior tooth eruption using an anterior bite plate. Both the intrusion arches and the bite plates were successful in correcting the deep overbite over a relatively short period of treatment, although by different mechanisms. The maxillary incisors in the intrusion group were significantly intruded during treatment, with a corresponding decrease in the lip–upper incisor measurement, from a mean of 5.4 mm (SD 2.0 mm) to 3.0 mm (SD 1.4 mm), as measured in relaxed-lip posture. The overbite correction in the bite plate group was achieved by a combination of lower incisor intrusion, significant flaring of the lower incisors, and a small opening rotation of the mandibular plane secondary to posterior tooth eruption. The clinical lip–upper incisor measurement was reduced by about 1 mm in the bite plate group.

The significant decrease of about 2.5 mm of maxillary incisor display with the lips at rest when using a maxillary intrusion arch[19] should be an alarming finding when patients with deep overbite and minimal incisor show are treated orthodontically. Any maxillary incisor intrusion must be made with due respect to (1) the patient's initial tooth

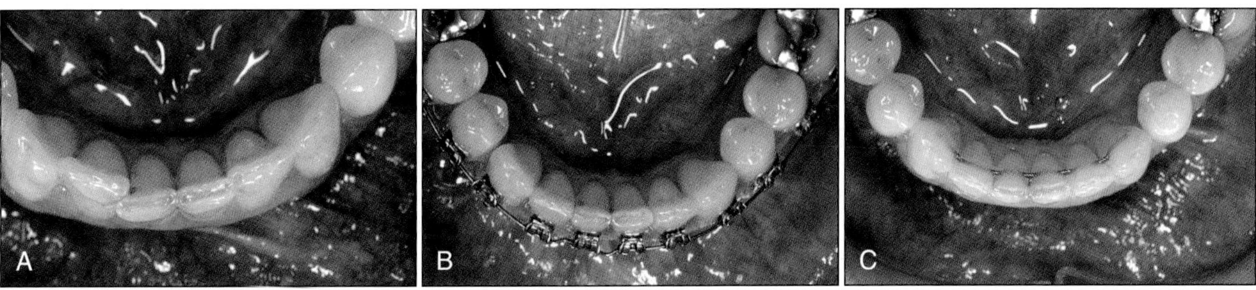

Fig. 8-1 Full correction of the crowded mandibular right central incisor (**A**) required marked archwire bends (**B**). **C**, Mesiodistal enamel reduction (stripping) was used to avoid incisor proclination and converted the contact points to small contact areas. The distal contact areas of the lateral incisors are purposely placed slightly labial to the mesial contact points of the canines and retained in these positions.

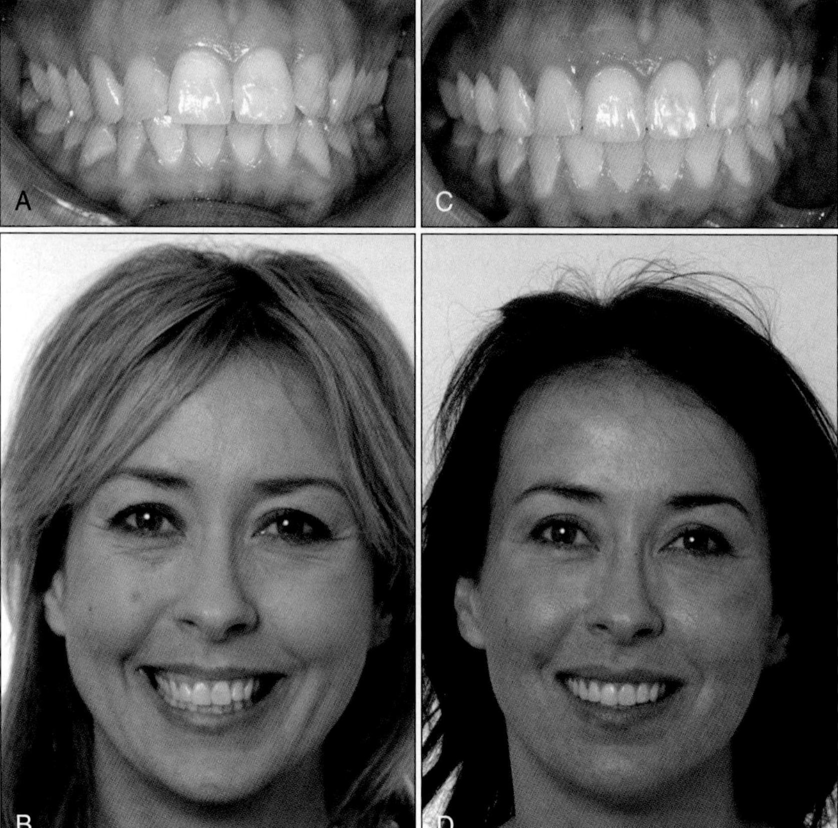

Fig. 8-2 Adult female patient with marked lingual tilt of all maxillary and mandibular teeth (**A**) and constricted smile with excessive gingiva-to-lip distance on the right side (**B**). **C,** Increased lingual root torque was provided by third-order bends in rectangular stainless steel archwires. Electrosurgery was performed from right second premolar to left lateral incisor. **D,** Posttreatment smile is radiant with symmetrical gingival exposure.

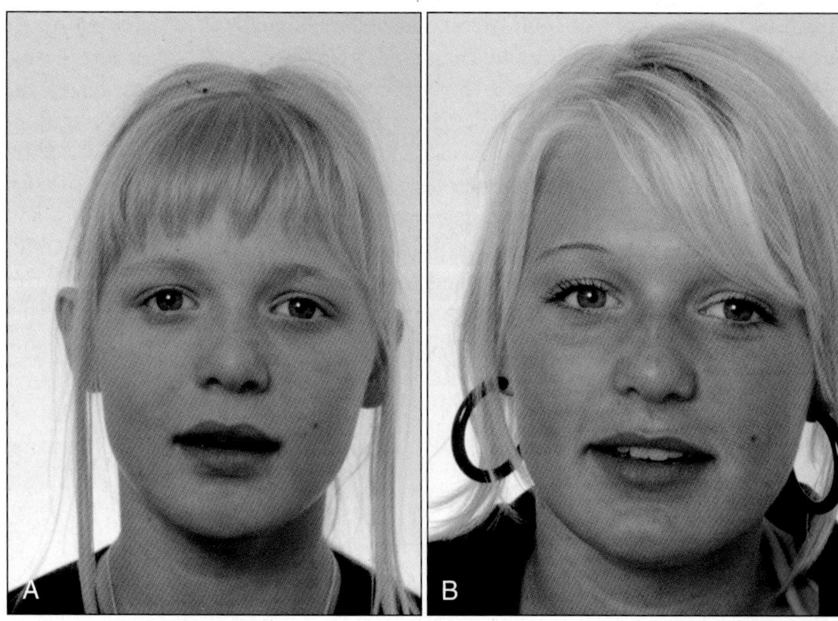

Fig. 8-3 **A,** Young girl with Class II, Division 1 malocclusion and deep overbite. Note minimal display of maxillary incisors with relaxed lips. During treatment the maxillary incisors were extruded and the deep bite corrected by mandibular incisor intrusion (as described in Fig. 8-4, *A* and *B*). **B,** The improved maxillary anterior tooth display with lips at rest is of esthetic importance when the patient is speaking.

display with relaxed lips, (2) the show of maxillary incisors with the patient speaking, and (3) the patient's age and gender. Maxillary incisor intrusion is therefore rarely indicated in the average orthodontic patient with deep anterior overbite.[20,21] Normative values for maxillary incisor display with relaxed lips, as observed during speech, are now available for all age groups.[22-24]

As a general rule, it is detrimental to make orthodontic patients look older than their chronologic age. In some deep overbite cases, when patients demonstrate little upper incisor with relaxed lips for their age group at the start of treatment (Fig. 8-3, *A*), the maxillary incisors may be purposely extruded during treatment (Fig. 8-3, *B*) to improve the esthetic appearance after appliance removal.[21] Similarly, if

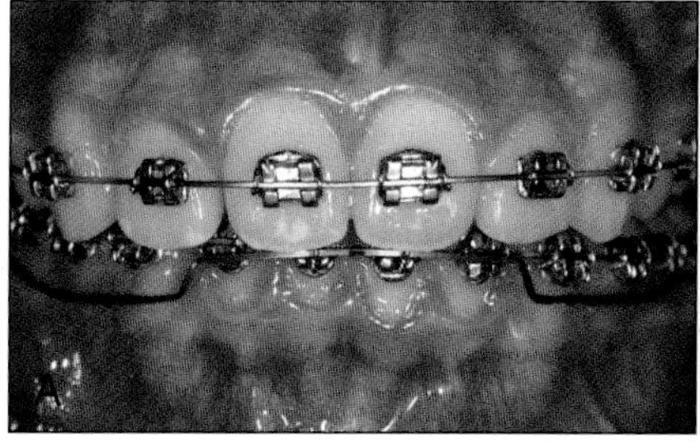

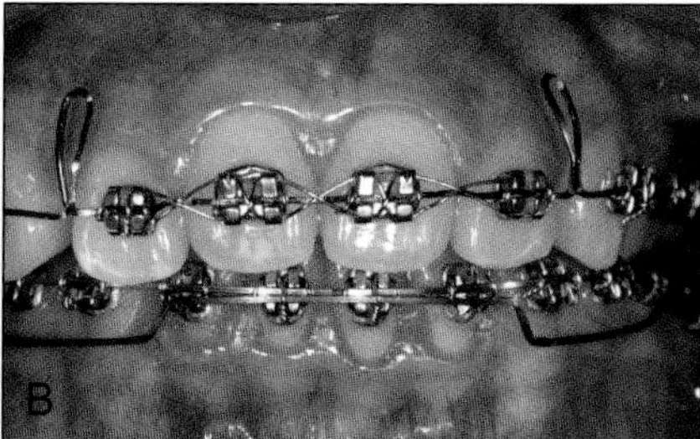

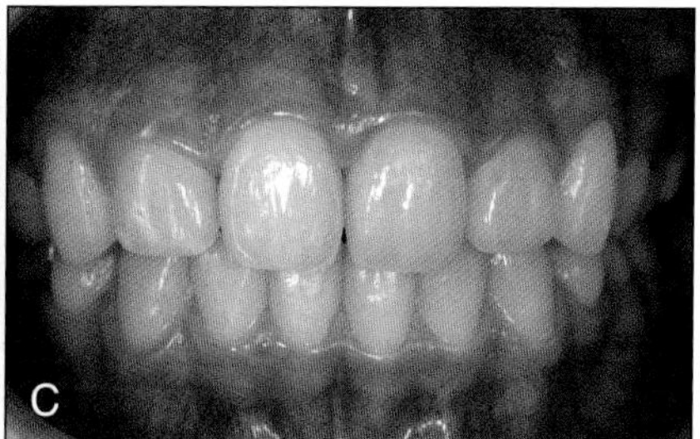

Fig. 8-4 Intrusion of mandibular incisors in patient with deep overbite, using CNA (beta III titanium) overlay base arch inserted in bonded double tubes on the mandibular first molars. The rate of lower incisor intrusion can be followed by registration of maxillary central incisor edge relative to archwire and brackets on the mandibular teeth (**A** and **B**). **C,** After intrusion and debonding.

finishing of the case involves incisal edge recontouring for esthetic purposes, it is advantageous to purposely extrude the maxillary incisors beyond what is normal for the patient's age before enameloplasty is performed.

Mandibular incisor intrusion can be achieved with mandibular utility arches,[25] segmented intrusion arches,[26-28] and overlay base arches[20,29] (Fig. 8-4). The rate of intrusion can be controlled by recording the position of the maxillary central incisor edge relative to fixed points on the mandibular appliances[21] (Fig. 8-4, *A* and *B*). Using overlay base arches, the mandibular incisor intrusion rate is about 0.5 mm per month. It is emphasized that it is not possible to intrude mandibular incisors effectively with one continuous archwire, such as in the straight-wire concept. Compared with a continuous archwire, segmented mechanics will produce more incisor intrusion and less molar extrusion.[25,30] Continuous-leveling archwires produce less true lower incisor intrusion, more premolar extrusion, and more incisor proclination[25,30] Such proclination of mandibular incisors may correlate with long-term overbite relapse.[31]

NEED TO USE TRANSPALATAL ARCHES AS SUPPLEMENTS TO LABIAL ARCHWIRES

When comparing Class II molar relationships by visual inspection of plaster models from the buccal and lingual sides, the Class II conditions are generally more pronounced when the occlusion is viewed from the buccal aspect.[32] This results from the mesial rotation of the molars. Because the occlusal surface of the first permanent molar is trapezoidal in shape, more mesiodistal space is used in the dental arch when this tooth rotates mesially on the lingual root as the axis. The implication is that in the majority of Class II cases, proper derotation of the maxillary first molars should be part of a sound treatment plan. A complete and controlled derotation of the maxillary molars in all Class I and II cases is difficult, if not impossible, with labial archwires only. Even if the buccal tubes are greatly offset distally, it is difficult to derotate the upper first molars properly with labial archwires only, because of the insufficient power of the terminal ends.

The superiority of a transpalatal (TP) arch in proper molar control is obvious[33] (Fig. 8-5, *B* and *C*; see also Fig. 8-6, *B*). The reason for this difference is that the solidity of a heavy (.036-inch) TP arch dominates the labial arch force systems. Even over-derotation of the molars can be obtained clinically by adding rotation adjustment bends in the TP arch.[33]

The custom-made TP arch[34-36] (see Fig. 8-5, *B*) is fundamental in the author's treatment technique and has been used in almost every patient the author has treated over the past 10 years. It is effective for (1) maxillary molar derotation, (2) maxillary arch width control and lateral expansion, (3) adding buccal root torque to upper first molars, (4) reinforcing posterior anchorage, (5) vertical control of upper molar eruption, (6) securing and maintaining maxillary arch form control throughout treatment, and (7) correcting mesiodistal asymmetries.[34]

The main differences between the author's design and the traditional Goshgarian-type TP arch design are in the amount and shape of the wire in the palatal loop. The middle loop is larger and longer than the single Coffin loop of the Goshgarian arch. Together, the large anterior loop and the two smaller posterior loops of the custom-made TP arch act similar to the acrylic button of the TP arch with a large acrylic button, dubbed the "vertical holding appliance" (VHA) by Nanda.[37] When the VHA is used for 1 to 2 years, a significant effect is caused by the tongue on the vertical movement of the first molars (mean effect up to 1 mm of intrusion).[37] The effect of the tongue is likely greater on the custom-made TP arch than on a conventional Goshgarian arch,[38] where the Coffin loop is much smaller. Even on a Goshgarian palatal arch, however, the effect of tongue function has been found to be effective for vertical control of the maxillary molars.[38-41]

Increasing the length of the wire will increase springiness and range, lower the load-deflection rate, and make the forces more constant and precise.[35] Compared with Goshgarian-type arches, the author's design produces lower and more constant moments for derotation.[35] The two small, distal-directed loops give the arch obvious flexibility, which makes the engagement into the attachments easier with less

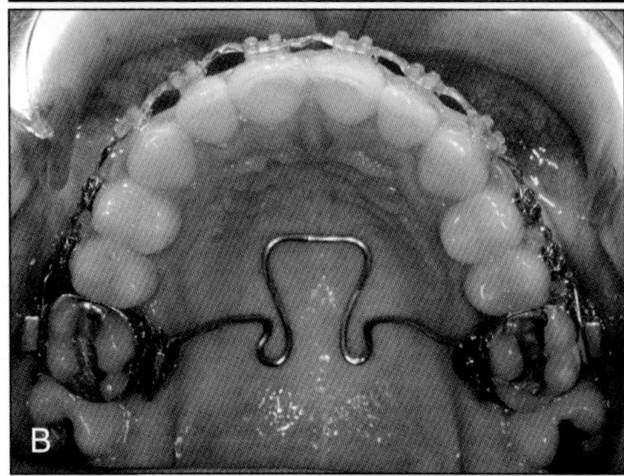

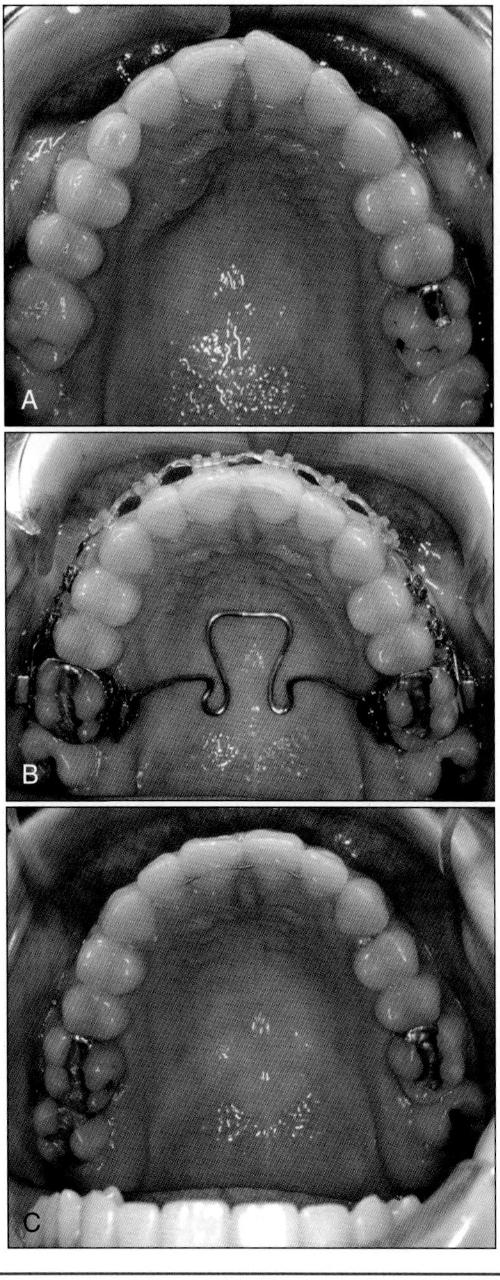

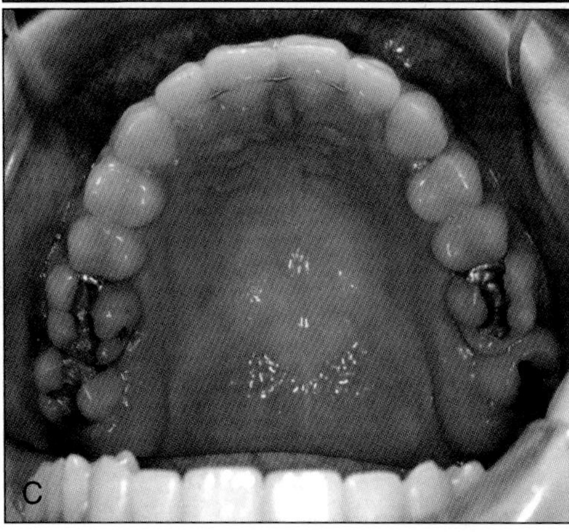

Fig. 8-5 **A,** Female adolescent patient with Class II, Division 1 malocclusion and typically mesially rotated first molars. The patient also had an impacted maxillary right canine and overlapping central incisors. **B,** Derotation of the first molars into proper Class I molar relationship was achieved with the custom-designed transpalatal arch, made in .036-inch blue Elgiloy wire. **C,** At appliance removal, the fully corrected central incisors were retained with a four-unit lingual retainer.

loss of activation. It takes less time to derotate molars with this design than with traditional Goshgarian arches.[36,37,42]

When only labial archwires are used, the Class II correction in young patients becomes more difficult than when a high-pull headgear is used together with the TP arch. The TP arch is used to add buccal root torque to the first molars, derotate the molars, and expand the intermolar distance as required. Both the high-pull headgear and the custom-made TP arch exert intrusive effects on the molars and the maxillary complex. The vertical control is an important ingredient in the treatment of sagittal discrepancies.[39,43] The explanation is that the mechanical inhibition of vertical maxillary growth leads to a greater anterior component of the available mandibular growth.[44] In addition, the effective molar derotation obtained with the TP arch plus the distally directed pull of the headgear contribute significantly to the Class II correction.

NEED FOR DIFFERENTIATED LONG-TERM RATHER THAN PERMANENT RETENTION

Provided that a careful wire-bending and bonding technique is used, the different bonded retainers generally have excellent outcomes over at least 10 to 15 years.[45] Patient acceptance is also satisfactory.[45,46] In particular, adult patients appreciate that the stability of the treatment results are ensured without need for their active cooperation.

There is a risk in using retainers for life when all six or eight teeth in a segment are bonded, because the patient may not notice if one (or more) of the bonds comes loose after some time in retention. Many patients have difficulty keeping the retainer area clean, despite instruction in hygiene. This almost creates an experimental caries model that may even provoke the need for endodontic treatment.

As discussed elsewhere,[45,47] many advantages exist with a more selective approach to orthodontic retention, in which 3-3 retainers bonded in thick (.030- to .036-inch) stainless steel or gold-coated wires bonded to the lower canines only (Fig. 8-6, *A*), four-unit retainers (Fig. 8-6, *B*; see also Fig. 8-5, *C*), short labial retainers (Fig. 8-6, *C*), and different forms of wire extensions into the occlusal fissures of premolars[45,47] are used for extended periods. Retention periods of up to 10 years are now recommended by most clinicians.[14,47-50] Long retention periods are favorable in many patients while waiting for the patient's third molars to erupt; and long retention counters the effects of postpubertal growth activity and maxillomandibular adjustments, which may continue well into the second decade and longer.[48,51,52]

Particularly in young and adolescent patients, the solid mandibular 3-3 retainer (see Fig. 8-6, *A*) is more hygienic and much safer to use than retainers bonded to all six anterior teeth.[45,47] Every patient will notice immediately when a lower retainer comes loose if it is bonded only to the canines. The patient can then call for a rebonding appointment or remove the retainer with fingers. Being the simplest and safest of the bonded retainers, the 3-3 retainer is also useful in many adult patients with little pretreatment crowding or spacing of the teeth.

The author believes that the use of permanent retention should be restricted to orthodontic patients who really need it. This category may include adults with advanced periodontal tissue breakdown, in whom the bonded retainers serve the dual purpose of preventing unwanted tooth movements and acting as a periodontal splint. Also, patients with

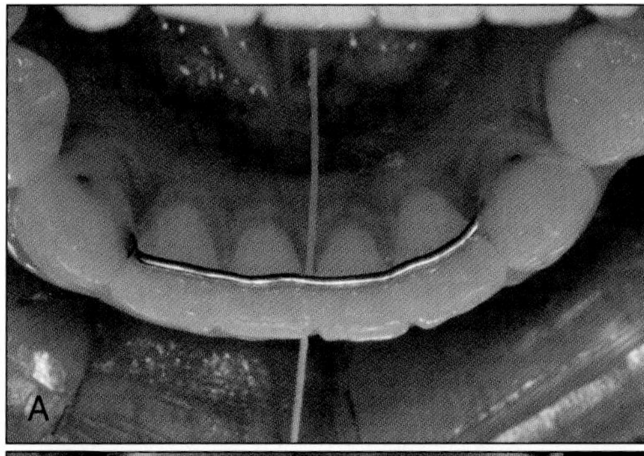

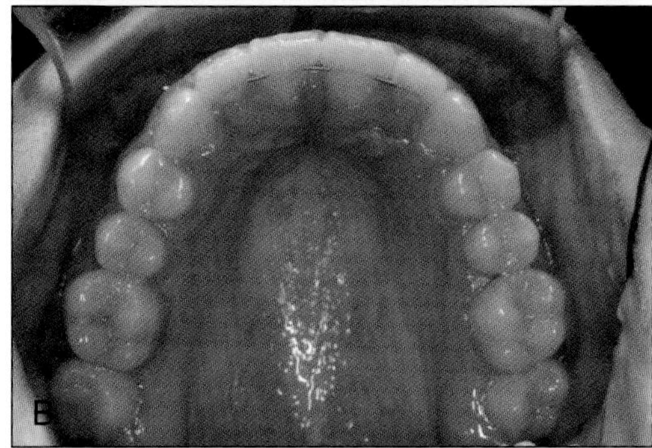

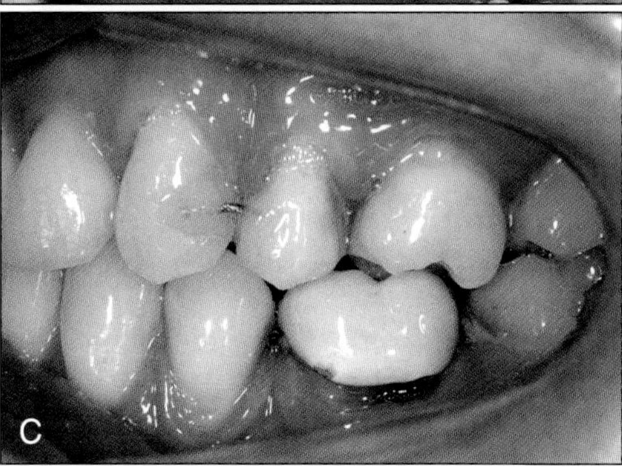

Fig. 8-6 Different types of bonded retainers: **A,** Gold-coated .030-inch-thick wire bonded only to the canines in a young girl. **B,** Four-unit gold-coated flexible spiral wire retainer made of .0215-inch five-stranded wire. **C,** Short labial wire segment from canine to second premolar to prevent reopening of space after extraction of first premolar in adult patient.

pretreatment marked median diastemas and adults with pronounced anterior crowding may need permanent stabilization of the treatment results. In some cases, it may be advantageous to use the bonded retainers for a prolonged retention period, then replace them with a removable retainer for nighttime wear on a long-term or more permanent basis.[45]

CONCLUSION

Clinicians need to challenge new and popular trends in orthodontics. Quality of orthodontic care depends on careful treatment planning and use of variable and customized mechanics. The prevailing myth that indiscriminate appliance-driven orthodontics represents progress has been rejected.

REFERENCES

1. Zachrisson BU: Use of self-ligating brackets, superelastic wires, expansion/proclination, and permanent retention: a word of caution, *World J Orthod* 7:198-206, 2006.
2. Weinstein S, Haack DC, Morris LY, et al: On an equilibrium theory of tooth position, *Angle Orthod* 33:1-26, 1963.
3. Proffit WR: Equilibrium theory revisited: factors influencing position of the teeth, *Angle Orthod* 48:175-186, 1978.
4. Proffit WR, Fields HW: Orthodontic treatment planning, limitations, controversies, and special problems. In Proffit WR, Fields HW Jr, editors: *Contemporary orthodontics,* ed 3, St Louis, 2000, Mosby, pp 240-293.
5. McLaughlin RP, Bennett JC: Finishing with the preadjusted orthodontic appliance, *Semin Orthod* 9:165-183, 2003.
6. Riedel RA: Post-pubertal occlusal changes. In McNamara JA, editor: *The biology of occlusal development,* monograph 7, Craniofacial Growth Series, Ann Arbor, 1977, Center for Human Growth and Development, University of Michigan, pp 113-140.
7. Riedel RA: A post-retention assessment of relapse, recidivism, adjustment, change, and stability. In Moorrees CFA, van der Linden FPGM, editors: *Orthodontics: evaluation and future,* The Netherlands, 1988, University of Nymegen, pp 281-306.
8. Gorman JC: The effects of premolar extractions on the long-term stability of the mandibular incisors. In Burstone CJ, Nanda R, editors: *Retention and stability in orthodontics,* Philadelphia, 1993, Saunders, pp 81-95.
9. Sadowsky C, Schneider BJ, BeGole EA, Tahir E: Long-term stability after orthodontic treatment: nonextraction with prolonged retention, *Am J Orthod Dentofacial Orthop* 106:243-249, 1994.
10. Paquette DE, Beattie JR, Johnston LE: A long-term comparison of nonextraction and premolar extraction edgewise therapy in "borderline" Class II patients, *Am J Orthod Dentofacial Orthop* 102:1-14, 1992.
11. Franklin GS: A longitudinal study of dental and skeletal parameters associated with stability of orthodontic treatment, 1995, University of Toronto (thesis).
12. Felton JM, Sinclair PM, Jones DL, Alexander RG: A computerized analysis of the shape and stability of mandibular arch form, *Am J Orthod Dentofacial Orthop* 92:478-483, 1987.
13. De La Cruz A, Sampson P, Little RM, et al: Long-term changes in arch form after orthodontic treatment and retention, *Am J Orthod Dentofacial Orthop* 107:518-530, 1995.
14. Zachrisson BU: Important aspects of long-term stability, *J Clin Orthod* 31:562-583, 1997.
15. Hopkins JB, Murphy J: Variations in good occlusions, *Angle Orthod* 41:64-68, 1971.
16. Zachrisson BU: Buccal uprighting of canines and premolars for improved smile esthetics and stability, *World J Orthod* 7:406-412, 2006.
17. Spear FM, Kokich VG, Mathews DP: Interdisciplinary management of anterior dental esthetics, *J Am Dent Assoc* 137:160-169, 2006.
18. Rationale for lower anterior veneers, *CRA Foundation Newslett* 30(issue 6):1, 2006.
19. Lindauer SJ, Lewis SM, Shroff B: Overbite correction and smile aesthetics, *Semin Orthod* 11:62-66, 2005.
20. Zachrisson BU: Esthetic factors involved in anterior tooth display and the smile: vertical dimension, *J Clin Orthod* 32:432-445, 1998.

21. Zachrisson BU: Facial esthetics: guide to tooth positioning and maxillary incisor display, *World J Orthod* 8:308-314, 2007.
22. Vig RG, Brundo GC: The kinetics of anterior tooth display, *J Prosthet Dent* 39:502-504, 1978.
23. Dong JK, Jin TH, Cho HW, Oh SC: The esthetics of the smile: a review of some recent studies, *Int J Prosthdont* 12:9-19, 1999.
24. Peck S, Peck L, Kataya M: Some vertical lineaments of lip position, *Am J Orthod Dentofacial Orthop* 101:519-524, 1992.
25. Al Qabandi A, Sadowsky C, Sellke T: A comparison of continuous archwire and utility archwires for leveling the curve of Spee, *World J Orthod* 3:159-165, 2002.
26. Burstone CJ: Lip posture and its significance in treatment planning, *Am J Orthod* 53:262-284, 1967.
27. Burstone CJ, Nanda R: JCO interviews Charles J. Burstone, DDS, MS. Part 1. Facial esthetics, *J Clin Orthod* 41:79-87, 2007.
28. Shroff B, Yoon WM, Lindauer SJ, Burstone CJ: Simultaneous intrusion and retraction using a three-piece base arch, *Angle Orthod* 67:455-462, 1997.
29. Zachrisson BU: Mechanical intrusion of maxillary incisors: a treatment strategy to be abandoned? *World J Orthod* 3:358-364, 2002.
30. Weiland FJ, Bantleon HP, Droschl H: Evaluation of continuous arch and segmented arch leveling techniques in adult patients: a clinical study, *Am J Orthod Dentofacial Orthop* 110:647-652, 1996.
31. Simons ME, Joondeph DR: Change in overbite: a ten-year postretention study, *Am J Orthod* 64:349-367, 1973.
32. Zachrisson BU: Clinical use of custom-made transpalatal arches: why and how, *World J Orthod* 5:260-267, 2004.
33. Liu D, Melsen B: Reappraisal of Class II molar relationships diagnosed from the lingual aspect, *Eur J Orthod* 23:457, 2001.
34. Ten Hoeve A: Palatal bar and lip bumper in nonextraction treatment, *J Clin Orthod* 19:272-291, 1985.
35. Gündüz E, Zachrisson BU, Hönigl KD, et al: An improved transpalatal bar design. Part I. Comparison of moments and forces delivered by two bar designs for symmetrical molar derotation, *Angle Orthod* 73:239-243, 2003.
36. Gündüz E, Crismani AG, Zachrisson BU, et al: An improved transpalatal bar design. Part II. Clinical upper molar derotation: case report, *Angle Orthod* 73:244-248, 2003.
37. DeBerardinis M, Stretesky T, Sinha P, Nanda RS: Evaluation of the vertical holding appliance in treatment of high-angle patients, *Am J Orthod Dentofacial Orthop* 117:700-705, 2000.
38. Wise JB, Magness WB, Powers JM: Maxillary molar vertical control with the use of transpalatal arches, *Am J Orthod Dentofacial Orthop* 106:403-408, 1994.
39. Hata M: Effect on the dentofacial complex of *Macaca irus* of functional tongue forces imparted on a palatal bar, *J Osaka Dent Univ* 27:51-66, 1993.
40. Yamawaki H, Kawamoto T: Effect of palatal bar on maxillary molars during swallowing, *Shika Igaku J Osaka Odontol Soc* 59:53-63, 1996.
41. Chiba Y, Motoyoshi M, Namura S: Tongue pressure on loop of transpalatal arch during deglutition, *Am J Orthod Dentofacial Orthop* 123:29-34, 2003.
42. Dahlquist A, Gebauer U, Ingervall B: The effect of a transpalatal arch for the correction of first molar rotation, *Eur J Orthod* 18:257-267, 1996.
43. Fotis V, Melsen B, Williams S, Droschl H: Vertical control as an important ingredient in the treatment of severe sagittal discrepancies, *Am J Orthod* 86:224-232, 1984.
44. Sinclair PM, Little RM: Dentofacial maturation of untreated normals, *Am J Orthod* 88:146-156, 1985.
45. Zachrisson BU, Büyükyilmaz T: Bonding in orthodontics. In Graber TM, Vanarsdall RL Jr, Vig KWL, editors: *Orthodontics: current principles and techniques,* ed 4, St Louis, 2005, Elsevier, pp 579-659.
46. Wong P, Freer TJ: Patients' attitudes towards compliance with retainer wear, *Aust Orthod J* 21:45-53, 2005.
47. Zachrisson BU: Differential retention with bonded retainers, *World J Orthod* 8:190-196, 2007.
48. Behrents RG: *The consequences of adult craniofacial growth,* monograph 22, Craniofacial Growth Series, Ann Arbor, 1989, Center for Human Growth and Development, University of Michigan.
49. Gorman JC, Smith RJ: Comparison of treatment effects with labial and lingual fixed appliances, *Am J Orthod Dentofacial Orthop* 99:202-209, 1991.
50. Sadowsky C, Schneider BJ, BeGole EA, et al: Long-term stability after orthodontic treatment: nonextraction with prolonged retention, *Am J Orthod Dentofacial Orthop* 106:243-249, 1994.
51. Iseri H, Solow B: Continued eruption of maxillary incisors and first molars in girls from 9 to 25 years studied by the implant method, *Eur J Orthod* 18:245-256, 1996.
52. Tallgren A: Changes in adult face height due to ageing, wear and loss of teeth and prosthetic treatment: a roentgen cephalometric study mainly on Finnish women, thesis, Finland, 1957, University of Helsinki.

PART II

Clinical Management of Sagittal and Vertical Discrepancies

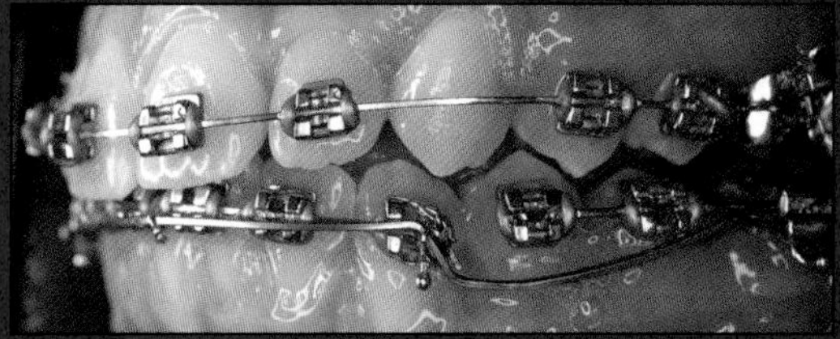

CHAPTER 9

Functional Treatment Objectives

William J. Clark

The rate of technological change in contemporary society is accelerating, and orthodontics is not exempt from this process. After a century of inconclusive evidence, the question of whether craniofacial growth can be modified by functional orthopedic techniques remains unresolved. A new paradigm for successful treatment presents a philosophical challenge: to combine the benefits of orthodontic and orthopedic techniques in the treatment of malocclusions that require a combination of dental and skeletal correction.

ORTHODONTICS AND DENTOFACIAL ORTHOPEDICS

What ambitions do orthodontists hold for the future? As implied by the definition of "orthodontics," are they satisfied simply to produce "straight teeth" within the strict confines of a genetic paradigm? Is there a scope for significant improvements in conventional orthodontic techniques, or has this aspect of orthodontic development been exhausted? Precision orthodontic techniques with conventional fixed appliances have simplified orthodontic correction and are frequently delegated to auxiliaries under supervision. If treatment objectives are confined to orthodontics, will specialists still be needed?

An essential distinction exists between the terms *orthodontics* and *dental orthopedics,* which vary fundamentally in their approach to the correction of dentofacial abnormalities. By definition, "orthodontic" treatment aims to correct dental irregularity. The alternative term "dental orthopaedics" was suggested by the late Sir Norman Bennett, and although it has a wider definition than "orthodontics," it still does not convey the objective of improving facial development. The broader description of *dentofacial orthopedics* conveys the concept that treatment aims to improve not only dental and orthopedic relationships in the stomatognathic system, but also facial balance. The adoption of a wider definition has the advantage of extending the horizons of the profession, as well as educating the public to appreciate the benefits of dentofacial therapy in more comprehensive esthetic terms.

Abnormal musculoskeletal development is frequently the cause of dental malocclusion. The treatment objective in the growing child with a resultant skeletal discrepancy changes from an *orthodontic* approach, aiming to correct the dental irregularity, to an *orthopedic* approach, where the objective is to correct the underlying skeletal abnormality. This difference in emphasis reflects the existence of two distinct schools of thought in evaluating the aims of orthodontic and dental orthopedic treatment.

After a century of investigating functional orthopedic techniques, opinions still vary regarding their effectiveness in promoting or modifying dentofacial growth and development. In the evolution of orthodontic technique, geographical location has been a significant factor. Functional orthopedic techniques were developed mainly in Europe during the twentieth century, and in the past, Europeans had greater experience with these techniques than their colleagues around the world. In many countries, fixed-appliance techniques have been the basis of orthodontic training programs, often with limited exposure to the teachings and practice of orthopedics, depending on the prevailing philosophy of treatment.

The orthopedic response to functional therapy has frequently been questioned on the basis of results published in the literature. The majority of studies during the twentieth century relate to part-time wear of functional appliances. Inevitably, there is a time lag between the development of

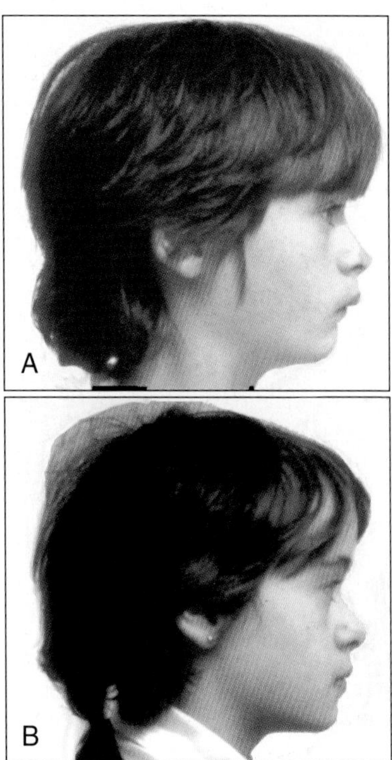

Fig. 9-1 **A,** Pretreatment, and **B,** posttreatment, photographs show the dramatic facial change that can be achieved after 6 months of treatment with a functional appliance. Treatment of severe Class II malocclusion is much more effective with an efficient functional appliance than with a conventional fixed appliance.

new clinical techniques and their acceptance by scientific investigation. *Evidence-based research* largely depends on statistical analysis of existing techniques and does not take into account future developments. However, this should not limit the ability to explore new horizons in orthodontics and dentofacial orthopedics.

Significantly, the title of the *American Journal of Orthodontics* was revised in 1985 to include dentofacial orthopedics. Its current title is the *American Journal of Orthodontics and Dentofacial Orthopedics* (AJODO). The American Dental Association (ADA) adopted the new name and definition for the specialty of "orthodontics and dentofacial orthopedics" in April 2003. These visionary changes can be attributed mainly to the efforts of Thomas M. Graber (mentor and former editor of AJODO) in recognizing the importance of dentofacial orthopedics as a means of correcting musculoskeletal discrepancies by functional orthopedic techniques. This represents the first official recognition within the specialty, and in the dental profession as a whole, of the importance of orthopedics in the field of orthodontics.

CONCEPT OF FUNCTIONAL THERAPY

The challenge of functional therapy is to maximize the genetic potential of growth of the individual and guide the growing face and developing dentition toward a pattern of optimal development (Fig. 9-1).

Review of Treatment Objectives

New research is providing convincing evidence to support the value of orthopedic techniques using full-time appliances to influence the functional environment of the developing dentition and to produce significant improvements in the pattern of facial growth and dental arch development.

The new challenge in the specialty is to improve orthopedic techniques in the treatment of skeletal and functional discrepancies and to relate this treatment to the holistic functional treatment objectives. It is essential to recognize the importance of using orthopedic techniques to achieve facial balance and harmony and to extend esthetic and functional objectives beyond a balanced functional occlusion.

Distraction osteogenesis illustrates the potential for modifying bone growth, and fixed functional techniques offer a new opportunity for noninvasive, osteogenic stimulation.

The next step in the evolution of orthopedic techniques is to resolve any remaining doubts regarding the efficacy of an orthopedic approach and to improve techniques in order to combine the benefits of orthodontic and orthopedic treatment.

Recent Research in Growth Modification

Do functional appliances produce supplementary growth of the mandible? This question has remained unanswered throughout the last century.

Remodeling of the condyle and the fossa in the temporomandibular joint (TMJ) was originally investigated in animal experiments[1] (Fig. 9-2). The potential for condylar growth and new bone formation in the glenoid fossa to change growth of the fossa to an anterior direction is now established in nonhuman primates. Anterior and inferior remodeling of the glenoid fossa was seen in a reverse direction compared with controls.[2,3] A study of juvenile *Macaca fascicularis* monkeys with Herbst treatment concluded the following:

- Increased condylar growth can be demonstrated cephalometrically with the Björk implant method and confirmed histologically.
- "The potential for condylar growth in juvenile non primates in the mixed dentition to induce increased mandibular length appears to be great."
- Histomorphometric analysis shows that the increased amount and area of new bone in the glenoid fossa are statistically significant compared with controls. This formation appears to increase with time.

Clinical Studies

Parallel clinical studies with magnetic resonance imaging (MRI) have since confirmed, first in Herbst treatment[4] and later in twin block therapy,[5,6] that similar clinical growth

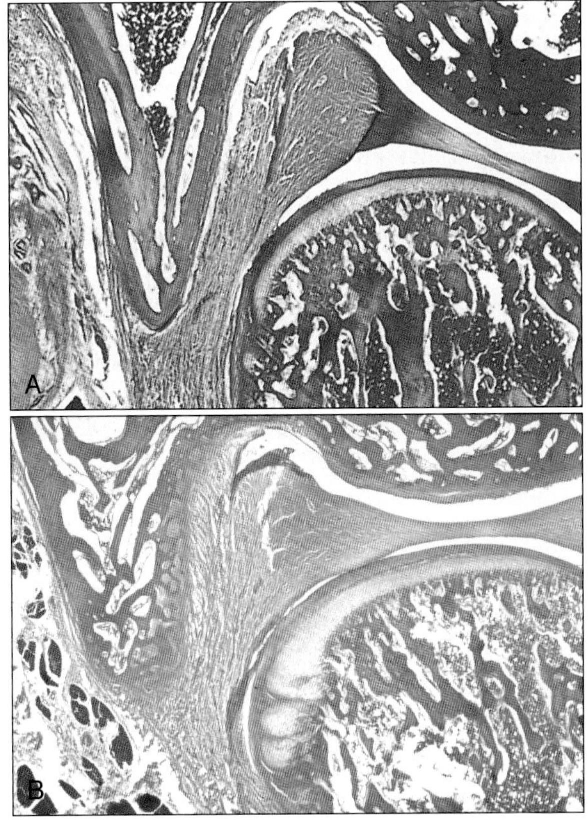

Fig. 9-2 Proliferation of condylar cartilage and bony remodeling in the articular fossa in **A,** experimental animals, compared with **B,** controls. (From Clark WJ: *Twin block functional therapy: applications in dentofacial orthopaedics,* ed 2, Edinburgh, 2002, Mosby Ltd.)

changes occur in response to mandibular propulsion with full-time functional appliances. Growth studies during and after twin block therapy compared matched controls from the Burlington Growth Centre and concluded the following[7,8]:

- Mandibular unit length increases almost three times as much in twin block patients as in controls.
- Approximately two thirds of the increase can be attributed to an increase in mandibular ramus height.
- Much of the skeletal improvement is related to an increase in mandibular length, and these changes largely are stable 3 years after treatment (Fig. 9-3).

An interesting pattern is observed in which the gonial angle frequently increases during the twin block stage of treatment, followed by an increase in corpus length during the posttreatment period. This may be interpreted as a change in condylar growth to a more distal direction during active mandibular propulsion, followed by remodeling of the mandibular ramus posttreatment to restore the original shape of the mandible.

This pattern of distal growth of the condyle is confirmed in a finite element scaling analysis[9] to determine the localiza-

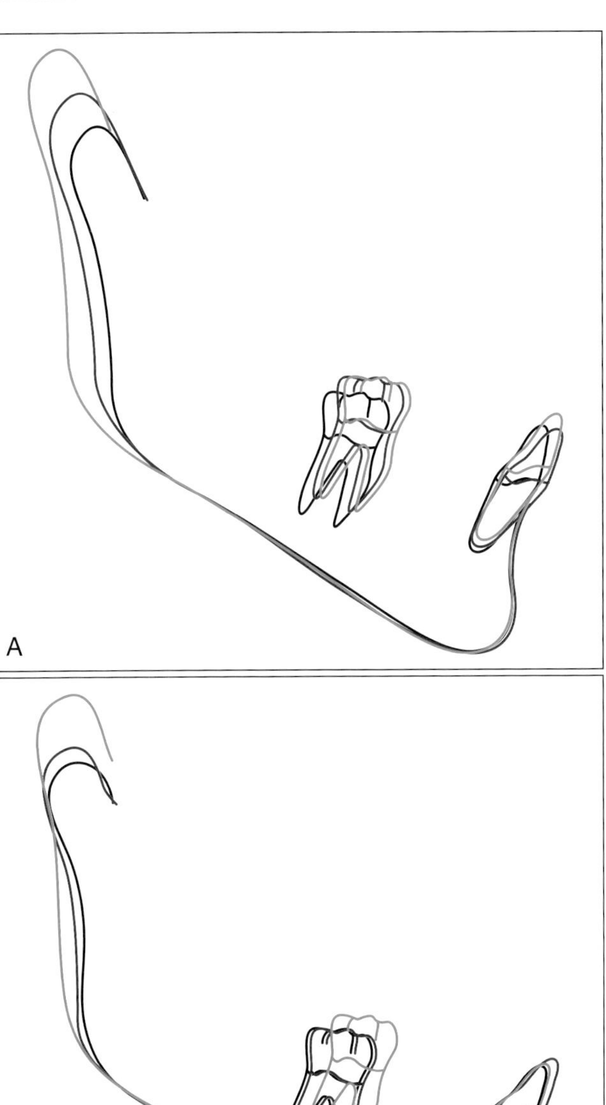

Fig. 9-3 **A,** Twin block treatment. **B,** Controls. *Treatment:* T_1 = 9 years, 1 month; T_2 = 10 years, 3 months; T_3 = 13 years, 1 month. *Control:* T_1 = 9 years, 1 month; T_2 = 10 years, 2 months; T_3 = 12 years, 11 months. This illustrates an important difference in response between twin block treatment and controls. In addition to extension of condylar length, the twin block sample clearly shows distal growth of the condyle compared to vertical growth in the controls. A change in direction of growth of the condyle contributes to forward positioning of the mandible in correction of mandibular retrusion. (From Clark WJ: *Twin block functional therapy: applications in dentofacial orthopaedics,* ed 2, Edinburgh, 2002, Mosby Ltd.)

tion of mandibular changes in patients treated by the author with the twin block appliance. In all four groups of prepubertal and postpubertal boys and girls, the distal area of the neck of the condyle showed the most significant growth changes. This may be interpreted as remodeling of the neck of the condyle as a result of lengthening or distal growth of the condyle.

A prospective study of twin block appliance therapy assessed by MRI in the University of Adelaide[5,6] confirmed the following:

- Condyles that were positioned at the crest of the eminence at the beginning of treatment had reseated back into the glenoid fossa after 6 months.

The clinical implication of this finding is that active functional therapy by forward mandibular propulsion should continue for a minimum of 6 months or preferably 9 months. This ensures that treatment continues for a sufficient time to allow adaptive skeletal growth changes to occur, and that these changes are reinforced before the functional appliance is removed. In addition, the author advises that functional therapy should be followed by a period of functional retention, with the mandible supported in a forward position, perhaps with a nighttime functional appliance. This protocol is successful in preventing "mandibular setback," which has been previously reported after functional treatment to advance the mandible.

Biological Research

Biological research is making rapid progress in identifying the controlling factors in growth modification. The landmark article "Functional appliance therapy accelerates and enhances condylar growth"[10] is not the optimistic evaluation of an enthusiastic clinician. Rather, it represents a revolution in scientific research techniques at the cellular and molecular level to examine and define the chemical and biological factors involved in growth modification.

Replicating mesenchymal cells have been identified in the condyle and glenoid fossa during mandibular forward positioning.[11] Scientific study confirms the importance of the genetic control factor. Patients with a high mesenchymal cell count would respond well to functional mandibular advancement, whereas a low cell count would produce a poor mandibular growth response.

In the future, the mesenchymal cell count from a blood sample may define a patient's potential to respond to functional mandibular advancement. Clinicians may be able to predict the individual patient's response to functional therapy with information from a blood test or salivary smear. Biological research can answer the questions that statistical studies have failed to resolve.

RESPONSE TO FUNCTIONAL THERAPY

It is universally accepted that genetic factors are of prime importance in determining an individual's response to functional therapy. This explains the variation in growth response in patients treated at different stages in the growth cycle.

Timing of Treatment

The best mandibular growth response is achieved when patients are treated during or slightly after the onset of the pubertal growth spurt. The optimum time to gain advantage is during a period of rapid growth. The timing of treatment is important, especially with a severe Class II skeletal discrepancy where the objective is to maximize the mandibular growth response using the proprioceptive stimulus of functional mandibular protrusion.

Investigations of treatment timing for twin block therapy[12] concluded that treatment in the late mixed-dentition phase or the early permanent-dentition phase produces more favorable effects, such as the following:

- Greater skeletal contribution to molar correction
- Large increments in mandibular length and ramus height
- More posterior direction of condylar growth

Following earlier research in this field, a skeletal maturation evaluation using the stages of cervical vertebrae development is recommended to determine the optimum timing to commence treatment[13-15] (Fig. 9-4).

DIAGNOSIS AND TREATMENT PLANNING

Photographic Records

In planning functional therapy to correct a mandibular retrusion, facial and dental photographs are an invaluable diagnostic aid to establish the objectives of treatment and to monitor progress. Photographs are used to predict the changes in facial appearance that will result from treatment. Profile and full-face photographs with the mandible in the retrusive position show the pretreatment appearance and are repeated with the mandible advanced to show the projected improvement in facial appearance (Fig 9-5).

An additional set of digital photographs improves motivation by showing the patient a preview of the end result. The patient is able to observe the rapid improvement in appearance experienced during the first few months of treatment.

Clinical Examination

Clinical examination provides a simple guideline in case selection for functional therapy in the treatment of Class II malocclusion. A retrusive mandible can be detected by examining the profile and the facial contours with the teeth in occlusion. The patient is instructed to close the incisors in a normal relationship by protruding the mandible, with the lips closed *lightly* together. The change in facial appearance is a preview of the anticipated result of functional treatment. If

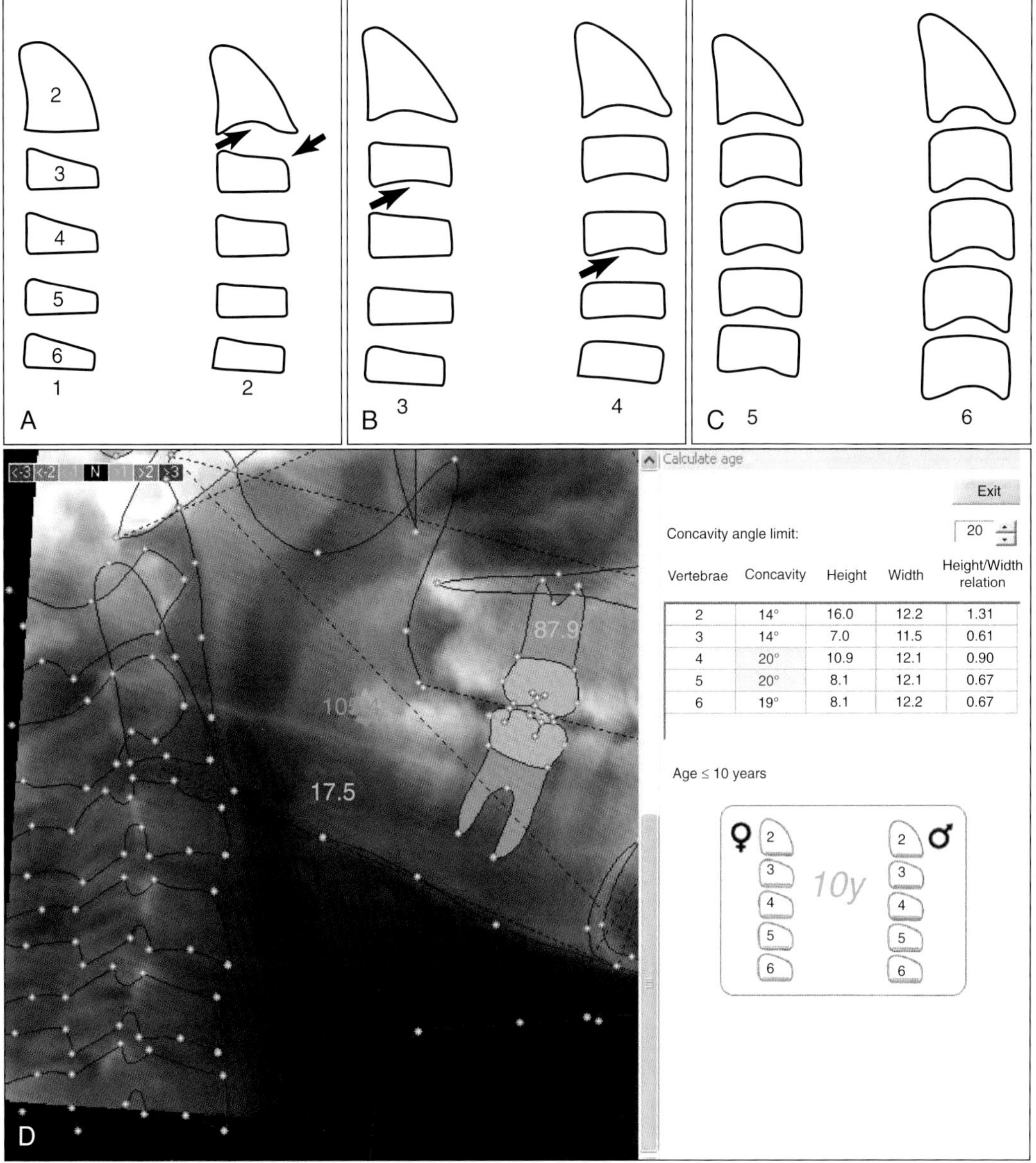

Vertebrae	Concavity	Height	Width	Height/Width relation
2	14°	16.0	12.2	1.31
3	14°	7.0	11.5	0.61
4	20°	10.9	12.1	0.90
5	20°	8.1	12.1	0.67
6	19°	8.1	12.2	0.67

Fig. 9-4 Developmental stages of cervical vertebrae. **A,** Prepubertal stages 1 and 2. *1,* Inferior borders of the bodies of all cervical vertebrae are flat. Superior borders are tapered from posterior to anterior. *2,* A concavity develops in the inferior border of the second vertebra. The anterior vertical height of the bodies increases. **B,** Pubertal peak stages 3 and 4. *3,* A concavity develops in the inferior border of the third vertebra. *4,* A concavity develops in the inferior border of the fourth vertebra. Concavities begin to form in the lower borders of the fifth and sixth vertebrae. The bodies of all cervical vertebrae are rectangular in shape. **C,** Postpubertal peak stages 5 and 6. *5,* Concavities are well defined in the lower borders of all six cervical vertebrae. The bodies are almost square, and spaces between the bodies are reduced. *6,* All concavities have deepened. The bodies are now higher than they are wide. **D,** Nemoceph Cervical Vertebrae Development Software Program. Cervical vertebrae are digitized to determine the age-related stage of development. (**A** to **C** modified from Franchi L, Baccetti T, McNamara JA Jr: *Am J Orthod Dentofacial Orthop* 18:335, 2000.)

the profile improves with the mandible advanced, this is a clear indication that functional mandibular advancement is the treatment of choice. If the profile does *not* improve by advancing the mandible and closing the lips, this is a *contra-indication* for mandibular advancement (see Fig. 9-5).

What you see is what you get

Clinical diagnosis has the advantage of providing an accurate prediction of the three-dimensional change in the facial contours as a result of mandibular advancement and is more important than lines and angles drawn on a cephalometric

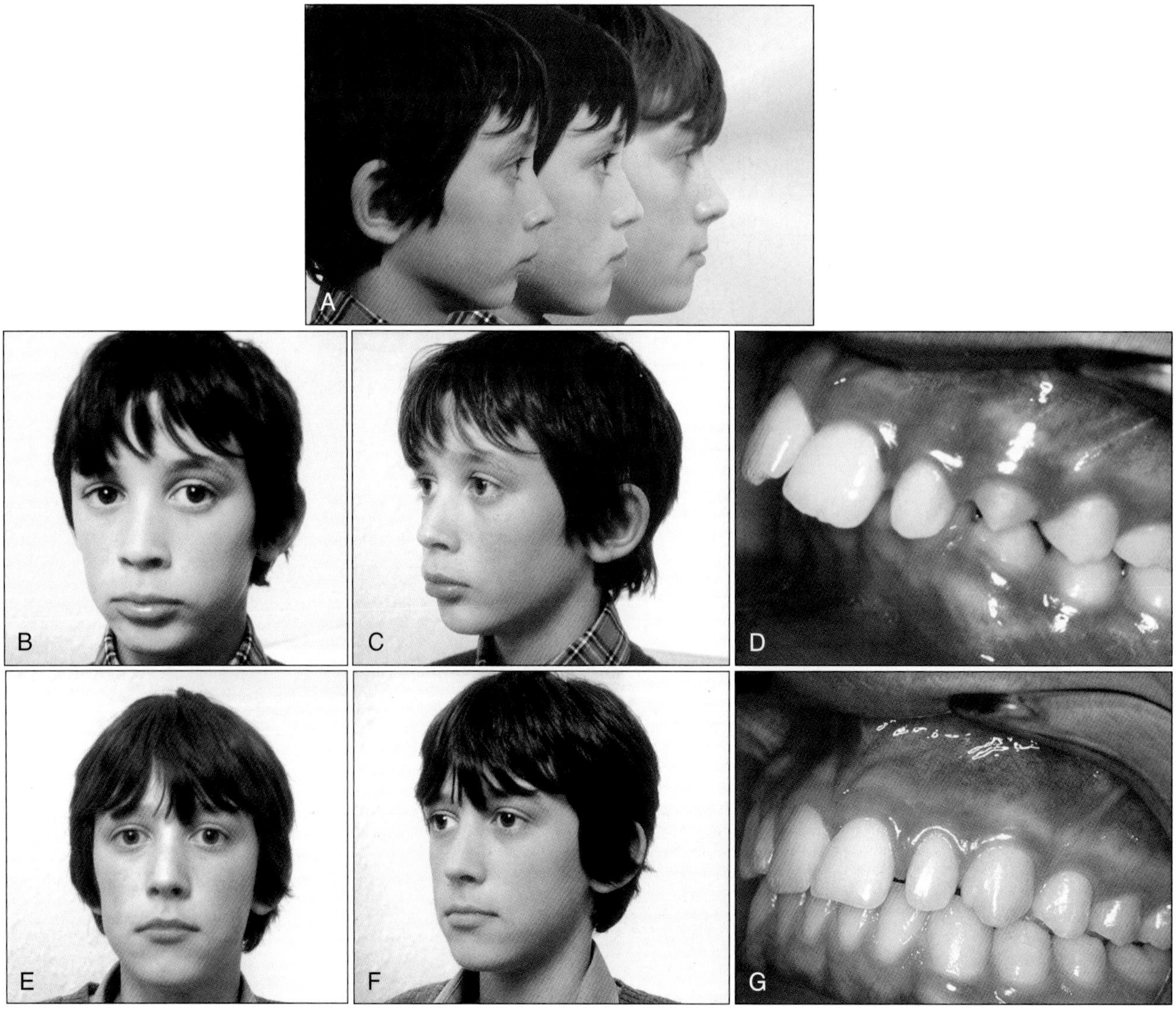

A

B

C

D

E

F

G

Fig. 9-5 Clinical examination provides the fundamental guideline in case selection for functional therapy. A retrusive mandible can be detected by examining the profile and the facial contours with teeth in occlusion. The patient then closes the incisors in normal relationship by protruding the mandible with lips closed. **A,** Left profile of this patient (age 14 years, 2 months) shows a retrusive mandible before treatment. Middle profile (also taken before treatment) with the mandible protruded to bring the incisors into the normal relationship, showing a preview of the anticipated response to functional mandibular advancement. Right profile (age 15 years, 1 month) confirms that appearance after treatment is very close to the predicted result. **B** and **C,** Facial views, and **D,** occlusion, before treatment. **E** and **F,** Facial appearance, and **G,** occlusion, after treatment, showing the change in appearance. (From Clark WJ: *Twin block functional therapy: applications in dentofacial orthopaedics,* ed 2, Edinburgh, 2002, Mosby Ltd.)

x-ray film. This does not negate or diminish the value of cephalometric analysis, but rather adds a three-dimensional view to support and confirm the diagnosis.

FUNCTIONAL TREATMENT OBJECTIVE

Photographic and cephalometric records are used to prepare a *functional treatment objective* (FTO), with less reliance on mean population growth increments. The *visual treatment objective* (VTO) is also used for orthodontic treatment planning. Similarly, a *surgical treatment objective* (STO) provides useful information for maxillofacial surgical procedures; no such program is yet available for planning functional treatment.

In collaboration with Nemotec, the author has developed a new software program to prepare a customized FTO to predict the result of treatment of Class II malocclusion by functional mandibular advancement.

Method

Profile photographs are taken before treatment, first with the mandible retruded, then with the mandible advanced to correct the overjet, with the lips closed together. Pretreatment photographs show an accurate prediction of the change in facial appearance on completion of functional therapy.

Photographic and cephalometric records can be used to estimate the anticipated response to functional mandibular advancement. The technique is similar to that used to prepare an STO by *morphing* techniques. The FTO provides an individual prediction based on the patient's postured position rather than relying entirely on morphing or mean growth values.

A tracing is prepared on a pretreatment cephalogram with the mandible in occlusion in the retruded position. The tracing is superimposed, first on the profile photograph with the mandible retruded, then on the protrusive profile photograph. The soft tissue outline on the postured photograph is used as a template to determine the change in position of the mandible, using the thickness of the soft tissues as a guide to estimate the corrected mandibular position. In addition, the incisor relationship and overjet correction are taken into account to anticipate the change in mandibular position. Allowance may also be made for dental movements, as employed in preparing a VTO.

The period of treatment with full-time functional appliances is typically 6 to 9 months to correct a distal occlusion. The need to refer to mean growth values is reduced in arriving at an estimate of the corrected mandibular position after functional therapy.

Case Reports

The following case reports illustrate a typical response to full-time functional therapy with twin block appliances followed by fixed-appliance therapy to detail the occlusion. The patients in cases #1 to #4 were treated by Dr. Forbes Leishman in his orthodontic practice in Aukland, New Zealand. Before settling in New Zealand, Dr. Leishman attended the first twin block course the author offered in his orthodontic practice in Scotland in 1979. An experienced clinician in twin block therapy, Leishman's protocol for the treatment of severe Class II, Division I malocclusion is to correct the Class II skeletal relationship first with twin blocks before completing treatment with fixed appliances. Cases #5, #6, and #7 were treated by the author.

Case #1 (Fig. 9-6)

A male patient age 12 years, 8 months has a severe dental Class II malocclusion with buccal occlusion of all the upper premolars, in addition to a 12-mm overjet and excessive overbite. Vertical collapse has occurred in this malocclusion because of the premolar crossbite. Although a convexity of 2 mm is within the range of "normal," this malocclusion requires careful management in view of the severity of the dental malocclusion.

Vertical control is important to encourage an increase in ramus height and eruption of the posterior teeth to offer vertical support. A combined orthopedic and orthodontic approach advances the mandible and simplifies the finishing phase with fixed appliances.

Excellent stability and improved facial esthetics were achieved; final records show the position out of retention at age 18 years, 1 month (3 years after treatment). Condylar extension and distal growth of the condyle improved facial appearance and resulted in a stable occlusal correction.

Period of treatment

Twin blocks	11 months
Bite plane	3 months
Fixed appliances	10 months
TOTAL	2 years, followed by retention

Case #2 (Fig. 9-7)

A female patient age 11 years, 5 months has a severe malocclusion treated in the early permanent-dentition phase (when surgery might have been considered as a possible solution). Altered incisal angulations contribute to an overjet of 15 mm and excessive overbite, with the lower incisors 4 mm lingual to the A-Po line. The large overjet can be partly attributed to unfavorable lip posture, because a severely trapped lower lip accentuates the problem.

A brachyfacial growth pattern and 8-mm convexity result mainly from mandibular retrusion, and at this age the potential for correction with the assistance of growth is favorable. The convexity is reduced to 3 mm with a fully corrected occlusion, and the improvement is maintained 3 years after completion of treatment.

This patient's improved facial appearance is the result of significant condylar extension and a change in the direction of condylar growth, resulting in forward positioning of the mandible. The gonial angle increases during the twin block phase as a result of accelerated distal growth of the condyle, and the corpus length increases in the posttreatment period.

Period of treatment

Twin blocks	9 months
Bite plane	5 months
Fixed appliances	12 months
TOTAL	2 years, 2 months, followed by retention

Case #3 (Fig. 9-8)

This female patient, at age 14 years, 9 months, was a "late starter" when twin blocks were fitted. (A clinician might consider surgery to assist correction in a girl who is past the pubertal growth phase and whose growth is virtually complete, especially when the pretreatment profile is poor.) The convexity of 5 mm results from maxillary protrusion because the mandible is well developed and exhibits typical brachyfacial growth. This gives the appearance of overclosure, resulting from reduced lower facial height. The upper incisors are severely proclined, with the lower lip trapped in an overjet of 13 mm. The lower incisors are retroclined, biting into the palate with an excessive overbite, and are positioned

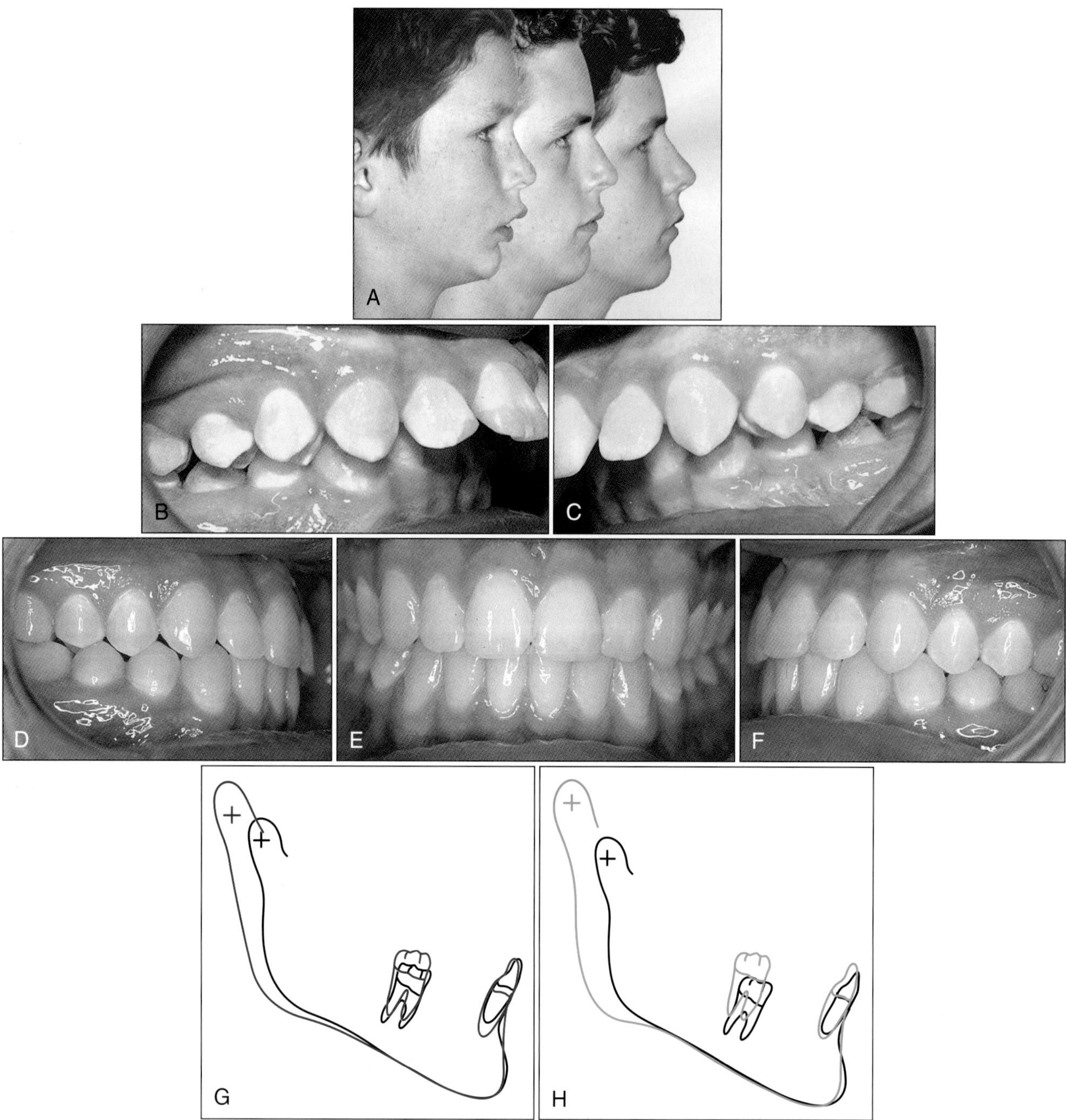

Fig. 9-6 Case #1. **A,** Treatment progress of severe Class II malocclusion with buccal occlusion of upper premolars, 12-mm overjet, and excessive overbite. Profiles at ages 12 years, 8 months (before treatment); 14 years, 8 months (after treatment); and 16 years, 6 months (out of retention). **B** and **C,** Occlusion before treatment. **D** to **F,** Occlusion after treatment. **G** and **H,** Mandibular superimpositions. Patient showed excellent mandibular response, with condylar extension and distal condylar growth. (Courtesy Dr. Forbes Leishman, Aukland, New Zealand. From Clark WJ: *Twin block functional therapy: applications in dentofacial orthopaedics,* ed 2, Edinburgh, 2002, Mosby Ltd.)

3 mm lingual to the A-Po line as a result of lower alveolar retrusion.

In this type of malocclusion the vertical correction is as important as sagittal correction. The profile improves with anterior repositioning of the mandible and adjustment of the blocks to allow vertical development of lower molars. The final orthodontic phase repositions the lower incisors in correct relationship to the anterior limit of the skeletal base (within range of +1 to +3 to A-Po line) to improve the contour of the lower lip. Final records show the position out of retention at age 20 years, 2 months.

The mandibular response in this patient may be more typical of a patient who is beyond the pubertal growth spurt. This is an example of forward positioning of the mandible

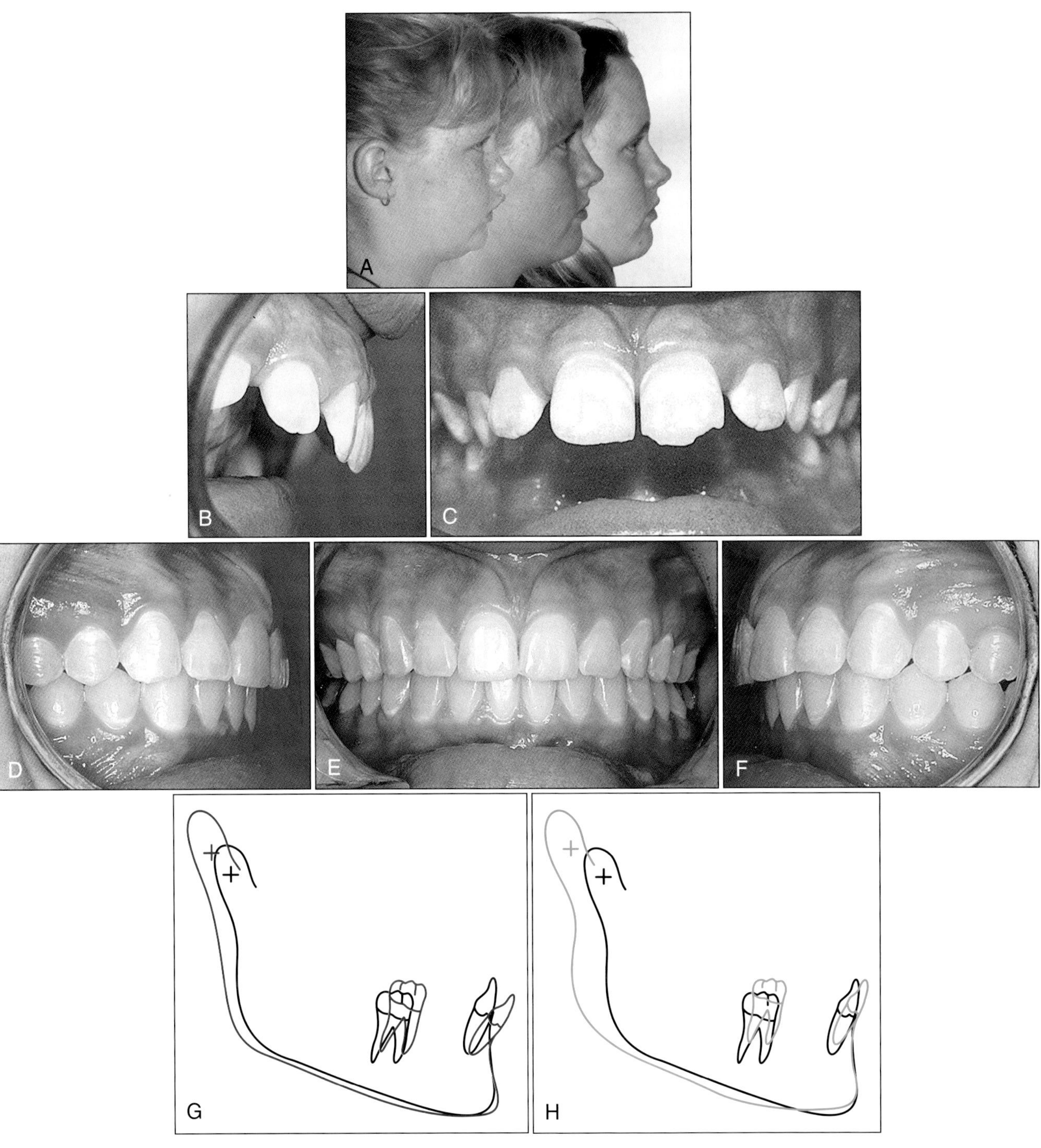

Fig. 9-7 Case #2. **A,** Treatment progress of severe malocclusion treated in early permanent dentition. Profiles at ages 11 years, 5 months (before treatment); 13 years, 9 months (after treatment); and 17 years (out of retention). **B** and **C,** Occlusion before treatment. **D** to **F,** Occlusion out of retention. **G** and **H,** Mandibular superimpositions. Patient showed excellent mandibular response, with condylar extension and distal condylar growth. (Courtesy Dr. Forbes Leishman, Aukland, New Zealand. From Clark WJ: *Twin block functional therapy: applications in dentofacial orthopaedics,* ed 2, Edinburgh, 2002, Mosby Ltd.)

caused by an alteration in the angle of condylar growth. Mandibular superimposition shows that the condyle has grown distally. This is confirmed by an increase in the gonial angle, and in this case this pattern is maintained out of retention.

It is important to appreciate that the facial appearance may improve considerably without significant extension of mandibular length. Distal growth of the condyle increases the effective length of the mandible and positions the mandible forward, although the mandibular

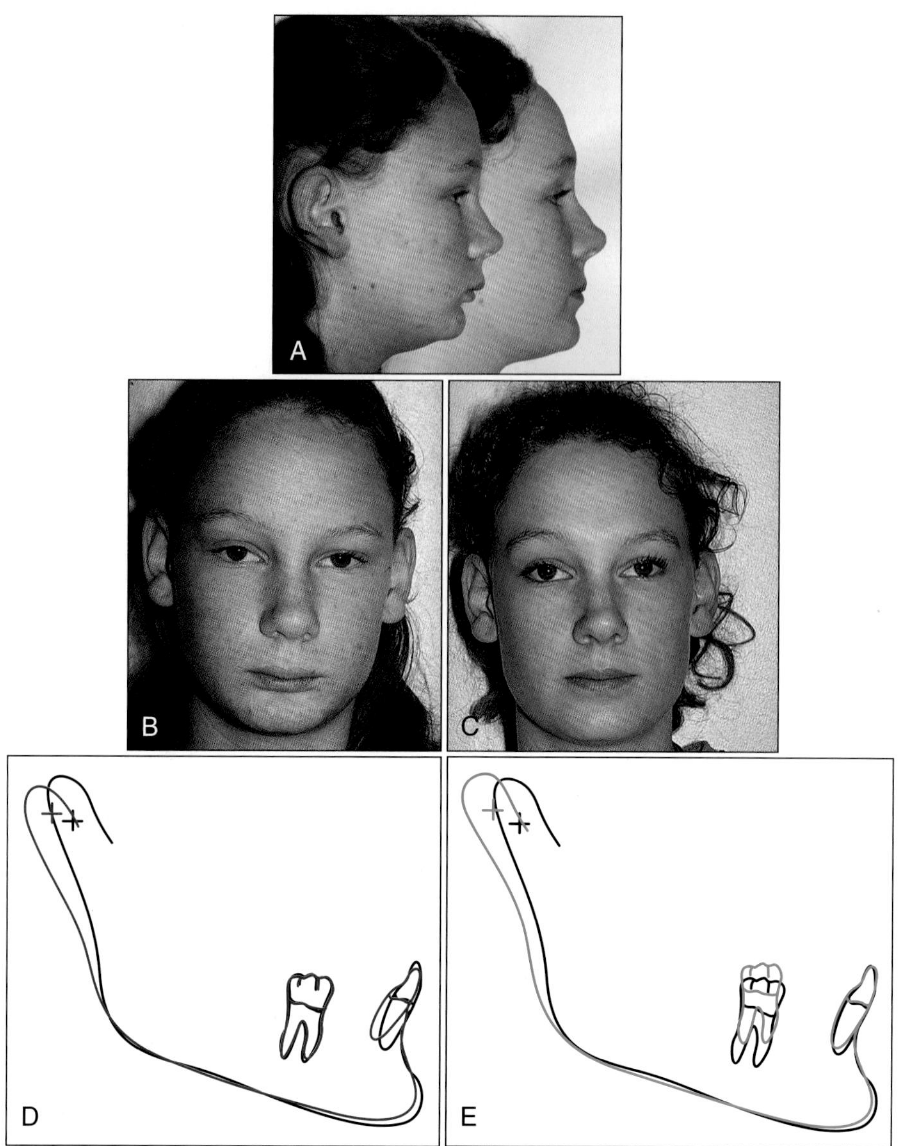

Fig. 9-8 Case #3. **A,** Treatment progress of patient who was a "late starter." Profiles at ages 14 years, 9 months (before treatment) and 20 years, 2 months (out of retention). Facial appearance before (**B**) and after (**C**) treatment. **D** and **E,** Mandibular superimpositions. Patient was treated later, beyond pubertal growth spurt, when growth in girls is slow. Improved facial appearance results from significant distal condylar growth, as confirmed by an increase in the gonial angle, without significant condylar extension. This case demonstrates that a change in the direction of condylar growth can contribute to correction of mandibular retrusion by forward repositioning of the mandible. (Courtesy Dr. Forbes Leishman, Aukland, New Zealand. From Clark WJ: *Twin block functional therapy: applications in dentofacial orthopaedics,* ed 2, Edinburgh, 2002, Mosby Ltd.)

length shows no significant change. Mandibular length is not the only factor in the forward positioning of the mandible as a result of functional mandibular protrusion.

Period of treatment

Twin blocks	15 months
Bite plane	3 months
Fixed appliances	12 months
TOTAL	2 years, 6 months, followed by retention

Case #4 (Fig. 9-9)
A female patient age 11 years presents with severe maxillary protrusion (main etiologic factor in this case) and a brachyfacial pattern, with a normal mandible and excessive overjet of 14 mm. The convexity of 6 mm results entirely from the maxillary protrusion, as confirmed by an SNA angle of 90 degrees.

This case demonstrates that maxillary protrusion may be treated effectively by mandibular advancement to produce

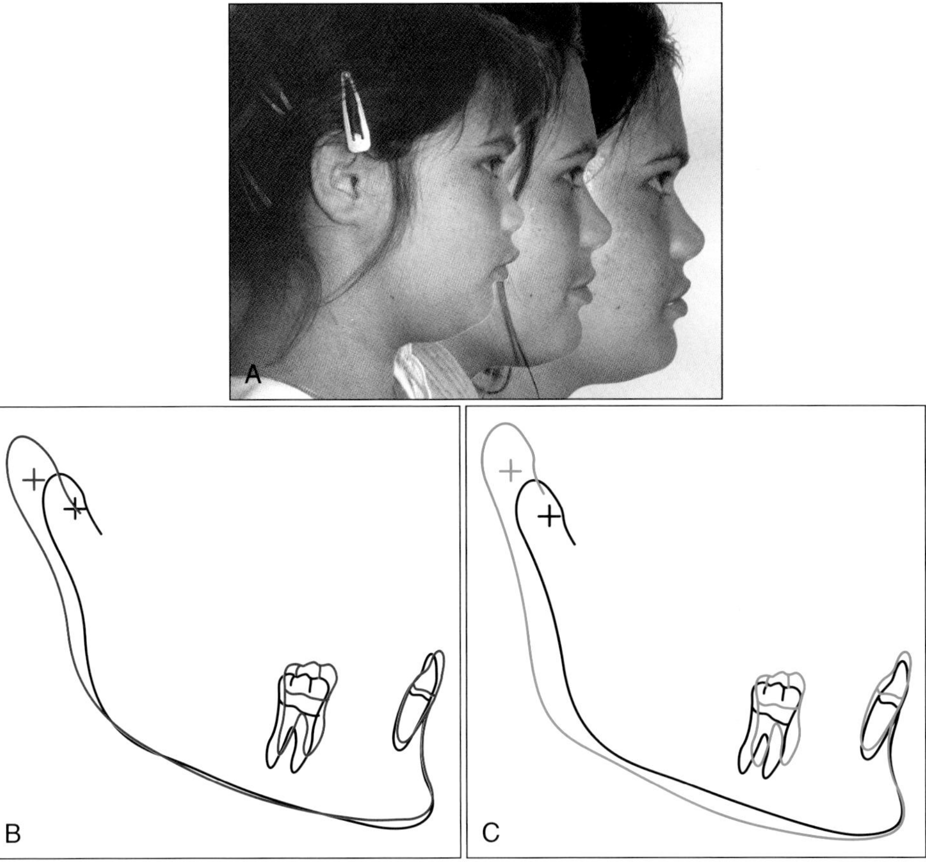

Fig. 9-9 Case #4. **A,** Treatment progress of patient with severe maxillary protrusion. Profiles at ages 11 years (before treatment); 13 years, 10 months (after treatment); and 16 years, 6 months (out of retention). **B** and **C,** Mandibular superimpositions. Patient showed excellent mandibular response, with condylar extension and distal condylar growth. (Courtesy Dr. Forbes Leishman, Aukland, New Zealand. From Clark WJ: *Twin block functional therapy: applications in dentofacial orthopaedics,* ed 2, Edinburgh, 2002, Mosby Ltd.)

an excellently balanced profile and good facial esthetics. It is important to confirm this before treatment by examining the profile with the mandible protruded to register a Class I relationship of the molars. This simple guideline is a preview of the end result and helps to confirm the diagnosis.

Correction is achieved by advancing the mandible to match the protrusive position of the maxilla. This produces a slightly prognathic straight profile with good facial balance and an esthetically pleasing result. The maxillary convexity reduced from 6 to 2 mm after 1 year's treatment, and excellent stability is maintained 3 years after completion of treatment, with a convexity of 1 mm.

This patient's improved facial appearance results from significant condylar extension and a change in the direction of condylar growth. The gonial angle increases during the twin block phase as a result of accelerated distal growth of the condyle. Typically the corpus length increases in the posttreatment period.

Period of treatment

Twin blocks	6 months
Harvold activator as retainer	5 months
Fixed appliances	21 months
TOTAL	2 years, 8 months, followed by retention

Case #5 (Fig. 9-10)

A female patient age 11 years, 4 months presents with a disfiguring Class II, Division 1 malocclusion, with an overjet of 17 mm and an excessive overbite. A combination of maxillary protrusion and mandibular retrusion has resulted in a severe distal occlusion and an equally severe transverse discrepancy, with buccal occlusion of the upper premolars and a traumatic occlusion of the lower incisors in the palate. The malocclusion is further complicated by the congenital absence of the second lower premolar on the left side,

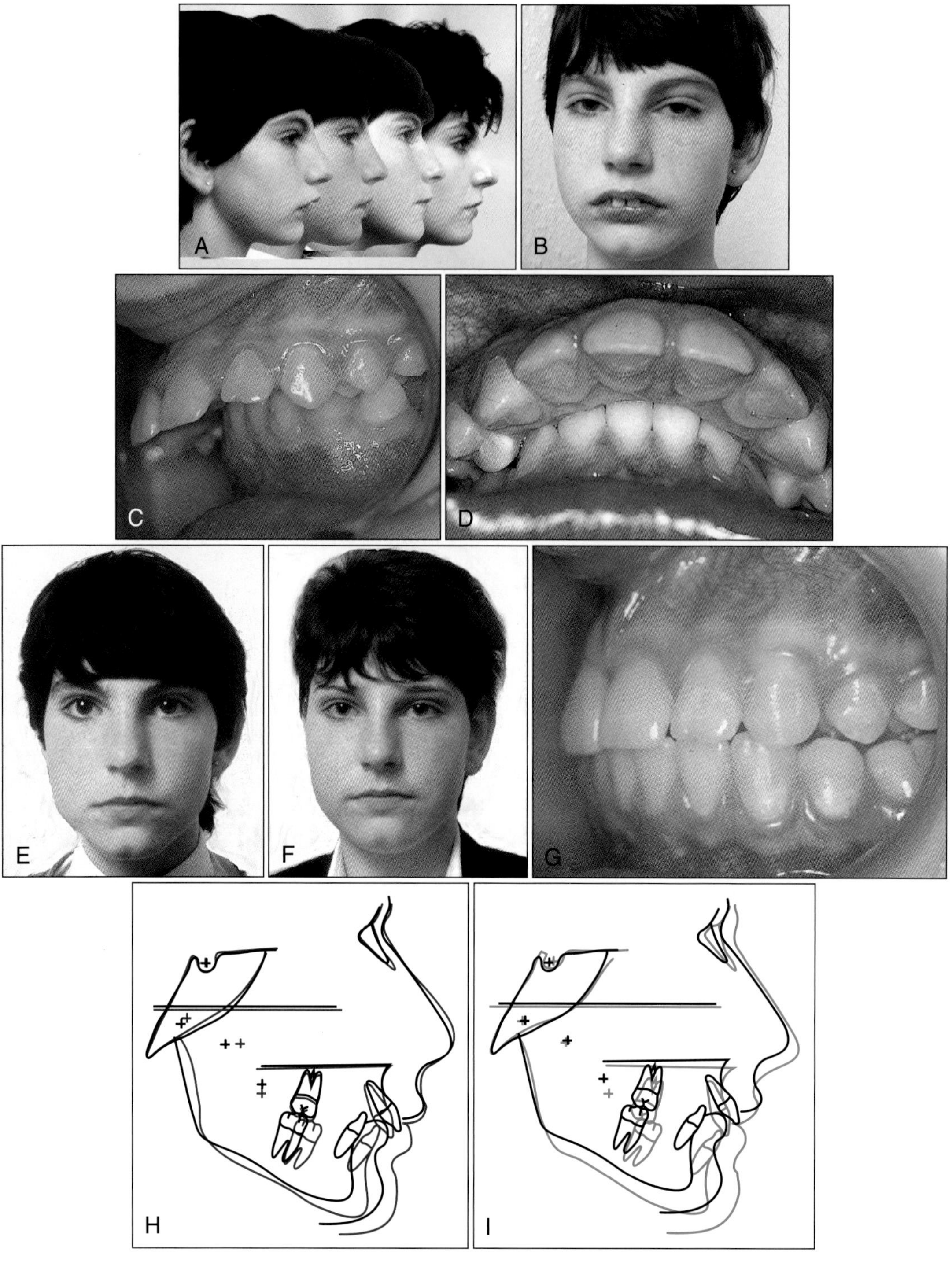

Fig. 9-10 Case #5. **A,** Treatment progress of patient with disfiguring Class II, Division 1 malocclusion with overjet of 17 mm and excessive overbite. Profiles at ages 11 years, 4 months (before treatment); 11 years, 7 months (3 months after treatment); 12 years, 3 months (11 months after treatment); and 18 years, 4 months. Facial appearance (**B**) and occlusion (**C** and **D**) views show a listless appearance, excessive overbite, and large overjet. **E,** Facial appearance at age 11 years, 8 months demonstrates a dramatic change. **F,** Facial appearance at age 12 years, 3 months. **G,** Occlusion at 18 years, 7 months. **H,** Basion superimposition to show changes before and after twin blocks. **I,** Changes consolidated after treatment. This case shows the correction of a severe malocclusion beyond the scope of conventional fixed technique. The rapid facial changes observed cannot be replicated in fixed therapy without mandibular propulsion. (From Clark WJ: *Twin block functional therapy: applications in dentofacial orthopaedics,* ed 2, Edinburgh, 2002, Mosby Ltd.)

resulting in displacement of the lower center line to the left. The dramatic facial and dental changes in this patient illustrate the benefits of a *functional* orthopedic approach to treatment versus a conventional orthodontic approach.

Before treatment, this patient has the typical listless appearance of many persons with severe Class II, Division 1 malocclusion. This has been described as "adenoidal facies" and is evident in the dull appearance of the eyes and poor skin tone. A large overjet with a distal occlusion is frequently associated with a backward tongue position and a restricted airway. These patients cannot breathe properly and, as a result, are subject to allergies and upper respiratory problems from inefficient respiratory function.

After 3 months' treatment the patient underwent a dramatic change in facial appearance that exceeds the parameters of orthodontic treatment in this time scale. The patient appears more alert, and there is a marked improvement in the eyes and complexion. This is a fundamental physiological change, extending beyond the limited objective of "correcting a malocclusion." The upper pharyngeal space increased from 5 mm before treatment to 20 mm after treatment. Increasing the airway achieves the crucially important benefit of improving respiratory function and may influence basal metabolism as a secondary effect. Increased space in the pharyngeal airway is a consistent feature of mandibular advancement with a full-time functional appliance. This is the most significant functional effect of advancing the mandible, as opposed to retracting the maxilla, in the treatment of Class II malocclusion.

Conventional fixed appliances with brackets cannot produce equivalent physiological changes in the treatment of patients with severe malocclusions. A functional approach achieves a rapid improvement in the facial appearance and can be followed by a simplified orthodontic phase of treatment to detail the occlusion.

The facial and intraoral photographs show the treatment progress at 11 months. A composite profile photographs shows the changes in appearance after 3 months, 11 months, and 5 years (see Fig. 9-12).

Period of treatment

Active phase, twin blocks	7 months
Support phase	6 months full-time wear
Orthodontic phase	12 months
TOTAL	2 years, 1 month

Case #6 (Fig. 9-11)

A male patient age 8 years, 9 months presents with disfiguring malocclusion in the early mixed dentition, with the upper incisors extremely vulnerable to trauma, resting completely outside the lower lip. The lower lip is trapped under an overjet of 15 mm. The lower incisors are biting into the soft tissue of the palate 5 mm lingual to the upper incisors. Early treatment is essential in this type of malocclusion to place the upper incisors safely under lip control. Mandibular retrusion accounts for a convexity of 9 mm, as evident in the profile. The maxilla is typically narrow, with a full-unit distal occlusion. The upper pharyngeal airway is severely restricted at 7 mm because of the mandibular retrusion.

Orthopedic correction to a Class I occlusion by twin blocks was followed by retention in the transition to permanent dentition before a second phase of orthodontic treatment with fixed appliances to detail the occlusion. The upper pharyngeal space increased from 7 to 11 mm after 1 year's treatment, then to 14 mm 2 years later, and finally to 21 mm after 6 years.

This case is an example of two-phase treatment with functional correction in mixed dentition, followed by fixed appliances in permanent dentition to detail the occlusion.

Period of treatment

Active phase, twin blocks	14 months
Support phase	9 months full-time wear
Transitional functional retention	2 years
Orthodontic phase	12 months
TOTAL	4 years, 11 months

Case #7 (Fig. 9-12)

A female patient age 11 years, 2 months presents with a severe Class II, Division 1 malocclusion that is complicated by crowding in the lower arch. The position of the lower incisors 4 mm lingual to the A-Po line compensates for the degree of crowding in the lower arch. The facial pattern is brachyfacial and retrognathic with mandibular retrusion. The dental relationship is severe Class II with a full-unit distal occlusion and an overjet of 13 mm and excessive overbite. The left lower canine is excluded from the arch buccally, with a resulting displacement of the lower center line to the left.

An overjet of 10 mm and a full-unit distal occlusion remain after arch development and are corrected with twin blocks. The profile photographs show that a dramatic change in facial balance is evident after only 8 weeks' treatment with twin blocks. After the rapid response the improvement was stable 18 months out of retention at age 14 years, 9 months.

This patient was first treated by arch development to resolve crowding before completing treatment with twin blocks. The composite profile photographs show progress from the start of twin block treatment, treatment after 8 weeks, and results 2 years after treatment. This confirms the rapid facial changes observed in the early stages of treatment.

This case demonstrates arch development before functional therapy and a combination of fixed and functional therapy.

Period of treatment

Arch development	11 months
Twin blocks	7 months
Retention	7 months
TOTAL	2 years, 1 month

CONCLUSION

Functional appliances have been criticized because of an unpredictable response and a lack of long-term influence on

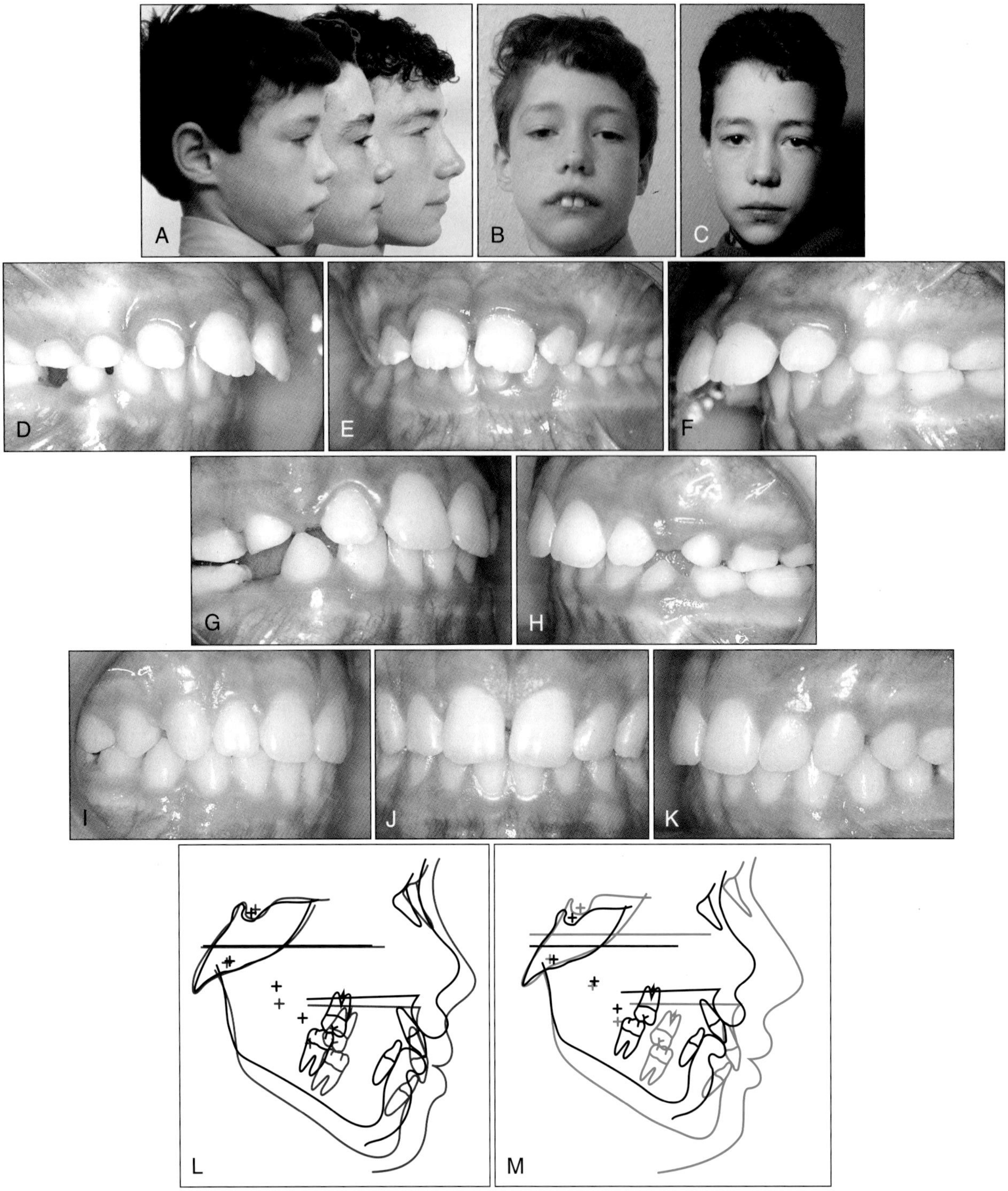

A B C D E F G H I J K L M

Fig. 9-11 Case #6. **A,** Treatment progress of patient with disfiguring malocclusion in early mixed dentition, with upper incisors vulnerable to trauma. Profiles at ages 8 years, 9 months (before treatment); 10 years, 1 month (after treatment); and 14 years, 11 months (out of retention). Facial appearance before (**B**) and after (**C**) treatment. **D** to **F,** Occlusion before treatment. **G** and **H,** Twin blocks were worn for 14 months. Occlusion after 8 months of treatment. **I** to **K,** Occlusion 1 year out of retention. **L,** Basion superimposition showing before and after treatment with twin blocks, ages 8 years, 9 months and 10 years, 1 month. **M,** Basion superimposition after treatment at age 11 years, 11 months. This case is an example of two-phase treatment with functional correction in mixed dentition, followed by fixed appliances in permanent dentition to detail the occlusion. The correction in the profile occurs during the functional phase, with an excellent mandibular growth response. (From Clark WJ: *Twin block functional therapy: applications in dentofacial orthopaedics,* ed 2, Edinburgh, 2002, Mosby Ltd.)

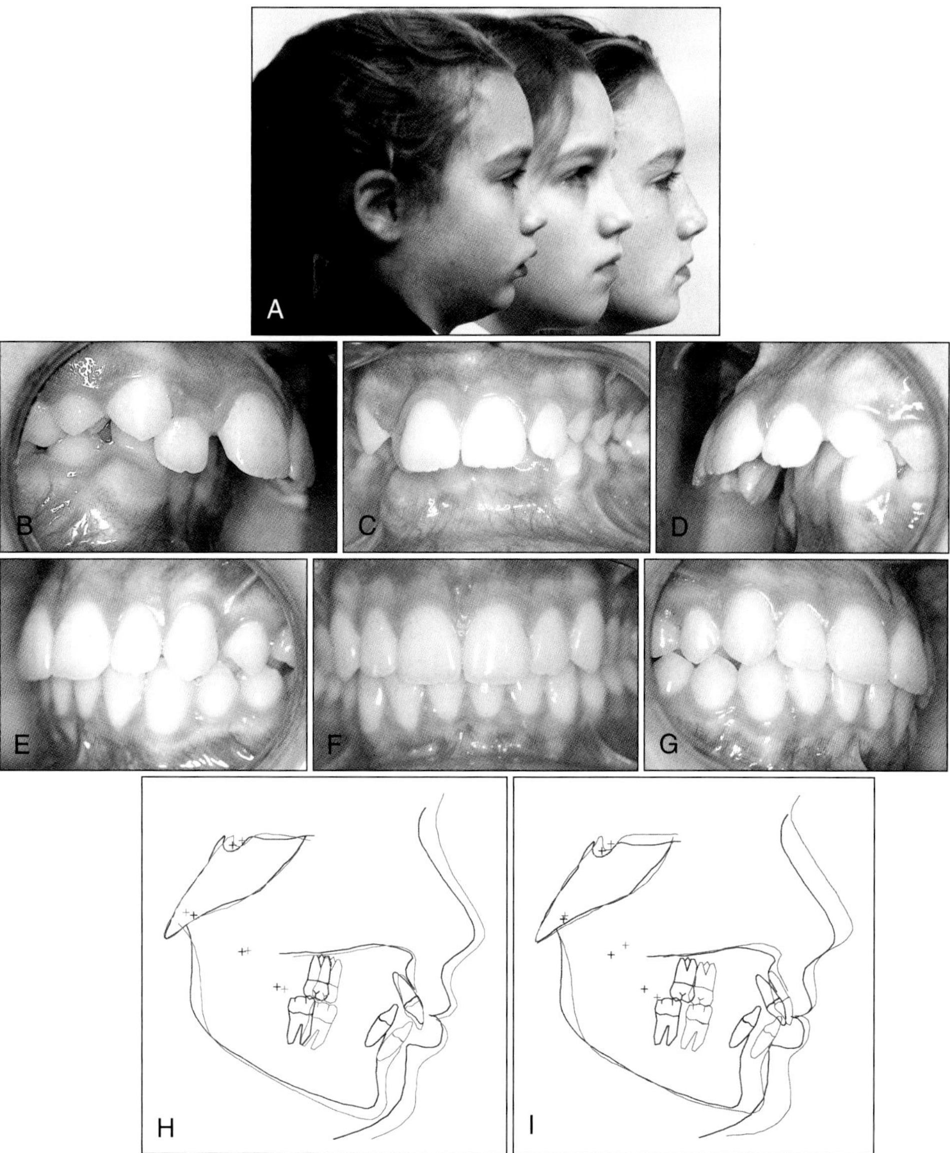

Fig. 9-12 Case #7. **A,** Treatment progress of patient with severe Class II, Division 1 malocclusion complicated by crowding in lower arch. Profiles at ages 11 years, 11 months (before twin block treatment, mandible retruded); 12 years, 2 months (after 8 weeks' treatment with twin blocks) and 14 years, 7 months (18 months out of retention). Rapid improvement results from early muscle adaptation in response to full-time functional mandibular advancement. Corrected profile after treatment is close to the predicted result. **B** to **D,** Occlusion before treatment. **E** to **G,** Occlusion 18 months out of retention. **H,** Basion superimposition to show growth changes during 8 months of twin block treatment. There is evidence of significant distal condylar growth, resulting in forward positioning of the mandible, as confirmed by an increase in the gonial angle. *Black line,* 11 years, 11 months; *red line,* 12 years, 7 months. **I,** Positive changes observed during twin block phase are consolidated 2 years later. The condyle grew significantly in a distal direction. *Black line,* 11 years, 11 months; *blue line,* 14 years, 7 months. (**A** to **G** from Clark WJ: *Twin block functional therapy: applications in dentofacial orthopaedics,* ed 2, Edinburgh, 2002, Mosby Ltd.)

facial growth. Although it is not possible to encourage the mandible to grow beyond the individual's genetic potential, environmental factors play a major role in perpetuating a severe Class II malocclusion. A distal occlusion exerts restraining occlusal forces on the mandibular dentition, and the maxillary dental arch is narrow from distal positioning of the lower dentition. These factors may not allow the mandible to grow to its full genetic potential. In severe class II malocclusion the tongue is back in the throat because it is contained within a retrusive lower dental arch. This pattern has negative effects on the health and metabolism of these patients.

Expanding the maxilla and advancing the mandible unlock the malocclusion. In functional terms, advancing the mandible advances the tongue and, as cephalometric records confirm, increases the airway. This is a fundamental physiological change with beneficial effects that can be seen clearly within 2 or 3 months of commencing treatment. In the hands of an experienced clinician, full-time functional appliances are more efficient in correcting severe Class II malocclusion than conventional fixed-appliance techniques without mandibular propulsion. This is especially true when treatment is timed to coincide with the pubertal growth spurt, but equally appropriate in early treatment.

The goal of functional therapy is to elicit a proprioceptive response in the muscles and ligaments, and as a secondary response, to influence the pattern of bone growth to support a new functional environment for the developing dentition. The best results are obtained by combining orthodontic and orthopedic techniques, and the future for the orthodontic specialty lies in advancing orthopedic techniques toward a holistic approach to reduce skeletal discrepancies and restore normal function in promoting normal growth and development.

A comprehensive description of the twin block technique is illustrated in the author's *Twin block functional therapy: applications in dentofacial orthopaedics* (ed 2, Edinburgh, 2002, Mosby Ltd.), with information on clinical management for the efficient use of the technique.

References

1. McNamara JA Jr, Bryan FA: Long-term mandibular adaptations to protrusive function: an experimental study in *Macaca mulatta*, *Am J Orthod Dentofacial Orthop* 92:98-108, 1987.
2. Voudouris JC, Woodside DG, Altuna G, et al: Condyle fossa modifications and muscle interactions during Herbst treatment. Part 1 New technological methods, *Am J Orthod Dentofacial Orthop* 123:604-613, 2003.
3. Voudouris JC, Woodside DG, Altuna G, et al: Condyle fossa modifications and muscle interactions during Herbst treatment. Part 2. Results and conclusions, *Am J Orthod Dentofacial Orthop* 124:13-29, 2003.
4. Ruf S, Pancherz H. Temporomandibular joint remodeling in adolescents and young adults during Herbst treatment: a prospective longitudinal magnetic resonance imaging and cephalometric radiographic investigation, *Am J Orthod Dentofacial Orthop* 115:607-618, 1999.
5. Chintakanon, K, Turker KS, Sampson W, et al: Effects of twin-block therapy on protrusive muscle functions, *Am J Orthod Dentofacial Orthop* 118:392-396, 2000.
6. Chintakanon K, Turker KS, Sampson W, et al: A prospective study of twin-block appliance therapy assessed by magnetic resonance imaging, *Am J Orthod Dentofac Orthop* 118:494-504, 2000.
7. Mills CM, McCulloch KJ: Treatment effects of the twin block appliance: a cephalometric study, *Am J Orthod Dentofacial Orthop* 114:15-24, 1998.
8. Mills CM, McCulloch KJ: Post treatment changes following successful correction of Class II malocclusions with the twin block appliance, *Am J Orthod Dentofacial Orthop* 118:24-33, 2000.
9. Singh GD, Clark WJ: Localization of mandibular changes in patients with Class II Division 1 malocclusion treated with twin block appliances: finite element scaling analysis, *Am J Orthod Dentofacial Orthop* 119:419-425, 2001.
10. Rabie ABM et al: Functional appliance therapy accelerates and enhances condylar growth, *Am J Orthod Dentofacial Orthop* 123:40-48, 2003.
11. Rabie ABM et al: Replicating mesenchymal cells in the condyle and the glenoid fossa during mandibular forward posturing, *Am J Orthod Dentofacial Orthop* 123:4-57, 2003.
12. Baccetti T, Franchi L, McNamara JA Jr: Treatment timing for twin block therapy, *Am J Orthod Dentofacial Orthop* 118:159-170, 2000.
13. O'Reilly M, Yanniello GJ: Mandibular growth changes and maturation of the cervical vertebrae: a longitudinal cephalometric study, *Angle Orthod* 58:179-184, 1988.
14. Hassel B, Farman A: Skeletal maturation evaluation using cervical vertebrae, *Am J Orthod Dentofacial Orthop* 107:58-66, 1995.
15. Franchi L, Baccetti T, McNamara JA Jr: Mandibular growth and cervical vertebrae maturation and body height, *Am J Orthod Dentofacial Orthop* 118:335-340, 2000.

CHAPTER 10

Hybrid Functional Appliances for Management of Class II Malocclusions

Tarisai C. Dandajena

Class II malocclusion can be managed in three different ways: extraction, nonextraction with distal movement of the maxillary teeth into Class I, and orthognathic surgery, which can be combined with extraction or nonextraction of teeth. Factors that might influence the treatment options include the severity of the Class II malocclusion and age of the patient. For the growing patient, nonextraction with growth modification may be the treatment of choice. Modification of growth is usually done by functional appliances, either removable or fixed.

TRADITIONAL FUNCTIONAL APPLIANCES

A variety of removable functional appliances have historically been used in the management of Class II malocclusion in the growing patient.

Headgear

Of all the functional appliances, headgear is the most common. Its use dates back to the nineteenth century.[1,2] The headgear restricts maxillary growth as well as distal movement of the maxillary first molars to which the headgear forces are applied. Forces from the headgear can be efficiently controlled, which makes it a versatile appliance. Success with the headgear largely depends on patient cooperation. Although the preadolescent patient is usually very compliant, teenage patients are the least likely to use the headgear effectively because of peer pressure. Also, the headgear should be used cautiously because of the risk of possible impaction of the unerupted maxillary second molars.[3]

Other Nonfixed Functional Appliances

Whereas the headgear can be used universally, other nonfixed functional appliances may not have this advantage. Certain criteria must be fulfilled for a patient to be treated with removable functional appliances. These criteria include low mandibular plane to Frankfort horizontal angle (FMA no greater than 30 degrees), upright mandibular incisors, and growth potential. Low FMA is most preferred because of the bite-opening effect of functional appliances during correction of Class II malocclusion. Functional appliances are usually contraindicated in high-angle patients because these appliances tend to open the bite.[4] In addition, because they rest against the mandibular incisors, these appliances can result in their proclination and thus are contraindicated in proclined and procumbent incisors as well.

Fixed Functional Appliances

The fixed functional appliances can be classified into three groups: fixed rigid, fixed flexible, and fixed hybrid.[5] The most used and historically prominent of the fixed rigid functional appliances is the Herbst.

Herbst appliance

The Herbst appliance (Dentauram, Ispringen, Germany) was first introduced in the early twentieth century and gained popularity in the 1980s after work by Pancherz. Considerable debate surrounds how correction of Class II malocclusion is achieved during use of the Herbst. Users of the appliance have argued in favor of growth modification. Research has shown that the Herbst, as with other functional appliances, does not "grow" mandibles but produces a "headgear effect" by distalizing the maxillary molars and restricting maxillary growth. There is no evidence to support enhanced mandibular growth from use of the Herbst. The results obtained from the Herbst may be no different from Class II elastics.

Interpretation of these studies requires caution. The basic tool used to assess changes in most studies is the lateral cephalogram, which has limited application in detecting condylar changes and is more suited to interpretation of large, gross changes. Computed tomography (CT) scans would be better suited for such assessment but are more expensive.

The Herbst appliance was initially developed for the growing patient. However, its applications to correct Class II malocclusion have been extended to adult patients. Other appliances in the same category as the Herbst include the *mandibular anterior repositioning appliance* (MARA) (AOA Orthodontic Appliances, Sturtevant, Wis.) and fixed twin block. Of the flexible fixed functional appliances, the most studied is the Jasper Jumper (American Orthodontics, Sheboygan, Wis.).

HYBRID FUNCTIONAL APPLIANCES

Recently, a new group of hybrid functional appliances have appeared in the orthodontic armamentarium. Unlike the rigid fixed functional appliances that lack flexibility, hybrid functional appliances contain the features of both rigid and flexible appliances. They are spring loaded, which allows greater flexibility of the mandible. Two such appliances include the Sabbagh Universal Spring (Dentaurum) and the Forsus Spring (3M Unitek, Monrovia, Calif.).

Sabbagh Universal Spring

Developed by Dr. Sabbagh in Germany, the Sabbagh Universal Spring (SUS) is a telescopic device similar to the Herbst externally but with a different mode of activation. The SUS consists of a telescopic rod fitted into a guide tube (Fig. 10-1, *A*). Inside the guide tube is a spring that can be adjusted to deliver different force levels, depending on the severity of the Class II malocclusion (Fig. 10-1, *B*). Its U-loop is designed to fit into the maxillary first molars while the lower end is tied to the archwire between the first premolar and the canine, or even between the canine and the lateral incisor.

Unlike the Forsus, the SUS is a true universal spring in that it does not have a left or right side. External springs can be added on to the appliance to increase its springiness. Dentaurum supplies springs for such a purpose, but any spring that fits into the telescopic rod can be used.

Indications

The SUS can efficiently treat a variety of Class II malocclusions. Currently, limited information is available in the literature on the use of the SUS. Studies conducted at the University of Oklahoma have shown that the appliance can be used in both adult and young patients to correct Class II

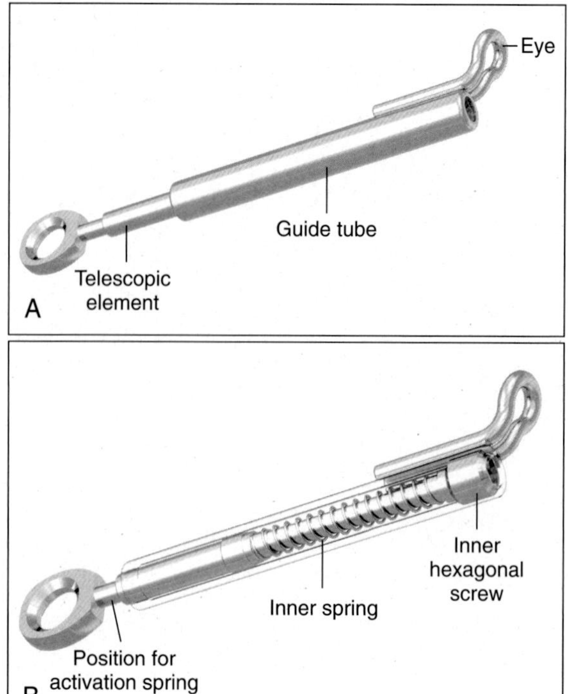

Fig. 10-1 The Sabbagh Universal Spring[2] (SUS[2]). **A,** Telescopic rod is fitted into the guide tube. **B,** Spring inside the guide tube can be adjusted to deliver different force levels. The research addressed in this chapter was conducted using the original version of the Sabbagh Universal Spring. (Courtesy Dentaurum, Ispringen, Germany.)

discrepancies. Treatment of the adult patient is based on the understanding that management of Class II malocclusion using the nonextraction protocol does not depend on restriction of maxillary growth or modification of mandibular growth; rather, it is mostly dentoalveolar.[6]

The SUS can be used in patients with high or low FMA because the appliance intrudes the buccal segments in the maxillary arch. In patients whose second molars have erupted, it is recommended that the arch wire be extended to include the maxillary second molars. The SUS delivers an intrusive force to the maxillary first molars, and failure to incorporate the maxillary second molars into the archwire may result in severe second-order discrepancy between the first and second molars after the first molar is moved distally and intruded.

Figure 10-2 shows a patient with bilateral Class II malocclusion who was treated with an SUS. Initially, the second molars were not included in the archwires, as shown by the vertical discrepancy between the first and second molars. This could have been avoided if the second molars had been either bonded or banded and included in the initial archwires used for distal movement of the maxillary arch.

As in the maxillary arch, the mandibular second molars also need to be included in the mandibular archwires to increase the anchorage in that arch. Although it is not necessary to use a full-size wire in the maxillary arch, a rigid full-size wire is recommended in the mandibular arch to avoid

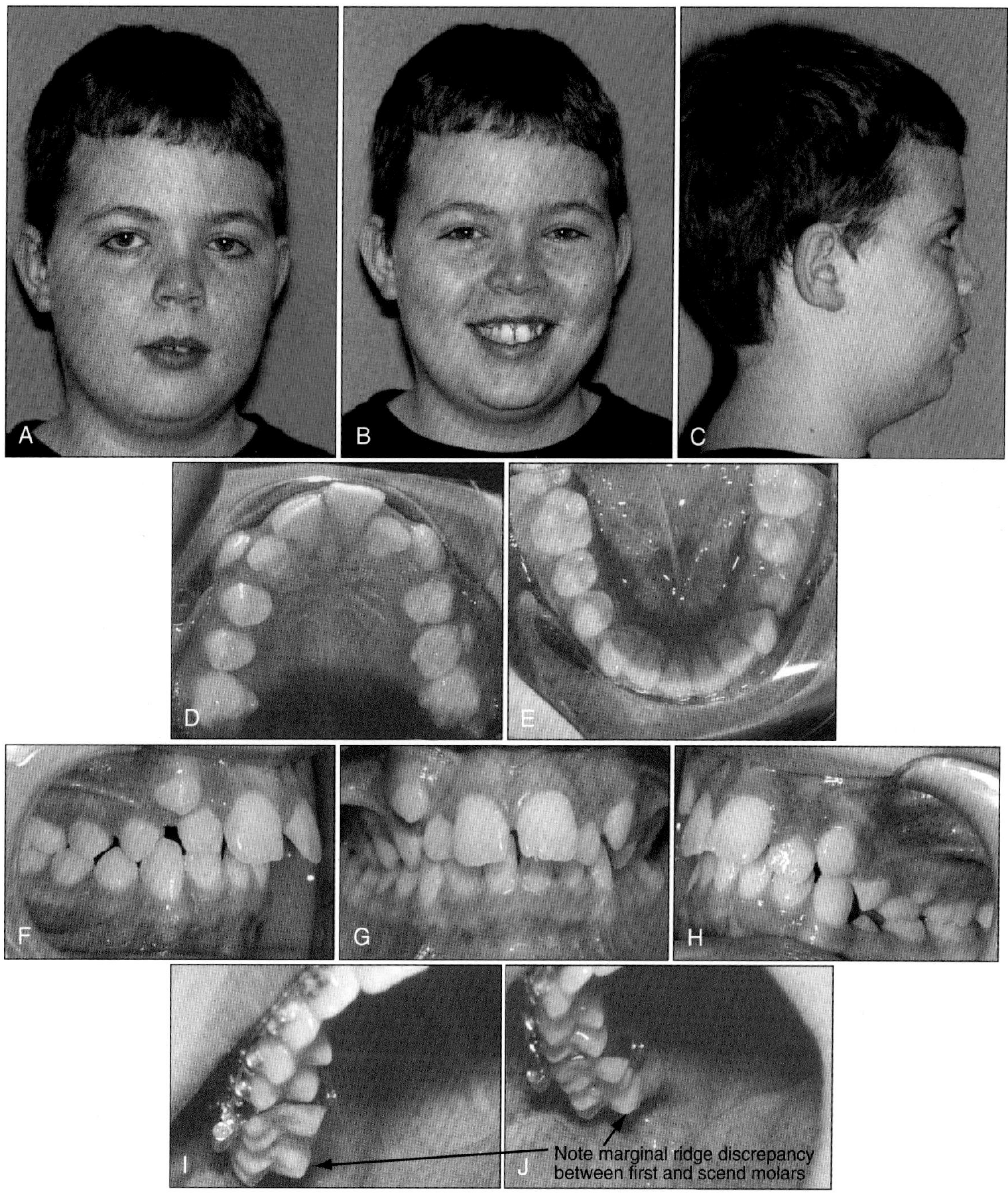

Fig. 10-2 Extrusion of the second molars when they are not included in the archwire. Pretreatment facial (**A-C**) and intraoral (**D-H**) photographs show a Class II malocclusion with deep curve of Spee and blocked right canine. **I** and **J**, Second molar extrusion.

Continued

proclination of the mandibular incisors. The author also recommends an omega loop mesial to the mandibular first or second molars to tie back the whole mandibular arch. If this is not done, the patient will likely develop spacing between the first premolars and the canines if the mesial part of the SUS is engaged between these two teeth.

A contraindication of functional appliances is proclination of the mandibular incisors, which may occur during use of the appliance. After the appliance is removed and during the recovery period, the mandibular incisors return to their previous position before delivery of the SUS. The same is true for the Forsus appliance.

Table 10-1 summarizes cephalometric measurements of patients treated with the SUS. The average time needed to correct the Class II malocclusion is 3 to 4 months. Depending on space available in the maxillary arch, no more than 6

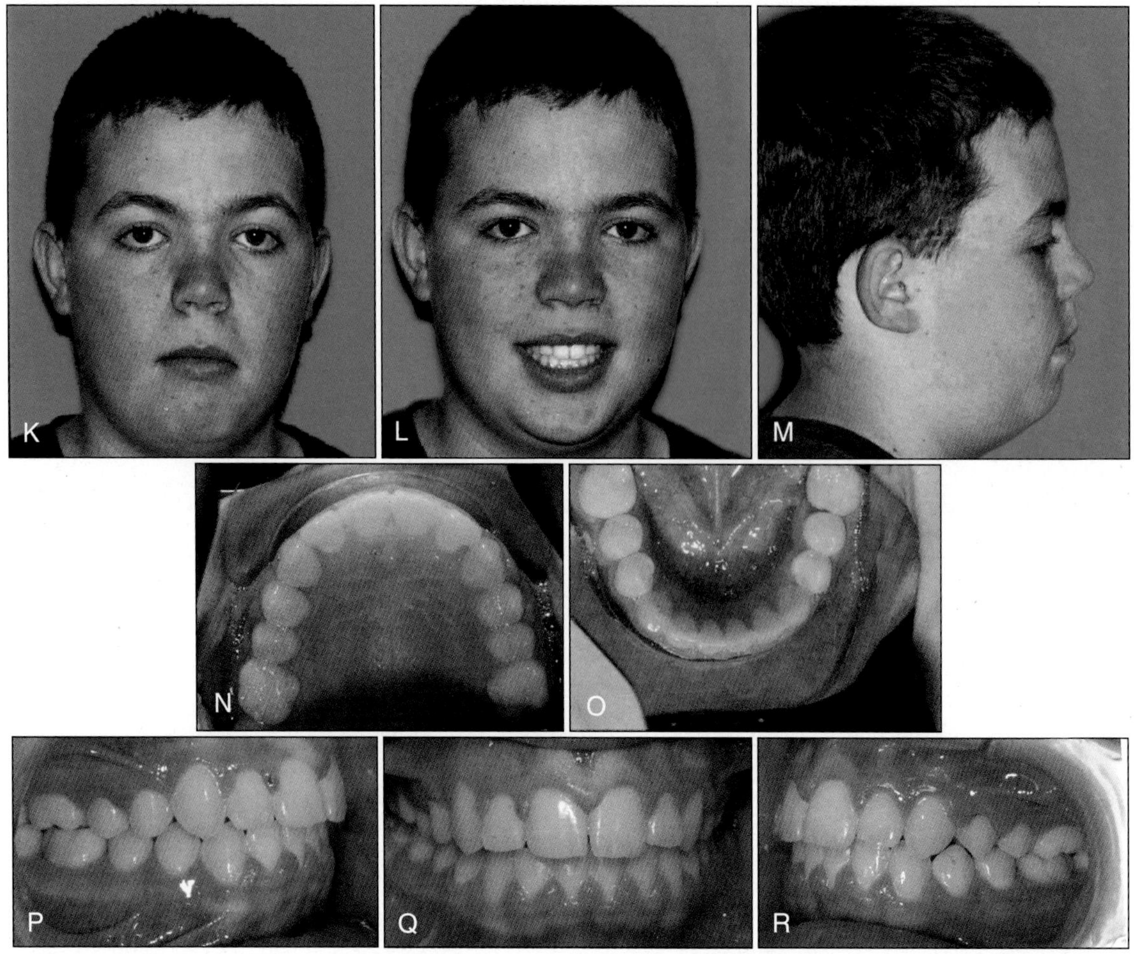

Fig. 10-2, cont'd Final facial (**K-M**) and intraoral (**N-R**) photographs.

months is required after Class II correction to detail and finish the treatment. Thus on average, a full-step Class II malocclusion is treated in 15 months.

The mandibular incisors proclined while using this appliance, an observation similar to that documented by Wieslander[7] with the Herbst. There was no significant change in the FMA, as also reported by Ruf and Pancherz[8] with their appliance. They further reported continued decrease in FMA years after removal of the Herbst appliance.

Another important feature of the SUS is that in those patients that present with crowding in the maxillary arch (e.g., blocked-out canines), the clinician does not need to create space for the blocked-out teeth before delivery of the SUS. The space for the blocked-out teeth is created during distal molar movement of the teeth posterior to the canines. Also, a full size wire is not needed in the maxillary arch to initiate maxillary molar distalization; this can be done even with nickel-titanium (Ni-Ti) wires. However, stainless steel (ss) wires are recommended for the mandibular arch.

Figure 10-3 shows a patient with Class II malocclusion who was treated with the SUS. The maxillary arch presented with crowding (blocked-out canines). Initial treatment involved alignment of the mandibular arch. The SUS was delivered while the mandibular arch was in a 17 × 25 ss archwire. No attempt was made to expand the maxillary arch to create space for the blocked-out canines. The maxillary archwire (16 × 22 TMA) extended from the second molar to second molar, excluding the canines. As the maxillary molars were moved distally, space was created initially between the first molars and second premolars, then between the premolars and canines. The SUS was kept in place until the premolars were retracted.

A notable advantage of the SUS is improvement of the profile. Figure 10-4 shows a patient who had been treatment-planned for surgery but was effectively treated with the SUS. The patient initially presented with full-step Class II, deep bite with gummy smile, and some mandibular anterior crowding. The maxillary arch was distalized as well as intruded with efficient control of the vertical dimension. His FMA increased by 1 degree, from 26 to 27 degrees. A

TABLE 10-1

Statistics for Group of Patients Treated with Sabbagh Universal Spring (SUS)*

	T1 (N = 7)				T2 (N = 6)				T3 (N = 7)			
Variable	**Mean**	**STD**	**LCL**	**UCL**	**Mean**	**STD**	**LCL**	**UCL**	**Mean**	**STD**	**LCL**	**UCL**
SNA	81.97	4.87	77.46	86.48	82.53	4.55	77.76	87.31	80.84	4.59	76.6	85.09
SNB	76.97	3.55	73.69	80.25	77.08	2.96	73.97	80.19	76.47	3.16	73.54	79.4
ANB	5	2.83	2.38	7.62	5.45	2.7	2.61	8.29	4.37	2.37	2.18	6.56
FMA	21.56	3.58	18.25	24.87	22.62	3.94	18.48	26.75	22.06	4.42	17.97	26.15
Facial angle	89.09	3.66	85.7	92.47	89.12	4.33	84.57	93.66	89.74	4.03	86.01	93.47
PPMP	24.26	2.88	21.6	26.92	25.32	3.19	21.97	28.66	23.86	3.21	20.89	26.83
ConvAng	8.1	6.58	2.01	14.19	8.92	5.97	2.65	15.18	6.33	5.89	0.88	11.78
U1NA (mm)	5.36	3.27	2.33	8.38	3.02	2.88	0	6.04	4.34	2.27	2.24	6.44
L1NB (mm)	5.81	2.3	3.69	7.94	7.27	1.81	5.37	9.17	7.1	1.67	5.56	8.64
L1APog (mm)	0.13	2.78	−2.44	2.7	2.22	2.47	−0.37	4.81	2.2	1.36	0.94	3.46
PogNB (mm)	2.26	1.29	1.06	3.45	2.1	1.37	0.66	3.54	2.74	1.76	1.11	4.37
AOBO (mm)	3.79	2.41	1.56	6.01	1.9	1.18	0.66	3.14	1.19	1.2	0.07	2.3
MePP (mm)	65.86	4.45	61.74	69.98	69.03	4.58	64.23	73.83	70.53	4.34	66.51	74.54
IMPA	90.94	4.97	86.34	95.54	98	5.95	91.75	104.25	94.06	4.59	89.81	98.31
ULE (mm)	−2.07	3.3	−5.12	0.98	−3	2.23	−5.34	−0.66	−4.36	2.75	−6.9	−1.81
LLE (mm)	−0.56	2.89	−3.23	2.12	−0.02	1.48	−1.57	1.54	−1.46	1.62	−2.96	0.04
DiffZ	1.64	2.75	−0.9	4.19	4.38	0.91	3.43	5.33	2.8	2.28	0.69	4.91
MdLth (mm)	110.71	3.69	107.3	114.13	113.72	5.65	107.79	119.65	115.7	4.46	111.57	119.83
MxLth (mm)	93.9	5.13	89.15	98.65	93.62	4.82	88.56	98.67	95.7	5.23	90.86	100.54

*Unless stated otherwise, all measurements are in degrees.

STD, Standard deviation; upper *(UCL)* and lower *(LCL)* 95% confidence level of the mean at T1, T2, and T3.

MdLth, Mandibular length from condylion (Co) to gnathion; *MxLth,* maxillary length from Co to A-point; *DiffZ,* difference between upper lip and lower lip Z-angles; a positive number indicates the upper lip was more protrusive compared with the lower lip; *ULE,* upper lip to E-line; *LLE,* lower lip to E-line.

notable change in this patient was the soft tissue profile; the Z-angle improved from 63.5 degrees to an ideal of 72 degrees. According to Merrifield,[9] an ideal Z-angle should be between 72 and 80 degrees. An assessment of patients treated with extraction and nonextraction has also shown that the Z-angle is an important discriminator between extraction and nonextraction and is a good parameter for assessing the soft tissue profile.[10]

The SUS can appropriately be used in the management of unilateral Class II malocclusions as well. Such use is most appropriate when there are midline discrepancies or crowding. Although it is possible to use the appliance unilaterally in such cases, the author recommends placement of a passive appliance on the contralateral side.

Anchorage control in extraction cases

Orthodontics has found the "holy grail" of extraction space closure in *temporary anchorage devices* (TADs).[11] The SUS can be efficiently used in cases requiring Group A anchorage in the maxillary arch and Group C anchorage in the mandibular arch.

Figure 10-5, *A* to *H,* illustrates a patient who presented with Class II malocclusion as well as bialveolar protrusion.[12] The treatment required extraction of the maxillary first premolars and mandibular second premolars, with maximum retraction of the maxillary anterior segments (Group A anchorage) and protraction of the mandibular buccal segments (Group C anchorage). To improve the profile, the clinician required an efficient way to minimize movement of the anchor segments.

The teeth in both arches were aligned using a 0.018 copper nickel-titanium (CNT) and a 16 × 22 CNT. Working wires in both arches were 18 × 25 ss. Power arms were welded onto the archwires distal to the canines in both arches. SUS devices were then placed on either side of the arches, and en masse retraction in the maxillary arch was initiated using retraction coil springs (GAC International, Bohemia, N.Y.). Protraction of the mandibular molars was done in the same way. Figure 10-5, *I* to *K,* demonstrate the armamentarium for en masse retraction using the SUS.

The patient was scheduled to report back every 6 weeks. At one point, the patient went on vacation for 3 months and

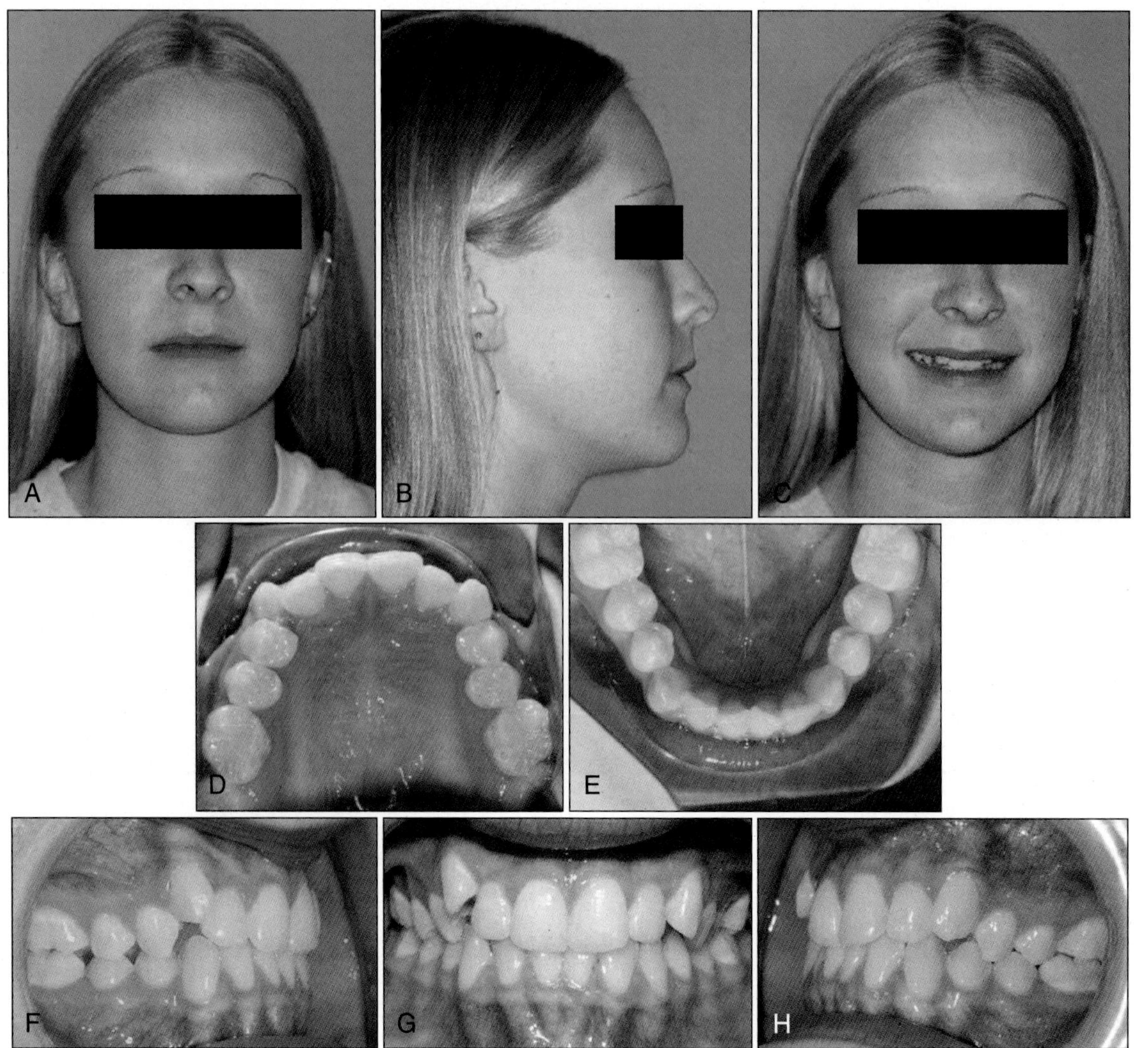

Fig. 10-3 Class II malocclusion with maxillary crowding. Pretreatment facial (**A-C**) and intraoral (**D-H**) photographs. Space for the blocked out canine was created by distalization of the maxillary first molars.

returned with all spaces closed but in Class III relationship. Figure 10-5, *L*, shows the cephalometric radiograph of that patient at that appointment; *M* and *N* show progress and final cephalograms. The SUS and retraction springs were removed, and some relapse was allowed to occur. Figure 10-5, *O* to *V*, show the final images of this patient, with acceptably good Class I relationship.

When the SUS is used for anchorage control, patients need to be monitored closely because they might develop Class III occlusion from Class II relationship. The same is true when the SUS is used for the correction of Class II malocclusion to Class I during nonextraction treatment.

Forsus Fatigue-Resistant Device

The Forsus fatigue-resistant device (Forsus Spring) is designed similar to the SUS (see Fig. 10-5). Unlike the SUS, however, the Forsus consists of a pushrod designed for either left or right side only. The clinician must select the correct length of the pushrod that can be used for the patient. Its activation is done through wedges placed on the pushrod.

Minimal research is available on the Forsus, but it possesses the same advantages as the SUS. Research conducted at the University of Oklahoma[13] compared the Forsus to an untreated group of subjects over 6 months. The research also compared two modalities of treatment with the Forsus. One group of patients was treated with en masse retraction of the maxillary arch while using a lip bumper in the mandibular arch to anchor the mandibular molars as well as avoid proclination of the mandibular incisors. In the second group the maxillary molars were first distalized with overcorrection to Class I, at which point the Forsus was removed.

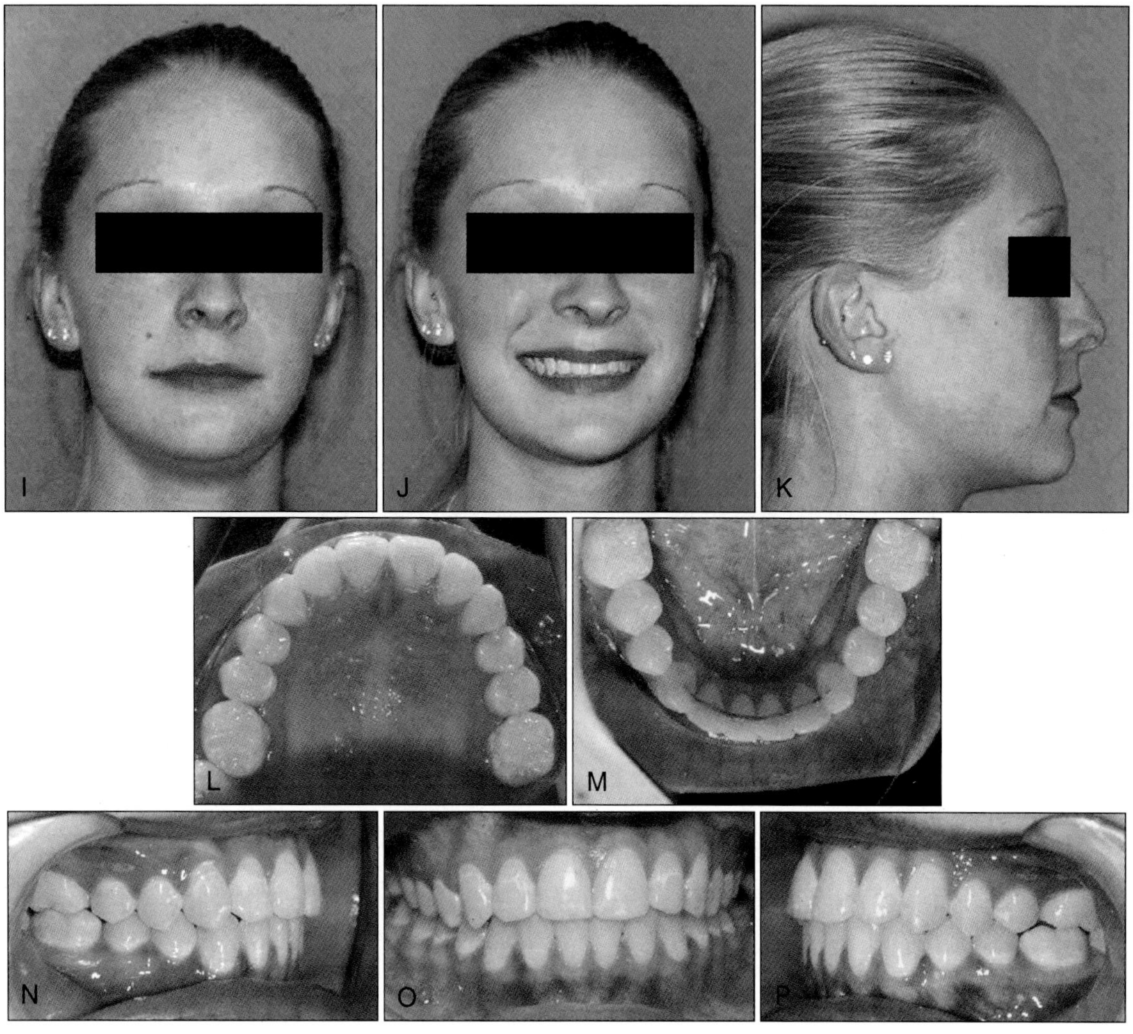

Fig. 10-3, cont'd Final facial (**I-K**) and intraoral (**L-P**) photographs.

The results showed no significant difference in mandibular incisor positions or mandibular molar inclination between the group treated using lip bumper for anchorage and the group without lip bumper. Correction to Class I was faster in the group for whom the initial goal was to distalize the maxillary molars only. The maxillary incisors were also more upright after the first phase of treatment in the group with the first molars distalized first.

CONCLUSION

The author has observed a greater tendency toward relapse in patients treated with en masse correction to Class I occlusion. Such response has not been observed in patients who had the maxillary molars distalized first, followed by the rest of the teeth mesial to the first molars. If the maxillary second molars are erupted, the author recommends that they be banded or bonded and included in the initial archwires. As previously discussed, the maxillary second molars will extrude if they are not included in the archwires. Extrusion of the second molars will delay treatment when a smaller-size wire is used again to align the second molars.

When crowding occurs in the maxillary arch and nonextraction treatment is planned, the author recommends distal movement of the molars to create room for the teeth that are blocked out. Use of auxiliaries such as lip bumper to enhance anchorage in the mandibular arch may not be necessary. It is recommended to apply lingual crown torque to the mandibular anterior teeth even in brackets with a prescription.

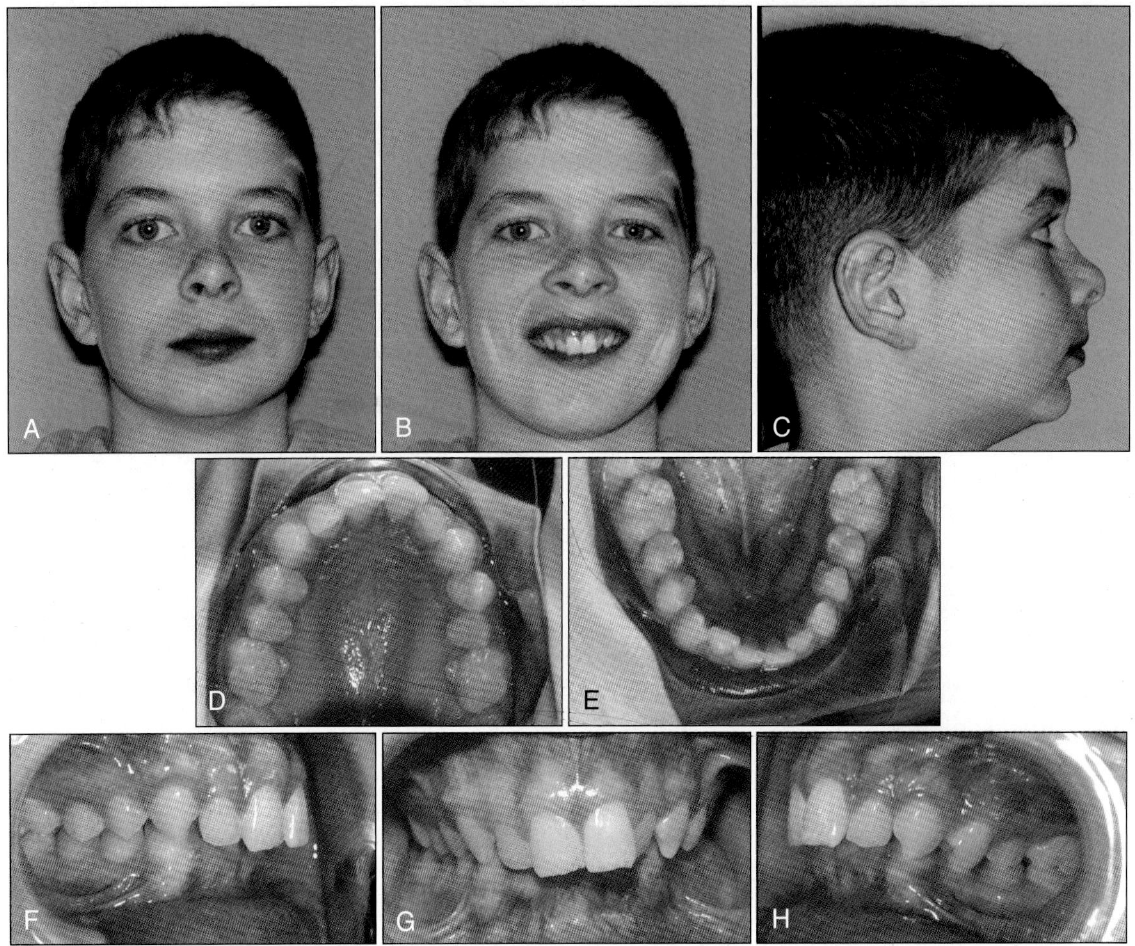

Fig. 10-4 Full-step Class II, Division 1 malocclusion with deep bite and maxillary crowding treated with the SUS. Pretreatment facial (**A-C**) and intraoral (**D-H**) photographs.

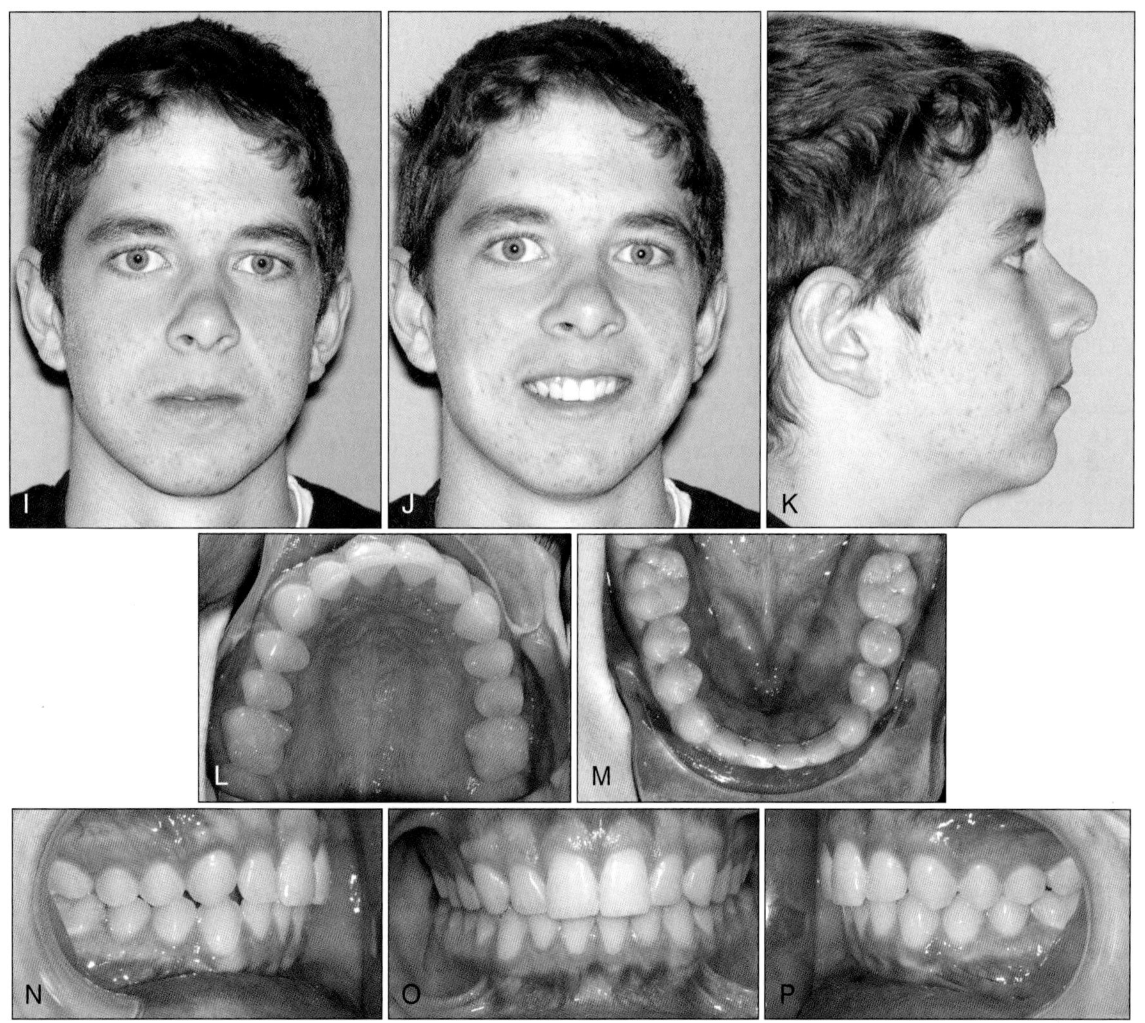

Fig. 10-4, cont'd Posttreatment facial (**I-K**) and intraoral (**L-P**) photographs.

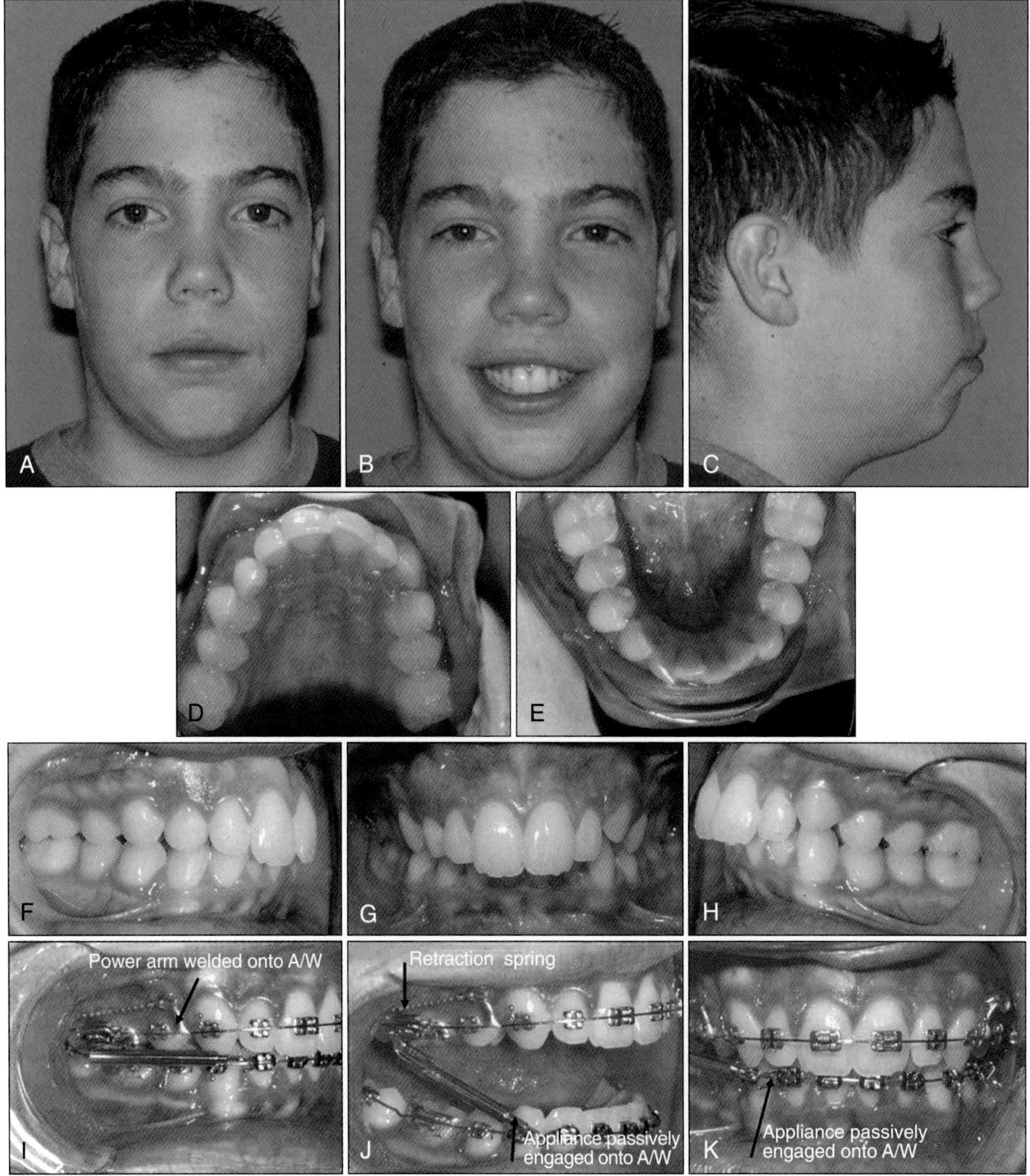

Fig. 10-5 Class II, Division 1 malocclusion that required Group A and Group C anchorage in mandibular arch. Pretreatment facial (**A-C**) and intraoral (**D-H**) photographs. **I** to **K,** Setup for en masse retraction using SUS for maximum anchorage. *A/W,* Archwire.

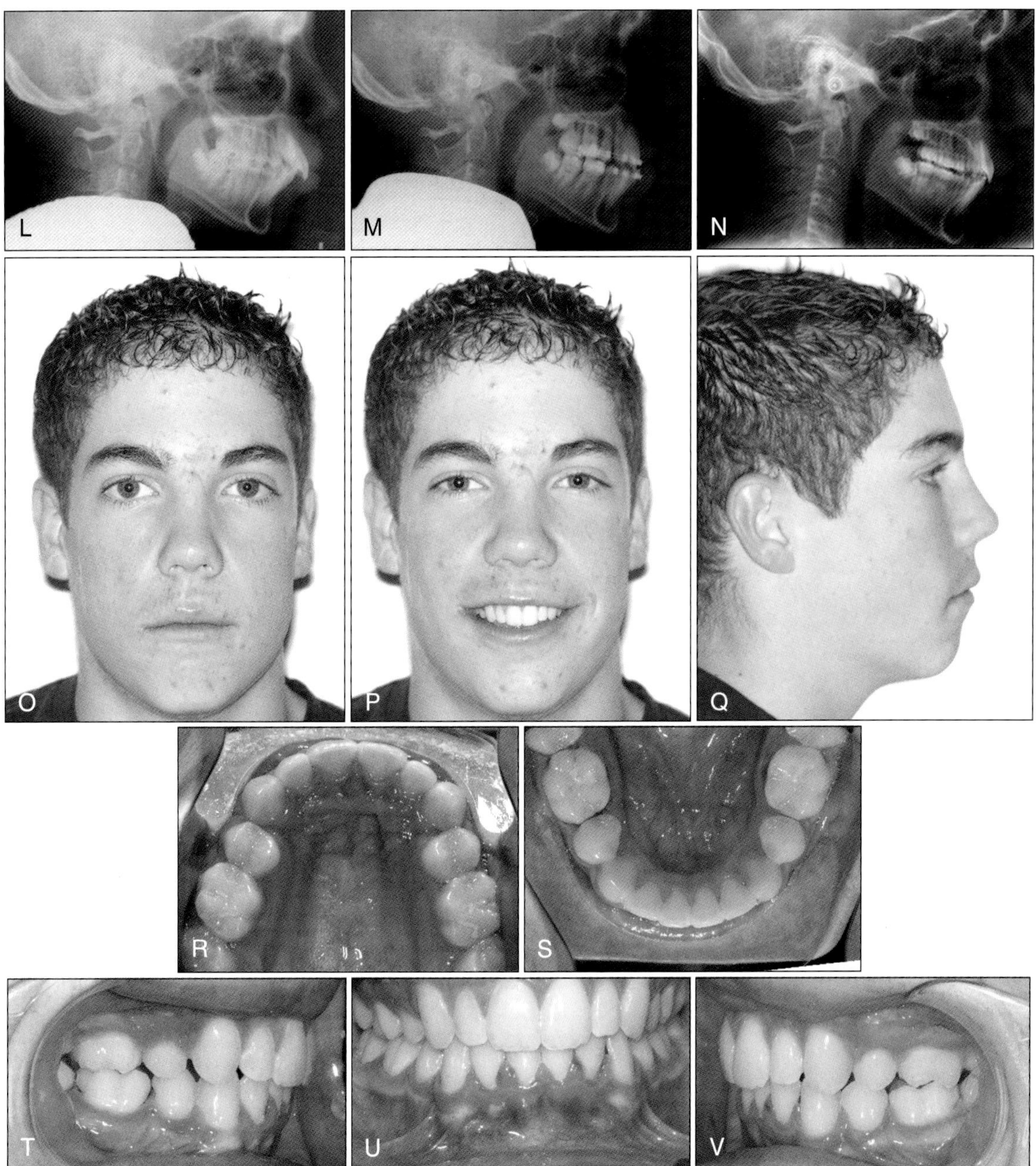

Fig. 10-5, cont'd **L** to **N**, Cephalograms of patient. SUS was used to retract the maxillary anterior segment en masse as well as protract the mandibular posterior segment. Pretreatment (**L**) and progress (**M**) cephalograms. The patient now presents with Class III occlusion. Springs were removed and occlusion allowed to settle. **N**, Cephalogram showing end of treatment. Final facial (**O-Q**) and intraoral (**R-V**) photographs. Patient was satisfactorily finished in Class I occlusion.

References

1. Kingsley NW: *Treatise on oral deformities*, New York, 1880, Appleton.
2. Angle EH: *Treatment of malocclusion of the teeth*, Philadelphia, 1907, SS White Dental Manufacturing.
3. Nanda RS, Dandajena TC, Nanda R: Biomechanical strategies for nonextraction Class II malocclusions. In Nanda R, editor: *Biomechanics and esthetic strategies in clinical orthodontics,* ed 2, Philadelphia, 2005, Saunders, pp 156-176.
4. Barton S, Cook PA: Predicting functional appliance treatment in Class II malocclusions—a review, *Am J Orthod Dentofacial Orthop* 112:282-286, 1997.
5. Ritto AK: Fixed functional appliances: trends for the next century, *Functional Orthodontist* 16:122-135, 1999.
6. Almeida M, Henriques FFC, Almeida RR, et al: Short-term treatment effects produced by the Herbst appliance in the mixed dentition, *Angle Orthod* 75:476-483, 2005.
7. Wieslander L: Long-term effect of treatment with the headgear-Herbst appliance in the early mixed dentition:

stability or relapse? *Am J Orthod Dentofacial Orthop* 104:319-329, 1993.

8. Ruf S, Pancherz H: The effect of Herbst appliance treatment on the mandibular plane angle: a cephalometric roentgenographic study, *Am J Orthod Dentofacial Orthop* 110:225-229, 1996.
9. Merrifield LL: The profile line as an aid in critically evaluating facial esthetics, *Am J Orthod* 52:804-822, 1966.
10. Erdinc AE, Nanda RS, Dandajena TC: Profile changes of patients treated with and without premolar extractions, *Am J Orthod Dentofacial Orthop* 132:324-331, 2007.
11. Graber TM: Have we finally found the Holy Grail of Orthodontics? *World J Orthod* 3:107, 2002.
12. Dandajena TC, Nanda RS: Bialveolar protrusion in a Zimbabwean sample, *Am J Orthod Dentofacial Orthop* 123:133-137, 2003.
13. Bedard A: Assessment of Class II correction with Forsus spring, thesis, Oklahoma City, Health Sciences Center, 2006, University of Oklahoma.

CHAPTER 11

Class II Combination Therapy: Molar Distalization and Fixed Functional Appliances

S. Jay Bowman

PATIENT COMPLIANCE IN ORTHODONTICS

Some degree of patient compliance is required for the success of any course of orthodontic treatment. Unfortunately, patient cooperation has diminished in all aspects of health care,[1] and orthodontics is no exception.[2]

Malocclusions featuring skeletal discrepancies (Class II and III) are most affected by lapses of cooperation because patients have been traditionally required to comply by wearing removable appliances, intermaxillary elastics, and extraoral traction in attempts to attain a Class I dental and skeletal relationship. Patient education and motivational techniques are at best temporarily successful in eliciting compliance with these traditional orthodontic biomechanics. The orthodontic specialist now apparently needs charisma and interpersonal skills in addition to tooth-regulation acumen.[3]

Behrents[4] suggests that compliance is the "most important factor in determining treatment success." Again, unfortunately, patient compliance has decreased.[1,2] Identifying patients who will be cooperative and then measuring their level of compliance is about as successful as picking lottery numbers.[5-7] It is also disconcerting that the dose-effect relationships between appliance wear and outcome are poorly correlated in orthodontics.[8] As a result, "noncompliant patient therapies" have become a popular topic in orthodontic continuing education, the literature, and the marketplace.

DEVELOPING A TREATMENT PHILOSOPHY

This chapter reviews a method of treatment for Class II malocclusions that requires only a single phase of mechanics and reduces reliance on patient compliance for consistent and predictable case completion.[9-15] Orthodontists have become preoccupied with improving their treatment efficiency and efficacy; however, treatment quality, stability, and patient comfort should not be compromised in this pursuit.

On-Time Finishing

Treatment mechanics less dependent on compliance may reduce "cases beyond estimates." The benefits of improving "on-time completion" percentages in clinical practice include limiting practice overhead and increasing goodwill with both parents and referrers. Reducing extended treatment times also limits "exposure time" for iatrogenic effects, potentially decreasing rates of root resorption, enamel decalcification scars, periodontal concerns, and the incidence of temporomandibular disorder (TMD) symptoms. Orthodontists may then focus attention on other patient compliance issues, such as oral hygiene, reducing scar formation,[16] appliance breakage, and missed appointments.

Moreover, noncompliance therapy is not only for patients identified as "noncompliant"; many patients might benefit from improved efficiency of traditional techniques.[17] Selecting methods for timely and consistent case completion is a logical goal for all patients, especially when the identification of a noncompliant patient seems unpredictable before the patient's involvement in actual treatment.

One-Phase Versus Two-Phase Treatment

Class II malocclusion has been described as "one of the most frequent treatment problems in orthodontic practice," with a frequency of 37% in preadolescent patients. The development of Class II appears to be promoted and maintained by both facial growth and dental eruption. A deficient mandible has been described as the most common reason, with less than 30% of Class II patients in a group of 8- to 10-year-old children displaying protrusive maxillae.[18] Although a sample of older patients might demonstrate fewer mandibular retrusions, factoring the effects of continued facial growth, the actual percentages might be considered academic, unless you elect to treat later.

It would then seem reasonable to expect that treatments designed to promote mandibular growth (e.g., functional appliances) rather than to restrict maxillary development (e.g., headgear) would be preferred. Consequently, functional jaw orthopedics (FJO) developed as the "growth industry of the 1980s," with the prevalence of two-phase treatment increasing to approximately 25% of all patients,[19] or one third of all children entering orthodontic treatment at its height of popularity. The strong belief in FJO stimulated the resurrection and creation of many orthodontic appliances, most of which were removable and required excellent patient compliance.

Unfortunately, two-stage treatments, designed to stimulate *extra* mandibular growth (i.e., functional appliances or arch development "bimaxillary expansion" devices), have little support in the literature.[8,20-22] The concerns with most two-phase systems include protracted treatment with long transition periods (often requiring additional appliances or "phase-one orthotics" to prevent immediate relapse), reduced stability, increased iatrogenic effects, and increased financial burden. Therefore a cost/benefit analysis is warranted: do the benefits of early intervention justify the costs of two-phase treatment?[20-22]

Gianelly[21] argued that "at least 90% of all growing patients can be successfully treated in only one phase by starting treatment in the late mixed dentition stage of development; identified by the exfoliation of all deciduous teeth except the second primary molars." In 1947, Hays Nance[23] shared a similar philosophy: "Active treatment in the mixed dentition period is desirable only in Class III cases, crossbites, and Class II cases wherein facial appearance is markedly affected." Unless we suspend disbelief, there are few, if any, long-term benefits specific to much of what passes for early treatment today.[22] Accordingly, treatment plans featuring a single phase of treatment may be preferable for the majority of patients presenting to an orthodontist's practice.

CLASS II CORRECTION

Contributions from both orthopedic and orthodontic factors are common to the resolution of Class II malocclusions.[24] Some treatment effects involve movement of the dentition, and others involve changes in bone (sutural adjustment and growth). To the consternation of FJO enthusiasts, traditional edgewise treatments (often involving extraoral traction and intermaxillary elastics) have demonstrated orthopedic effects that are much the same as those achieved by functional appliances.[20]

Some may be surprised that successful and dramatic orthodontic results were produced before the current preponderance of two-phase treatments that often feature routine "bimaxillary expansion" with jackscrew devices and removable "jaw-growing" appliances. These "modern" mechanics may be more a function of wishful thinking than necessity.

For at least 75% of Class II cases, two-phase functional/edgewise treatment yields results indistinguishable, in terms of facial, skeletal, and occlusal factors, from shorter and more efficiently applied one-phase edgewise therapy.[20] Therefore, the majority of two-stage treatments demonstrate no superior benefits compared with traditional treatment, especially for patients with less than 7 to 11 mm of overjet.[8,25] This suggests that the selection of two-phase functional treatment may well be a practice management decision rather than one based on biology.[20,26-29]

Choosing a Class II Treatment Modality

Indeed, if the final results from the various methods of Class II correction used in the past millennium of orthodontics were "created equal," it would be wiser to consider the potential effects of limited patient cooperation when selecting an appropriate appliance. Patients only have a limited quantity of "compliance," and it may not be expressed during preadolescence (perhaps compromising prolonged dual-stage strategies and their inherently protracted two phases of retention).[29]

Because selection of a cooperative patient cannot be guaranteed, it is important to ask if the treatment method chosen is simple, comfortable, and easy to comply with (i.e., the "Keep-It-Simple-Stupid" [KISS] principle). It may be beneficial to bring patients into the decision process and have them help select their own appliance. "If correction by the various mechanisms is virtually the same, what would you choose to 'wear' (Fränkel, Bionator, Bio-bloc, twin block, Herbst, jackscrew expanders, headgear), and would you prefer one or two phases of treatment?"

Some might opine that "you cannot develop a practice philosophy based on the scientific literature."[30] In the current environment, however, featuring evidence-based approaches, the author would argue that it is necessary to reference the literature when selecting treatment modalities designed to be the most effective, efficient, predictable, and comfortable for our patients.

CONTEMPORARY MOLAR DISTALIZATION

One type of Class II correction involves placing "mesially positioned" and rotated Class II maxillary molars into a Class I position. Devices to "distalize" maxillary molars have been developed and include compressed bulbous loops, jigs, springs, magnets, transpalatal arches, and headgears. One method was even patented to "develop" a nonexistent "premaxillomaxillary suture."[31]

Although the term *distalization* is a neologism, it has become a common descriptor for the biomechanics involved in moving maxillary first and second molars distally and into a Class I molar relationship.[32] More recent molar distalization techniques have included the use of repelling magnets,[33] bulbous superelastic wire loops,[34] and proprietary devices such as the Pendulum[35] (including such variations as Pendex, T-Rex, Pendulum K, AOA Orthodontic Appliances, Sturtevant, Wis.), Jones Jig (American Orthodontics, Sheboygan, Wis.)[36] (i.e., Lokar, Ormco Corp., Orange, Calif.), and Distal Jet (AOA Orthodontic Appliances)[37] (i.e., Keles Slider, Great Lakes Orthodontics, New York, N.Y.). Others are merely alternative means for the application of Class II intermaxillary elastic force (i.e., Bimetric Maxillary Distalizing Arch, Ormco Corp. or Carrière Distalizer, Clínica Carrière, Barcelona, Spain) and, as such, require absolute patient cooperation and may stress mandibular anchorage.

Most of these "continuous force" appliances are not cooperation dependent, may incorporate a modified Nance holding arch or transpalatal connection for some anchorage support, and can produce molar distalization of 1 to 2 mm per month, thereby converting the Class II malocclusion to a more easily resolvable Class I spacing problem in 5 to 9 months.[17] Because there appears to be no substantial advantage to initiating molar distalization methods before the late mixed dentition, these techniques preclude a two-stage regimen.[10,17,21,32]

Typical contraindications to distalization have been patients who feature one or more of the following: significant crowding, bimaxillary protrusion, obtuse mandibular angle, and open bite.[10]

BOX 11-1 Advantages of Distal Jet

- Esthetic
- Simple insertion and activation
- Intraoral conversion to a modified Nance holding arch[15,37,38,45]
- One appliance serves two purposes: distalizer and holding arch[38]
- Less molar tipping[42]
- Favorable premolar distal tipping[42]
- Minimal vertical effects[42]
- No bite plane or jackscrew required
- No compliance required
- Self-limiting

Comparative Analysis of Molar Distalizers

The Distal Jet design, clinical applications, and instructions for use have been described in detail.[10,15,37-45] The clinical effects of the device have also been rigorously documented. Boxes 11-1 and 11-2 outline the advantages of the Distal Jet and evidence-based recommendations.

Molar distalization and tipping

During the typical 5 to 7 months of molar distalization, the Distal Jet has been demonstrated to produce an average of 3.2 mm of distal movement of the maxillary first molar crown.[15] The corresponding amount of distal tip to the molar crown appears to range from 3 to 7 degrees. The magnitude of tipping, however, is often less than with other popular distalizing devices (e.g., Pendulum: 8-16 degrees; Jones Jig: 7-8; GMD: 7; Wilson modular technique: 8; cervical headgear/sagittal appliance: 13; repelling magnets: 7 degrees).[15,43] The reason is that the Distal Jet forces are applied more apically, through a couple (bayonet wire), closer to the center of resistance of the molars (Fig. 11-1).

BOX 11-2 Evidence-Based Recommendations for Distal Jet

1. Average starting age: 12 to 13 years.
2. Second molar eruption: slight advantage.[15,58]
3. Use 240-g nickel-titanium open-coil springs.[58]
4. Construct appliance from first premolars, and permit second premolars to drift distal due to effect of transseptal periodontal fibers.[42]
5. Bend "double-back" wire, inserted in the lingual sheath to rotate molars distally around the palatal root.[38]
6. Check parallelism of construction to occlusal plane and buccal dentition to produce or reduce expansion and bite opening.[42]
7. Level and align only the mandibular dentition with brackets during maxillary molar distalization.[43,44,47]

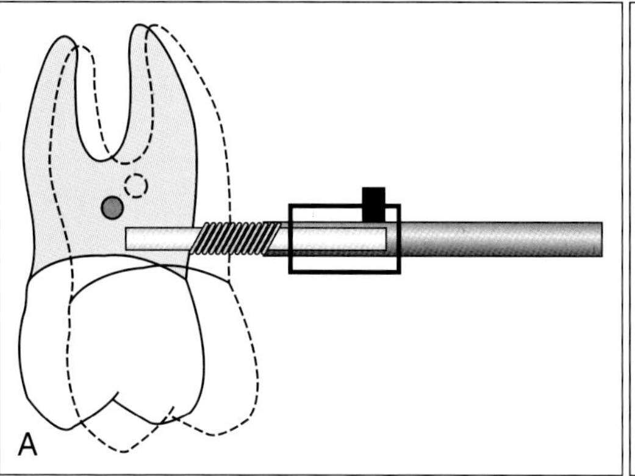

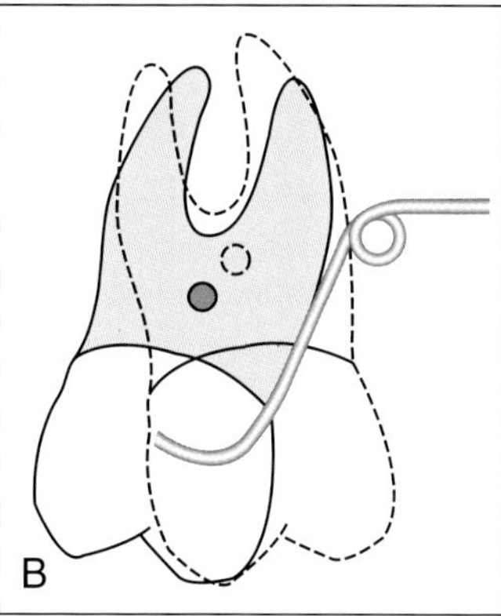

Fig. 11-1 **A,** Distal Jet tends to produce less distal tipping of the maxillary molars as forces are applied more apically, through a couple, closer to the center of resistance. **B,** Sweep arms of the Pendulum produce constriction of intermolar width (unless accompanied by active maxillary expansion) and greater distal tipping of molars.

Anchorage loss

As the molars are pushed back, spaces tend to open between the molars and premolars. Some of the space results from the distal movement of the molars, but some is also a result of mesial anchorage loss caused by the reciprocal forces applied to premolars (teeth included in the construction framework of Distal Jet appliance). The amount of anchorage loss with this appliance typically varied from 15% to 55% (measured at the premolars).[40,41] In fact, more anchorage loss was noted when the Distal Jet was combined with maxillary preadjusted bracket mechanics[46,47] (Fig. 11-2).

Specifically, an average 10-degree increase in incisal angulation was noted when leveling mechanics, using upper braces (preadjusted appliance), were accomplished concomitant with molar distalization.[46,47] Despite that a normal incisor angulation was achieved by the conclusion of treatment[40] (Fig. 11-2, *H-M*), there appears to be no advantage to placing maxillary brackets before completing molar distal movement.[44,46,47]

Creation of space

The total amount of space created during the Distal Jet molar distalization process ranged widely between 4.6 and 13.4 mm on each side of the dental arch.[42] On average, the space was somewhat less than the amount of space produced by the Pendulum (10-15 mm),[48-55] although that device yielded substantially more molar tipping.

Although maxillary premolars were moved mesially with all distalizers, they curiously tipped distally with the Distal Jet,[15] a finding that was different from other popular appliances. Initially, this effect seemed to make little sense until the biomechanics of the device were examined. Because the forces were applied closer to the center of resistance (via a couple) of the molars and premolars (i.e., more apically), there was more likelihood of mesial bodily movement of the premolars. Forces were applied to the acrylic Nance button in the premaxillary region of the palate such that it had a tendency to migrate occlusally, which caused it to slightly rotate down from the palate (Fig. 11-3). This, in turn, pro-

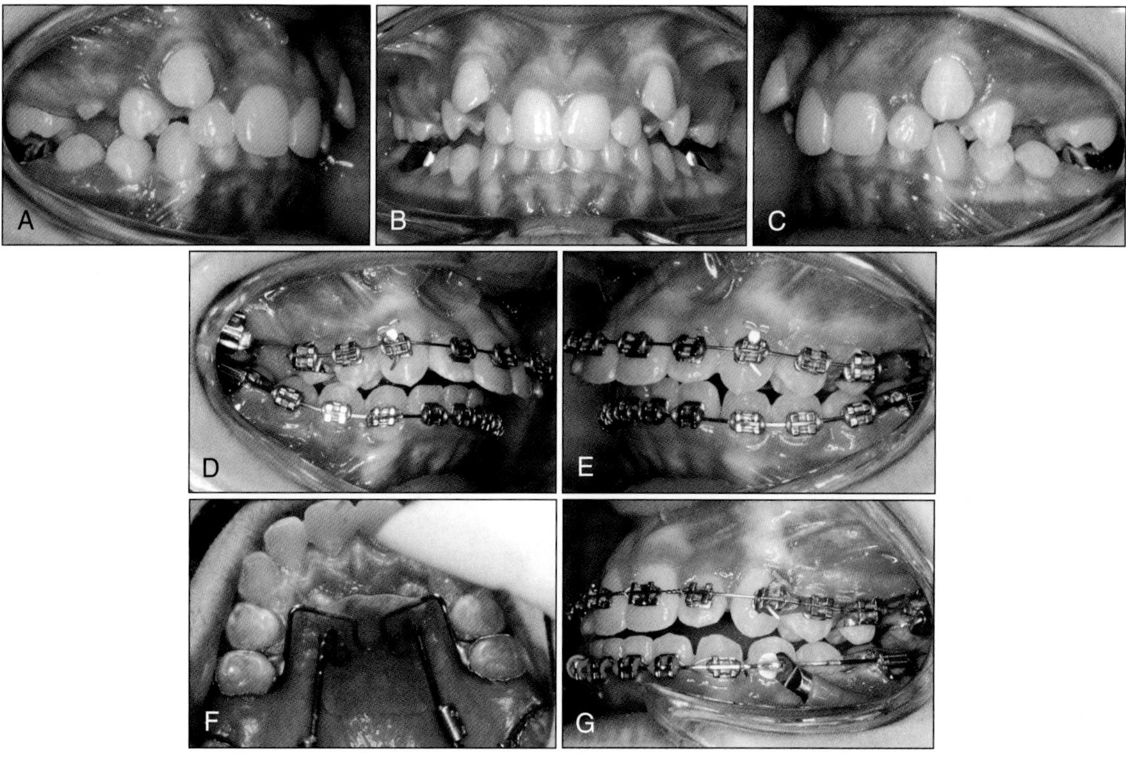

Fig. 11-2 **A** to **C,** Treatment initiated for 13-year-old patient with labially displaced maxillary canines. Fixed lingual arch preserved mandibular arch length, precluding mandibular expansion or extraction strategies. **D** and **E,** Original Distal Jet was used during concurrent leveling and alignment with Roth preadjusted appliance, resulting in flaring of the incisors and increased overjet. Although ideal incisor angulation was achieved by the conclusion of treatment, there appears to be no anchorage advantage to placing brackets on the maxillary teeth until the conclusion of distalization. **F** and **G,** After distalizing the upper molars to an overcorrected "super" Class I in 7 months, Jasper Jumpers were added to help preserve the new molar position during the 6 months of retracting the remaining maxillary teeth.

duced the mild, but favorable, distal cant of the premolars, contrasting greatly to the sometimes dramatic mesial flaring of premolars found with other devices (e.g., GMD, Jones Jig, Pendulum).[15,43,51,53-56] Excessive distal tipping of molars and mesial tipping of premolars, often seen with alternatives to the Distal Jet, are clinically significant for the following reasons:

- More molar tipping produces vertical changes (e.g., increases in mandibular plane and lower anterior face height).
- More "space" appears to be created (from tipping of molars and premolars), but actually the same amount of usable space (or distalization) is produced.
- Subsequent uprighting or paralleling of the tipped molar and premolar roots promotes anchorage loss and is redundant (i.e., a "round-trip").

When the effects of adverse molar and premolar tipping are accounted for in calculations of the space created during molar distalization, the Distal Jet and the Pendulum appeared equivalent in amount of "usable" distalization.[42] Unfortunately, later uprighting of molars and premolars must be accomplished with the Pendulum, and there was also more potential for adverse vertical effects caused by the molar tipping.[42] Unfortunately, the action of the Pendulum is also not self-limiting, unlike the Distal Jet appliance, and unattended use may produce adverse effects. In contrast, the Distal Jet produced no significant increase in vertical dimension (no molar extrusion, no change in mandibular or occlusal plane angles, no undesirable change in lower anterior face height), even for patients who initially presented with more obtuse mandibular plane angles.[42]

Timing of treatment

Most recommendations for the timing of distalization have been to treat "earlier," before the eruption of the second molars.[51,55,57] In the mixed dentition, less anchorage loss reportedly is produced because there are only the two first permanent molars to push distally.

The opposite response was found for the Distal Jet; namely, that waiting to treat until at least partial eruption of the second molars has occurred is a slight advantage.[15,58] No greater anchorage loss appeared to occur, and there was less adverse tipping of the first molar, because the center of resistance of the molar was moved occlusally when it was "braced" against the erupting second molar (Fig. 11-4). Graber[59] reported the same effect when using the cervical headgear for distalizing.

If the contribution of greater amounts of molar tipping (when second molars are unerupted) were included in calculations of efficiency in studies examining other distalizing devices, similar conclusions (e.g., starting treatment later) may have been attributed to these devices as well.[55]

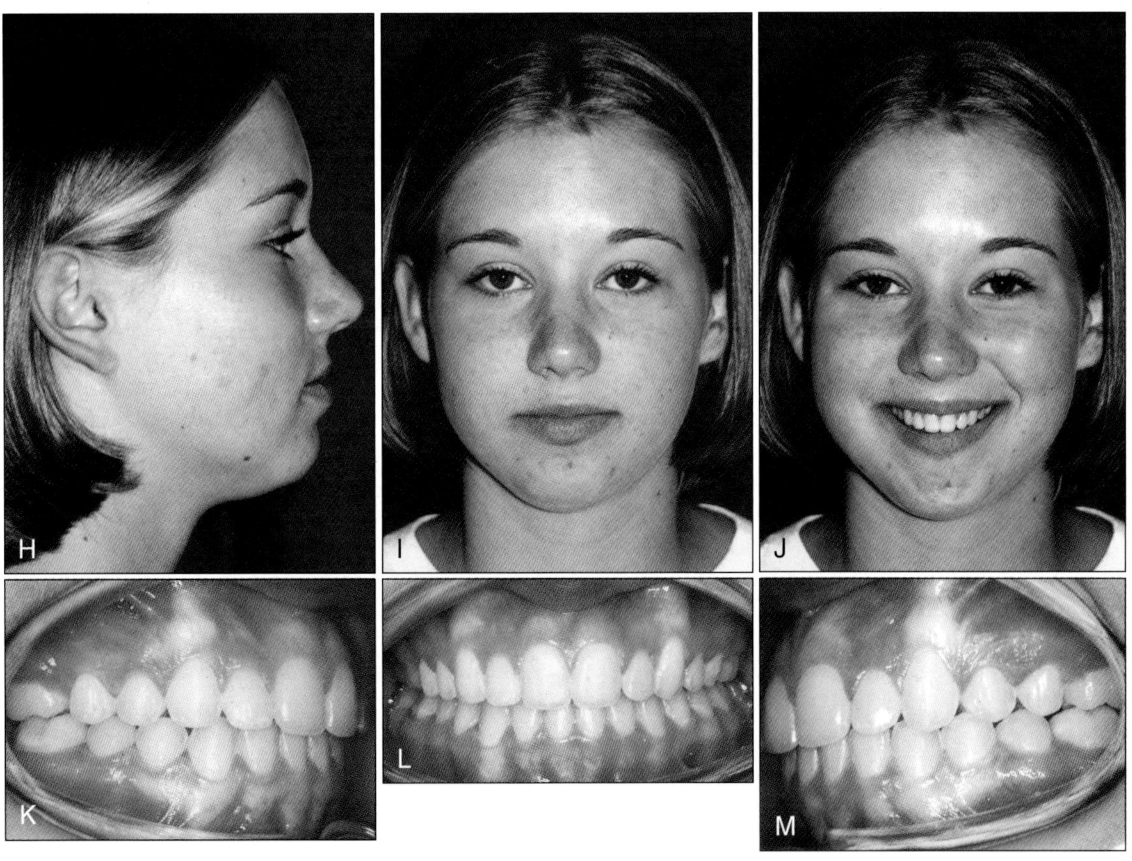

Fig. 11-2, cont'd **H** to **M,** Final facial (**H-J**) and intraoral (**K-M**) photographs. Total treatment time was 25 months.

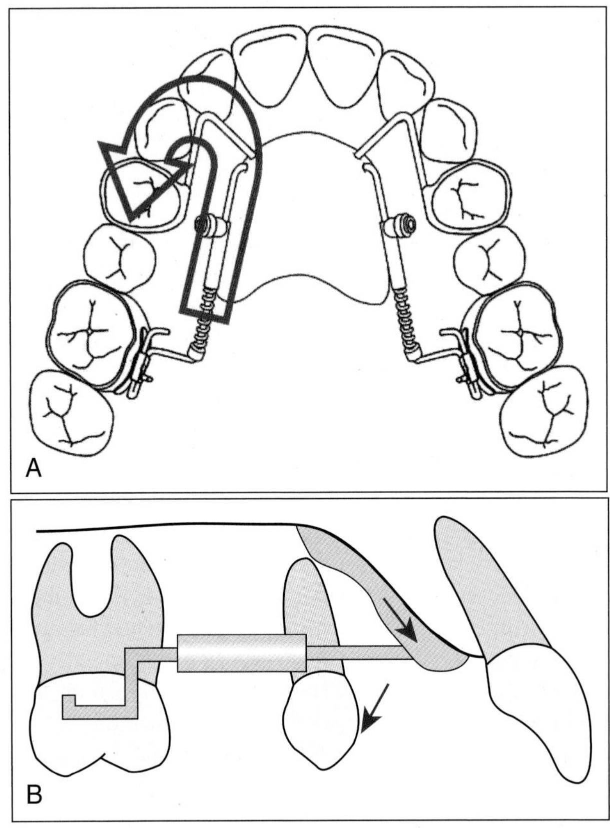

Fig. 11-3 **A** and **B,** In contrast to other molar distalizers, Distal Jet tends to produce distal tipping of the maxillary first premolars due to forces pushing the acrylic button up the slope of the premaxilla; rotating the premolars distally.

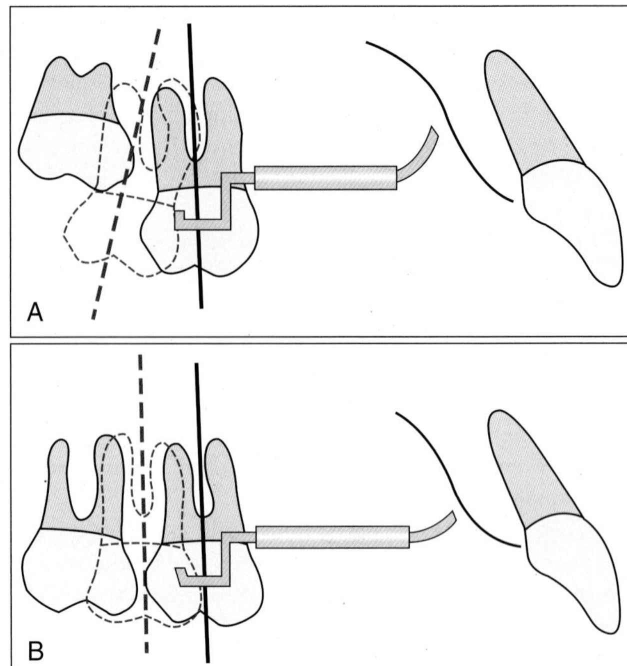

Fig. 11-4 **A,** When second molars are unerupted (early treatment with Distal Jet), there is a tendency for more molar tipping. The first molar "trips" over the unerupted second molar as the center of resistance is moved apically. Although more space may appear to be produced (implying more effective distalization), subsequent uprighting of the molars is required. **B,** There are similar amounts of distal molar movement and anchorage loss when the second molars are partially or totally erupted. The first molar is "braced" against the second molar, moving the center of resistance more inferiorly, thereby, producing less molar tipping.

Molar rotation and expansion

Lemons and Holmes[60] reported that a majority of patients with Class II malocclusions exhibit maxillary first molars that are rotated mesially around the palatal root. In other words, the palatal root may be in a normal, Class I position despite giving the clinical appearance of Class II when the first molar is viewed from the buccal surface. The implication is that, in some cases, simply producing a distal rotation of the molar will produce a Class I molar relationship for many patients.

Molar distalizing appliances that produce forces on the lingual surfaces of the upper molars (Distal Jet, Pendulum, GMD)[43] may produce additional inappropriate mesial rotation. A simple preventive solution has been described for the Distal Jet.[15,38] Before delivering the device, a utility pliers is used to bend the double-back wire (inserted into lingual sheath on maxillary first molar band) to produce a distal molar counterrotation (Fig. 11-5), similar to the bend described by McNamara and Brudon[61] for adjusting transpalatal arches. In this manner, the Distal Jet may produce some corrective molar rotation before or during concurrent molar distalization. Also, most preadjusted appliance prescriptions have some degree of corrective molar rotation built into them as well.

Some degree of maxillary expansion reportedly is required for the correction of Class II malocclusions.[17,35] Unfortunately, this implies that some type of active palatal expansion is required in the treatment of Class II, when in the absence of posterior crossbite, separating the midpalatal suture is not a prerequisite.[27] Although the Pendulum requires a jackscrew to counteract the adverse constriction of molars that it produces, the Distal Jet yields an average of 3 to 4 mm of expansion (across the molars without a jackscrew) simply because of the divergent nature of its construction[15,41-43] (Fig. 11-6).

FIXED FUNCTIONAL APPLIANCES

Orthopedic change, most often attributed only to functional appliances, is an undeniably important factor of Class II correction for the growing patient. Mandibular protraction or advancement is the one feature that is common to all functional appliances. Johnston[62] described this jaw advancement as "taking out an installment loan" against future growth. Holding the mandible forward is the assumption of that loan, while eventual condylar growth and

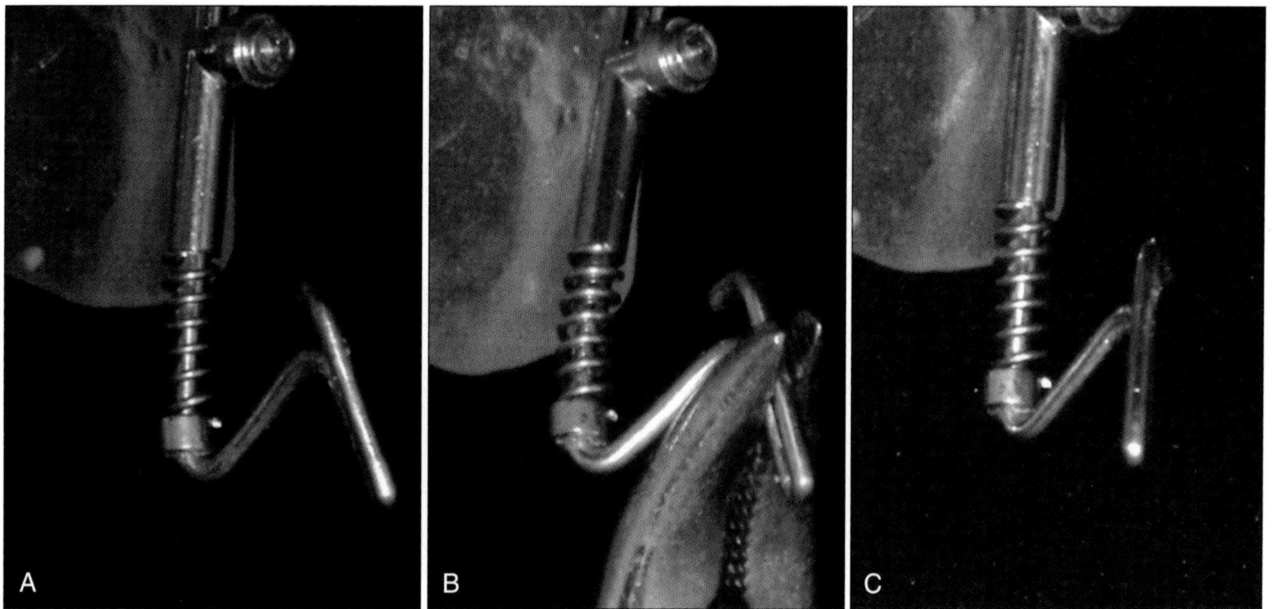

Fig. 11-5 Before seating Distal Jet, double-back portion of its bayonet wire (**A**) (inserted into lingual sheath on first molar band) may be bent with a utility pliers (**B**) (toe-in) to counteract the mesial rotation of the maxillary molar during distalization (**C**).

remodeling "pays back" the loan over time. Fixed functional appliances, such as the Herbst (Dentaurum, Ispringen, Germany)[63] or Jasper Jumpers (American Orthodontics, Sheboygan, Wis.),[64] are able to produce mandibular protraction independent of patient compliance.

Variations of the Herbst have proliferated, as has its popularity as the functional appliance of choice by an increasing number of specialists. This once stimulated the recommendation that "100% of orthodontists should think about using the Herbst,"[65] despite the concerns for significant clinical problems (discomfort, restriction of function, breakage, laboratory repairs).[66]

Herbst-type treatment effects, including both benefits and advantages, have been thoroughly reported (e.g., Herbst,[63,67-72] Jasper Jumper[28,73-75]). It appears that fixed functional mechanics are less ideal when used prior to the late mixed dentition because of a significant relapse potential.[63] Even in the permanent dentition, the Herbst appliance unfortunately requires either a two-stage system or, at best, a compromise in edgewise mechanics during its application.[17,76]

Auxiliary appliances, designed to mimic the Herbst, have the versatility of being added to traditional edgewise mechanics (e.g., Adjustable Bite Corrector [Ortho Plus Inc., Santa Rosa, Calif.], Twin Force Bite Corrector [Ortho Organizers, Carlsbad, Calif.], Eureka Spring [Eureka Spring Inc., San Luis Obispo, Calif., MALU [Saga Dental Supply AIS, Kongsvinger, Norway], Forsus [3M Unitek, Monrovia, Calif.], Jasper Jumpers, Millennium Distal Mover [American Orthodontics GmbH, Lemgo, Germany]). Consequently, it might be preferable to add a fixed functional auxiliary to augment a single phase of traditional appliance mechanotherapy.

Regrettably, all fixed functional devices also tend to produce adverse labial flaring of mandibular incisors.[77,78] This may result in a detrimental effect in lower lip eversion or profile fullness, a reduction in the amount of possible mandibular advancement, and inherent instability. Although both Herbst and Jasper Jumpers are subject to breakage, repair of Jasper Jumpers is a short clinical procedure that requires no laboratory procedures and is therefore more akin to "changing a flat tire" than an "overhaul of the transmission" process common with Herbst repairs.

COMPARING MOLAR DISTALIZERS WITH FIXED FUNCTIONAL APPLIANCES

When the effects of pushing upper molars back were compared with treatments that advance the mandible, the results were surprisingly similar.[79] In other words, methods to effect change in one jaw (distalizing maxillary molars) tended to produce the same final results as methods designed to protract the mandible (Herbst appliance). However, some might say, "You're treating the wrong jaw," with devices applied to the maxilla (cervical headgears, distalizers, Class II intermaxillary elastics). They may insist that some type of growth modification device or FJO is required to resolve the problem of the "small mandible."

When samples of patients treated with either molar distalization or fixed functional appliance were compared, the amount of mandibular growth contributing to the

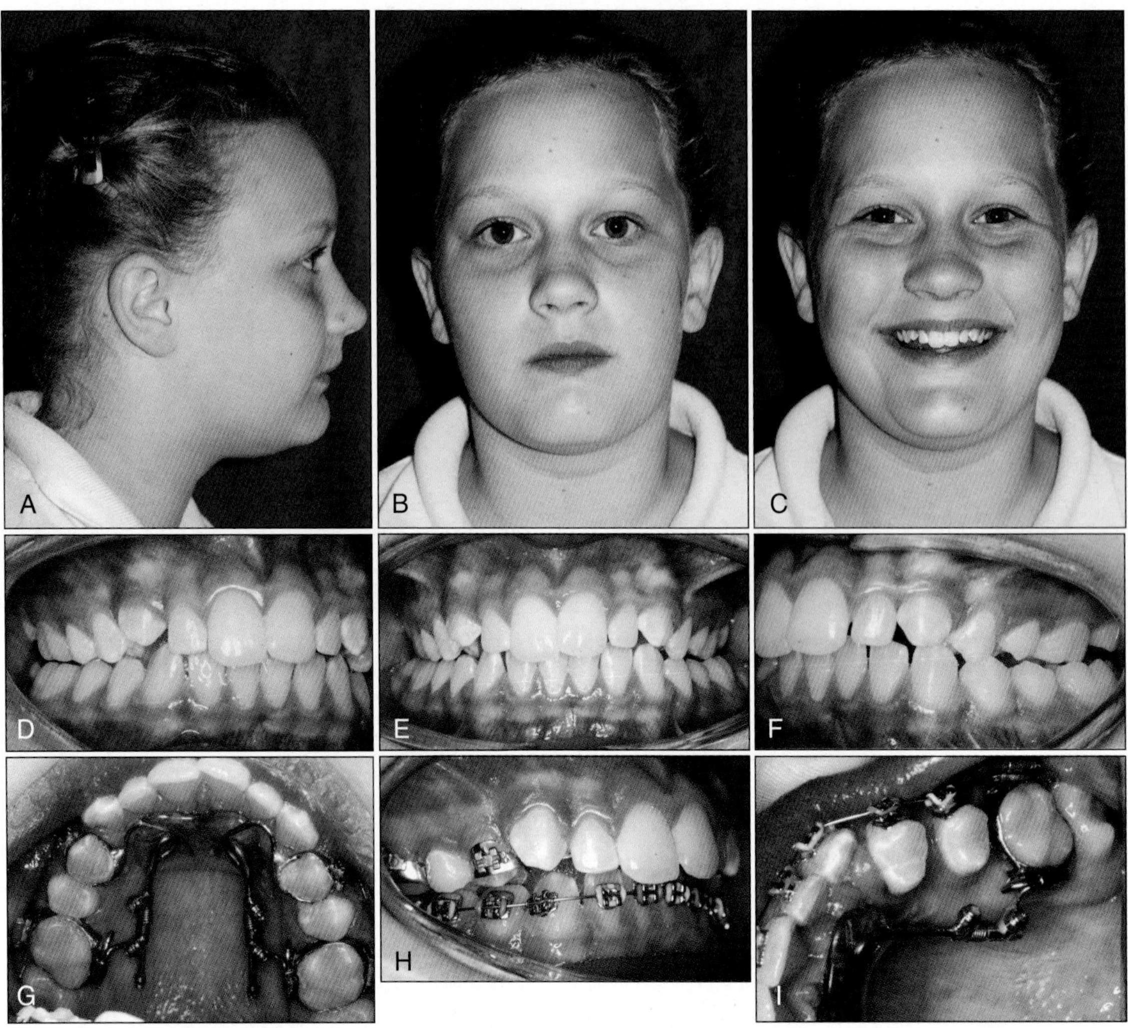

Fig. 11-6 Treatment was initiated for 11-year-old girl with Class II malocclusion with posterior crossbite. Pretreatment facial (**A-C**) and intraoral (**D-F**) photographs. **G** to **I,** Molar distalization with Bowman Modification was accomplished in 6 months while the lower teeth were also leveled and aligned. The crossbites were resolved because of molar expansion inherent to the divergent nature of the appliance design. No active palatal expansion was required. Maxillary preadjusted (Butterfly System[97]) appliances were added after Bowman Modification was converted into a modified Nance holding arch. Jasper Jumpers supported 4 months of anterior space closure.

correction of the Class II discrepancy was found to be the same.[79] Although growth and tooth movement are both important aspects of correction, the interruption of dentoalveolar compensation may be the real key to the resolution of Class II, at least for growing patients. Therefore, if maxillary molars are moved distally, there appears to be some interruption of this compensation mechanism, wherein mandibular growth can also contribute to the correction of the skeletal difference, similar to that produced by holding the mandible forward with a bite-jumping device.

Watson[80] correctly noted that, for distalization, much of the actual Class II "correction came during the final phase of fixed appliance therapy with headgear, mandibular repositioning appliances, and Class II elastics." This is also true when fixed functional appliances are utilized as the primary corrective device; the mandible is held forward for a period of time by the device; it is released (or retained with some type of "bite orthotic"); and then solid intercuspation (accentuated with intermaxillary elastics) is maintained until condylar growth "catches up."[62] This type of concern led directly to the combined use of both mechanisms (distalization and functional) for some patients.

Unfortunately, both molar distalization and fixed functional appliances have the side effect of anchorage loss, mesial reciprocal movement of upper anteriors (distalizers), or mesial flaring of lower anteriors (fixed functionals). The recent advent of temporary anchorage devices (TADs) or miniscrews may help to limit those concerns.[15,81-86]

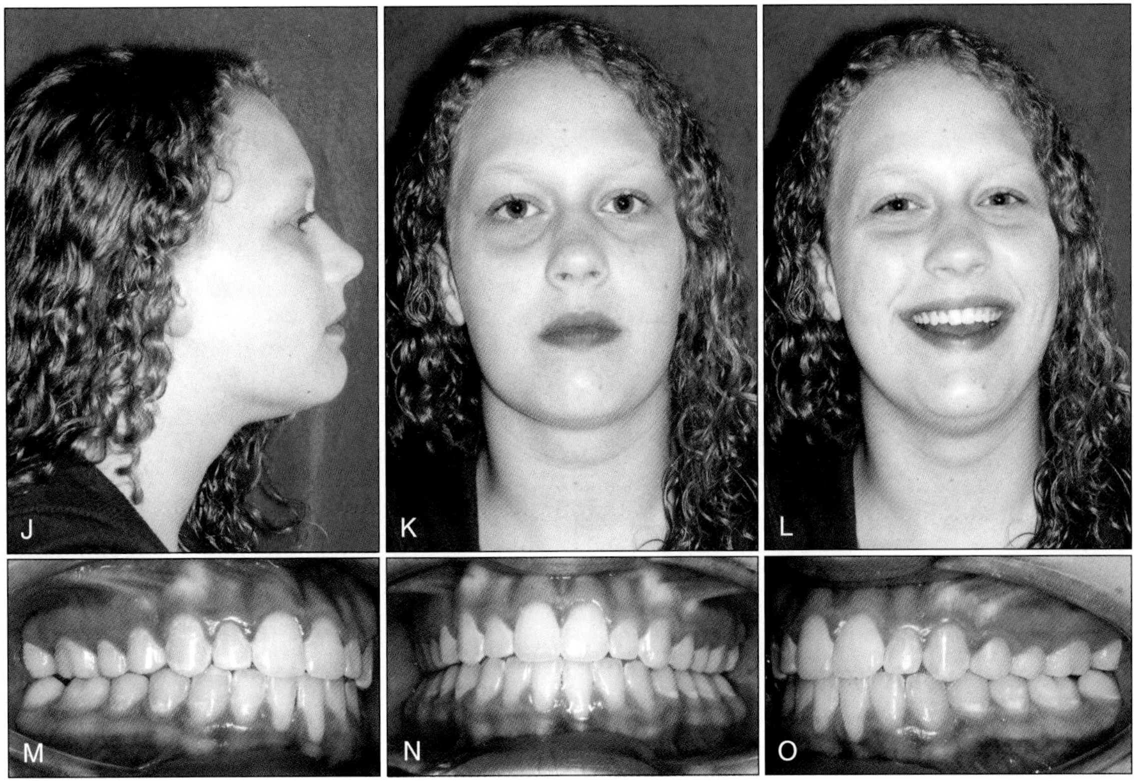

Fig. 11-6, cont'd **J** to **O**, Limited compliance (several missed appointments with long period of inactivity) extended treatment to 34 months. Note the favorable facial changes (**J-L**). Anterior mucogingival defect will require periodontal graft.

ADDING MINISCREW ANCHORAGE

Improving anchorage support for either molar distalization or mandibular advancement may assist in reducing the iatrogenic effects of each. The inclusion of TADs—miniscrews inserted into the alveolar bone and attached to existing force systems—appears to be a relatively simple way to improve the predictability of these mechanics.[15,81-86]

Initial attempts of using miniscrews with the Distal Jet focused on placing the implants in the anterior palate as part of the construction of the device[83] (Fig. 11-7). Unfortunately, the bone adjacent to the midsagittal suture is not ideal (especially for adolescents), and although there are no roots to contend with, the persistent, intermittent forces from the tongue, consistently "worrying" the implant, may contribute to more frequent failure of the miniscrew. In addition, when miniscrews are designed to be integral to the construction of any device, it is a concern. Failure (i.e., loosening caused by periimplant inflammation) may not be easily discerned when the screw is part of the appliance. If the miniscrew must be removed, often a new distalizing appliance must fabricated; it is probably not desirable to place another miniscrew immediately into the same, failed site. To help avoid these concerns, the TAD may be placed posterior to the appliance and tied to it with a stainless steel ligature wire (Fig. 11-7, *C*). In this arrangement, the screw is independent from appliance construction, its retention can be easily evaluated, and the screw can be removed and replaced without fabricating a new device.

Inserting miniscrew implants in the interradicular space between the maxillary first molar and second premolar or between the two premolars, either on the buccal or lingual surface (Fig. 11-7, *D*) of the alveolus, is another option.[15,81,82,84] The TADs are then connected to attachments on the first premolars to resist anchorage loss from reciprocal forces of the Distal Jet appliance. Unfortunately, after the completion of distal molar movement, the miniscrews often need to be removed and possibly placed in another location (e.g., between first and second molar or just mesial to the distalized first molar) to avoid interference from the miniscrew with the roots of the second premolars during retraction of the remaining maxillary teeth.

Another alternative is to place the TADs in the infrazygomatic crest, apical to the buccal roots of the maxillary first molar. Although buccal access provides more direct visualization for the insertion of the miniscrew, precise positioning to avoid the root apices could be required. Furthermore, the miniscrew will often need to be inserted into the buccal mucosa instead of the attached gingival margin. This may occasionally require a "stab" incision (to avoid winding tissue around threads of screw) and the possibility of more tissue irritation, discomfort, and mucosal overgrowth of the screw in the buccal vestibule. In this case, surgical exposure would be required for later removal of the screw.

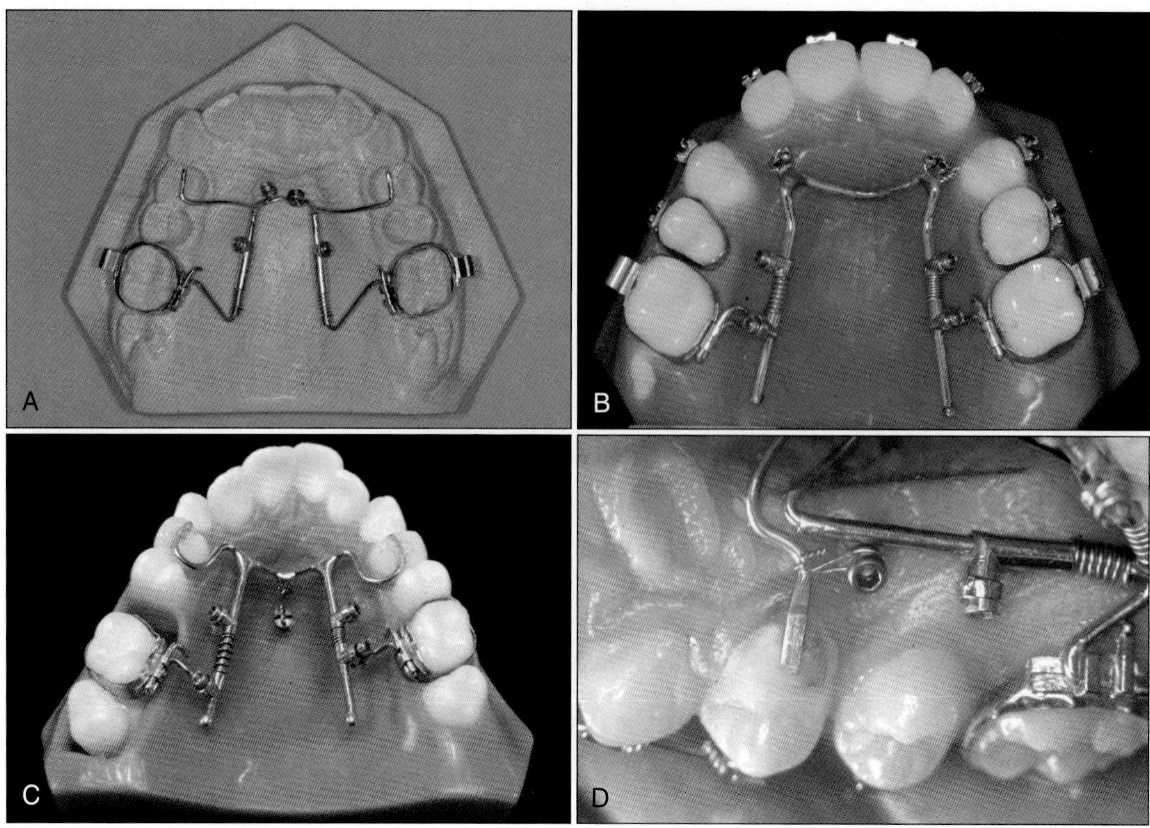

Fig. 11-7 **A,** Modified Distal Jet abutted against two temporary anchorage device (TAD) miniscrews inserted adjacent to midpalatal suture. Light-cured adhesive can be applied over the heads of the screws and the wire for stability. **B,** Bowman Modification with two TADs inserted, between canines and first premolars. **C,** Bowman Modification with TAD inserted adjacent to midpalatal suture. TAD is tied with stainless steel ligature to the appliance for anchorage support. **D,** Alternative site for TAD placement is in palatal alveolus between the maxillary first and second premolars. (**A** courtesy Dr. Gero Kinzinger; **D** courtesy Dr. Stefano Velo.)

Anka[87] suggests that a more favorable TAD insertion point may be on the palatal side of the alveolar ridge, between the maxillary first molars and second premolars. If the screw is angled occusally (30-45 degrees from perpendicular) to the sloping surface of the alveolus (Fig. 11-8), sufficient thickness of cortical bone has been found: from 1.7 ± 0.5 mm to 2.2 ± 0.4 mm for adults.[88] In an anecdotal examination of a series of adolescent patients presenting for tomographic evaluation, Sonis[89] also noted a similar amount of cortical bone (~1.7 mm) present in the adolescent group of patients, who would most often benefit from this method of Class II treatment.

The root of the maxillary second premolar is most often angled buccally, and the first molar has only one (more distally positioned) palatal root, resulting in the following (Fig. 11-8, *B-D*):

- There is less potential for iatrogenic damage from screw insertion because substantial space exists between the roots of these two teeth.
- A miniscrew can be inserted more distally, closer to palatal root (farther from second premolar root).
- The second premolar root is more likely to miss the lingually positioned miniscrew during its spontaneous distal movement (from the effects of transseptal fibers) and subsequent retraction.

In other words, the screw may not need to be removed after distalization of the molars, the premolars may move posteriorly on their own, and the remaining teeth then retracted using support from the same original screws.

The attached gingiva on the lingual alveolus is also more favorable than on the buccal surface, and the Distal Jet pieces help to protect or block the TADs from intermittent forces from the tongue, although concern for oral hygiene is still paramount. Note that this version of the Distal Jet appliance (Horseshoe Jet) completely relies on the TADs for anchorage (i.e., there are no premolar support wires or acrylic button). Therefore, if a TAD fails, it must be replaced, or no distalization will occur. Because there is more favorable bone/attached gingiva and less likelihood of touching a root at this insertion point, a lower incidence of TAD failure may result as well.

In terms of anesthesia, only a profound topical anesthetic (e.g., 20% TAC Alternate or EMLA), and in some patients infiltration with a typical dental anesthetic, is required for insertion of the screws. This is in contrast to the often painful incisive foramen injection required for anterior palate placement of TADs or the more difficult access when placing screws in the midpalate or anterior palate.

The Horseshoe Jet eliminates the acrylic Nance button by tying the anchoring TADs to hooks on the horseshoe-shaped tracking wire using stainless steel ligature wire (see Fig. 11-8, *A*). In this manner, TAD-supported anchorage from the Horseshoe Jet is available during both molar distalization and subsequent retraction of the remaining maxillary teeth. Simply locking the distal lock on the tracking wire stops the active distalization process (open-coil spring is not removed). Retraction of the remaining maxillary dentition is then maintained by indirect anchorage (first molars) from the TAD-supported Horseshoe Jet tracking wire. One screw-anchored appliance serves both purposes.

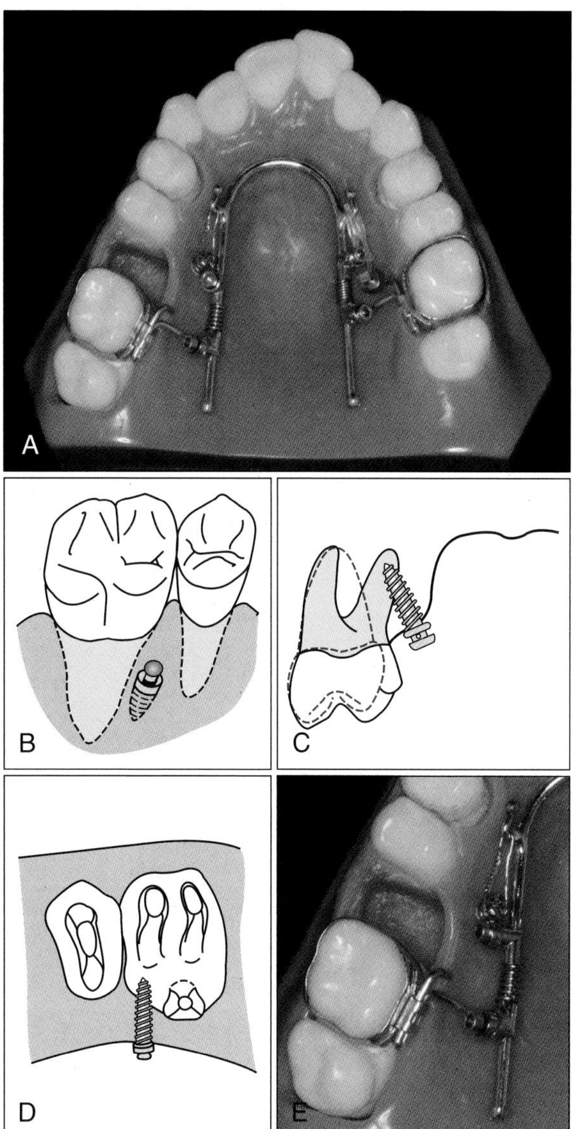

Fig. 11-8 **A,** Horseshoe Jet is supported by two TADs inserted on the lingual slope of the maxillary alveolus, tied with stainless steel ligatures to hooks on the tracking wire. **B,** The miniscrews are inserted at an angle to the alveolus. **C** and **D,** Because the root of the second premolar is angled buccally and the first molar has only one palatal root, there is less concern for iatrogenic damage to the roots when inserting the implants and during subsequent retraction of the second premolar. **E,** During distalization, the mesial locking collar may be rotated buccally and abutted against the distal of the TAD or can be simply tied with stainless steel ligature or elastic ties. Once molar distalization is complete, the distal hex screw is locked, and now the device serves as TAD-supported anchorage for retraction of the remaining upper teeth.

CLASS II COMBINATION THERAPY

The concept of Class II combination therapy[10] incorporates mechanics that require less patient cooperation with the intent of improving the predictability in completing Class II treatment. The technique combines orthodontics and orthopedic effects, performed in a single phase of fixed appliance therapy.[9-15]

Class II combination therapy starts with maxillary molar distalization (e.g., Distal Jet), occasionally followed by fixed functional auxiliaries (e.g., Jasper Jumpers) and/or Class II elastics. After maxillary molars are moved distally, a Nance holding arch is placed (or simply converted from Distal Jet)[38] from the first molars and braced against the anterior palate. Jasper Jumpers or other fixed functional auxiliaries are occasionally added for additional anchorage support to the maxillary first molars during subsequent retraction of the remaining dentition, while any potential orthopedic benefits are derived as well.

Stage I

Conservative space management in the late mixed dentition sets the stage. A mandibular lingual arch may be required to maintain mandibular first molar position. In at least 75% of crowded mixed-dentition patients (with favorable facial profiles), the leeway or transitional "E" space can be used to resolve mandibular anterior crowding of 3 to 4 mm,[90] with favorable stability[91] and without inherent unstable arch development or expansion[92,93] (Fig. 11-9).

Full-fixed appliances are placed in the lower arch to initiate this one-stage comprehensive care. A molar distalization device (e.g., Distal Jet) is fabricated and delivered for the upper arch.[38,45] The activation collars of the Distal Jet are unlocked, moved distal to compress superelastic coil springs, and then locked to hold this activation. This process is repeated every 5 to 6 weeks until a "super" Class I or overcorrected molar relationship is achieved.[17,57] Mandibular leveling and alignment are done concurrently during the maxillary distalization process so that a full-dimension archwire is in place by the time either Class II elastics or Jasper

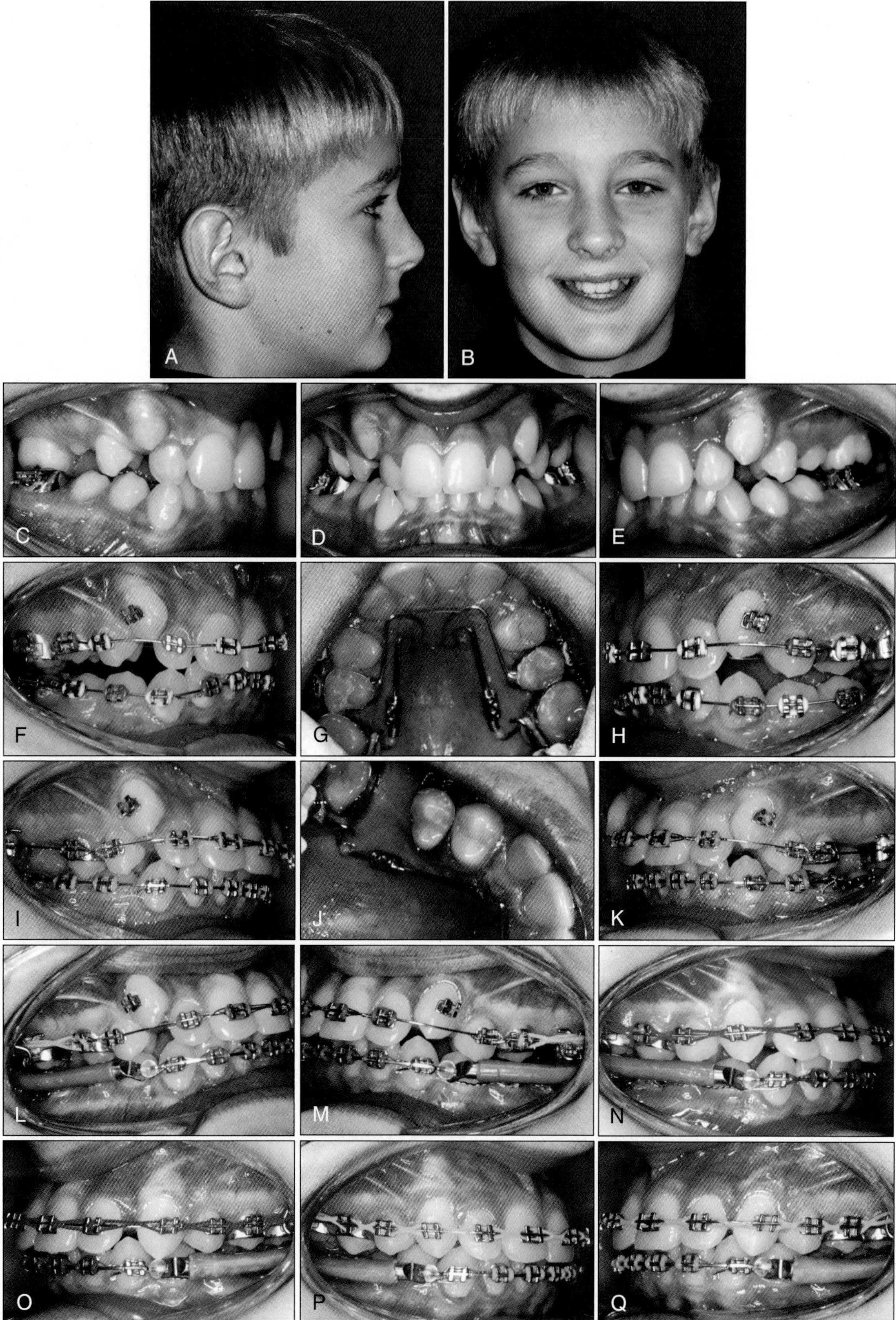

Fig. 11-9 Treatment was initiated for 12-year-old boy whose compliance, especially with oral hygiene, was an issue. Pretreatment facial (**A** and **B**) and intraoral (**C-E**) photographs. **F** to **H,** Preadjusted appliance was placed during distalization using Distal Jet. **I** to **K,** After overcorrection into a "super" Class I molar relationship in 7 months (note space produced between molars and premolars), Distal Jet was converted into a modified Nance holding arch. **L** and **M,** To ensure maintenance of the new upper molar position, fixed functional appliances (Jasper Jumpers) were installed onto a mandibular, full-size, rectangular archwire. **N** to **Q,** Sliding mechanics were used to close the remaining maxillary spaces.

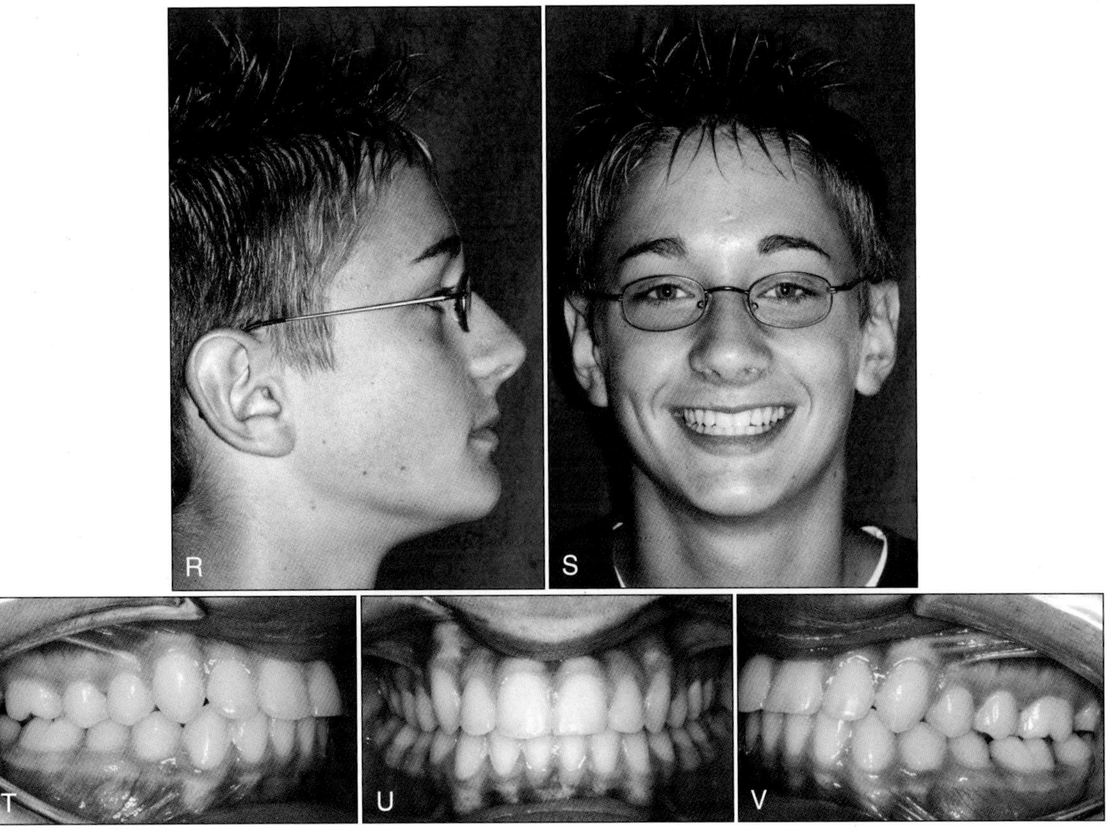

Fig. 11-9, cont'd **R** to **V**, Posttreatment facial (**R** and **S**) and intraoral (**T-V**) photographs. Treatment was completed in 30 months.

Jumpers might be used to help maintain the new, distal position of the maxillary molars.

As an option, short, Class II intermaxillary elastics may be added to brackets or bonded buttons on the maxillary first premolars to help reduce anchorage loss. Side effects must be considered in this arrangement (extrusion of upper premolars and lower molars, loss of mandibular anchorage or incisor flaring), and the results are compliance dependent (Fig. 11-10).

Stage II

The new distal position of the maxillary molars is maintained by a Nance holding arch, fabricated from the molars to the anterior palate.[10,15,38] An advantage of the Distal Jet appliance is that this device can also be converted to a modified Nance intraorally (i.e., one device serves two purposes).[45] Once the molars have been moved distally, the superelastic springs are removed using Weingardt pliers. The activation collars are slid distal to the "stop" on the bayonet wire and locked in place to help prevent mesial migration of the molars. The supporting wires from the acrylic palatal button to the premolars are then sectioned using a crosscut bur in a high-speed handpiece (Fig. 11-11).

Stage III

If needed, fixed functional auxiliaries (e.g., Jasper Jumpers) are added[10,94,95] to help maintain the maxillary molar position during subsequent retraction of the remaining maxillary teeth (using sectional,[96] sliding, or closed-loop mechanics[9,10-12,15]) and may provide an orthopedic effect (Fig. 11-12). Typically, fixed functional appliances may be required only if distalization was incomplete (e.g., broken distalizer), overjet increase was substantial (poor anchorage control), additional molar correction is desired, or poor patient compliance with intermaxillary elastics is anticipated.

One or more of the following options may assist in preventing the potential for iatrogenic labial tipping of the mandibular incisors inherent with fixed functionals[77,78]:

- A mandibular lingual arch and/or, full-dimension archwire with lingual crown torque for the anterior teeth.[57]
- From 5 to 10 degrees of lingual crown torque incorporated into the prescription for the anterior brackets (e.g., Butterfly System[97]).
- A torquing auxiliary, with uprighting springs added to cuspid bracket vertical slots to push the crowns distally.
- Previously prepared (Tweed) anchorage.
- J-hook headgear applied to the mandible.

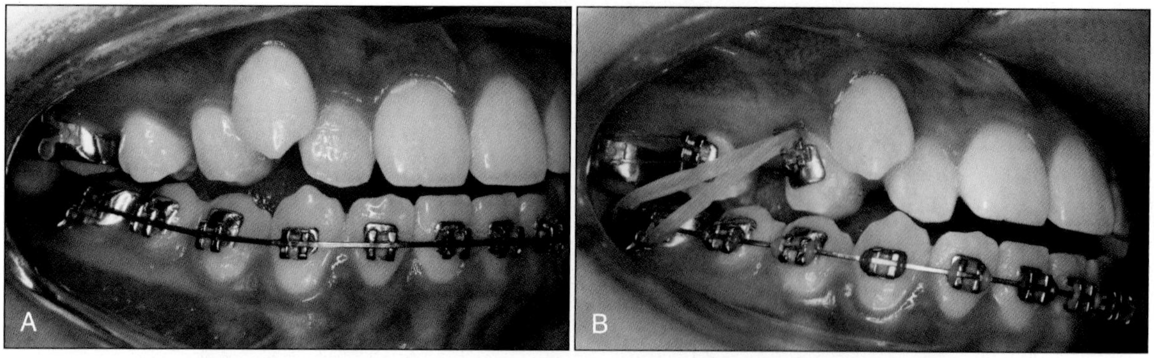

Fig. 11-10 **A** and **B,** Optional support from Class II intermaxillary elastics can be added to reduce anchorage loss during distalization with Distal Jet. Elastics are worn from brackets or buttons bonded onto the maxillary first premolars.

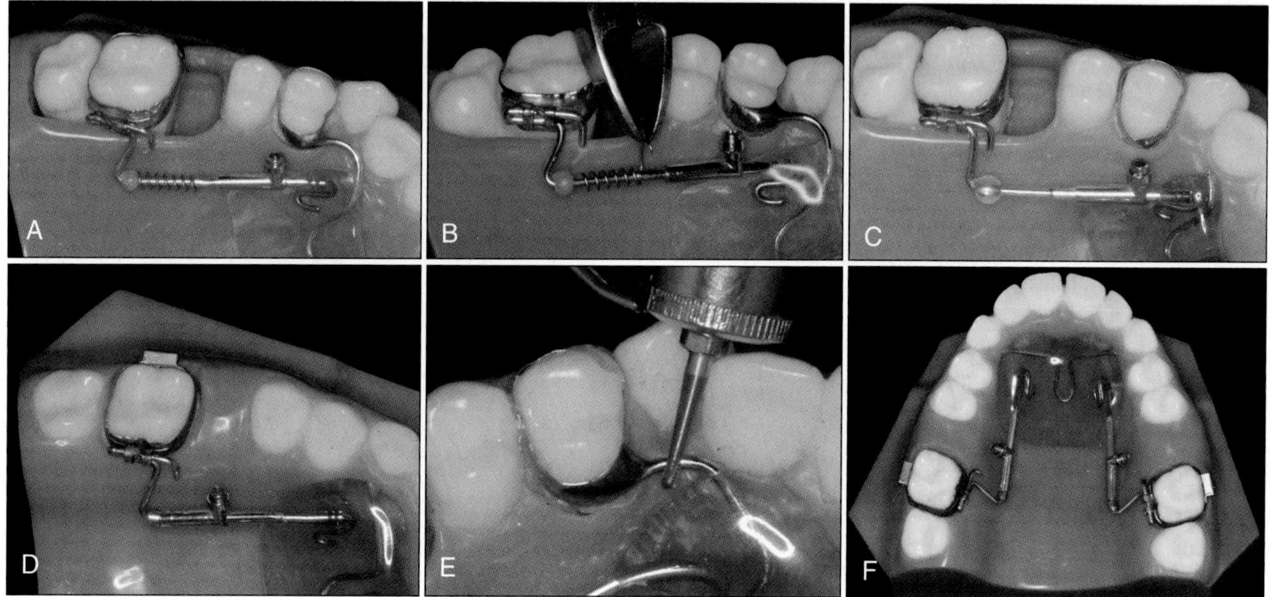

Fig. 11-11 **A,** After molar distalization is complete, activation collar on Distal Jet is unlocked and moved mesially. **B** and **C,** Superelastic coil spring is removed. **D,** Collar is then moved back to the stop on the bayonet wire, and a hex screw is locked onto the tube. **E,** The premolar supporting wires are sectioned adjacent to the palatal acrylic button using a cross-cut fissure bur in a high-speed handpiece. **F,** Completed conversion to a modified Nance holding arch.

- Lip bumper (e.g., Bumper Jumper[10]) or TADs (miniscrews) placed for support in the mandibular alveolus.

As the maxillary molar position is maintained, the premolars are permitted to "drift" distally from the effects of transseptal fibers,[32] or are actively retracted[10,96] using sectional[96] or full-arch sliding mechanics[12] or even bypassing the retraction of cuspids and premolars with a utility arch[10] ("floating back"[17]). This is followed by closed-loop or sliding mechanics to close the remaining anterior space.[10] Unfortunately, friction and "poking" terminal wire ends (that create painful patient emergencies) may plague sliding mechanics.

Approximately 4 to 6 months is required to achieve complete maxillary space closure and to derive any orthopedic benefits before Jasper Jumpers and/or Class II elastics are completely discontinued. It is important that solid intercuspation be maintained (e.g., delta or triangle intermaxillary elastics) to hold the Class I occlusion to avoid relapse during the finalization of treatment. Second molars are subsequently bracketed, followed by cusp seating, artistic positioning wire bends and repositioning of brackets, and other finishing procedures.

Treatment times for patients receiving Class II combination therapy have been reported to average 26 months,[40]

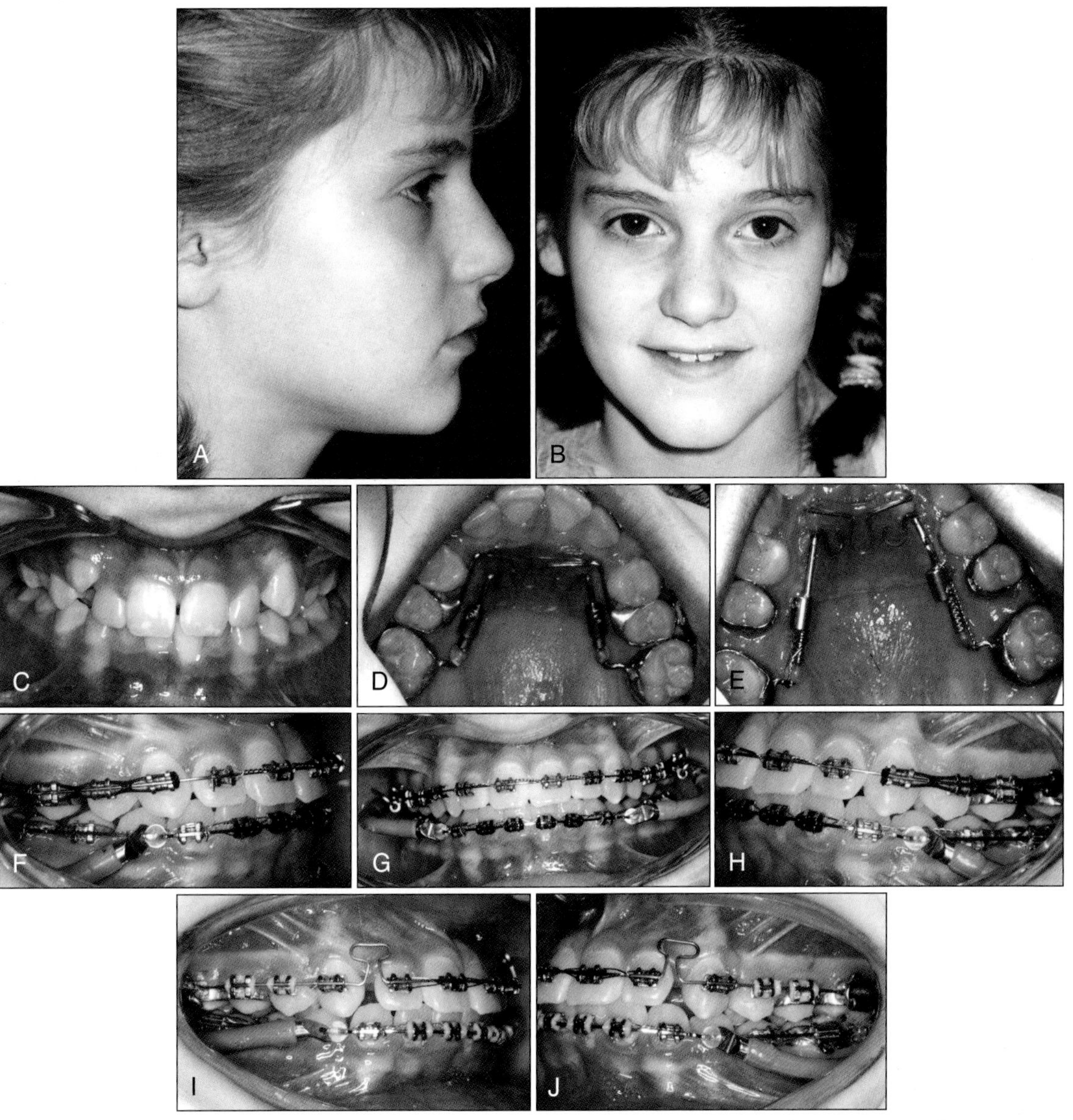

Fig. 11-12 Treatment was initiated for 12-year-old girl who was treated with original version of the Distal Jet and preadjusted appliances. Pretreatment facial (**A** and **B**) and intraoral (**C**) photographs. **D** and **E,** Molar distalization was completed in 5 months, and device was converted into a modified Nance holding arch. **F** to **J,** Subsequent retraction of remaining upper teeth was accomplished in 6 months (supported by Jasper Jumpers). Treatment was completed in 19 months.

Continued

shorter (by about 4 months) than for patients treated with a Herbst or Pendulum appliance[79] in a typical two-stage treatment.[98] These treatment times are also comparable to a sample of mixed-extraction/nonextraction patients treated with Damon "self-ligated" brackets examined at Temple University (25 months),[99] those treated with conventionally ligated brackets (23 months;[100] 23 months[101]), and two samples of consecutively treated patients using the author's Butterfly System[97] (N = 323, 25 months; N = 295, 25 months).[102]

Perhaps with the addition of miniscrew anchorage (TADs), Class II combination therapy will be accomplished with (1) less anchorage loss during molar distalization, (2) more predictability for the treatment of some adult patients, (3) less need for a fixed functional appliance for postdistal-

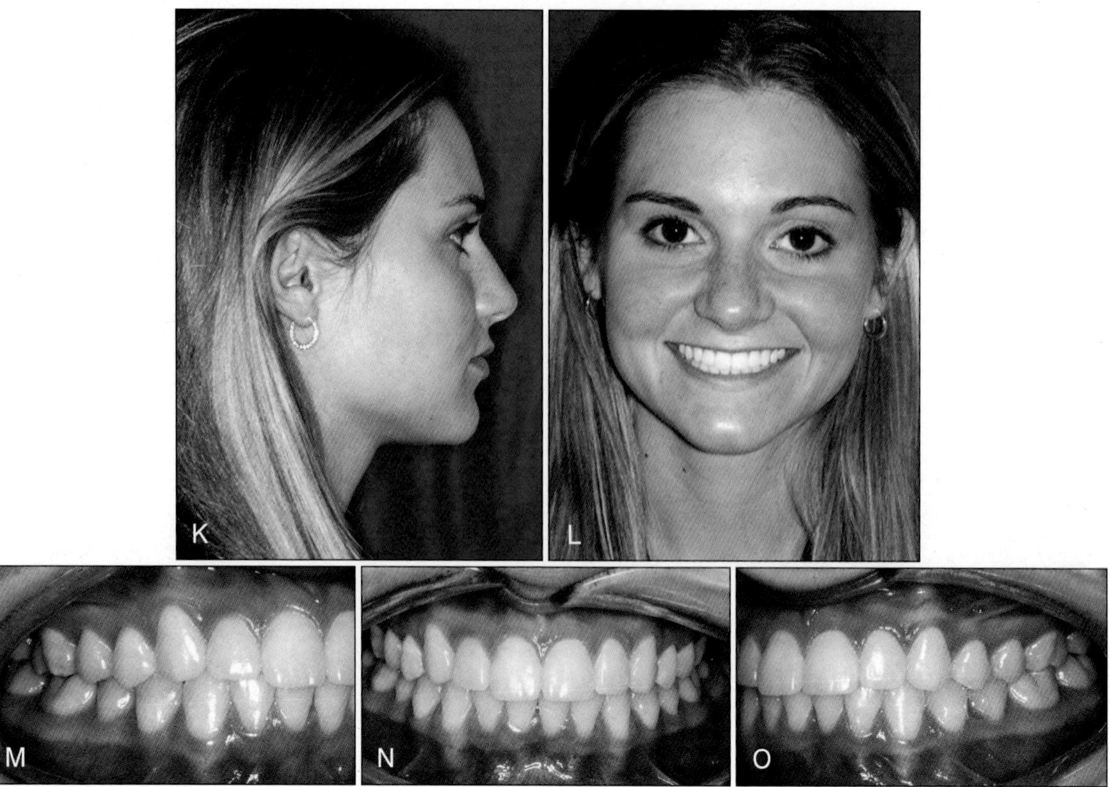

Fig. 11-12, cont'd **K** to **O,** Facial (**K** and **L**) and intraoral (**M-O**) photographs show the results 6 years after completion of treatment.

ization anchorage support, and (4) shorter treatment times.[103]

Bowman Modification

An alternate laboratory modification of the Distal Jet, the Bowman Modification (Fig. 11-13), simplifies appliance construction, insertion, and eventual conversion to a modified Nance holding arch. The tube/piston portion of the original Distal Jet design is replaced with a more rigid, solid tracking wire. The double-back bayonet wire is laser-welded to a second activation collar, with the locking screw angled toward the lingual cusp of the first molar to permit easy intraoral access for the hex wrench. Occlusal rests may be bonded with light-cured flowable composite on first premolars, rather than using the typical supporting arms that are soldered to first premolar bands. These bonded occlusal rests also provide some bite opening to facilitate initial distalization.

To activate the Bowman Modification, the distal hex screw (located in the collar, laser-welded to the bayonet wire, which is inserted into the lingual sheath of the first band) is loosened one-quarter turn (counterclockwise) to permit distal translation of the molar. The mesial activation collar is then moved back to compress the superelastic open-coil spring, and the hex screw is locked down on the tracking wire to maintain this activation (Figs. 11-14 and 11-15).

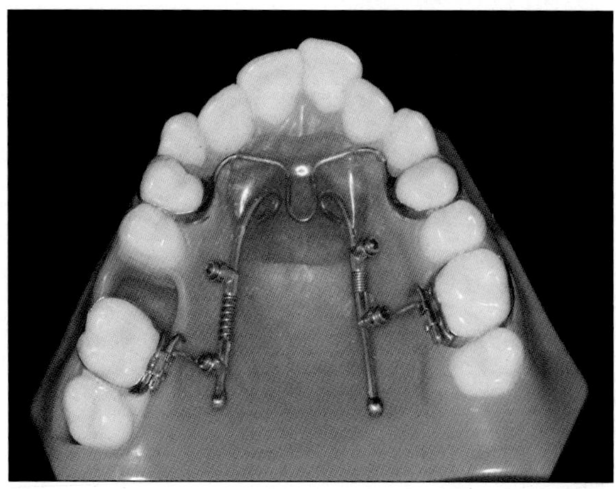

Fig. 11-13 Bowman Modification is a laboratory modification of Distal Jet. The tube and piston of the original design are replaced with a solid tracking wire. Anchorage support from an acrylic palatal button and transpalatal support arms are soldered to bands or constructed to occlusal rests, bonded with light-cured adhesive, onto the first premolars. The simplified and more rigid construction is easier to seat, and device is self-limiting.

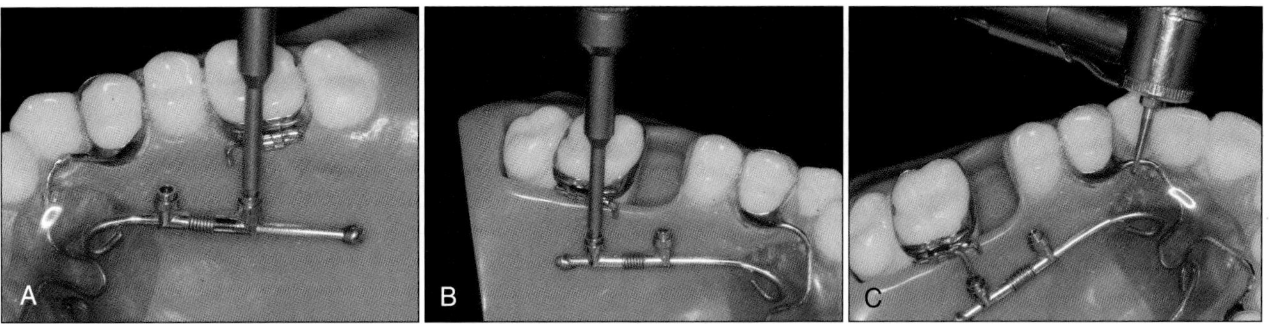

Fig. 11-14 **A,** To begin distal molar movement with Bowman Modification, the posterior hex screw is loosened one-quarter turn clockwise. The anterior activation collar is pushed back to compress the superelastic coil spring and the hex screw locked onto the tracking wire. **B,** Only after achieving a Class I molar relationship is the posterior hex screw locked down onto the tracking wire. Double hex screws prevent movement of the molar. **C,** The premolar supporting wires are sectioned adjacent to the palatal acrylic button. Note that the superelastic coil springs are not removed. The resulting holding arch is more rigid because there is no tube/piston.

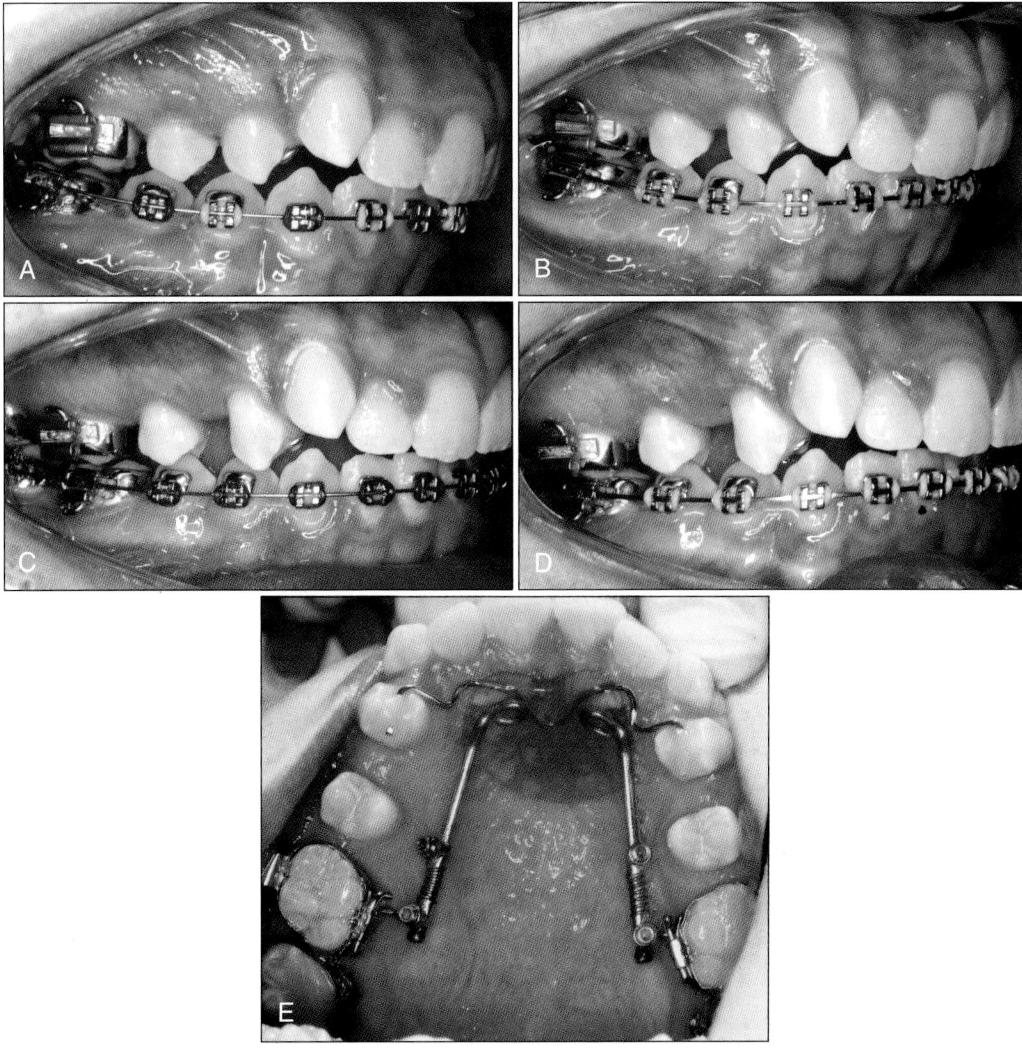

Fig. 11-15 **A,** Bowman Modification used with lower fixed appliances (Butterfly System[97]) for 13-year-old patient with Class II malocclusion. Note that bonded occlusal rests function as a bite plane. **B** to **E,** Little anchorage loss noted when molar distalization is accomplished in 8 months without upper braces. Lower dentition is leveled and aligned by the completion of distalization.

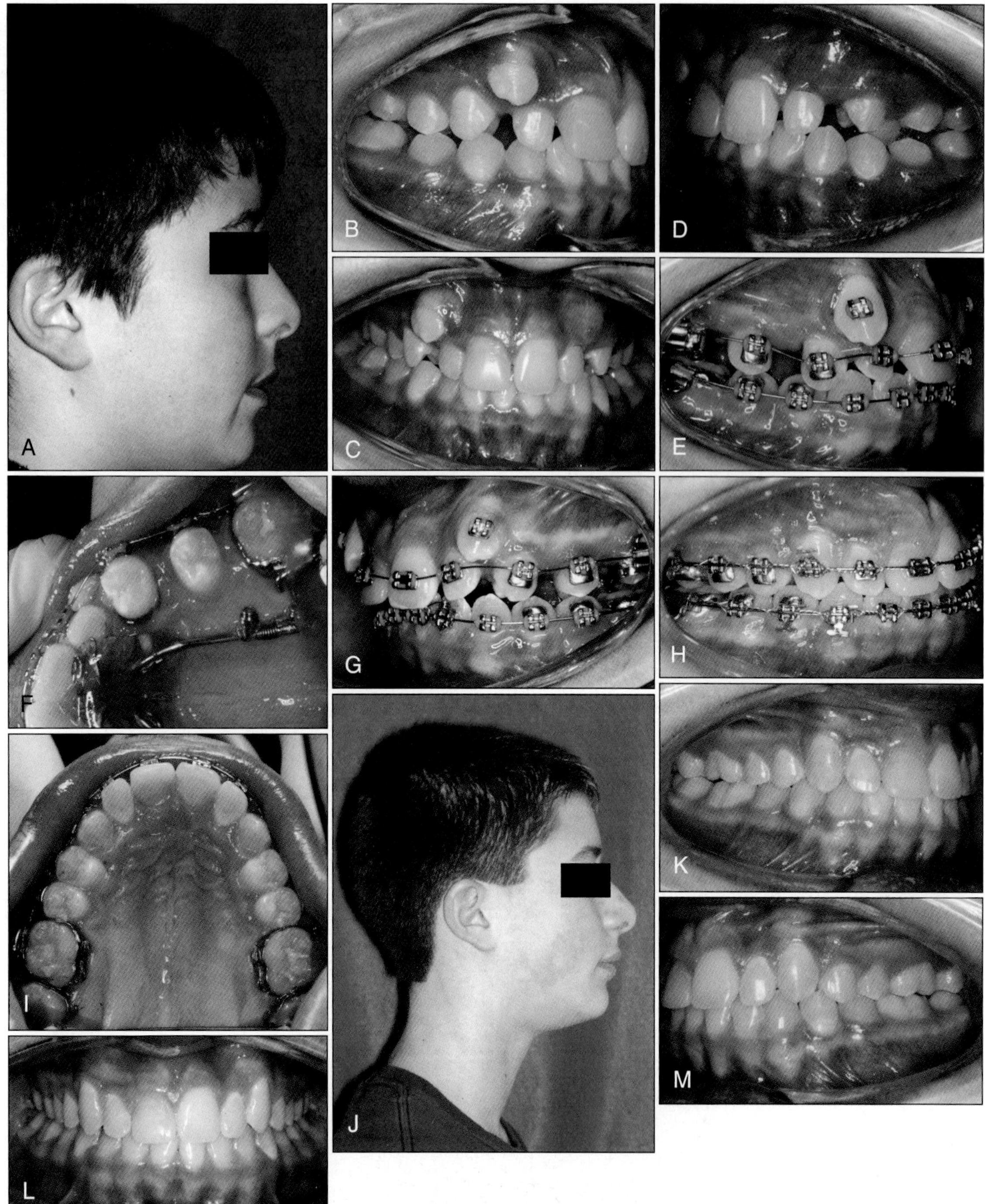

Fig. 11-16 A 12-year-old boy with a mild Class II molar relationship, significant maxillary discrepancy, and favorable facial profile. Pretreatment facial (**A**) and intraoral (**B-D**) photographs. Treatment initiated with Bowman Modification and mandibular preadjusted appliances. **E** to **I,** At the completion of molar distalization, the hex screws were locked and the premolar supporting wires sectioned at the acrylic button. Maxillary braces were placed and space consolidation accomplished. **J** to **M,** Posttreatment facial (**J**) and intraoral (**K-M**) photographs. Total treatment completed in 24 months. Extraction of maxillary first premolars could be considered a viable treatment alternative in this type of situation.

Only when sufficient molar distalization has been achieved is the distal hex screw locked onto the tracking wire. Next, the supporting arms to the first premolars are sectioned, at the acrylic button, with a crosscut fissure bur in a high-speed handpiece using water-spray cooling. Maxillary preadjusted brackets may now be placed (Fig. 11-16 and 11-17; see also Fig. 11-13.)

In contrast to the standard Distal Jet, the Bowman Modification construction has the following advantages:

- More rigid
- Not subject to separation at the tube/piston parts of the original appliance
- Double-locked to hold the new molar position
- Designed so that the coil spring does not have to be removed

CONCLUSION

Class II combination therapy is an adjunct to traditional fixed appliances in an attempt to reduce dependency on unpredictable patient compliance and to complete treatment in a timely and consistent manner.

ACKNOWLEDGMENT

This chapter is dedicated to Dr. Aldo Carano, one of the developers of the Distal Jet appliance. He was a friend, colleague, and collaborator and will be sorely missed.

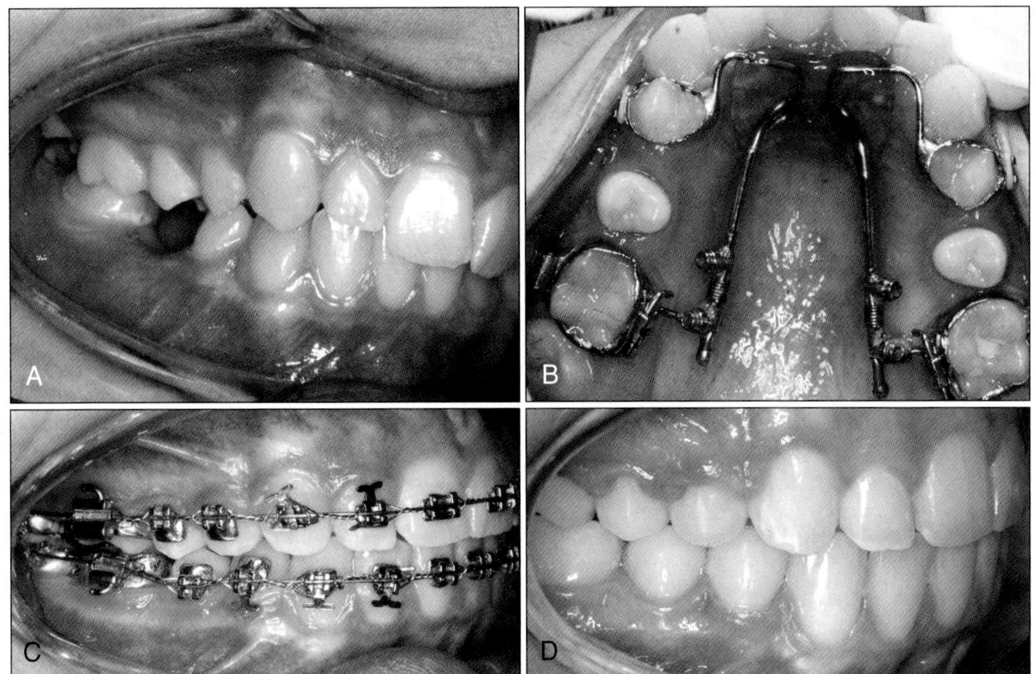

Fig. 11-17 **A,** Intraoral photo of 13-year-old patient who was treated at the point of exfoliation of mandibular second primary molars. **B,** Adequate molar distalization achieved in 7 months using Bowman Modification. Concurrent leveling and aligning of the lower teeth was achieved with a preadjusted appliance. **C,** Device was then converted into a modified Nance holding arch by simply locking the distal hex screw and sectioning the premolar support wires. Retraction of remaining maxillary teeth was accomplished using sliding mechanics, supported with intermaxillary elastics (no fixed functional appliances were used). **D,** Treatment was completed in 26 months.

References

1. Koltun A, Stone GC: Past and current trends in patient noncompliance research: focus on diseases, regimes-programs, and provider-disciplines, *J Compl Health Care* 1:21-32, 1986.
2. Sahm G, Bartsch A, Witt E: Reliability of patient reports on compliance, *Eur J Orthod* 12:438-446, 1990.
3. Sinha PK, Nanda RS, McNeil DW: Perceived orthodontist behaviors that predict patient satisfaction, orthodontist-patient relationship, and patient adherence in orthodontic treatment, *Am J Orthod Dentofacial Orthop* 110:370-377, 1996.
4. Behrents RG: Iatrogenic problems associated with the clinical practice of orthodontics. In McNamara JA Jr, Trotman C, editors: *Orthodontic treatment: the management of unfavorable sequelae*, Monograph 31, Craniofacial Growth Series, Ann Arbor, 1996, Center for Human Growth and Development, University of Michigan, pp 1-28.
5. Nanda RS, Kieri MJ: Prediction of cooperation in orthodontic treatment, *Am J Orthod Dentofacial Orthop* 102:15-21, 1992.
6. Cureton SL, Regennitter FJ, Yancy JM: Clinical versus quantitative assessment of headgear compliance, *Am J Orthod Dentofacial Orthop* 104:277-284, 1993.
7. Sahm G, Bartsch A, Witt E: Micro-electronic monitoring of functional appliance wear, *Eur J Orthod* 12:297-301, 1990.
8. Tulloch JFC, Proffit WR, Phillips C: Influence on the outcome of early treatment for Class II malocclusion, *Am J Orthod Dentofacial Orthop* 111:533-542, 1997.
9. Bowman SJ: Class II correction and orthodontics for the noncompliant patient, *Gutta Percha Clarion,* Kalamazoo Valley District Dental Society Newsletter, Spring 1993, pp 13-17.
10. Bowman SJ: Class II combination therapy: molar distalization and fixed functionals to reduce reliance upon compliance for predictable case completion, *J Clin Orthod* 32:611-620, 1998.
11. Bowman SJ: Class II combination therapy: a case report, *J Orthod* 27:213-218, 2000.
12. Bowman SJ: Alternatives after molar distalization, *Am Orthod Good Pract* 1:2-3, 2000.
13. Bowman SJ: The Distal Jet appliance: Class II correction by maxillary molar distalization, *Belgisch Tijdschrift Orthod* 3:65-72, 2002.
14. Bowman SJ: Distalizacion molar y aparatos fijos funcionales: combinación de terapia de Clase II, *Colegio Cirujanos Dent* 1:36-39, 2004.
15. Carano A, Bowman S: Non-compliance Class II treatment with the Distal Jet. In Papadopoulos MA, editor: *Orthodontic treatment for the Class II noncompliant patient: current principles and techniques,* Edinburgh, 2006, Elsevier, pp 265-289.
16. Bowman SJ: Scar tactic: fluoride varnishes to reduce decalcification stains in orthodontic patients, *Orthod Prod,* March 2002, pp 32-35.
17. Hilgers JJ: The era of hyper-efficient orthodontics, Ann Arbor, September 1997, University of Michigan (seminar).
18. McNamara JA Jr: Components of Class II malocclusion in children 8-10 years of age, *Angle Orthod* 51:177-202, 1981.
19. Gottlieb EL, Nelson AH, Vogels II: 1990 study of orthodontic diagnosis and treatment procedures. Part 2, *J Clin Orthod* 25:223-230, 1991.
20. Liveratos FA, Johnston LE Jr: A comparison of one-stage and two-stage nonextraction alternatives in matched Class II samples, *Am J Orthod Dentofacial Orthop* 108:118-131, 1995.
21. Gianelly AA: One- versus two-phase treatment, *Am J Orthod Dentofacial Orthop* 108:556-559, 1995.
22. Bowman SJ: One-stage versus two-stage treatment: are two really necessary? *Am J Orthod Dentofacial Orthop* 113:111-116, 1998.
23. Nance HN: The limitations of orthodontic treatment. I. Mixed dentition: diagnosis and treatment, *Am J Orthod* 33:177-233, 1947.
24. Johnston LE Jr: A comparative analysis of Class II treatment methods. In McNamara JA Jr, Carlson DS, Vig PS, Ribbens KA, editors: *Science and clinical judgment in orthodontics,* Monograph 19, Craniofacial Growth Series, Ann Arbor, 1986, University of Michigan, pp 103-148.
25. Barton S, Cook PA: Predicting functional appliance treatment outcome in Class II malocclusions: a review, *Am J Orthod Dentofacial Orthop* 112:282-286, 1997.
26. McNamara JA Jr: Long-term adaptations to changes in transverse dimension in juveniles and adolescents. When to treat? Making decisions: a symposium on early treatment, American Association of Orthodontists Early Treatment Symposium, Las Vegas, January 2005.
27. Gianelly AA: Rapid palatal expansion in the absence of crossbites: added value? *Am J Orthod Dentofacial Orthop* 124:362-365, 2003.
28. Weiland FJ, Ingervall B, Bantleon HP, Droschl H: Initial effects of treatment of Class II malocclusion with the Herren activator, activator-headgear combination, and Jasper Jumper, *Am J Orthod Dentofacial Orthop* 112:19-27, 1997.
29. Keeling SD, King GJ, Wheeler TT, McGorry S: Timing of Class II treatment: rationale, methods, and early results of an ongoing randomized clinical trial. In Trotman C, McNamara JA Jr, editors: *Orthodontic treatment outcome and effectiveness,* Monograph 30, Craniofacial Growth Series, Ann Arbor, 1995, University of Michigan, pp 81-112.
30. Roth R: Personal communication.
31. Witzig JW, Spahl TJ. In *The clinical management of basic maxillofacial orthopedic appliances.* Vol I. *Mechanics,* Littleton, Mass, 1987, PSG Publishing, pp 236-238.
32. Cetlin NM, Ten Hoeve A: Nonextraction treatment, *J Clin Orthod* 17:396-413, 1996.
33. Gianelly AA, Vaitas AS, Thomas WM: The use of magnets to move molars distally, *Am J Orthod Dentofacial Orthop* 96:161-167, 1989.
34. Locatelli R, Bednar J, Deitz VS, Gianelly AA: Molar distalization with superelastics NiTi wire, *J Clin Orthod* 26:277-279, 1992.
35. Hilgers JJ: The Pendulum appliance for Class II noncompliance therapy, *J Clin Orthod* 26:700-713, 1992.
36. Jones R, White J: Rapid Class II molar correction with an open-coil jig, *J Clin Orthod* 26:661-664, 1992.
37. Carano A, Testa M: The Distal Jet for upper molar distalization, *J Clin Orthod* 30:374-380, 1996.
38. Bowman SJ: Modifications of the Distal Jet, *J Clin Orthod* 32:549-556, 1998.
39. Patel AN. Analysis of the Distal Jet appliance for maxillary molar distalization, Oklahoma City, 1999, University of Oklahoma (master's thesis).

40. Ngantung V, Nanda R, Bowman S: Post-treatment evaluation of the Distal Jet appliance, *Am J Orthod Dentofacial Orthop* 120:178-185, 2001.
41. Huerter G: A retrospective evaluation of maxillary molar distalization with the Distal Jet appliance, St Louis, 2000, Center for Advanced Dental Education, Saint Louis University (master's thesis).
42. Bolla E, Muratore F, Carano A, Bowman S: Evaluation of maxillary molar distalization with the Distal Jet, *Angle Orthod* 72:481-494, 2002.
43. Ferguson DJ, Carano A, Bowman SJ, et al: A comparison of two maxillary molar distalizing appliances with the Distal Jet, *World J Orthod* 6:382-390, 2005.
44. Chiu PP, McNamara JA Jr, Franchi L: A comparison of two intraoral molar distalization appliances: Distal Jet versus Pendulum, *Am J Orthod Dentofacial Orthop* 128:353-365, 2005.
45. Carano A, Testa M, Bowman S: The Distal Jet: simplified and updated, *J Clin Orthod* 36:586-590, 2002.
46. Guiterrez VME: Treatment effects of the Distal Jet appliance with and without edgewise therapy, St Louis, 2001, Center for Advanced Dental Education, Saint Louis University (master's thesis).
47. Bowman CJ: Molar distalization: what method produces the least amount of flaring of the front teeth? Kalamazoo, Mich, 2003, Kalamazoo Academy (sixth-grade science project).
48. Ghosh J, Nanda RS: Evaluation of an intraoral maxillary molar distalization technique, *Am J Orthod Dentofacial Orthop* 110:639-646, 1996.
49. Chaqués-Asensi J, Kalra V: Effects of the Pendulum appliance on the dentofacial complex, *J Clin Orthop* 35:254-257, 2001.
50. Byloff FK, Darendeliler MA: Distal molar movement using the Pendulum appliance. Part I. Clinical and radiological evaluation, *Angle Orthod* 67:249-260, 1997.
51. Bussick TJ, McNamara JA Jr: Dentoalveolar and skeletal changes associated with the Pendulum appliance, *Am J Orthod Dentofacial Orthop* 177:333-343, 2000.
52. Kinzinger G, Wehrbein H, Diedrich P: Molar distalization with a modified Pendulum appliance: in vitro analysis of the force systems and an in vivo study in children and adolescents, *Angle Orthod* 75:484-493, 2005.
53. Runge ME, Martin JT, Bukai F: Analysis of rapid maxillary molar distal movement without patient cooperation, *Am J Orthod Dentofacial Orthop* 115:153-157, 1999.
54. Brickman CD, Sinha PK, Nanda RS: Evaluation of the Jones Jig appliance for distal molar movement, *Am J Orthod Dentofacial Orthop* 118:526-534, 2000.
55. Kinzinger GSM, Fritz UB, Sander FG, Diedrich RP: Efficiency of a Pendulum appliance for molar distalization with a Pendulum appliance, *Am J Orthod Dentofacial Orthop* 125:8-23, 2004.
56. Papadopoulos MA, Mavropoulos A, Karamouzos A: Cephalometric changes following simultaneous first and second molar distalization using a non-compliance intraoral appliance, *J Orofac Orthop* 65:123-136, 2004.
57. Gianelly AA: *Bidimensional technique: theory and practice,* Islandia, NY, 2000, GAC International.
58. Maginnis JJ: Treatment effects of the Distal Jet with 180 gram and 240 gram springs, St Louis, 2002, Center for Advanced Dental Education, Saint Louis University (master's thesis).
59. Graber TM: Extraoral force-fact and fallacies, *Am J Orthod* 41:490, 1955.
60. Lemons FF, Holmes CW: The problem of the rotated maxillary first permanent molar, *Am J Orthod* 47:246-272, 1961.
61. McNamara JA Jr, Brudon WL: Transpalatal arch. In *Orthodontics and dentofacial orthopedics,* Ann Arbor, Mich, 2001, Needham Press, pp 199-209.
62. Johnston LE Jr: Functional appliances: a mortgage on mandibular position, *Aust Orthod J* 14:154-156, 1996.
63. Pancherz H: The effects, limitations, and long-term dentofacial adaptations to treatment with the Herbst appliance, *Semin Orthod* 3:232-243, 1997.
64. Jasper JJ: Jasper Jumper: a fixed functional appliance, *Am Orthod,* December 1987.
65. McNamara JA Jr: Orthodontics at Michigan Seminar, Ann Arbor, November 1995, University of Michigan.
66. Sanden E, Pancherz H, Hansen K: Complications during Herbst appliance treatment, *J Clin Orthod* 38:130-133, 2004.
67. Franchi L, Baccetti T: Prediction of individual mandibular changes induced by functional jaw orthopedics followed by fixed appliances in Class II patients, *Angle Orthod* 76:950-954, 2006.
68. Popowich K, Nebbe B, Heo G, et al: Predictors for Class II treatment duration, *Am J Orthod Dentofacial Orthop* 127:293-300, 2005.
69. Wieslander L: Long-term effect of treatment with the headgear-Herbst appliance in the early mixed dentition: stability or relapse? *Am J Orthod Dentofacial Orthop* 104:319-329, 1993.
70. Pancherz H, Fäckel U: The skeletofacial growth pattern pre- and post-dentofacial orthopedics: a long-term study of Class II malocclusions treated with the Herbst appliance, *Eur J Orthod* 12:209-218, 1990.
71. Pancherz H: The nature of Class II relapse after Herbst appliance treatment: a cephalometric long-term investigation, *Am J Orthod Dentofacial Orthop* 100:220-233, 1991.
72. Hansen K, Koutsonas TG, Pancherz H: Long-term effects of Herbst treatment on the mandibular incisor segment: a cephalometric and biometric investigation, *Am J Orthod Dentofacial Orthop* 112:92-103, 1997.
73. Nalbantgil D, Arun T, Sayinsu K, Isik F: Skeletal, dental and soft-tissue changes induced by the Jasper Jumper appliance in late adolescence, *Angle Orthod* 75:426-436, 2005.
74. Jasper JJ, McNamara JA Jr: The correction on interarch malocclusions using a fixed force module, *Am J Orthod Dentofacial Orthop* 108:641-650, 1995.
75. May TW, Chada J, Ledoux W, et al: Skeletal and dental changes using a Jasper Jumper, *J Dent Res* (IADR Suppl), 1992.
76. Dischinger T: Edgewise Herbst appliance, *J Clin Orthod* 29:738-742, 1995.
77. Rothenberg J, Campbell ES, Nanda R: Class II correction with the twin force bite corrector, *J Clin Orthod* 38:232-240, 2004.
78. Ruf S, Hansen K, Pancherz H: Does orthodontic proclination of lower incisors in children and adolescents cause gingival recession? *Am J Orthod Dentofacial Orthop* 114:100-106, 1998.
79. Burkhardt DR, McNamara JA Jr, Baccetti T: Maxillary molar distalization or mandibular enhancement: a cephalometric comparison of comprehensive orthodontic treatment including the Pendulum and the Herbst appliances, *Am J Orthod Dentofacial Orthop* 123:108-116, 2003.

80. Watson WG Distal Jet versus Pendulum appliance, *Am J Orthod Dentofacial Orthop* 129:3, 2006 (letter).
81. Velo S, Rotunno E, Cozzani M: The implant Distal Jet, *J Clin Orthod* 41:88-93, 2007.
82. Carano A, Velo S: The miniscrew anchorage system. In Cope J, editor. *OrthoTADs: the clinical guide and atlas,* Dallas, 2007, Under Dog Media, pp 231-243.
83. Kinzinger GSM, Diedrich PR, Bowman SJ: Upper molar distalization with a miniscrew-supported Distal Jet, *J Clin Orthod* 40:672-678, 2006.
84. Bowman SJ: A spike in the ice: altering the extraction decision with mini-screws. 106th American Association of Orthodontists Annual Session, Las Vegas, 2006.
85. Kinzinger G, Wehrbein H, Byloff FK, et al: Innovative anchorage alternatives for molar distalization: an overview, *J Orofac Orthop* 66:397-413, 2005.
86. Chang H, Hsiao H, Tsai C, Roberts WE: Bone-screw anchorage for Pendulum appliances and other fixed mechanics, *Semin Orthod* 12:284-293, 2006.
87. Anka G: Personal communication, 2007.
88. Deguchi T, Nasu M, Murakami K, et al: Quantitative evaluation of cortical bone thickness with computed tomographic scanning for orthodontic implants, *Am J Orthod Dentofacial Orthop* 129:721.e7-e12, 2006.
89. Sonis AL: Unpublished data, 2007.
90. Gianelly AA: Leeway space and the resolution of crowding in the mixed dentition, *Semin Orthod* 1:118-194, 1995.
91. Dugoni SA, Lee JS, Varela J, Dugoni AA: Early mixed dentition treatment: postretention evaluation of stability and relapse, *Angle Orthod* 65:311-320, 1995.
92. Little RM, Reidel RA, Stein A: Mandibular arch length increase during the mixed dentition: Postretention evaluation of stability and relapse, *Am J Orthod Dentofacial Orthop* 97:393-404, 1990.
93. O'Grady PW, McNamara JA Jr: A long-term evaluation of the mandibular Schwartz appliance and the acrylic splint expander in early mixed dentition patients, Ann Arbor, 2003, University of Michigan (master's thesis).
94. Blackwood HO: Clinical management of the Jasper Jumper, *J Clin Orthod* 15:755-760, 1991.
95. Schwindling F: *Jasper Jumper color atlas,* Waldstrasse, Germany, 1997, Edition Schwindling-Zahnarzicher Fachverlag.
96. Bolla E, Doldo T, Giorgetti R: Distal movement of maxillary canines and premolars with sectional mechanics following Distal Jet application to molars, *Prog Orthod* 5:72-89, 2004.
97. Bowman SJ, Carano A: The Butterfly System, *J Clin Orthod* 38:274-287, 2004.
98. Angelieri F, de Almedia RR, Almeida MR, Fuziy A: Dentoalveolar and skeletal changes associated with the Pendulum appliance followed by fixed orthodontic treatment, *Am J Orthod Dentofacial Orthop* 129:520-527, 2006.
99. Eberting JJ, Straja SR, Tuncay CR: Treatment time, outcome, and patient satisfaction comparisons of Damon and conventional brackets, *Clin Orthod Res* 4:228-234, 2001.
100. Fink DF, Smith RJ: The duration of orthodontic treatment, *Am J Orthod Dentofacial Orthop* 102:45-51, 1992.
101. Skidmore KJ, Brook KJ, Thomason WM, Harding WJ: Factors influencing treatment time in orthodontic patients, *Am J Orthod Dentofacial Orthop* 129:230-238, 2006.
102. Bowman SJ: Unpublished data, 2002, 2005.
103. Bowman SJ: Thinking outside the box with mini-screws. In McNamara JA Jr, Ribbens KA, editors: *Microimplants as temporary anchorage in orthodontics,* Monograph 34, Craniofacial Growth Series, Ann Arbor, 2008, University of Michigan.

CHAPTER 12

Maxillary Deficiency Syndrome

James A. McNamara, Jr.

One of the major concepts that has emerged during the author's 40+ years of clinical practice in orthodontics concerns the diagnosis and treatment of what can be termed *maxillary deficiency syndrome.*[1] In fact, maxillary transverse and/or sagittal deficiency may be one of the most pervasive skeletal problems in the craniofacial region, especially in patients of European ancestry. Many of the individual characteristics or symptoms of this condition have been well recognized in orthodontics, but rarely are they combined conceptually. However, it may be possible to produce a greater treatment effect on the skeletal structures of the maxillary complex than in the mandible, particularly with regard to the management of the transverse dimension.

MANIFESTATIONS OF MAXILLARY TRANSVERSE DEFICIENCY

The manifestations of maxillary transverse deficiency are encountered by the orthodontist on a daily basis, but usually they are not quantified. As part of an initial evaluation of a patient, it is recommended that the distance between the closest points of the maxillary first molars (i.e., *transpalatal width*) be measured[2] (Fig. 12-1). Typically, a maxillary arch with a transpalatal width of 35 to 39 mm can accommodate a dentition of average size without crowding or spacing. However, maxillary arches less than 31 mm in transpalatal width may be crowded and thus in need of orthopedic expansion in growing individuals or surgically assisted expansion in adults.[3] Other factors that must be considered when making the extraction/expansion decision include facial type, soft tissue profile, and level of muscle tonus.

Transverse Skeletal Imbalances

A major conceptual leap is from using *rapid maxillary expansion* (RME) in the correction of posterior crossbite to using RME in patients *without crossbite.* Orthodontists traditionally have used RME to correct posterior crossbites, but little else. In contrast to the aggressive approaches often taken in treating skeletally based anteroposterior and vertical problems,[4-8] many orthodontists have been reluctant to change arch dimensions transversely. However, the transverse dimension of the maxilla may be the most adaptable of all the regions of the craniofacial complex. Many, if not most, transverse skeletal imbalances in the maxilla are ignored or simply not recognized, and thus the treatment options for such patients are necessarily more limited than if these imbalances were considered.

Crowding and Protrusion

Other than crossbite, two of the most common problems encountered by the orthodontist are crowding (Fig. 12-2, *A*) and protrusion (Fig. 12-2, *B*) of the teeth, both of which result from discrepancies between the size of the teeth and the size of the bony bases. Howe et al.[3] have shown that dental crowding appears to be related more to a deficiency in arch perimeter than to teeth that are too large. A primary factor in dental crowding often is maxillary transverse and/or sagittal deficiency. If the position of the maxillary dentition reflects the skeletal discrepancy, crossbite results; on the other hand, if maxillary constriction is camouflaged by the dentition, and both dental arches are constricted, crowding in the absence of crossbite is observed.

It is well recognized that one of the limiting factors in the management of tooth-size/arch-size problems is available space in the mandibular dental arch. Unfortunately, true orthopedic expansion of the lower arch is not possible, unless recently developed distraction osteogenesis techniques are used. Interestingly, it has been the author's observation that the position of the mandibular dentition may be influenced more by maxillary skeletal morphology than by the size and shape of the mandible.[9] For example, after RME in the mixed dentition, there is not only expansion of the maxillary dental arch with the acrylic splint expander (Fig. 12-3), but also subsequent spontaneous widening of the lower dental arch in some patients after expansion. In other patients with constricted mandibular dentitions and crowding of the lower incisors, the author often uses a removable lower Schwarz expansion appliance (Fig. 12-4) to upright the lower posterior teeth that have erupted into occlusion in a more lingual orientation because of the associated constricted maxilla. Widening the mandibular dental arch *orthodontically* before expanding the maxilla *orthopedically* allows for greater widening of the maxilla by "decompensating" the positions of the mandibular teeth (Figs. 12-5 and 12-6).

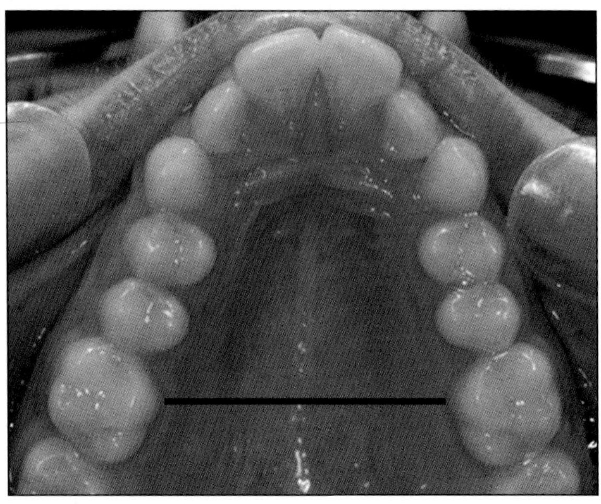

Fig. 12-1 Transpalatal width is measured from the closest points on the lingual surfaces on the maxillary first molars. Normal transpalatal width is 35 to 39 mm in the permanent dentition and 33 to 35 mm in the mixed dentition.

Other Clinical Signs of Maxillary Deficiency

Crossbite and dental crowding are two easily recognizable clinical signs that could be the result of maxillary deficiency. Other effects of maxillary deficiency, however, are not as easily identifiable and often not detected. For example, laterally flared maxillary posterior teeth (Fig. 12-7) may camouflage a maxillary skeletal transverse deficiency. These patients have what appears to be a normal posterior occlusion, although on closer inspection the maxilla is narrow (e.g., intermolar width <31 mm), and the curve of Wilson is accentuated. The lingual cusps of the maxillary posterior teeth extend below the occlusal plane, often leading to balancing interferences during function. Even though there is no crossbite, such patients are candidates for RME before comprehensive edgewise therapy.

Another clinical manifestation of maxillary deficiency is dark spaces at the corner of the mouth (Fig. 12-8). Vanarsdall[10] has used the term "negative space" to refer to the shadows that occur in the corners of the mouth during smiling in some patients having a narrow, tapered maxilla and a mesofacial or brachyfacial skeletal pattern. Regardless of whether teeth are extracted, the maxilla can be widened by means of RME, increasing transpalatal width and eliminating or reducing the dark spaces in the "buccal corridors." This type of orthopedic intervention results in what many consider a more pleasing frontal facial appearance. Using RME for esthetic purposes (e.g., "broadening the smile") will become an increasingly recognized indication for RME in patients with narrow dental arches.

CLASS III MALOCCLUSIONS

It is not surprising that certain types of sagittal malocclusions also are associated with maxillary deficiency. One of the major components of Class III malocclusion is maxillary

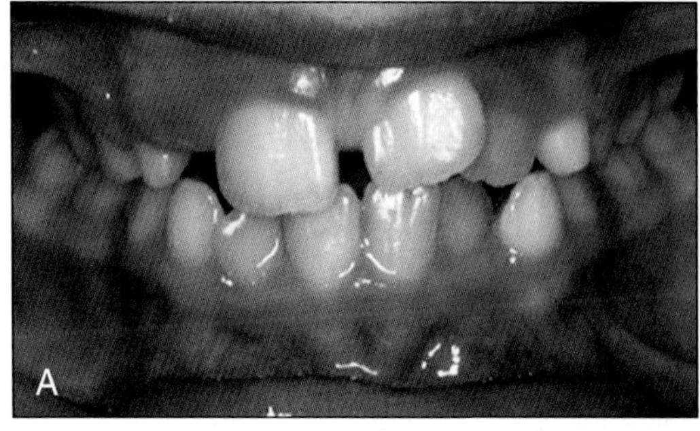

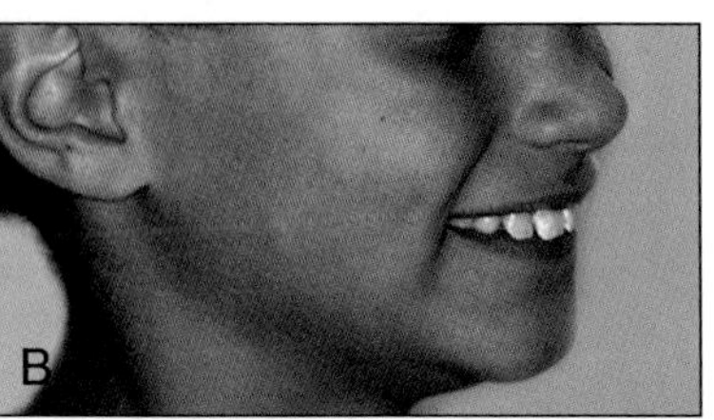

Fig. 12-2 **A,** Crowding is a common observation in mixed-dentition patients. This patient presented with crowded lower incisors and an unerupted upper-right lateral incisor. **B,** Protrusion of the maxillary dentition is evident in this patient.

skeletal retrusion, a condition that occurs in almost half of all Class III patients.[11] The most efficient and effective treatment for Class III problems in the early mixed dentition appears to be RME (Fig. 12-9) combined with the orthopedic facial mask (Fig. 12-10), although the recent utilization of anchor plates and intermaxillary traction by DeClerck[12] shows significant promise in Class III patients with severe anteroposterior problems.

In some mixed-dentition patients with only mild skeletal imbalances, however, simply widening the maxilla without initiating facial mask treatment may lead to a spontaneous correction of anterior crossbite and the resolution of the Class III molar relationship.[13] In patients with more severe problems, modest maxillary skeletal advancement combined with a similar amount of maxillary dentoalveolar advancement can be induced by RME combined with facial mask therapy.[14-16] The most common surgical treatment for this condition in the mature patient at present is the LeFort I osteotomy, a procedure during which the maxilla can be both advanced and widened, instead of reliance on surgical procedures that involve the mandible.

CLASS II MALOCCLUSIONS

Counterintuitively, certain Class II malocclusions also may be associated with maxillary deficiency. From a sagittal perspective, *maxillary skeletal protrusion* occurs only in about 5% to 10% of Class II patients of European ancestry, whereas as many as 30% of Class II patients may have *maxillary skeletal retrusion*, often associated with an obtuse nasolabial angle and a steep mandibular plane angle.[16] Further, many Class II malocclusions, when evaluated clinically, have no obvious maxillary transverse constriction. When the study models of the patient are "hand-articulated" into a Class I canine relationship, however, a unilateral or bilateral crossbite results. In fact, Tollaro et al.[17] have shown that a Class II patient with what appears to be a normal buccolingual relationship of the posterior dentition usually has a 3-mm to 5-mm transverse discrepancy between the maxilla and mandible.

It appears that most Class II malocclusions in mixed-dentition patients are associated with maxillary constriction. When a clinician is initiating treatment in the mixed dentition, the first step in the treatment of mild to moderate Class II malocclusions, characterized at least in part by mild mandibular skeletal retrusion and maxillary constriction (e.g., intermolar width ≤30 mm in the early mixed dentition), should be orthopedic expansion of the maxilla. The maxillary posterior teeth can be left in an overexpanded position, with contact still being maintained between the upper lingual cusps and the buccal cusps of the lower posterior teeth.[2] The occlusion subsequently is stabilized using a removable palatal

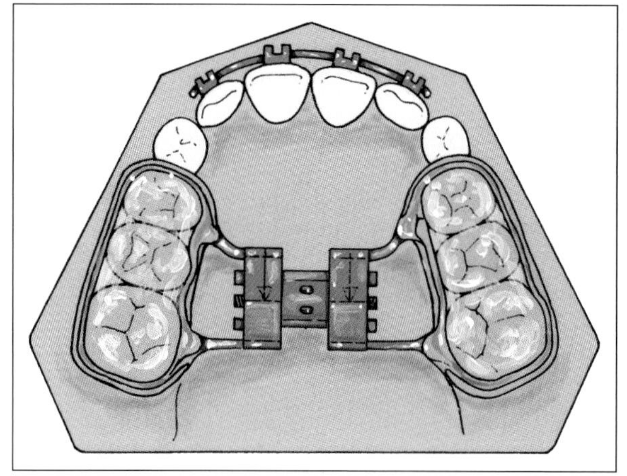

Fig. 12-3 An acrylic splint expander that is bonded to the maxillary posterior teeth is the appliance of choice in the mixed-dentition patient with a narrow maxilla. (Modified from McNamara JA Jr, Brudon WL: *Orthodontics and dentofacial orthopedics,* Ann Arbor, Mich, 2001, Needham Press.)

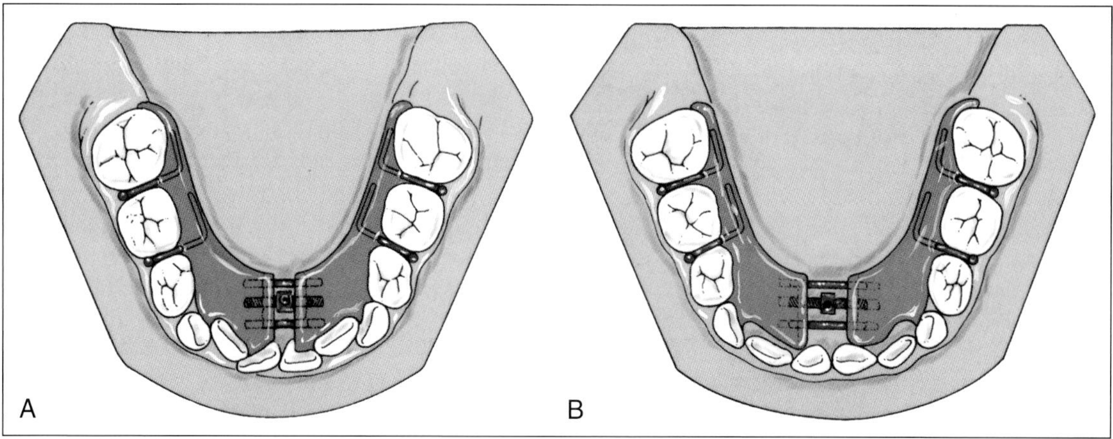

Fig. 12-4 Lower removable Schwarz appliance. **A,** After initial placement. **B,** After 5 months of active treatment. The lower posterior teeth have been uprighted, and a modest amount of arch space has been gained in the lower anterior region. (From McNamara JA Jr, Brudon WL: *Orthodontics and dentofacial orthopedics,* Ann Arbor, Mich, 2001, Needham Press.)

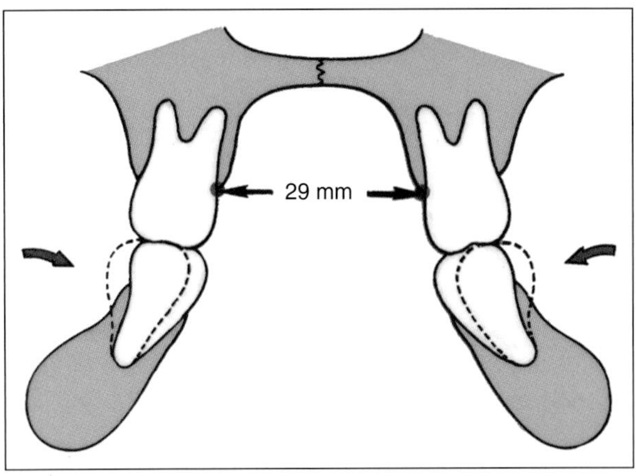

Fig. 12-5 Lateral bialveolar constriction. Frontal view of a patient with maxillary constriction whose mandibular molars, instead of erupting into a posterior crossbite relationship *(dashed lines)*, have erupted lingually. The buccal occlusion appears normal, and no crossbite is evident. (From McNamara JA Jr, Brudon WL: *Orthodontics and dentofacial orthopedics,* Ann Arbor, Mich, 2001, Needham Press.)

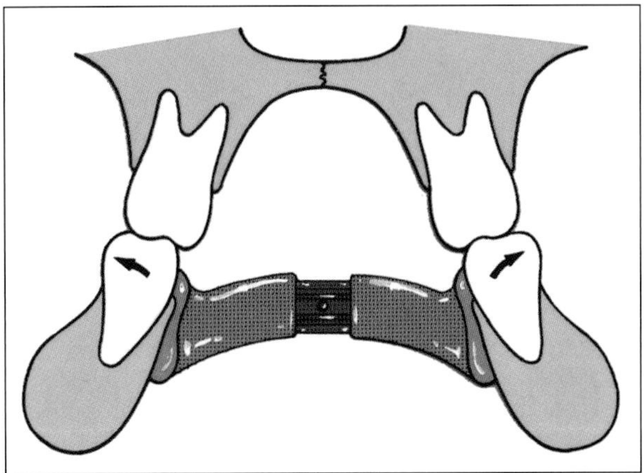

Fig. 12-6 A lower Schwarz appliance can be used to upright the lower dentition, producing a tendency toward a posterior crossbite. The maxilla subsequently can be expanded further because the mandibular dental arch has been widened initially. (From McNamara JA Jr, Brudon WL: *Orthodontics and dentofacial orthopedics,* Ann Arbor, Mich, 2001, Needham Press.)

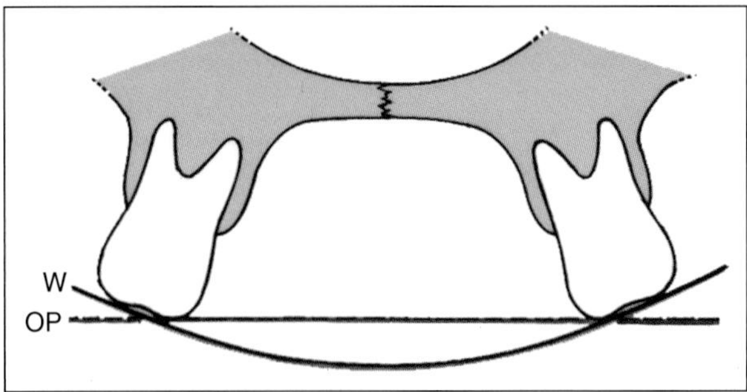

Fig. 12-7 Maxillary constriction can lead to an accentuated curve of Wilson *(W)*. When this condition exists, the lingual cusps hang down, often leading to balancing interferences. A flat occlusal plane *(OP)* often is a treatment objective. (From McNamara JA Jr, Brudon WL: *Orthodontics and dentofacial orthopedics,* Ann Arbor, Mich, 2001, Needham Press.)

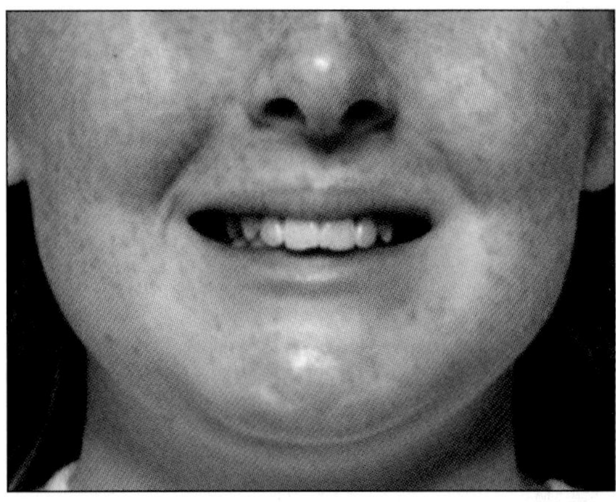

Fig. 12-8 Maxillary constriction can be evidenced by black spaces appearing at the corners of the mouth during smiling. (From McNamara JA Jr, Brudon WL: *Orthodontics and dentofacial orthopedics,* Ann Arbor, Mich, 2001, Needham Press.)

plate in the mixed dentition or, alternatively, full orthodontic appliances combined with a transpalatal arch in the permanent dentition.

Spontaneous Correction of Class II Malocclusion

An interesting (and somewhat surprising) observation following initial efforts to expand Class II patients in the early mixed dentition was the occurrence of a spontaneous correction of the Class II malocclusion during the retention period. Such patients had either an end-to-end or full-cusp Class II molar relationship. Generally, these patients did not have severe skeletal imbalances but typically were characterized clinically as having either mild-to-moderate mandibular skeletal retrusion or an orthognathic facial profile. At the time of expander removal, these patients had a strong tendency toward a buccal crossbite with only the lingual cusps of the upper posterior teeth contacting the buccal cusps of the lower posterior teeth. After expander removal, a maxillary maintenance plate was used for stabilization. Several appointments later, the tendency toward a buccal crossbite often disappeared, and some of the patients now had a solid Class I occlusal relationship.

It should be noted that the shift in molar relationship in these patients occurred before the transition from the lower second deciduous molars to the lower second premolars, the point at which an improvement in Angle classification sometimes occurs in untreated subjects because of the forward movement of the lower first molars into the leeway space.

A large prospective clinical study[18] of full-cusp and end-to-end Class II patients treated with early orthopedic expansion of the maxilla from the author's private-practice database currently is underway. The initial analysis of the serial lateral cephalograms of these patients indicates that a spontaneous improvement in Class II molar relationship is a common occurrence.

This spontaneous correction has forced us to rethink our approach to Class II molar correction treatment. Traditionally, clinicians have viewed a Class II malocclusion as primarily a sagittal and vertical problem. Experience with the post-RME correction of the Class II problem in growing patients indicates that many Class II malocclusions have a strong transverse component. The overexpansion of the maxilla, which subsequently is stabilized with a removable palatal plate, disrupts the occlusion. The patient apparently becomes more inclined to position the jaw slightly forward,[19] thus eliminating the tendency toward a buccal crossbite and at the same time improving the sagittal occlusal relationship. Presumably, subsequent growth and remodeling of the structures of the temporomandibular joint make this initial postural change permanent.

Spontaneous Class II correction, if it is going to occur, usually happens during the first 6 to 12 months of the post-RME period. The Class II correction can be enhanced further at the end of the mixed-dentition period by way of a transpalatal arch that not only maintains the maxillary leeway space, but also can be activated sequentially to produce molar rotation and uprighting.[2] At this point, if the occlusion still has a Class II component, additional treatment approaches may be indicated (e.g., functional jaw orthopedics, Forsus appliance, Class II elastics).

The phenomenon of spontaneous correction after RME treatment combined with routine use of a transpalatal arch is now part of our mixed-dentition treatment protocol. We have found that the need for subsequent functional jaw orthopedics has decreased substantially in our practice during the last decade.

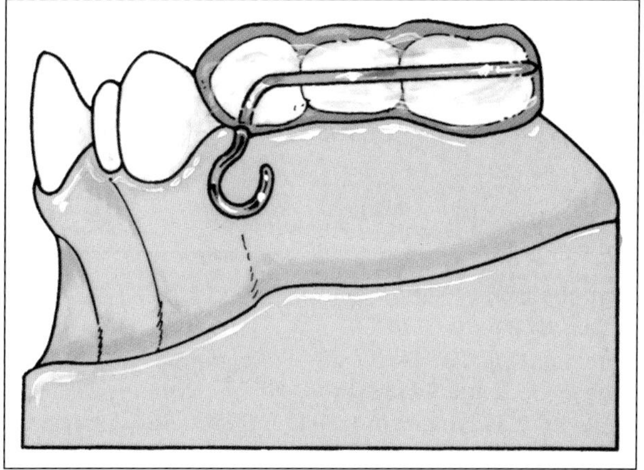

Fig. 12-9 Facial mask hooks have been added to the acrylic splint expander to allow for the attachment of elastics. (From McNamara JA Jr, Brudon WL: *Orthodontics and dentofacial orthopedics,* Ann Arbor, Mich, 2001, Needham Press.)

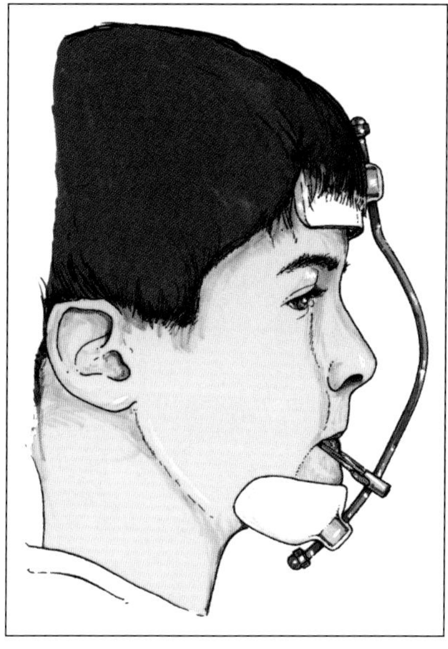

Fig. 12-10 The orthopedic facial mask of Petit often is used in patients with Class III malocclusion. (From McNamara JA Jr, Brudon WL: *Orthodontics and dentofacial orthopedics,* Ann Arbor, Mich, 2001, Needham Press.)

CONCLUSION

The various orthodontic problems discussed in this chapter are all linked to maxillary deficiency in the transverse or the sagittal dimension, or in both. Signs of maxillary deficiency include much more than anteroposterior crossbite and crowding of the maxillary dentition. Signs of maxillary deficiency often appear together in maxillary deficiency syndrome. A proven orthopedic appliance, the rapid maxillary expander, can be incorporated easily into treatment plans directed toward a variety of orthodontic conditions. RME is useful in correcting both Class II and Class III problems as well as in resolving mild to moderate tooth-size/arch-perimeter discrepancies. In addition, RME can be used to "broaden the smile" while improving nasal airway function in some patients.[20] Many or most of these signs appear in the same patient with maxillary deficiency, with rapid maxillary expansion available as an adjunct to fixed-appliance treatment, a procedure that presumably will be incorporated into orthodontic treatment protocols with increasing frequency in the future.

ACKNOWLEDGMENT

This chapter is written to honor Dr. Ram S. Nanda, Professor Emeritus and former Chair of the Department of Orthodontics at the University of Oklahoma. The Nanda family has made important contributions to orthodontics, with his brothers Dr. Ravindra Nanda Chair of Orthodontics at the University of Connecticut and the late Dr. Surender K.

Nanda a fellow faculty member for many years at the University of Michigan. It is my pleasure to write this chapter in honor of Dr. Ram Nanda's significant lifetime contributions to our specialty.

References

1. McNamara JA Jr: Maxillary transverse deficiency, *Am J Orthod Dentofacial Orthop* 117:567-570, 2000.
2. McNamara JA Jr, Brudon WL: *Orthodontics and dentofacial orthopedics*, Ann Arbor, Mich, 2001, Needham Press.
3. Howe RP, McNamara JA Jr, O'Connor KA: An examination of dental crowding and its relationship to tooth size and arch dimension, *Am J Orthod* 83:363-373, 1983.
4. Toth LR, McNamara JA Jr: Treatment effects produced by the twin block appliance and the FR-2 appliance of Fränkel compared to an untreated Class II sample, *Am J Orthod Dentofacial Orthop* 116:597-609, 1999.
5. Burkhardt DR, McNamara JA Jr, Baccetti T: Maxillary molar distalization or mandibular enhancement: a cephalometric comparison of the Pendulum and Herbst appliances, *Am J Orthod Dentofacial Orthop* 123:108-116, 2003.
6. Freeman DC, McNamara JA Jr, Baccetti T, Franchi L: Long-term treatment effects of the FR-2 appliance of Fränkel, *Am J Orthod Dentofacial Orthop* (in press).
7. Freeman CS, McNamara JA Jr, Baccetti T, Franchi L: Treatment effects of the Bionator and high-pull facebow combination followed by fixed appliances in patients with increased vertical dimension, *Am J Orthod Dentofacial Orthop* 131:184-195, 2007.
8. Schulz SO, McNamara JA Jr, Baccetti T, Franchi L: Treatment effects of bonded RME and vertical pull chin cup followed by fixed appliances in patients with increased vertical dimension, *Am J Orthod Dentofacial Orthop* 128:326-336, 2005.
9. McNamara JA Jr: *The role of the transverse dimension in orthodontic diagnosis and treatment*, Monograph 36, Craniofacial Growth Series, Ann Arbor, 1999, Center for Human Growth and Development, University of Michigan.
10. Vanarsdall RL Jr: Personal communication, 1992.
11. Guyer EC, Ellis E, McNamara JA Jr, Behrents RG: Components of Class III malocclusion in juveniles and adolescents, *Angle Orthod* 56:7-30, 1986.
12. DeClerck H: Unpublished data, 2007.
13. McNamara JA Jr: An orthopedic approach to the treatment of Class III malocclusion in young patients, *J Clin Orthod* 21:598-608, 1987.
14. McGill JS, McNamara JA Jr: Treatment and post-treatment effects of rapid maxillary expansion and facial mask therapy. In McNamara JA Jr, editor. *Growth modification: what works, what doesn't and why*, Monograph 36, Craniofacial Growth Series, Center for Human Growth and Development, Ann Arbor, 1999, University of Michigan.
15. Westwood PV, McNamara JA Jr, Baccetti T, et al: Long-term effects of early Class III treatment with rapid maxillary expansion and facial mask therapy, *Am J Orthod Dentofacial Orthop* 123:306-320, 2003.
16. McNamara JA Jr: Components of Class II malocclusion in children 8-10 years of age, *Angle Orthod* 51:177-202, 1981.
17. Tollaro I, Baccetti T, Franchi L, Tanasescu CD: Role of posterior transverse interarch discrepancy in Class II, Division 1 malocclusion during the mixed dentition phase, *Am J Orthod Dentofacial Orthop* 110:417-422, 1996.
18. Guest SS, McNamara JA Jr, Baccetti T, Franchi L: Improving Class II malocclusion as a "side-effect" of rapid maxillary expansion: a prospective clinical study, Submitted for publication, 2008.
19. Wendling LK, McNamara JA Jr, Franchi L, Baccetti T: Short-term skeletal and dental effects of the acrylic splint rapid maxillary expansion appliance, *Angle Orthod* 75:7-14, 2005.
20. Hartgerink DV, Vig PS, Abbott DW: The effect of rapid maxillary expansion on nasal airway resistance, *Am J Orthod Dentofacial Orthop* 92:381-389, 1987.

CHAPTER 13

Effective Maxillary Protraction for Class III Patients

■ *Peter Ngan and Hong He*

CLASS III MALOCCLUSION

Definition

Angle first published his classification of malocclusion in 1899, which was based solely on the dental arch relationship using study cast.[1] Class I occlusion occurred when the mesiobuccal cusp of upper first permanent molars occluded on the buccal groove of the lower first molar. Class III malocclusion occurred when the lower teeth occluded mesial to the width of one bicuspid, or even more in extreme cases.

The advent of cephalometric radiology in 1931 allowed clinicians to discern the underlying skeletal pattern of the Class III malocclusion.[2] Tweed[3] divided Class III malocclusions into (1) pseudo–Class III malocclusions with normally shaped mandibles and underdeveloped maxilla and (2) skeletal Class III malocclusions with large mandibles. Moyers[4] divided Class III *mesiocclusion* into three distinct types: osseous, muscular, and dental. The first condition is an abnormal osseous growth pattern, the second an acquired muscular reflex pattern of mandibular closure, and the third a problem in dental positioning.

Prevalence

Class III malocclusion is a less frequently observed clinical problem than Class II or Class I malocclusion, occurring in less than 5% of the U.S. population.[5,6] The prevalence is greater in Asian populations. The estimated incidence of Class III malocclusion among the Korean, Japanese, and Chinese is 4% to 14% because of the large percentage of patients with maxillary deficiency.[7-9] However, a study on Chinese children age 9 to 15 years that divided subjects into those with "pseudo" and "true" Class III malocclusions found a much lower prevalence of these disorders, 2.3% and 1.7%, respectively.[10]

In the African-American population the incidence of Class III malocclusion has been shown to be 6.3%.[11] Class III malocclusions are more prevalent in Hispanic than in African or Caucasian groups. Prevalence of Class III malocclusion in Latino Americans has been shown to be about 9.1%, similar to the 8.3% in Mexican Americans reported by the NHANES survey.[12]

As for the components of Class III malocclusion, a study of Class III surgical patients demonstrated that the combination of underdeveloped maxilla and overdeveloped mandible was most common at 30.1%, whereas those with a normal maxilla and overdeveloped mandible constituted 19.2% of the sample.[13] Most Korean patients, however, had a normal maxilla and overdeveloped mandible (47.7%), with fewer patients having an underdeveloped maxilla and overdeveloped mandible (13.5%).[14]

Etiology

Class III skeletal growth has a multifactorial basis that is influenced by genetics, function, deformities, size, and position of bones. According to Enlow,[15] the facial bones that contribute to a Class III skeletal pattern may include the anterior and posterior cranial base, the nasomaxillary complex, and the ramus and corpus of the mandible. Only a few types of Class III malocclusion are caused by specific interferences with growth. These interferences may be caused by habits or related to growth patterns. Accordingly, individuals with postural habits of the mandible and mouth breathing may present with a Class III type of malocclusion.[16] This investigation also demonstrated that interferences in occlusal function, such as reverse overjet, can alter the direction and shape of the mandible.

The more severe Class III cases are caused by a combination of inherited traits, which are made worse by environmental factors.[17] According to Park and Baik,[18] the etiology of Class III malocclusion can be classified into three types on the basis of the position of the maxilla relative to the craniofacial skeleton. *Type A* individuals have a normal maxilla and overgrown mandible, which is classified as true mandibular prognathism. *Type B* individuals have maxillary and mandibular excess, but the mandible has grown more than the maxilla; they present with an acute nasolabial angle and an anteriorly positioned A point. *Type C* individuals have hypoplasia of the maxilla; their facial profile is concave with an excessively large nasolabial angle, which is frequently camouflaged by dentoalveolar compensation.

Patients with Class III malocclusion may present with various combinations of other abnormal skeletal and dental patterns. The most common skeletal features include a shortened anterior cranial base, more obtuse gonial angle, anteriorly positioned glenoid fossa, decrease in cranial base flexure, sagittal discrepancy of the maxilla and/or mandible, and increase in anterior lower facial height. Dental findings usually include Angle Class III molars and canines, retroclined mandibular incisors, proclined maxillary incisors, and an edge-to-edge incisor relationship or negative overjet.

Differential Diagnosis

The differential diagnosis in skeletal Class III malocclusions plays a major role in the success of treatment results. The timing of orthodontic treatment has always been somewhat controversial,[19] and the prognosis is always guarded until growth is completed. Variations in magnitude and expression of Class III malocclusion can present with some difficulty during diagnosis. As mentioned earlier, a patient may present with a combination of one or more dentofacial deformities, such as true mandibular prognathism or maxillary retrognathism. To differentiate the underlying cause of a Class III malocclusion, a simplified method of evaluating patients has been suggested.[20-22]

First, it is important to question both the patient and the parents about the presence of a large jaw or anterior crossbite among family members. If a close relative required orthognathic surgery, the patient under examination may also exhibit a severe skeletal discrepancy.

Second, it is important to assess the presence of a functional shift. The relationship of maxilla to mandible should be evaluated to determine whether a discrepancy exists between centric relation and centric occlusion. Anterior repositioning of the mandible may be caused by abnormal tooth contact that forces the mandible forward. These patients tend to present with a Class I skeletal pattern, normal facial profile, and Class I molar relation in centric relation, but a Class III skeletal and dental pattern in centric occlusion. Early correction of this "pseudo" Class III condition may provide for a more favorable environment for future growth.

Third, a lateral cephalometric radiograph is required to complete the diagnosis and assist the clinician in treatment planning. A cephalometric analysis is needed to record quantitatively the severity of the Class III malocclusion and to determine the underlying cause of the deformity. Cephalometric measurements that relate the maxilla to the mandible (e.g., ANB, Wits, and linear measurements of difference between condylion to A point and condylion to gnathion) are particularly helpful in quantifying the severity of the malocclusion (Table 13-1).

Discriminant analysis has shown that Wits appraisal is most decisive in distinguishing camouflage treatment from surgical treatment.[23] The average Wits for camouflage treatment was −4.6 ± 1.7 mm and for surgical treatment was −12.1 ± 4.3 mm. Accordingly, on the basis of the Wits appraisal, the severity of skeletal Class III patients can been labeled as *red, green,* and *yellow* categories.[24] Patients with a Wits appraisal greater than 12 mm are labeled "red" and may eventually require orthognathic surgery to correct the skeletal deformity. Patients with a Wits appraisal smaller than 4 mm are labeled "green" and most likely can be camouflaged by orthodontic tooth movement. Patients with a Wits appraisal between 4 and 12 mm are labeled "yellow" and require further analysis, such as serial radiographs and a growth treatment response vector (GTRV) analysis,[25] before a decision can be made whether to camouflage the malocclusion or wait for completion of growth before surgical treatment is implemented.

Fourth, a thorough clinical assessment may be the most important evaluation for the diagnosis when the objective of treatment planning is to optimize facial esthetics.[26] The anteroposterior skeletal base relationship and the vertical facial proportions should be assessed while the patient is sitting upright in natural head position. Any profile disharmonies should be recorded. Similarly, the transverse dimension should be assessed at this point along with any facial and dental asymmetries. The temporomandibular joints,

TABLE 13-1

Cephalometric Variables and Standards for Class III Patients

Intermaxillary Cephalometric Variables	Standard (Age 6-18 years)
Wits analysis	0 mm
Maxillary-mandibular difference	23 mm (12 years old)
ANB angle	2 degrees
Zero meridian	
Maxilla	+2.3 mm
Pogonion	0 mm

associated musculature, and oral mucosa should also be examined.

The following discussion highlights diverse approaches for using maxillary protraction for the treatment of Class III malocclusions.

PROTRACTION OF MAXILLA

Patients with developing Class III malocclusion can be treated using chin cap, facemask, removable functional appliances, or fixed appliances.[27-30] *Protraction facemask* has been used in the treatment of patients with Class III malocclusions and a maxillary deficiency.[28,31-33] The facemask has an adjustable anterior wire that can accommodate a downward and forward pull on the maxilla with elastics. To minimize the tipping of the palatal plane, the protraction elastics are attached near the maxillary canines with a downward and forward pull of 30 degrees from the occlusal plane.[34] Maxillary protraction usually requires 300 to 600 g of force per side, depending on the age of the patient. Patients are instructed to wear the appliance for 12 hours a day.

In the mixed dentition, a banded or bonded *expansion appliance* can be fabricated as anchorage for maxillary protraction. Patients with an increased lower face height can benefit from using a bonded expansion appliance, which provides a temporary bite-plane effect. Additionally, a bonded maxillary appliance can be used in patients with a deep overbite and overclosure of the mandible to facilitate the jumping of the anterior crossbite.[35] The expansion appliance is activated twice daily (0.25 mm per turn) by the patient or parent for 7 to 10 days. In patients with a more constricted maxilla, activation of the appliance is carried out for 2 weeks or more.

Facial Sutures

Several facial sutures play an important role in the development of the nasomaxillary complex, including the frontomaxillary, nasomaxillary, zygomaticotemporal, zygomaticomaxillary, pterygopalatine, intermaxillary, ethmomaxillary, and lacrimomaxillary sutures (Fig. 13-1).

Animal studies have shown that the maxillary complex can be displaced anteriorly with significant changes in the facial sutures.[36-38] Maxillary protraction, however, does not always result in forward movement of the maxilla. With the same line of force, different midfacial bones are displaced in different directions depending on the moments of force generated at the sutures.[39] The center of resistance of the maxilla is located at the distal contacts of the maxillary first molars, one half the distance from the functional occlusal plane to the inferior border of the orbit.[40] Protraction of the maxilla below the center of resistance produces counterclockwise rotation of the maxilla, which may not be favorable for patients with open-bite tendency.[41]

Crossbite and Overjet/Overbite Correction

Clinically, anterior crossbite can be corrected with 3 to 4 months of maxillary expansion and protraction depending on the severity of the malocclusion. Improvement in overbite and molar relationship can be expected with an additional 4 to 6 months of treatment.

A prospective clinical trial found that overjet correction resulted from forward maxillary movement (31%), backward movement of the mandible (21%), labial movement of the maxillary incisors (28%), and lingual movement of the mandibular incisors (20%).[42] Overcorrection of the overjet and molar relationship was highly recommended to anticipate unfavorable mandibular growth. Overbite was improved by eruption of the posterior teeth. The total facial height was increased by inferior movement of the maxilla and downward and backward rotation of the mandible.

According to several clinical studies, the mean forward movement of the maxilla with 6 to 8 months of maxillary protraction is about 1 to 3 mm.[28,31,32,43,44] A meta-analysis on the effectiveness of protraction facemask treatment found that the average change in Wits appraisal was 4 to 6 mm and the average horizontal A-point movement was 1 to 3 mm.[45]

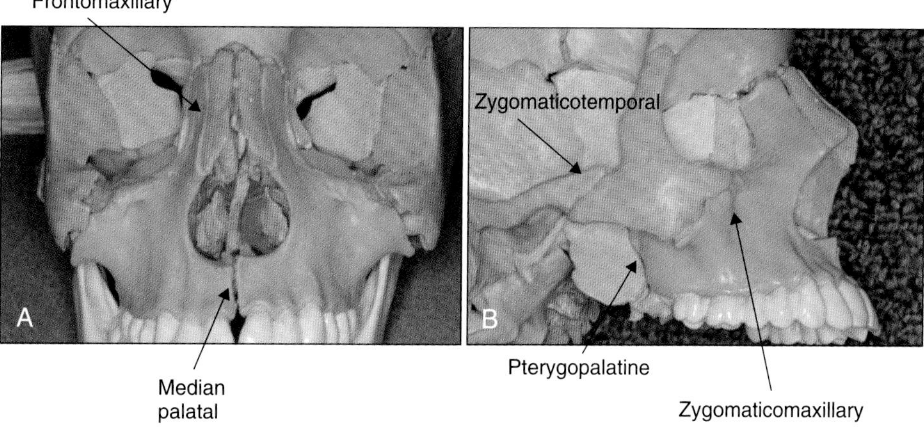

Fig. 13-1 Facial sutures that play an important role in the development of the nasomaxillary complex. **A,** Anterior view. **B,** Lateral view.

Timing of Treatment

A critical question in maxillary protraction concerns the best time to start facemask treatment. The main objective of early facemask treatment is to enhance forward displacement of the maxilla by sutural growth. Histological studies have shown that the midpalatal suture is broad and smooth during the "infantile" stage (8-10 years of age) and becomes more squamous and overlapping in the "juvenile" stage (10-13 years).[46-47] Biologically, the circum-maxillary sutures are smooth and broad before age 8 years and become more heavily interdigitated around puberty.[48]

These findings relate to observations in clinical studies showing that maxillary protraction is effective in the primary, mixed, as well as early permanent dentitions. Several studies suggest that a greater degree of anterior maxillary displacement can be found when treatment is initiated in the primary or early mixed dentition.[31,32]

The optimal time to intervene a Class III malocclusion is at the initial eruption of the maxillary incisors. A positive overjet/overbite at the end of the facemask treatment appears to maintain the anterior occlusion.

Another important question is whether the results of early protraction treatment can be sustained when subsequent mandibular growth occurs during the pubertal growth spurt. In a prospective clinical trial, protraction facemask treatment starting in the mixed dentition was stable 2 years after removal of the appliances.[42] This probably resulted from the overcorrection and the use of a functional appliance as retainer for 1 year. When these patients were followed for another 2 years, 15 of the 20 patients maintained a positive overjet.[42] In patients who relapsed to a negative overjet, the mandible outgrew the maxilla in the horizontal direction. When these patients were followed for another 4 years (8 years after treatment, until about 17.5 years of age), 14 of the 20 patients (67%) maintained a positive overjet.[49] For the patients who relapsed to a reverse overjet, the mandible outgrew the maxilla by four times, compared with twice that in the stable group.

These results suggest that in a random clinical trial when patients are followed until after completion of pubertal growth, two of three patients (67%) will have a favorable outcome. About one third of the patients might be candidates for orthognathic surgery later in life because of unfavorable growth pattern. Patients treated by protraction facemask either in the early mixed dentition or in the late mixed dentition and permanent dentition and followed up after a second phase of fixed-appliance therapy demonstrated ongoing improvements in the former group but not in the latter group at the end of phase II treatment.[50] Specifically, 1.8 mm of additional forward movement of the maxilla was noted in the early treatment group compared with the controls. In the late mixed-dentition group, no significant difference in forward movement of maxilla was found after puberty compared with the controls.

USE OF ONPLANTS TO IMPROVE ANCHORAGE

Orthodontic anchorage is defined as the resistance to undesirable tooth movement. Many conventional means to enhance orthodontic anchorage are less than ideal because they rely on either structures (teeth) that are potentially mobile or patient compliance in wearing headgear or elastics. Furthermore, these conventional means of anchorage are usually not adequate to withstand heavy forces such as those used for orthopedics.

On the other hand, palatal implants and onplants have shown success as temporary anchorage devices (TADs) because they offer maximal anchorage by virtue of osseointegration and can be removed after completion of orthodontic treatment.[51-55] Palatal implants and onplants can be connected by transpalatal arches to move segments of teeth or used in patients with insufficient dental anchorage because of tooth loss or periodontal disease.

The use of onplants for orthodontic or orthopedic anchorage is a relatively new area of research, and investigations are limited. In 1995, Block and Hoffman[51] reported on the successful use of an onplant, a subperiosteal disk, as an orthodontic anchorage in an experimental study in dogs and monkeys. It is a relatively flat, disk-shaped fixture of 7.7 mm (Nobel Biocare, Göteborg, Sweden) with a textured, hydroxyapatite-coated surface for integration with bone.

Unlike implants, onplants require only a simple surgical procedure to insert and to remove, which makes them more versatile as anchorage units in orthodontics. Also unlike implants, which are placed in freshly prepared bony sockets in alveolar bone, onplants are osseointegrated on relatively inactive bony surfaces. They can be placed on patients in various stages of dental eruption. Onplants are surgically placed on the flat part of the palatal bone near the maxillary molar region. The abutment is made in such a way that it can be connected to a transpalatal bar for tooth movement or anchorage.

The success of using onplants as orthodontic anchorage clinically depends on the amount of force it can withstand. Preclinical studies in monkeys and dogs showed that onplants can be used as stable anchorage to move teeth and can serve as abutments for distraction osteogenesis of the mandible.[1] In these experiments, onplants provided 3.06 newtons (N) of continuous force and 711 N of shear force.[51] Clinically, onplants have been applied successfully to close space orthodontically,[56] help move molars distally,[57] erupt teeth occlusally,[58] and provide anchorage for forward protraction of the maxilla.[59]

Clinical Procedure

After local anesthesia of the palate, a paramarginal incision is made in the palatal mucosa from the premolar area toward the midline (Fig. 13-2, *A-C*). The tissue is tunneled under, in full-thickness fashion, past the midline to the eventual implantation site. The onplant is then inserted into the

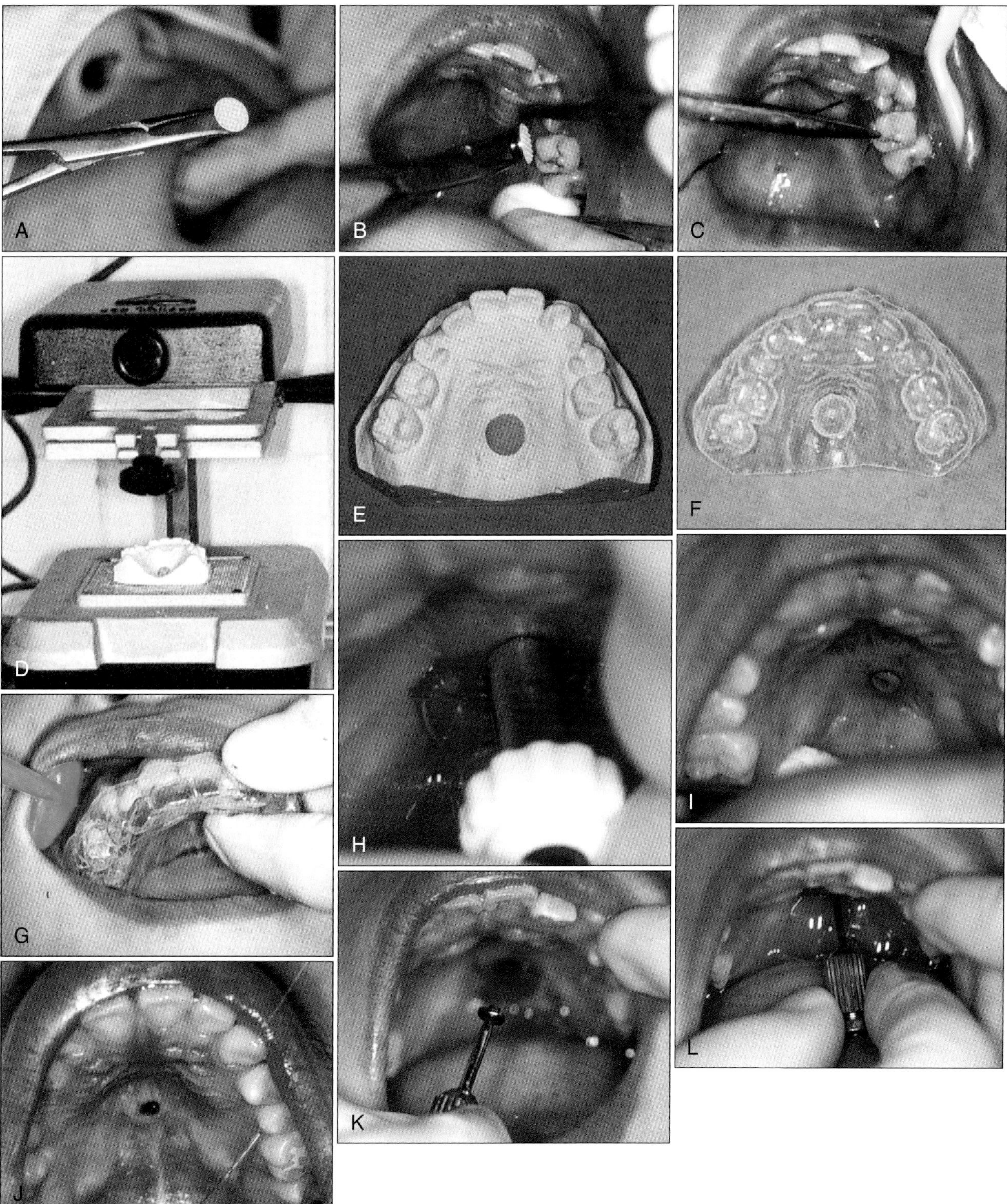

Fig. 13-2 Procedure for onplant anchorage in maxillary protraction. **A** to **C**, Surgical placement of onplant. **A**, Hydroxyapatite (HA) surface of onplant. **B**, Onplant is inserted into the tunnel with the HA surface directly on bone surface. **C**, Onplant is slid toward the palatal midline and tissue sutured. **D** to **G**, Fabrication of Vacuformed stent. **D**, Vacuform. **E**, Placement of putty material where onplant is positioned. **F**, Finished stent. **G**, Insertion of stent. **H** to **K**, Onplant exposed after osseointegration. **H**, Tissue punch. **I** and **J**, Removal of tissues above onplant. **K**, Removal of covering cap on onplant. **L** to **O**, Insertion of transmucosal abutment and heeling cap. **L**, Screwdriver for inserting transmucosal abutment.

Continued

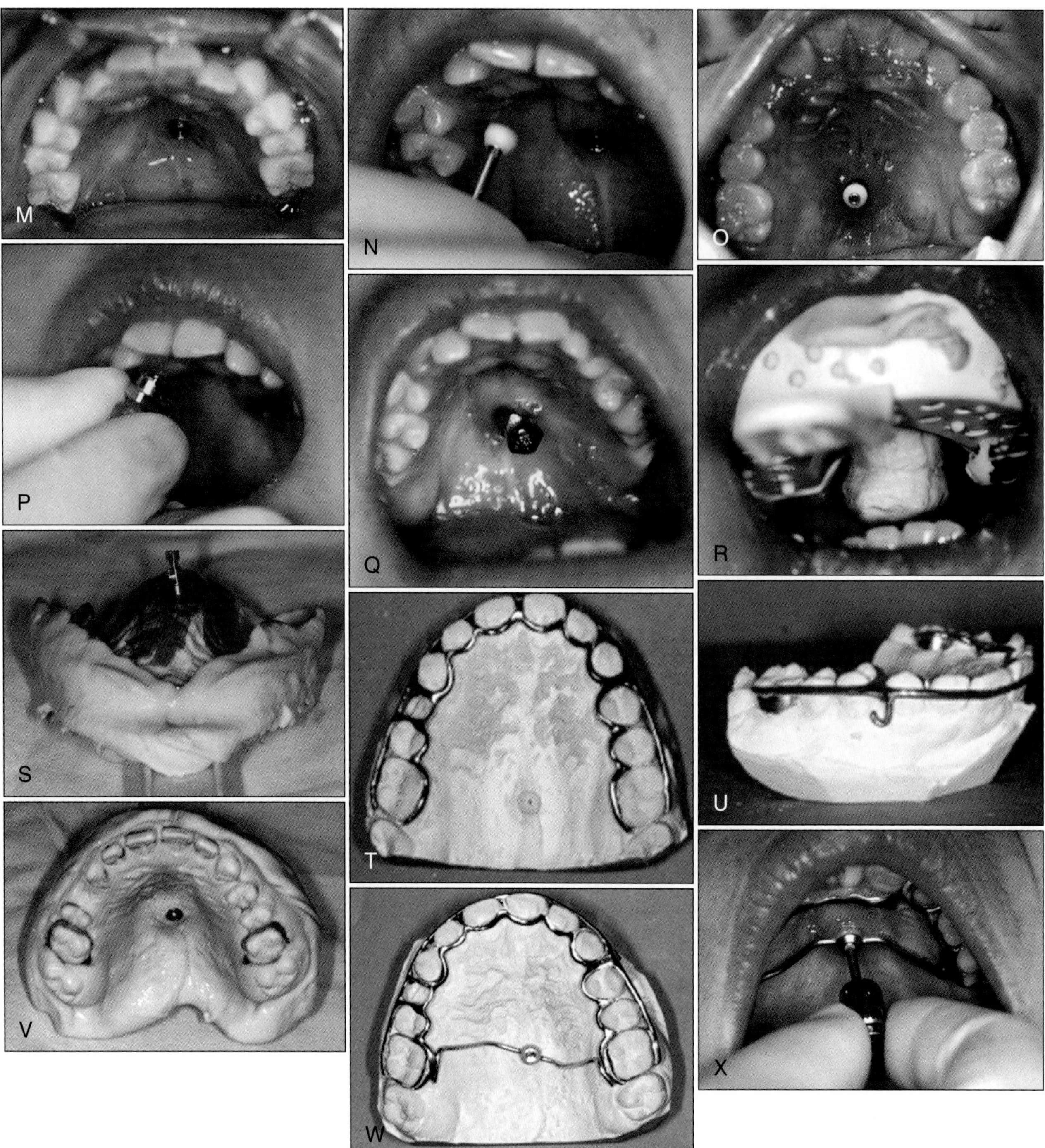

Fig. 13-2, cont'd **M,** Abutment in place. **N,** Insertion of healing cap. **O,** Healing cap in place. **P** to **S,** Transfer of abutment position to stone cast. **P,** Insertion of impression coping. **Q,** Impression coping in place. **R,** Impression to transfer the abutment position. **S,** Simulating implant is used to pour the working cast. **T** and **U,** Fabrication of silver splint. **T,** Silver splint on stone cast. **U,** Side view of silver splint on stone cast. **V** to **X,** Connection of silver splint to onplant with transpalatal bar. **V,** Impression with bands on posterior molars. **W,** Soldering transpalatal bar to silver splint on stone cast. **X,** Connection of appliance to onplant in patient.

tunnel and slid into position with the hydroxyapatite surface directly on the bone, close to the palatal midline. A Vacu-formed stent is worn by the patient 24 hours a day for 10 days to place pressure on the onplant (Fig. 13-2, *D-G*). This step is crucial to minimize movement of the onplant during osseointegration, which takes 3 to 4 months.

Once integration is achieved, the transmucosal abutment is placed by exposing the onplant using a tissue punch (Fig. 13-2, *H-K*). The cover screw is then removed and an abutment screw with healing cap placed (Fig. 13-2, *L-O*). To transfer the abutment position to a stone cast, an open-tray impression is taken by exposing the onplant, removing its cover screw, and securing an impression coping (Fig. 13-2, *P-R*). A simulating implant is used to pour the working cast (Fig. 13-2, *S*). A transpalatal arch is attached to the onplant and soldered to a silver-cast splint (Fig. 13-2, *T* and *U*), which connects all the maxillary teeth (Fig. 13-2, *V-X*).

Case Study

Figure 13-3 shows an 8-year-old girl who presented with a concave facial profile, crowding of the anterior teeth, and an anterior crossbite *(A-G)*. Cephalometric radiograph showed a Class III malocclusion and a deficient maxilla *(H)*. Panoramic radiograph revealed an impacted maxillary left canine *(I)*.

The patient was treated with a maxillary protraction facemask using an onplant as skeletal anchorage (Fig. 13-4). A Petit facemask (Ormco Corporation, Orange, Calif.) was fitted with elastics that delivered approximately 400 g of force on each side. The force was directed from the canine area 30 degrees from the occlusal plane to counteract the anticlockwise rotation of the palatal plane. The patient was instructed to wear the facemask for 12 hours per day.

Traction was continued for 12 months until sufficient clinical movement of the maxilla had been achieved to improve the midface esthetics (Fig. 13-5). At the end of the protraction period, the onplant was removed using a surgical elevator (Fig. 13-6).

All surgical procedures were carried out under local anesthesia. The perionplant soft tissue healed uneventfully within 2 weeks. The patient's acceptance of the surgical effects was positive, and postoperative pain and discomfort were negligible.

Phase II comprehensive orthodontic treatment was performed at the end of the patient's pubertal growth period. Figure 13-7 shows the substantial improvements in the skeletal and dental relationships at the completion of orthodontic treatment.

SUTURAL DISTRACTION TO DISARTICULATE MAXILLA

Sutural expansion and protraction induce new bone growth by mechanically stretching the sutures.[60-63] The craniofacial sutures are osteogenic tissues between opposing membranous bones. Experimental separation of craniofacial sutures in animals, with traction forces, resembles the sutural activity noted during normal growth, although more marked. The response to mechanical traction includes a widening of the sutures, changes in the orientation of fiber bundles, an increase in the number of osteoblasts, and deposition of osteoid on both sutural bone surfaces.

Clinically, maxillary expansion can disarticulate the maxilla to allow a more favorable forward movement of the maxilla. A well-disarticulated maxilla seems to be critical when using tooth-borne devices for orthopedic effects. A protocol of weekly, alternate rapid maxillary expansion and constriction of the maxilla to disarticulate the maxilla without overexpanding has been proposed previously.[64-66] Usually, it requires 7 to 9 weeks to loosen the maxilla. An average of 5.8 mm of forward movement of the maxilla at the A point was noted when using this method.[65]

Case Study

Figure 13-8 shows an 8-year-old boy treated with a double-hinged rapid maxillary expander (U.S. Patent No. 6334771 B1) and a protraction facemask *(A-F)*. This double-hinged expander is designed to expand and rotate each half of the maxilla outward for greater anterior displacement, with less risk of bone resorption behind the maxillary tuberosities *(G-K)*.

The maxilla was expanded 1 mm per day (four turns) for 1 week, then constricted 1 mm per day for the next week. This process was repeated for 7 weeks, until sufficient disarticulation had been achieved. The facemask was then fitted with a protraction force of 400 g per side produced by elastic ($\frac{3}{8}$ inch, 14 ounces) connected from the hook of the expansion appliance to the facemask. The patient was instructed to wear the facemask for 12 hours each day for 6 months.

Clinically, mobility of the maxilla was noted at the end of the expansion protocol. The anterior crossbite was corrected within 2 to 3 months of maxillary protraction. Overcorrection of the maxilla to an overjet of 3 to 4 mm was continued to anticipate excessive growth of the mandible during retention (Fig. 13-8, *L-Q*).

CONCLUSION

Orthodontic treatment of patients with Class III malocclusion using maxillary protraction can be effective with the help of temporary anchorage devices such as palatal implants or onplants. Distraction of the maxillary sutures in young patients allows more efficient forward movement of the maxilla. Future innovative method of maxillary protraction may include the use of miniplates and less invasive TAD such as miniscrews.

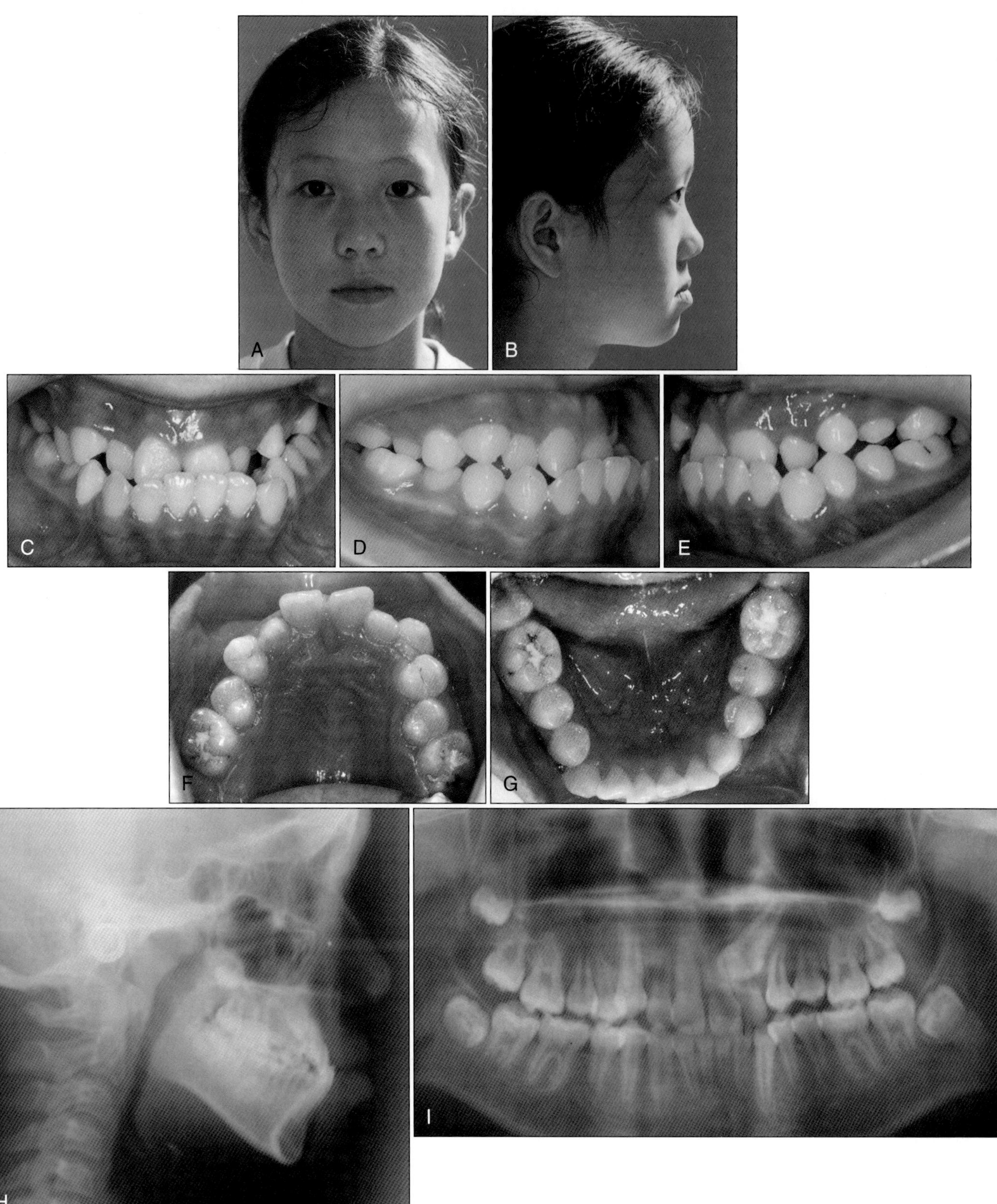

Fig. 13-3 Maxillary protraction for 8-year-old girl with Class III malocclusion. **A** to **G**, Pretreatment extraoral and intraoral photographs. **A,** Frontal facial view. **B,** Lateral facial profile. **C,** Frontal intraoral view. **D,** Right intraoral lateral view. **E,** Left intraoral lateral view. **F,** Maxillary occlusal view. **G,** Mandibular occlusal view. **H** and **I,** Pretreatment radiographs. **H,** Lateral cephalogram. **I,** Panoramic radiograph.

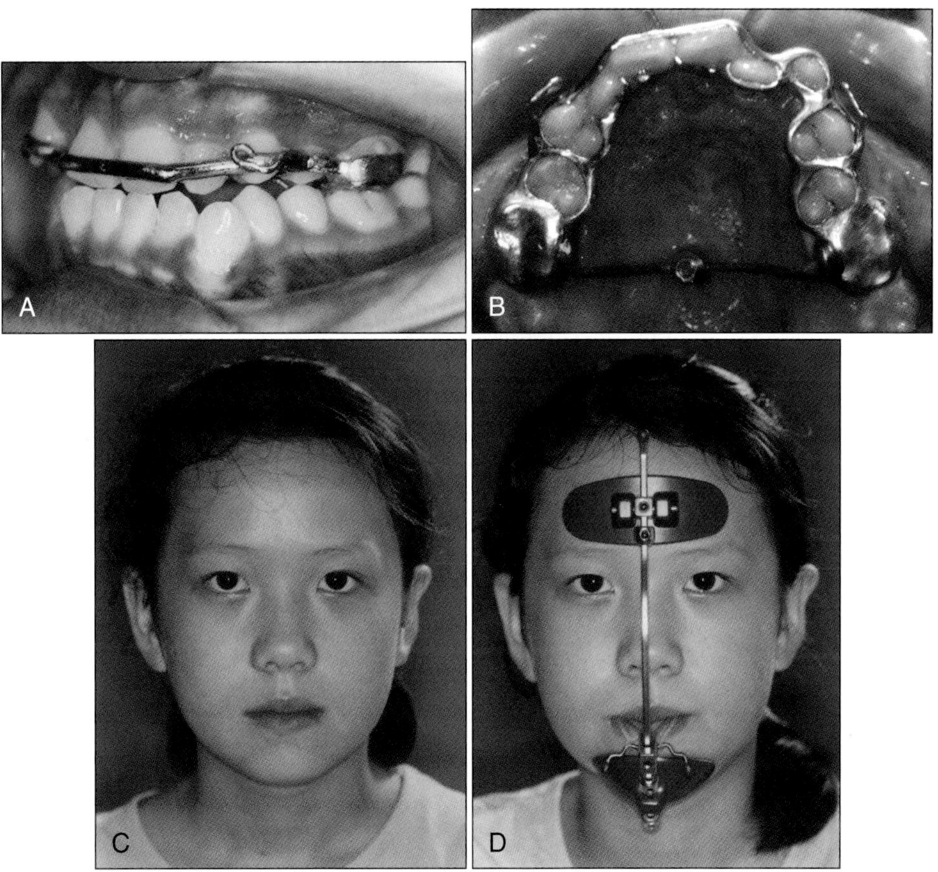

Fig. 13-4 Same patient as in Figure 13-3. **A** and **B**, Placement of onplant and connection with silver splint with transpalatal bar. **A**, Left buccal view. **B**, Maxillary occlusal view. **C** and **D**, Facial changes in patient after maxillary protraction. **C**, Anterior view after facemask treatment. **D**, Anterior view with facemask.

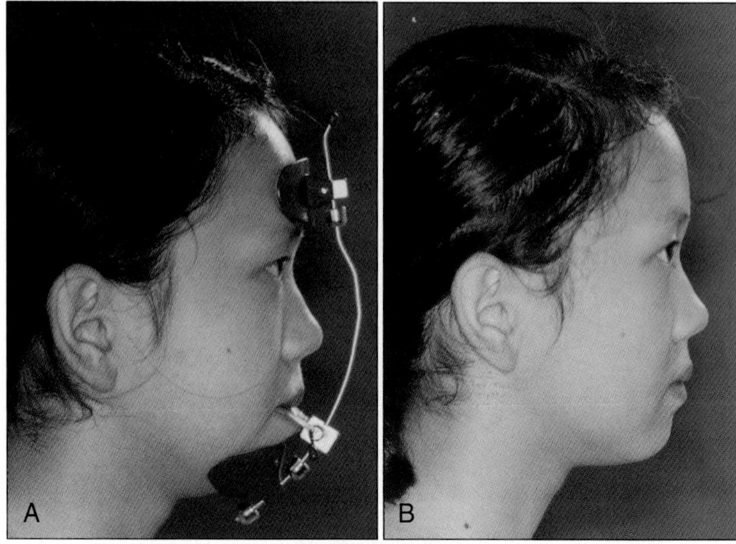

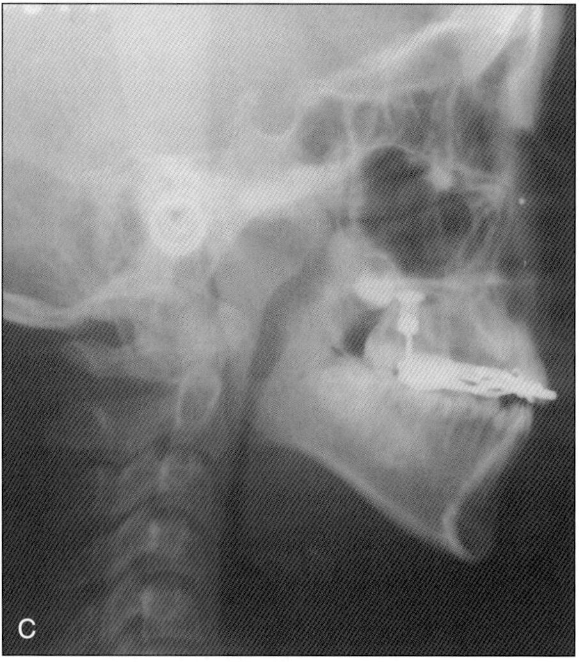

Fig. 13-5 Same patient as in Figures 13-3 and 13-4. **A,** Lateral profile with facemask. **B,** Lateral profile after facemask treatment. **C,** Lateral cephalometric radiograph showing position of onplant after maxillary protraction.

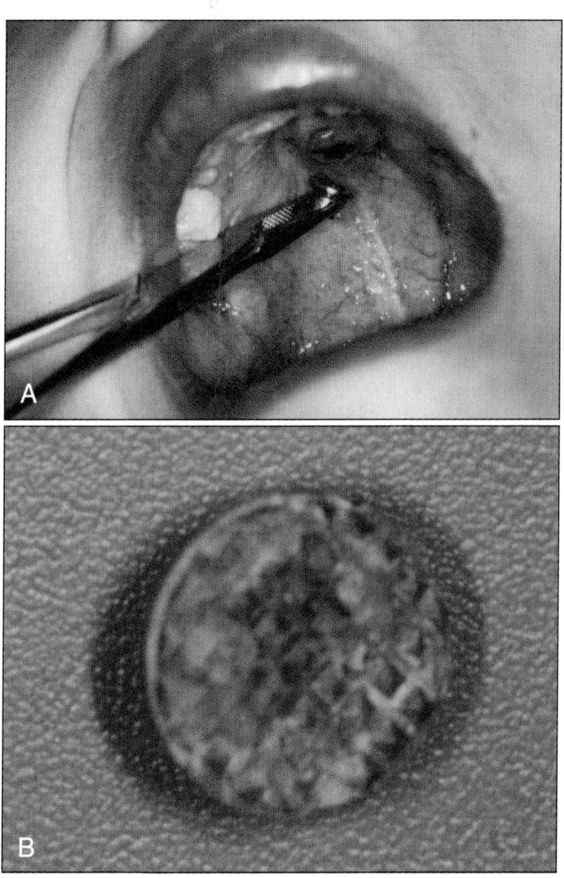

Fig. 13-6 Removal of onplant after facemask treatment in same patient. **A,** Removal of onplant. **B,** Surface of onplant that integrates with bone.

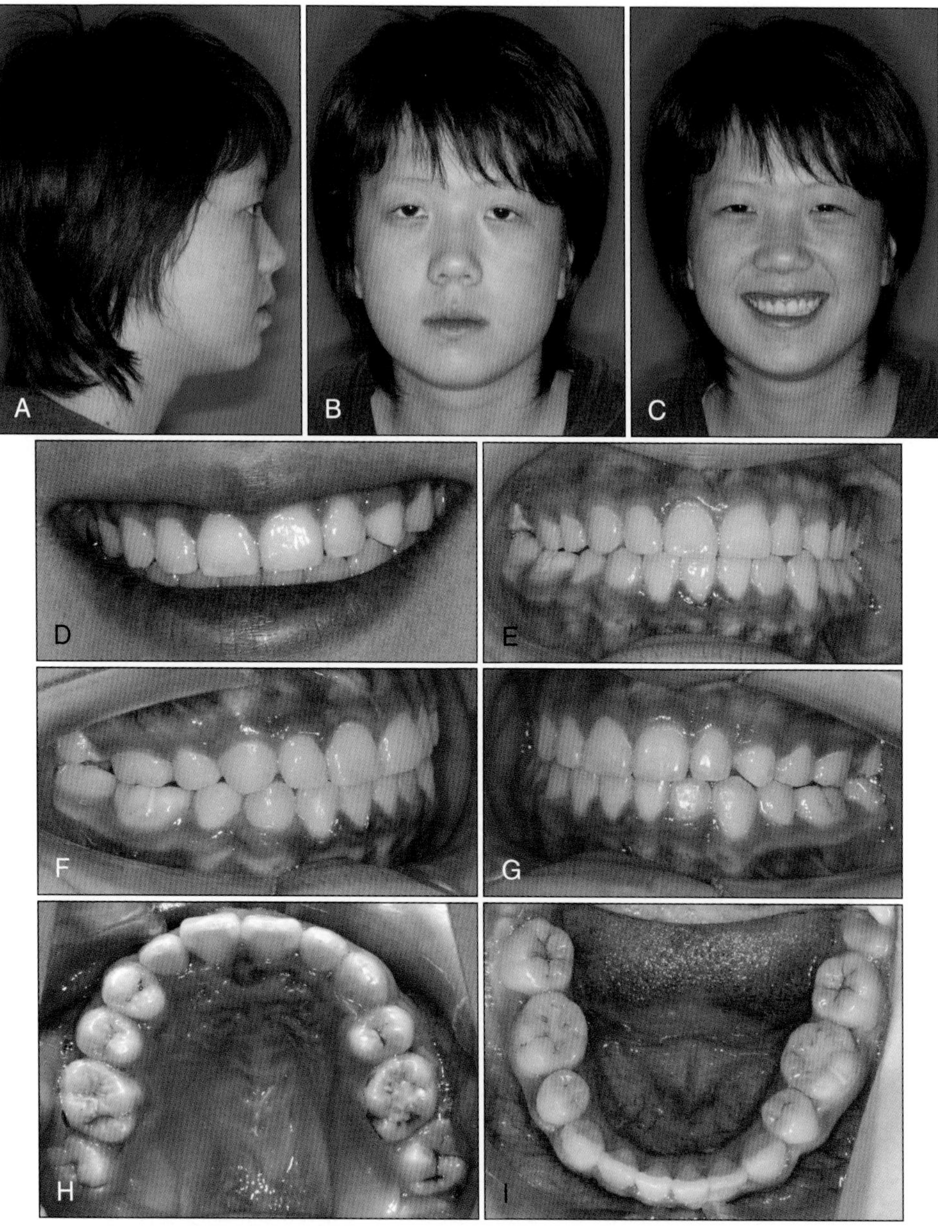

Fig. 13-7 Same patient as in Figures 13-3 to 13-6 after treatment. **A** to **I,** Posttreatment extraoral and intraoral photographs. **A,** Lateral profile. **B,** Anterior profile. **C,** Anterior smiling profile. **D,** Anterior smiling view. **E,** Anterior view. **F,** Right lateral view. **G,** Left lateral view. **H,** Maxillary occlusal view. **I,** Mandibular occlusal view.

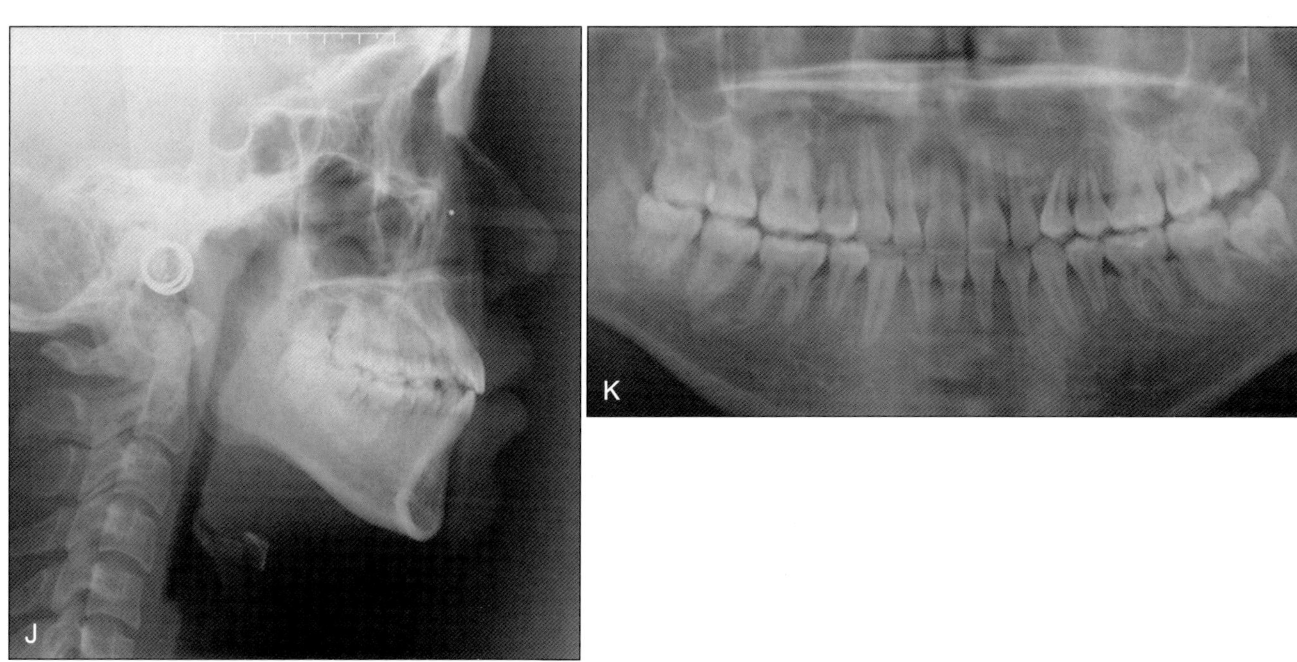

Fig. 13-7, cont'd **J** and **K**, Posttreatment radiographs. **J**, Lateral cephalogram. **K**, Panoramic radiograph.

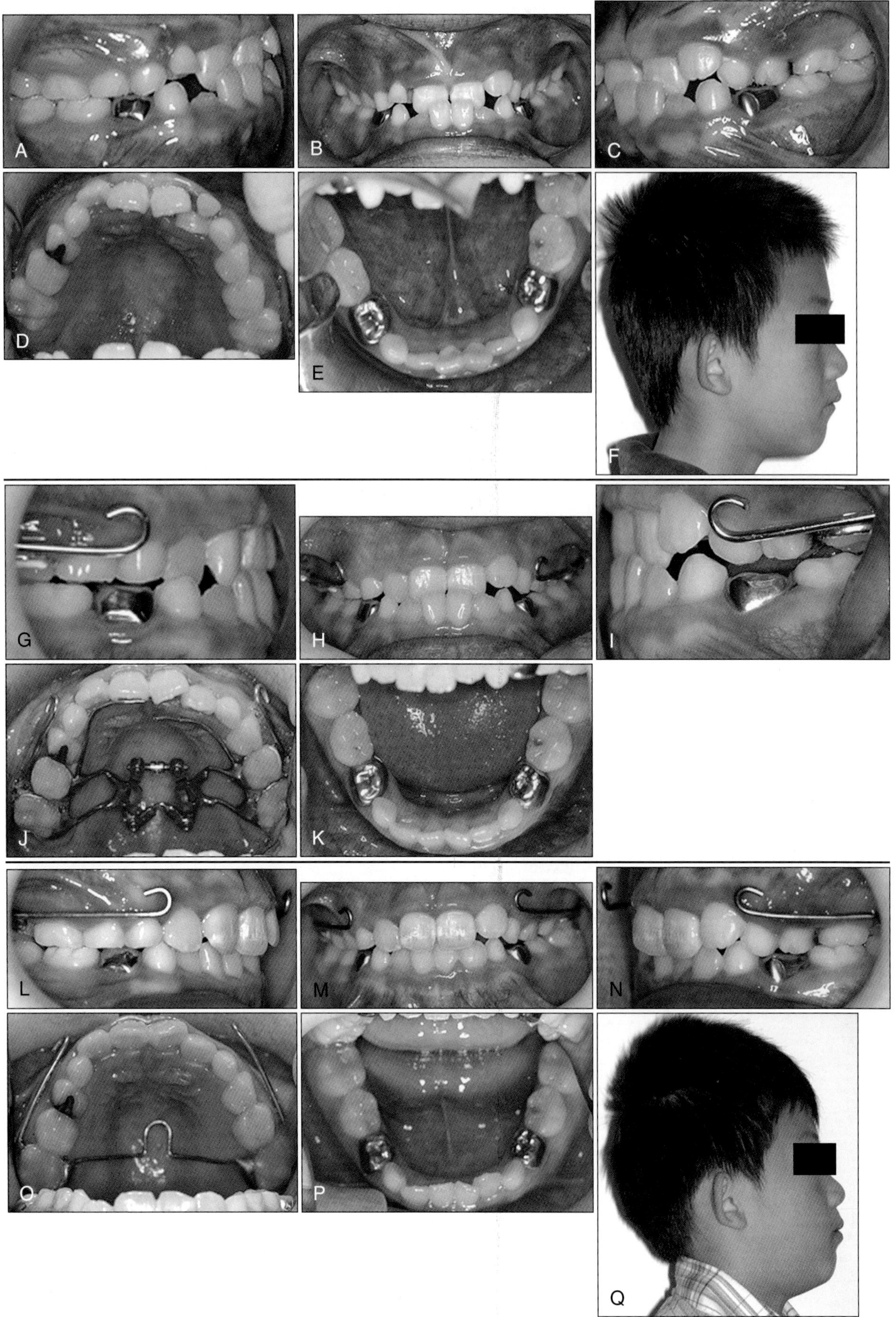

Fig. 13-8 Use of double-hinged maxillary expander and protraction facemask for 8-year-old boy with Class III malocclusion. **A** to **F,** Pretreatment extraoral and intraoral photographs. **G** to **K,** Progress intraoral photographs. **L** to **Q,** Posttreatment extraoral and intraoral photographs. (Patient was treated by Dr. Thuy Do-Delatour.)

References

1. Angle EH: Classification of malocclusion, *Dent Cosmos* 41:248, 1899.
2. Broadbent BH: A new X-ray technique and its application to orthodontia, *Angle Orthod* 1:45-46, 1931.
3. Tweed CH: *Clinical orthodontics,* vol 2, St Louis, 1966, Mosby.
4. Moyers R: *Handbook of orthodontics,* ed 3, Chicago, 1997, Year Book Medical Publishers, pp 564-570.
5. Hill IN, Blayney IR, Wolf W: The Evanston Dental Caries Study. XIX. Prevalence of malocclusion of children in a fluoridated and control area, *J Dent Res* 38:782-794, 1959.
6. Proffit WR, Fields HW Jr, Moray LJ: Prevalence of malocclusion and orthodontic treatment need in the United States: estimates from the NHANES III survey, *Int J Adult Orthod Orthog Surg* 13:97-106, 1998.
7. Baik HS, Kim KH, Park Y: Distribution and trend in malocclusion patients, *Kor J Orthod* 25:87-100, 1995.
8. Ishii H, Morita S, Takeuchi Y, et al: Treatment effect of combined maxillary protraction and chincap appliance in severe skeletal Class III cases, *Am J Orthod Dentofacial Orthop* 92:304-312, 1987.
9. Allwright WC, Burndred WH: A survey of handicapping dentofacial anomalies among Chinese in Hong Kong, *Int Dent J* 14:505-519, 1964.
10. Lin JJ: Prevalence of malocclusion in Chinese children age 9-15, *Clin Dent Chin* 5:57-65, 1985.
11. Garner LD, Butt MH: Malocclusion in black American and Nyeri Kenyanes, *Angle Orthod* 55:139-149, 1985.
12. Silva RG, Kang DS: Prevalence of malocclusion among Latino adolescents, *Am J Orthod Dentofacial Orthop* 119:313-315, 2001.
13. Ellis E, McNamara JA: Components of adult Class III malocclusion, *J Oral Maxillofac Surg* 42:295-305, 1984.
14. Baik HS, Han HK, Kim DJ, Proffit WR: Cephalometric characteristics of Korean Class III surgical patients and their relationship to plans for surgical treatment, *Int Adult Orthod Orthog Surg* 15:119-128, 2000.
15. Enlow DH: *Handbook of facial growth,* ed 2, Philadelphia, 1982, Saunders.
16. Rakosi T, Schilli W: Class III anomalies: a coordinated approach to skeletal, dental, and soft tissue problems, *J Oral Surg* 39:860-870, 1981.
17. Proffit WR, Fields HW Jr: *Contemporary orthodontics,* ed 3, St Louis, 2000, Mosby, pp 134-141.
18. Park JU, Baik SH: Classification of Angle Class III malocclusion and its treatment modalities, *Int J Adult Orthod Orthog Surg* 16:19-29, 2001.
19. Franchi L, Baccetti T, McNamara JA: Postpubertal assessment of treatment timing for maxillary expansion and protraction therapy followed by fixed appliances, *Am J Orthod Dentofacial Orthop* 126:555-568, 2004.
20. Turley PK: Treatment of Class III malocclusion with maxillary expansion and protraction, *Semin Orthod* 13:143-157, 2007.
21. Battagel JM: The aetiological factors in Class III malocclusion, *Br J Orthod* 15:347-370, 1993.
22. Ngan P, Hu AM, Fields HW: Treatment of Class III problems begins with differential diagnosis of anterior crossbites, *Pediatr Dent* 19:386-395, 1997.
23. Stellzig-Eisenhauer A, Lux CJ, Schuster G: Treatment decision in adult patients with Class III malocclusion: orthodontic therapy or orthognathic surgery? *Am J Orthod Dentofacial Orthop* 122:27-38, 2002.
24. Musich D: Severity of Class III malocclusion using the WITS appraisal, 2007 (personal communication).
25. Ngan P, Wei SHY: Early treatment of Class III patients to improve facial aesthetics and predict future growth, *Hong Kong Dent J* 1:24-30, 2004.
26. Ngan P: Treatment of Class III malocclusion in the primary and mixed dentitions. In Bishara SE, editor: *Textbook of orthodontics,* Philadelphia, 2001, Saunders, pp 375-411.
27. Mitani H, Fukazawa H: Effects of chin cup force on the timing and amount of mandibular growth associated with anterior reverse occlusion (Class III malocclusion) during puberty, *Am J Orthod Dentofacial Orthop* 9:454-463, 1986.
28. Petit H: Adaptations following accelerated facial mask therapy in clinical alteration of the growing face. In McNamara JA Jr, Ribbens KA, Howe RP, editors: Monograph 14, Craniofacial Growth Series, Ann Arbor, 1983, Center for Human Growth and Development, University of Michigan.
29. Ulgen M, Firatli S: The effects of Frankel's function regulator on the Class III malocclusion, *Am J Orthod* 105:561-567, 1994.
30. Hagg U, Tse A, Bendeus M, Rabie AB: A follow-up study of early treatment of pseudo Class III malocclusion, *Angle Orthod* 74:465-472, 2004.
31. Nartallo-Turley PE, Turley P: Cephalometric effects of combined palatal expansion and facemask therapy on Class III malocclusion, *Angle Orthod* 68:217-224, 1998.
32. Baccetti T, McGill JS, Franchi L, et al: Skeletal effects of early treatment of Class III malocclusion with maxillary expansion and facemask therapy, *Am J Orthod Dentofacial Orthop* 113:333-343, 1998.
33. Delaire J: Maxillary development revisited: relevance to the orthopaedic treatment of Class III malocclusions, *Eur J Orthod* 19:289-311, 1997.
34. Ngan P, Hagg U, Yiu C, Wei SHY: Treatment response and long-term dentofacial adaptations to maxillary expansion and protraction, *Semin Orthod* 3:255-264, 1997.
35. Ngan P, Cheung E, Wei S: Comparison of protraction facemask response using banded and bonded expansion appliances as anchorage, *Semin Orthod* 13:175-185, 2007.
36. Kambara T: Dentofacial changes produced by extraoral forward force in *Macaca irus, Am J Orthod* 71:249-277, 1977.
37. Nanda R: Protraction of maxilla in rhesus monkeys by controlled extraoral forces, *Am J Orthod* 74:121-141, 1978.
38. Jackson GW, Kokich VG, Shapiro PA: Experimental and postexperimental response to anteriorly directed extraoral force in young *Macaca nemestrina, Am J Orthod* 75:318-333, 1979.
39. Staggers JA, Germane N, Legan HL: Clinical considerations in the use of protraction headgear, *J Clin Orthod* 26:87-91, 1992.
40. Lee KG, Ryu YK, Park YC, Rudolph DJ: A study of holographic inferometry on the initial reaction of the maxillofacial complex during protraction, *Am J Orthod Dentofacial Orthop* 111:623-632, 1997.
41. Hata S, Itoh T, Nakagawa M, et al: Biomechanical effects of maxillary protraction on the craniofacial complex, *Am J Orthod Dentofacial Orthop* 91:305-311, 1987.

42. Ngan P, Yiu C, Hu A, et al: Cephalometric and occlusal changes following maxillary expansion and protraction, *Eur J Orthod* 20:237-254, 1998.
43. Baik HS: Clinical results of the maxillary protraction in Korean children, *Am J Orthod Dentofacial Orthop* 108:583-592, 1995.
44. Da Silva Filho OG, Magro AC, Capoiozza Filho L: Early treatment of the Class III malocclusion with rapid maxillary expansion and maxillary protraction, *Am J Orthod Dentofacial Orthop* 113:196-203, 1998.
45. Kim JH, Viana MA, Graber TM, et al: The effectiveness of protraction face mask therapy: a meta-analysis, *Am J Orthod Dentofacial Orthop* 119:675-685, 1999.
46. Melsen B, Melsen F: The postnatal development of the palatomaxillary region studied on human autopsy material, *Am J Orthod* 82:329-342, 1982.
47. Melsen B: Palatal growth studied on human autopsy material: a histologic microradiographic study, *Am J Orthod* 68:42-54, 1975.
48. Fields HW Jr, Proffit WR: Skeletal problems. In Proffit WR, Fields HW Jr: *Contemporary orthodontics,* ed 3, St Louis, 2000, Mosby, pp 511-512.
49. Hagg U, Tse A, Bendeus M, Rabie AB: Long-term follow-up of early treatment with reverse headgear, *Eur J Orthod* 25:95-102, 2003.
50. Westwood PV, McNamara JA Jr, Baccetti T, et al: Long-term effects of Class III treatment with rapid maxillary expansion and facemask therapy followed by fixed appliances, *Am J Orthod Dentofacial Orthop* 123:306-320, 2003.
51. Block MS, Hoffman DR: A new device for absolute anchorage for orthodontics, *Am J Orthod Dentofacial Orthop* 107:251-258, 1995.
52. Gray JB, Steen ME, King CJ, et al: Studies on the efficacy of implants as orthodontic anchorage, *Am J Orthod* 83:311-317, 1983.
53. Fritz U, Ehmer A, Diedrich P: Clinical suitability of titanium micro-screws for orthodontic anchorage: preliminary experiences, *J Orofac Orthop* 65:410-418, 2004.
54. Nojima K, Komatsu K, Isshiki Y, et al: The use of an osseointegrated implant for orthodontic anchorage to a Class II Div 1 malocclusion, *Bull Tokyo Dent Coll* 42:177-183, 2001.
55. Giancotti A, Greco M, Docimo R, Arcuri C: Extraction treatment using a palatal implant for anchorage, *Aust Orthod J* 19:87-90, 2003.
56. Armbruster PC, Block MS: Onplant-supported orthodontic anchorage, *Atlas Oral Maxillofac Surg Clin North Am* 1:53-74, 2001.
57. Bondemark L, Feldmann I, Feldmann F: Distal molar movement with an intra-arch device provided with the onplant system for absolute anchorage, *World J Orthod* 3:117-124, 2002.
58. Janssens F, Swennen G, Dujardin T, et al: Use of an onplant as orthodontic anchorage, *Am J Orthod Dentofacial Orthop* 122:566-570, 2002.
59. He H, Ngan P, Han GL, et al: Use of onplants as stable anchorage for facemask treatment: a case report, *Angle Orthod* 75:453-460, 2005.
60. Droshl H: The effect of heavy orthopedic forces on the sutures of the facial bones, *Angle Orthod* 45:26-33, 1975.
61. Engstrom C, Thilander B: Premature facial synostosis: the influence of biomechanical factors in normal and hypocalcemic young rats, *Eur J Orthod* 78:35-47, 1985.
62. Line L: Tissue reactions incident to widening of facial sutures: an experimental study in the *Macaca mulatta, Trans Eur Orthod Soc* 48:487-497, 1972.
63. Braun S, Bottrel JA, Lee KG, et al: The biomechanics of rapid maxillary sutural expansion, *Am J Orthod Dentofacial Orthop* 118:257-261, 2000.
64. Liou EJW: Effective maxillary orthopedic protraction for growing Class III patients: a clinical application simulates distraction osteogenesis, *Prog Orthod* 6:36-53, 2005.
65. Liou EJW, Tsai WC: A new protocol for maxillary protraction in cleft patients: repetitive weekly protocol of alternate rapid maxillary expansions and constrictions, *Cleft Palate Craniofac J* 42:121-127, 2005.
66. Liou EJW: Toothborne orthopedic maxillary protraction in Class III patients, *J Clin Orthod* 39:68-75, 2005.

CHAPTER 14

Etiological and Therapeutic Considerations with Open Bite

Kazunori Yamaguchi

Patients with open bite often complain of functional disorders, such as difficulties in cutting and chewing food with the upper and lower incisors (Fig. 14-1), as well as speech difficulty. Clinicians need to understand the factors causing this dentofacial skeletal problem and design therapeutic solutions accordingly.

CLASSIFICATION OF OPEN BITE

There are three types of open bite (Fig. 14-2). The finger-sucking habit during childhood impedes normal eruption of the anterior teeth and alveolar growth and induces *dentoalveolar open bite.* Prevention of the deleterious habit should be helpful in improving this type of open bite. *Skeletal open bite* with a long face can be divided into two types, one caused by clockwise rotation of the mandible, and the other by skeletal deformation, such as tipping of the maxilla and diversion of the gonial angle of the mandible.

Open bite is always accompanied by a tongue-thrusting habit. It appears that individuals with a long face have weaker contraction of the mandibular elevator muscles, lower electromyographic (EMG) activity of the muscles during maximum voluntary clenching, and lower occlusal force than the corresponding values of short-face individuals.[1-5]

Mechanisms of Skeletal Open Bite

The main mechanism responsible for skeletal open bite is a proportional discrepancy between the anterior and posterior facial heights. The vertical height of the nasomaxillary complex, the ramus height, and the posterior teeth are important factors that determine the mandibular vertical position. Any elongation or extrusion of the posterior teeth will result in a clockwise rotation of the mandible (see Fig. 14-2).

MASTICATION AND VERTICAL POSITION OF POSTERIOR TEETH

Magnitude and duration of force application are important factors for the stability of tooth position. The occlusal contact and the eruptive or extrusive movement of the tooth determine the vertical position of the posterior teeth. The *magnitude* of tooth contact force on the posterior teeth depends on the strength of muscular activity. The *duration* of daily tooth contact varies between 1 and 3 hours, depending on the duration of mastication, swallowing, and sleeping.[6-8]

Unless the magnitude and duration of occlusal contact force are sufficient to prevent elongation of the posterior teeth, they will extrude, resulting in open bite. For example, the food features or the food-intake habits of young people, such as consumption of soft diet within a short eating time and irregular meal intake, could result in reduced tooth contact of the posterior teeth and subsequent development of vertical occlusal problems.

The author's investigation was based on a questionnaire for dental students age 18 to 26 years. It showed that 55% of male and 81% of female students regularly eat three meals a day. Male students reported spending 48.1 minutes and female students 60.0 minutes eating food over three meals (Table 14-1).

Taking these findings into consideration, one can hypothesize that intensifying the vertical effect on the posterior teeth by increasing the degree and duration of the occlusal contact is a useful strategy (1) to promote healthy development of occlusion in growing children and (2) to obtain a stable outcome after orthodontic or orthognathic treatment.

Several studies have described methods to intensify muscle activity based on isometric muscle exercise.[9-12] As

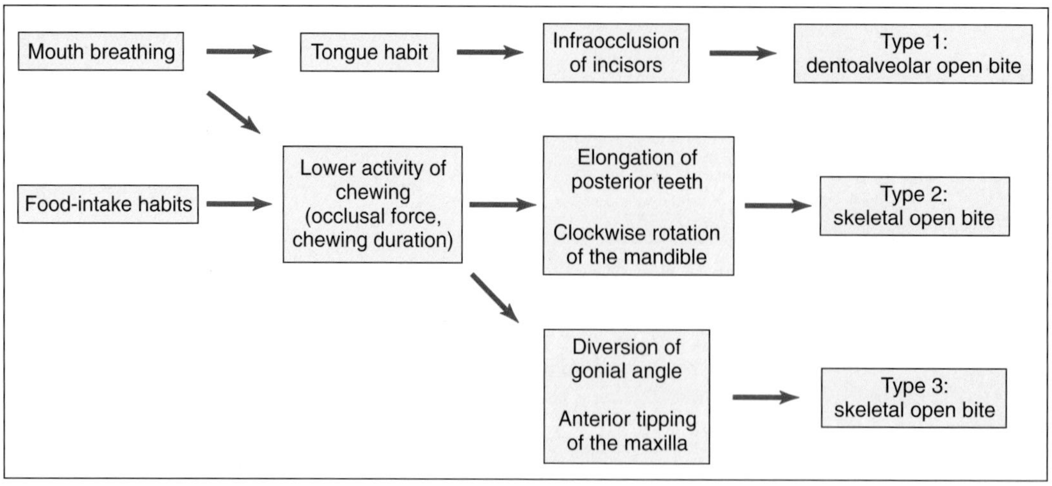

Mouth breathing → Tongue habit → Infraocclusion of incisors → Type 1: dentoalveolar open bite

Food-intake habits → Lower activity of chewing (occlusal force, chewing duration) → Elongation of posterior teeth / Clockwise rotation of the mandible → Type 2: skeletal open bite

Diversion of gonial angle / Anterior tipping of the maxilla → Type 3: skeletal open bite

Fig. 14-1 Etiological factors and morphological features of open bite.

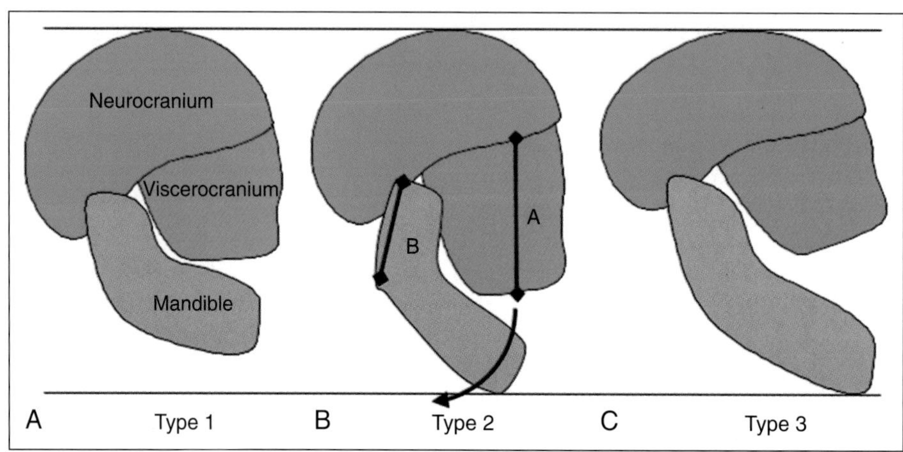

Fig. 14-2 Classification of open bite. **A,** Type 1: Dentoalveolar open bite. Finger-sucking habit impedes normal eruption of the anterior teeth and alveolar growth. Correction of the deleterious habits should improve this type of open bite. **B,** Type 2: Skeletal open bite with a long face caused by clockwise rotation of the mandible. **C,** Type 3: Skeletal open bite caused by skeletal deformation such as tipping of the maxilla and diversion of the gonial angle of the mandible.

TABLE **14-1**

Questionnaire Results: Duration of Meal for Dental Students

	Breakfast (min)	Lunch (min)	Dinner (min)	Total Time (min)
Male (n = 49)	7.6	18.8	21.8	48.1
Female (n = 49)	11.5	21.2	27.3	60.00
MEAN (n = 76)	8.8	19.3	23.2	51.4

reported by several investigators, isometric clenching increases the contraction force of the elevator muscle of the mandible and the bite force on the posterior teeth.[13-16] Some studies were done to examine only the muscular activity and bite force.[17-20] Muscle exercise was used to intensify the vertical effects on the teeth by increasing the magnitude and duration of the occlusal contact.[21-29]

Clenching Exercise Using Soft Bite Block

In one study, 24 healthy adult volunteers performed isometric clenching at maximum voluntary contraction against a soft bite block for 3 seconds with 5 seconds of rest over a 15-minute session, with at least two sessions per day over 8 weeks (Fig. 14-3).[30] The occlusal contact area and pressure were recorded using Dental Prescale film and analyzed by the Occluzer (FPD 703, Fuji Film, Tokyo, Japan). The upper soft bite block was adjusted to make full contact with the lower teeth in a nonrestrained mandibular position, to prevent negative reflection caused by possible interference of a single tooth.

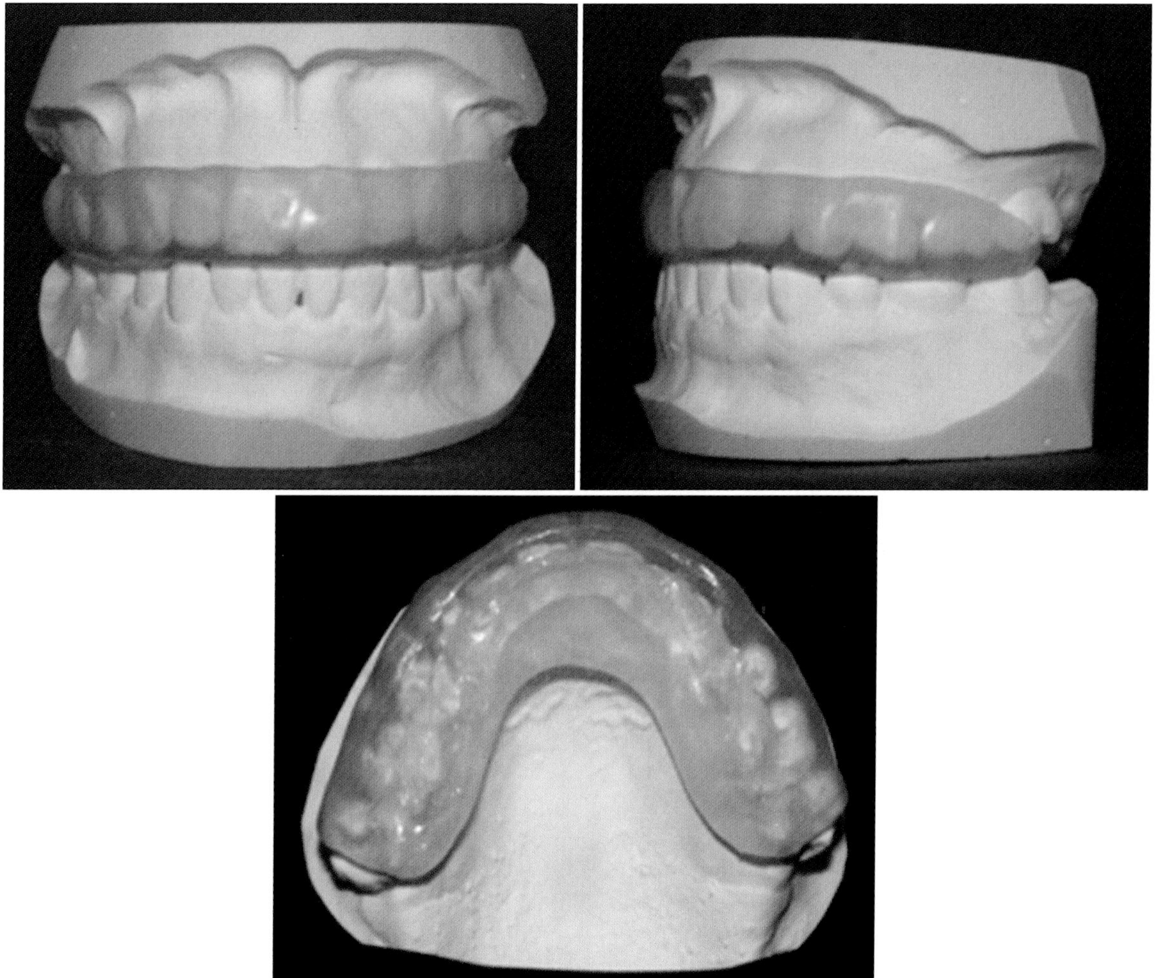

Fig. 14-3 Soft bite plate for clenching exercise. Upper soft bite block was adjusted to make full contact with lower teeth. (From Uchida M, Yamaguchi K, Nagano S, Ichida T: *Orthod Waves* 64:29-37, 2005.)

Subjects who complained about discomfort on the dentition and temporomandibular joint during muscle training were excluded from the study. It was presumed that the contact pressure during clenching the bite block at voluntary contraction was equivalent to the pressure on biting a Dental Prescale sheet. Although the occlusal parameters, including occlusal contact area and occlusal force, were higher in men than in women, the total contact force was 1122 ± 398 newtons (N), and the average contact pressure was 35.9 ± 4.7 megapascals (MPa)/mm^2 at baseline (Table 14-2).[30] Therefore the degree of occlusal contact force on the posterior teeth during clenching the bite block was more than the optimal force for tooth movement. The vertical force on the posterior teeth was not continuous but intermittent.

With regard to the duration of the muscle-training program, Petrofsky and Laymon[31] reported an effective training protocol that involved electrical stimulation of the quadriceps muscles, in which training was conducted for 15 or 30 minutes each day. Thompson et al.[14] stated that isometric clenching against a soft maxillary splint for five 1-minute sessions per day over a 6-week period increased the maximum bite force. Tzakis et al.[15] studied the influence of 30 minutes of intense chewing for 5 days on the masticatory function and showed that such a protocol had variable short-term effects on masticatory function. Kihara[8] reported that the average time of daily tooth contact at the first molar was 67 minutes, and that the mean frequency of daily tooth contact was about 4270 times in normal adult men.

It seems that isometric clenching on a bite plate for 30 minutes a day over 8 weeks prolongs the time of tooth contact and intensifies the vertical effect on dentition. In a preliminary study, the author's group found that it was very difficult for subjects to clench their teeth persistently over 30 minutes every day over 1 week. Instead, the subjects were asked to perform isometric clenching at maximum voluntary contraction against a soft bite block for 3 seconds with 5 seconds' rest for 15-minute sessions, with at least two sessions per day over 8 weeks. Recording of occlusal parameters was repeated three times with 3-minute intervals, and repeated over 5 days in the control group and every week for 8 weeks in the exercise group. This protocol increased the total, anterior, and posterior occlusal contact areas to 135.8%, 219.8%, and 129.6% relative to the baseline values, respectively, following the 8-week exercise (Fig. 14-4, *A*), and also significantly increased the anteroposterior balance of occlusal contact area (Fig. 14-4, *B*).[30] The same 8-week exercise did not alter the mesiolateral balance of occlusal contact area (Fig. 14-4, *C*) or the contact pressure (Fig. 14-5).

TABLE 14-2

Occlusal Parameters: Standard Values in Healthy Adult Volunteers

	Occlusal Force (N)	Occlusal Contact Area (mm^2)	Occlusal Pressure (MPa/ mm^2)
Men	1223.7	35.2	35.8
Women	895.8	26.99	36
TOTAL	1122.2	32.6	35.9

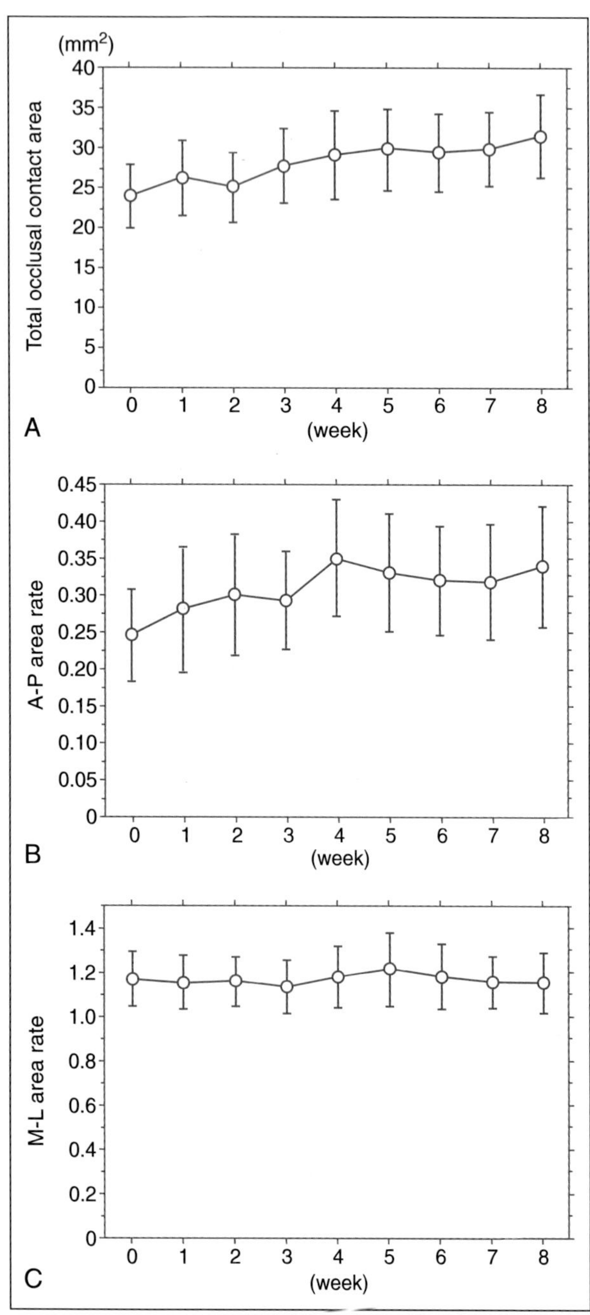

Fig. 14-4 Changes in contact area during voluntary clenching: **A,** total occlusal contact area; **B,** anteroposterior *(A-P)* area rate; **C,** mediolateral *(M-L)* area rate. The mean values of total occlusal contact area and anteroposterior area increased progressively during the muscle-training period. (From Uchida M, Yamaguchi K, Nagano S, Ichida T: *Orthod Waves* 64:29-37, 2005.)

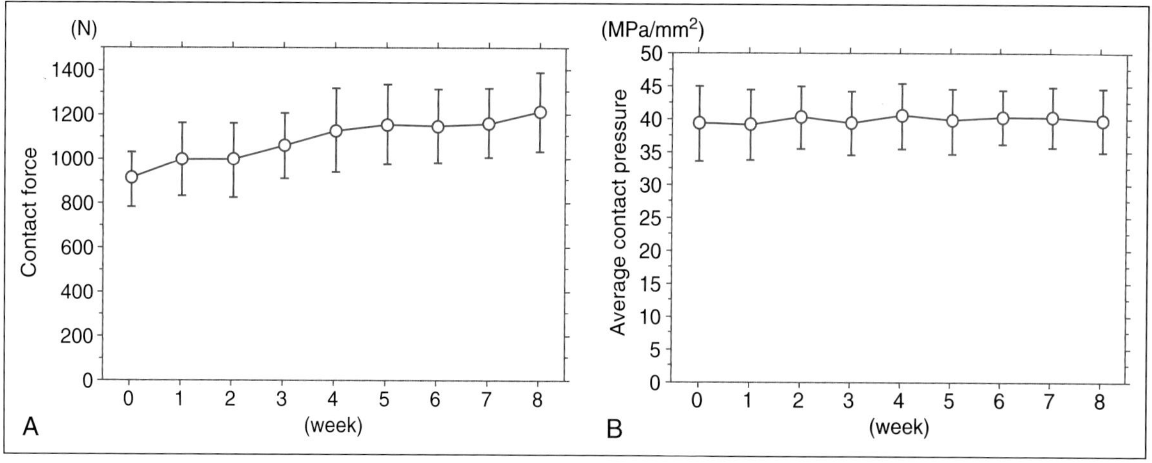

Fig. 14-5 Changes in **A,** contact force, and **B,** average contact pressure. Occlusal contact force increased progressively during the muscle-training period. There was no significant change in the average occlusal contact pressure. (From Uchida M, Yamaguchi K, Nagano S, Ichida T: *Orthod Waves* 64:29-37, 2005.)

Chewing Gum Exercise

The author's results indicated that isometric muscle exercise for 8 weeks increased occlusal contact area and advanced the balance of occlusal contact area. The questionnaire study on muscle exercise using a soft bite plate revealed that it was very difficult for subjects to continue the clenching exercise using the soft bite plate for 8 weeks. It was necessary to find a more comfortable and effective exercise protocol.

The habit of chewing gum is popular in many countries, especially after the introduction of sugarless chewing gum. The most frequent answer to the question, "What do you think is the purpose of chewing a gum?" was that chewing a gum was refreshing, enhanced concentration, and released stress[32] (Fig. 14-6). These findings indicated that chewing gum is not a stressful but rather a stress-releasing habit.

Because a more comfortable training protocol is more likely to be continued, the "chewing gum exercise" was designed. This involved chewing gum for 30 to 45 minutes per day over 4 weeks. Fifty dental students were enrolled in this study. The same occlusal parameters were estimated at the end of the exercise and 1 month later. At the end of the chewing gum exercise, the total occlusal force increased to 140% (Fig. 14-7), total contact area increased to 125%, but the occlusal pressure remained the same, relative to baseline values (before the exercise). One month after the end of the exercise, the increased occlusal force and occlusal contact area decreased to 105% and 103% of baseline, respectively.[33]

These results suggest that the chewing gum exercise is effective in increasing the occlusal contact and occlusal force. In addition, at the end of the protocol, most of the subjects answered "yes" to the question, "Do you think masticatory exercise using a chewing gum is comfortable to continue the training program?"

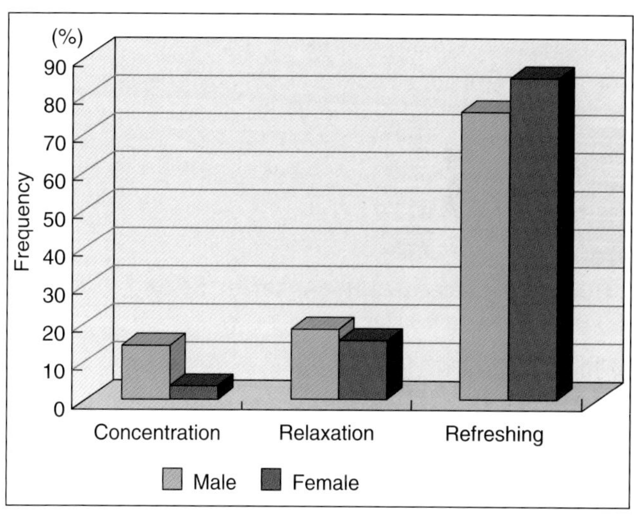

Fig. 14-6 Results from a questionnaire regarding the purpose of chewing gum. The most frequently cited purpose of chewing gum was refreshing, enhanced concentration, and release from stress.

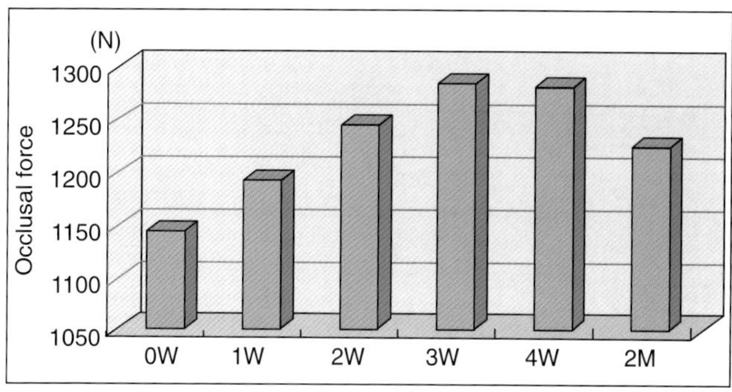

Fig. 14-7 Changes in occlusal force during and after chewing exercise. Occlusal contact force increased progressively during the 4-week chewing exercise but decreased 1 month later. *N,* Newtons; *W,* week(s); *M,* months.

Preserving Vertical Effect on Posterior Teeth After Correction of Open Bite

In the treatment of open bite or edge-to-edge bite, intrusion of the posterior teeth or maintenance of the posterior occlusal height is usually achieved by increasing the vertical effect on the posterior teeth using high-pull headgear, bite block, or metal implant.[34-38] Unless the magnitude and duration of occlusal contact force is sufficient to prevent elongation of the posterior teeth after active treatment, the posterior teeth will extrude again and result in recurrence of the open bite. This makes it imperative to preserve the vertical effect on the posterior teeth after active orthodontic and orthognathic surgical treatment of the open bite. The "chewing gum exercise" is one method that can ensure long-term stability in such patients.

MOUTH BREATHING

There has been an increased focus on mouth breathing in recent years not only in orthodontics, but also in the field of dentistry, as an integral part of oral health promotion. Breathing through the nose provides many benefits, such as warming and humidification of the inspired air before its delivery to the pharynx, larynx, bronchi, and lungs.[39] In addition, the warm air protects the oral mucosa compared with cool or dry air.

Breaking Posterior and Anterior Seals

For nasal breathing, the soft palate establishes a tight contact with the tongue to close the oropharyngeal isthmus, and the lips usually make a light contact without excessive contraction of the lower lip. When nasal resistance increases above certain level, the anterior and posterior seals are broken, and nasal breathing is switched to mouth breathing[40,41] (Fig. 14-8). High nasal resistance is typically seen in patients with common cold, chronic rhinitis, tonsillar or adenoidal hypertrophy, or a narrow nasopharyngeal airway.

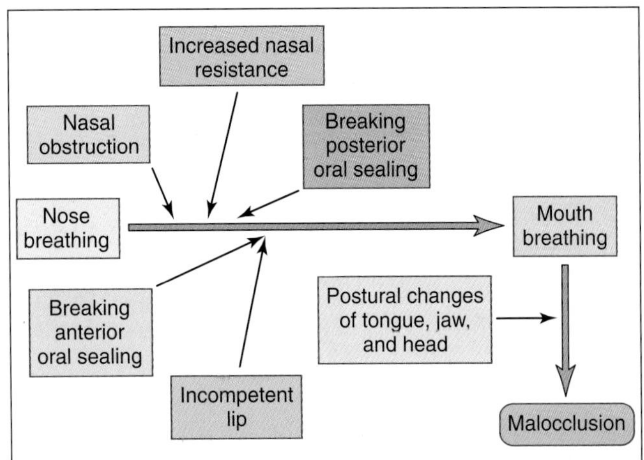

Fig. 14-8 Etiology and effect of mouth breathing.

To break the posterior oral seal, the soft palate is elevated toward the posterior pharyngeal wall, and the tongue sags posteriorly. The soft palate plays an important role in regulating airflow through the nose and mouth, although the posterior sealing function of the soft palate varies among patients.

Again, the lips usually establish a light contact without excessive contraction of the lower lip. The seal can be broken by (1) an incompetent lip, caused by the anteroposterior relationship between the upper and lower incisors and the vertical dimension of the dentofacial complex,[42-44] and (2) mouth breathing. For mouth breathing to occur, both the anterior and posterior seals should be broken.

Epidemiological Study

When studying the effects of mouth breathing on dentofacial growth in humans, many investigators focus on the etiological factors and symptoms of mouth breathing and examine airflow from the nose clinically using mirror and cotton fly tests. In a preliminary study, students at the author's school were asked 17 questions on the etiological factors and symptoms of mouth breathing. Two studies reported that the incidence of mouth breathers among 500 patients was 19%, and 6% had allergic rhinitis.[45,46] In our study, 34% of students complained of stuffy nose, 28% were known to snore during sleep, and 30% had allergic rhinitis (Fig. 14-9).

Subjects with stuffy nose are likely to open their lips at rest or during sleep (Fig. 14-10). Subjects with open lips at rest seem to complain of stuffy nose, snoring, and allergic rhinitis. The questionnaire results indicated that stuffy nose, snoring, and nasal allergy are the main mechanisms associated with obstructed nasal airway, and many subjects with stuffy nose who report snoring and nasal allergy tend to open the lips voluntarily at rest.

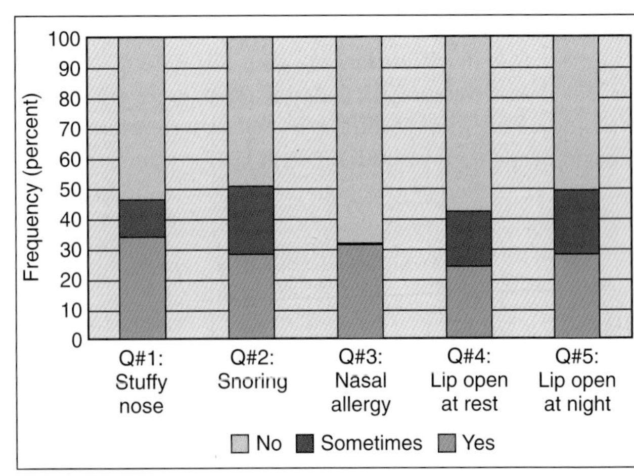

Fig. 14-9 Questions on breathing related to nasal problems. In the author's study, 34% of students complained of stuffy nose, 28% students were known snorers, and 30% had allergic rhinitis.

It should be emphasized that clinical tests based on questionnaire could yield misleading results, especially when they include only a brief interview with the patient or parents. There is a need to establish an objective diagnosis of mouth breathing.[47]

Functional Features of Mouth Breathing and Relationship to Malocclusion

The systematic changes in the soft tissues of the oronasal airway that allow mouth breathing should be the main factors that affect normal growth of dentofacial structures (Fig. 14-11). In experimental studies, switching from nasal to oral breathing often results in anterior reversed occlusion and/or open bite.[48-52]

The author conducted an experimental study in which mouth breathing was induced by nasal obstruction. Mouth breathing rapidly induced anterior reversed occlusion or anterior open bite when it was enforced in young animals with deciduous dentition during the period of change of upper and lower incisors (Fig. 14-12). In comparison, in adult subjects, such anterior reversed occlusion occurred 18 months after switching to mouth breathing.[52] In young monkeys the nasomaxillary complex showed downward growth, and the mandible showed clockwise rotation (Fig. 14-13).[52] The clockwise rotation of the nasomaxillary complex and mandible seem to induce open bite.

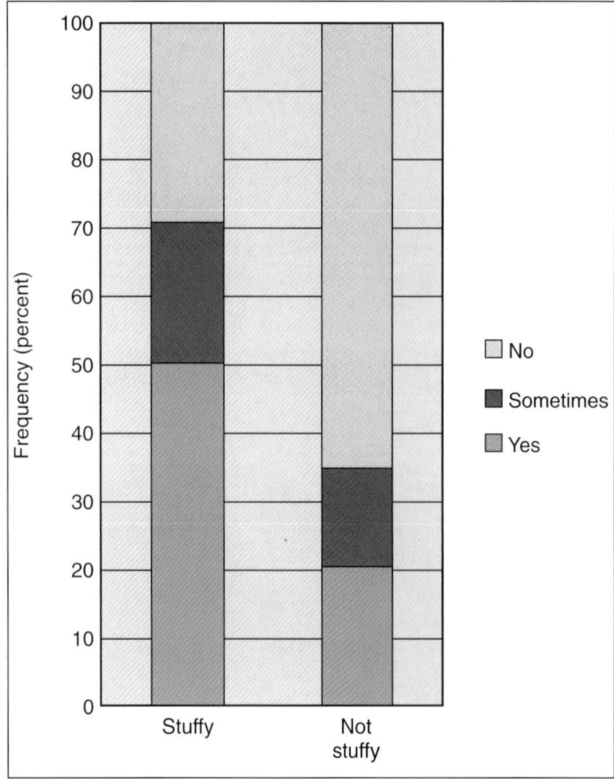

Fig. 14-10 Questions on nasal symptoms and lip sealing. In subjects with stuffy nose, percentage of those with voluntary open lips was significantly higher than those without stuffy nose. The result indicates that subjects complaining of stuffy nose are likely to have open lips at rest or at night.

Disordered Chewing Rhythm and Lip-Sealing Function

The author has found that duration of gum chewing depended on the lip-sealing function; the duration was shorter when chewing with the lips in contact compared with chewing with the lips apart (Fig. 14-14).[53] Although the pattern generator in the brainstem governs chewing-related muscle contraction, many factors may alter the chewing pattern and cycle.

Throckmorton et al.[54] studied changes in the masticatory cycle before and after treatment of posterior unilateral crossbite and found that a longer chewing cycle was shortened to become equal to the control values after treatment. Miyawaki et al.[55] stated that the mean duration of the chewing cycle decreased after surgical orthodontic treatment. Sohn et al.[56] reported that the duration of muscle activity and the incidence of silent periods of the masseter muscle during chewing significantly decreased after treatment. In an experimental study in rabbits, Matsuka et al.[57] reported that the animals exhibited a prolonged chewing cycle after placement of bite-raising splints. Karkazis and Kossioni[58] indicated that the duration of the chewing cycle, the chewing rate, and the relative contraction time during chewing were significantly higher for chewing of carrots than that for nonadhesive chewing gums. Papargyriou et al[59] reported that chewing cycle duration, the opening and occlusal time of the chewing cycle, increased during development.

During chewing, the lips act to seal the mouth so as to prevent food leakage from the oral cavity. Chewing with the lips in contact is an involuntary act, and chewing with the lips apart is a voluntary movement in subjects with competent or incompetent lips. It is expected that the open-lip posture during chewing affects chewing movement, and that the chewing cycle is shortened during the nonactive phase of masseter activity. In chewing food with the lips apart, it is difficult to achieve the chewing task without the cooperation of the tongue, cheek, and dentition. There should be profound tongue activity and limited mandibular movement when chewing food with the lips apart.[53]

Chewing and Breathing Through the Mouth

Mouth breathers have another disadvantage related to the chewing function. They must maintain a patent oral airway at rest and during food chewing, in addition to opening the lips at rest and during chewing of food. In subjects with competent lips, nasal breathing occurs while the lips are lightly in contact during regular and constant chewing activity, without breaking the chewing rhythm (Fig. 14-15). In mouth breathers with nasal obstruction, the anterior seal is broken, the mandible is lowered, and the tongue moves posteriorly at rest to maintain a patent oral airway. For this reason, such individuals stop the chewing activity when

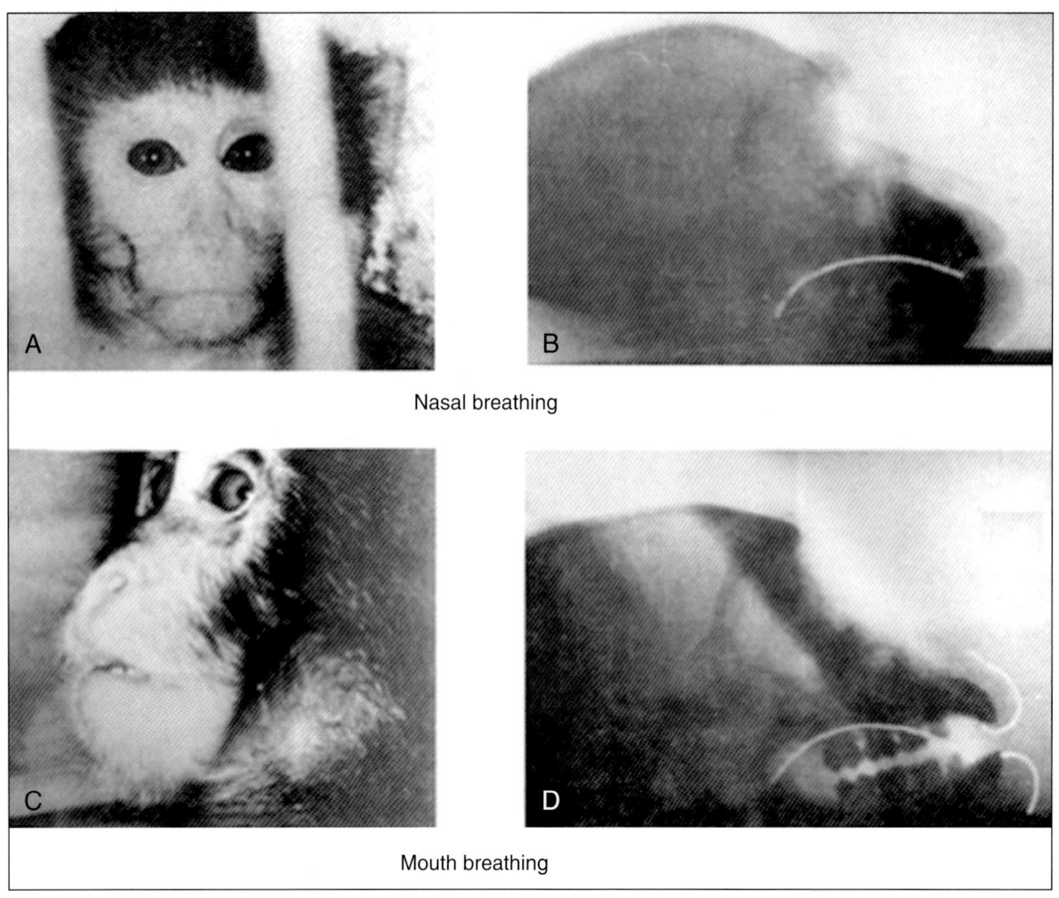

Fig. 14-11 Experimental mouth-breathing study in monkeys. **A** and **B**, Nasal breathing. **C** and **D**, Mouth breathing. Mouth breathing is controlled by the researcher. The anterior and posterior oral seals are broken, and mouth breathing is induced by nasal obstruction (From Yamaguchi K: *Nippon Kyosei Shika Gakkai Zasshi* 39:24-45, 1980.)

breathing through the mouth. The duration of chewing is shorter in mouth breathing induced by nasal obstruction. The respiratory rate in adults is 16 to 18 breaths/min but faster in younger individuals (20-30 breaths/min).

The author found that the duration of chewing with the nose obstructed for 10 strokes ranged from 6 to 7 seconds. Adult subjects would breathe at least once or twice during chewing for 10 strokes. As shown in Figure 14-16, subjects should halt chewing movement for a very short time for inspiration or expiration, and thus miss one or two breaths. The duration of chewing with the nose closed was significantly shorter compared with that for lips-closed chewing in subjects with incompetent lips.

Clinical Implications

Considered together, these findings suggest that the duration of chewing decreases and the chance for tooth contact in the posterior region diminishes in mouth breathers. Consequently, decreased tooth contact may reduce the vertical effect on the posterior teeth. Habitual mouth breathing will develop open bite or initiate vertical abnormal occlusion. Mouth breathing is induced by respiratory abnormalities of the nasopharyngeal airway (e.g., hypertrophy of adenoid and inflammation of the nasal mucosa). Orthodontists and pedodontists should identify mouth breathing in children at early stages of growth, and appreciate the deleterious effects of mouth breathing on the orofacial structure. It is important to diagnose mouth breathing, provide adequate information on possible treatment, and refer the individual for ears-nose-throat (ENT) assessment.

CONCLUSION

Clinicians need to consider causative factors in providing effective therapeutic strategies (e.g., gum chewing, mouth breathing) for functional disorders associated with open bite.

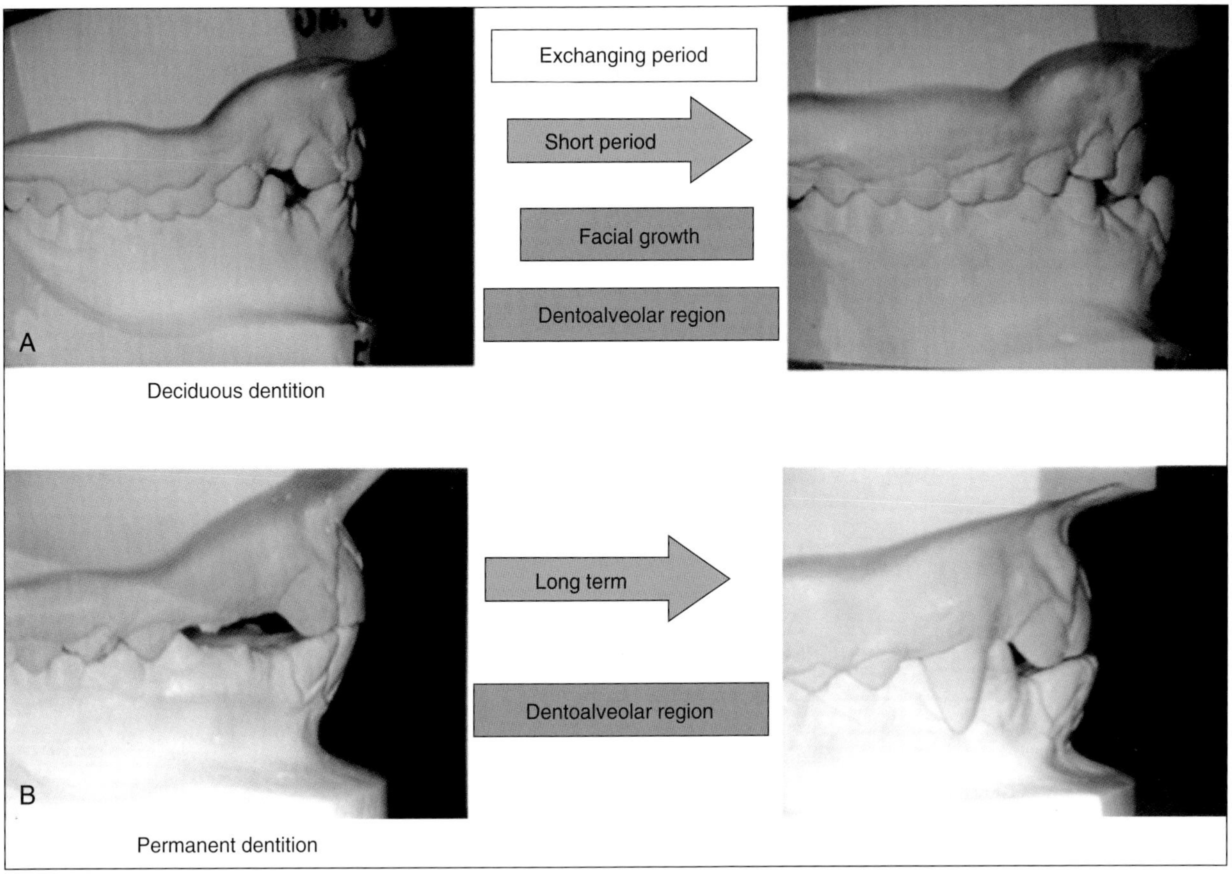

Exchanging period
Short period
Facial growth
Dentoalveolar region
A
Deciduous dentition
Long term
Dentoalveolar region
B
Permanent dentition

Fig. 14-12 Occurrence of malocclusion in young and adult monkeys. **A,** Deciduous dentition. **B,** Permanent dentition. Mouth breathing rapidly induced, anterior reversed occlusion when enforced in young animals with deciduous dentition during period of change of upper and lower incisors. In comparison, in adult subjects, such anterior reversed occlusion was noted 18 months after switching to mouth breathing. (From Yamaguchi K: *Nippon Kyosei Shika Gakkai Zasshi* 39:24-45, 1980.)

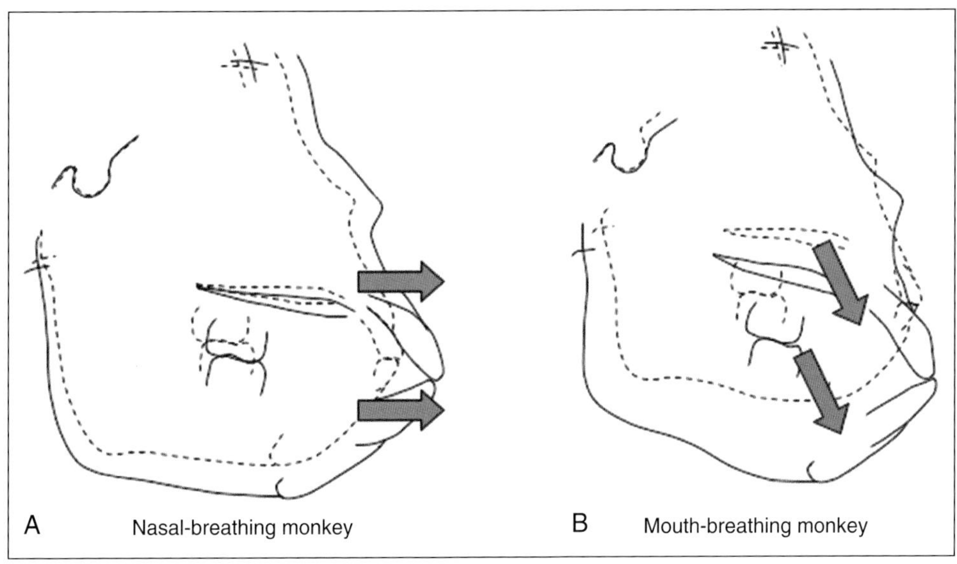

Fig. 14-13 Changes in growth direction of nasomaxillary complex in monkeys. **A,** Nasal breather. **B,** Mouth breather. In young monkeys, maxillary complex and mandible showed clockwise rotation. The clockwise rotation of the nasomaxillary complex and mandible may explain the open bite. (From Yamaguchi K: *Nippon Kyosei Shika Gakkai Zasshi* 39:24-45, 1980.)

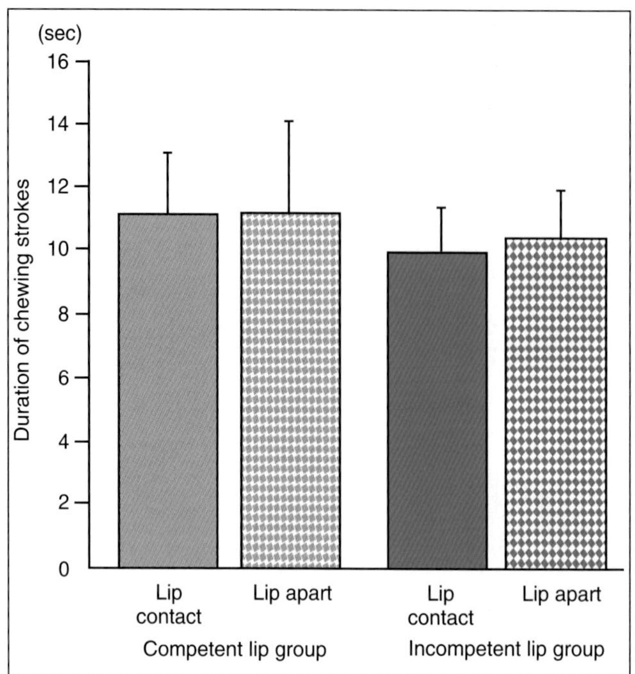

Fig. 14-14 Duration of 15 chewing strokes with the lips in contact and apart. (Modified from Tomiyama N, Ichida T, Yamaguchi K: *Angle Orthod* 74:31-36, 2004.)

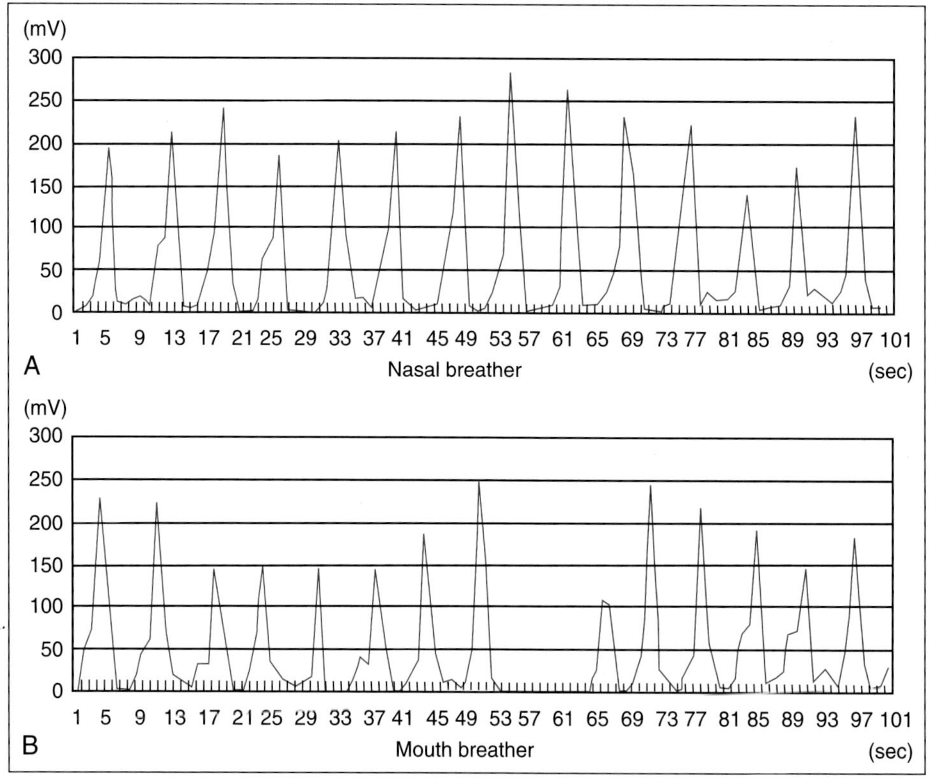

Fig. 14-15 Chewing rhythm in different breathing modes **A,** Nasal breathing. **B,** Mouth breathing.

REFERENCES

1. Bakke M, Michler L: Temporalis and masseter muscle activity in patients with anterior open bite and craniomandibular disorders, *Scand J Dent Res* 99:219-228, 1991.
2. Proffit WR, Fields HW: Occlusal forces in normal- and long-face children, *J Dent Res* 62:571-574, 1983.
3. Throckmorton GS, Finn RA, Bell WH: Biomechanics of differences in lower facial height, *Am J Orthod* 77:410-420, 1980.
4. Serrao G, Sforza C: Relation between vertical facial morphology and jaw muscle activity in healthy young men, *Prog Orthod* 4:45-51, 2003.
5. Kasai K: Soft tissue adaptability to hard tissues in facial profiles, *Am J Orthod Dentofacial Orthop* 113:674-684, 1998.
6. Sheppard IM, Marcus N: Total time of tooth contact during mastication, *J Prosthet Dent* 12:460-463, 1962.
7. Powell RN, Zander HA: The frequency and distribution of tooth contact, *J Dent Res* 44:713-717, 1965.
8. Kihara M: A study on factors related to stability of vertical position of the teeth, *J Kyushu Dent Soc* 28:511-528, 1975.
9. Hakkinen K, Komi PV, Alen M: Effect of explosive-type strength training on isometric force and relaxation time: electromyographic and muscle fibre characteristics of leg extensor muscles, *Acta Physiol Scand* 125:587-600, 1985.
10. Hakkinen K, Alen M, Komi PV: Changes in isometric force and relaxation time: electromyographic and muscle fibre characteristics of human skeletal muscle during strength training and detraining, *Acta Physiol Scand* 125:573-585, 1985.
11. Pavone E, Moffat M: Isometric torque of the quadriceps femoris after concentric, eccentric and isometric training, *Arch Physiol Med Rehabil* 66:168-170, 1985.
12. McDonagh MJ, Hayward CM, Davies CT: Isometric training in human elbow flexor muscles: the effects on voluntary and electrically evoked forces, *J Bone Joint Surg* 65:355-358, 1983.
13. Kiliaridis S, Tzakis MG, Carlsson GE: Effects of fatigue and chewing training on maximal bite force and endurance, *Am J Orthod Dentofacial Orthop* 107:372-378, 1995.
14. Thompson DJ, Throckmorton GS, Buschang PH: The effects of isometric exercise on maximum voluntary bite forces and jaw muscle strength and endurance, *J Oral Rehabil* 28:909-917, 2001.
15. Tzakis MG, Kiliaridis S, Carlsson GE: Effect of a fatigue test and chewing training on masticatory muscles, *J Oral Rehabil* 21:33-45, 1994.
16. Christensen LV, Mohamed SE, Rugh JD: Isometric endurance of the human masseter muscle during consecutive bouts of tooth clenching, *J Oral Rehabil* 12:509-514, 1985.
17. Raadsheer MC, Van Eijden TM, Van Ginkel FC, Prahl-Andersen B: Contribution of jaw muscle size and craniofacial morphology to human bite force magnitude, *J Dent Res* 78:31-42, 1999.
18. Van Spronsen PH, Koolstra JH, Van Ginkel FC, et al: Relationships between the orientation and moment arms of the human jaw muscles and normal craniofacial morphology, *Eur J Orthod* 19:313-328, 1997.
19. Van Eijden TM: Jaw muscle activity in relation to the direction and point of application of bite force, *J Dent Res* 69:901-905, 1990.
20. Garcia-Morales P, Buschang PH, Throckmorton GS, English JD: Maximum bite force, muscle efficiency and mechanical advantage in children with vertical growth patterns, *Eur J Orthod* 25:265-272, 2003.
21. Ohkura K, Harada K, Morishita S, Enomoto S: Changes in bite force and occlusal contact area after orthognathic surgery for correction of mandibular prognathism, *Oral Surg Oral Med Oral Pathol* 91:141-145, 2001.
22. Shinogaya T, Kimura M, Matsumoto M: Effects of occlusal contact on the level of mandibular elevator muscle activity during maximal clenching in lateral positions, *J Med Dent Sci* 44:105-112, 1997.
23. Kikuchi M, Korioth TW, Hannam AG: The association among occlusal contacts, clenching effort, and bite force distribution in man, *J Dent Res* 76:1316-1325, 1997.
24. Shinogaya T, Sodeyama A, Matsumoto M: Bite force and occlusal load distribution in normal complete dentitions of young adults, *Eur J Prosthod Restor Dent* 7:65-70, 1999.
25. Kumagai H, Suzuki T, Hamada T, et al: Occlusal force distribution on the dental arch during various levels of clenching, *J Oral Rehabil* 26:932-935, 1999.
26. Gabriel DA, Basford JR, An KN: Neural adaptations to fatigue: implications for muscle strength and training, *Med Sci Sports Exerc* 33:1354-1360, 2001.
27. Makofsky HW, Sexton TR, Diamond DZ, Sexton MT: The effect of head posture on muscle contact position using the T-Scan system of occlusal analysis, *Cranio* 9:316-321, 1991.
28. Chapman RJ, Maness WL, Osorio J: Occlusal contact variation with changes in head position, *Int J Prosthod* 4:377-381, 1991.
29. Sodeyama A, Shinogaya T, Matsumoto M: Reproducibility of maximal bite force distribution over dentition, *Kokubyo Gakkai Zasshi* 65:339-343, 1998.
30. Uchida M, Yamaguchi K, Nagano S, Ichida T: Daily clenching exercise enhances the occlusal contact, *Orthod Waves* 64:29-37, 2005.
31. Petrofsky JS, Laymon M: The effect of aging in spinal cord–injured humans on the blood pressure and heart rate responses during fatiguing isometric exercise, *Eur J Appl Physiol* 86:479-486, 2002.
32. Masumoto N, Yamaguchi K, Fujimoto S: Is chewing exercise improving occlusal contact? Questionnaire on manner of food taking. Presented at 66th Congress of Japanese Orthodontic Society, 2007.
33. Masumoto N, Yamaguchi K, Uchida M, Fujimoto S: Chewing exercise is improving occlusal contact: increasing chance of occlusal contact by daily chewing gum. Presented at 66th Congress of Japanese Orthodontic Society, 2007.
34. Throckmorton GS, Ellis E 3rd: The relationship between surgical changes in dentofacial morphology and changes in maximum bite force, *J Oral Maxillofac Surg* 59:620-627, 2001.
35. Athanasiou AE: Number and intensity of occlusal contacts following surgical correction of mandibular prognathism, *J Oral Rehabil* 19:145-150, 1992.
36. Hoppenreijs TJ, Van der Linden FP, Freihofer HP, et al: Occlusal and functional conditions after surgical correction of anterior open bite deformities, *Int J Adult Orthod Orthog Surg* 11:29-39, 1996.
37. Umemori M, Sugawara J, Mitani H, et al: Skeletal anchorage system for open-bite correction, *Am J Orthod Dentofacial Orthop* 115:166-174, 1999.
38. Erverdi N, Keles A, Nanda R: The use of skeletal anchorage in open bite treatment: a cephalometric evaluation, *Angle Orthod* 74:381-390, 2004.

39. Tanaka Y, Morikawa T, Honda Y: An assessment of nasal functions in control of breathing, *J Appl Physiol* 65:1520-1524, 1988.
40. Rodenstein DO, Stanescu DC: Soft palate and oronasal breathing in humans, *J Appl Physiol* 57:651-657, 1984.
41. Stanescu DC, Rodenstein DO: The role of the soft palate in respiration, *Rev Mal Respir* 5:21-29, 1988.
42. Yamaguchi K, Nanda RS, Ghosh J, Tanne K: Morphological differences in individuals with lip competence and incompetence based on electromyographic diagnosis, *J Oral Rehabil* 27:893-901, 2000.
43. Iwahashi F, Yamaguchi K, Nokita T, et al: Activity of the lips associated with simulated upper incisors position, *Orthod Waves* 63:7-14, 2004 (English edition).
44. Nokita T, Yamaguchi K, Tamura H, Imamura F: The lip sealing function correlates with increased facial height, *Orthod Waves* 64:8-15, 2005.
45. Corruccini RS, Flander LB, Kaul SS: Mouth breathing, occlusion, and modernization in a North Indian population: an epidemiologic study, *Angle Orthod* 55:190-196, 1985.
46. Samolinski B, Szczesnowicz-Dabrowska P: Relationship between inflammation of upper and lower respiratory airways, *Otolaryngol Pol* 56:49-55, 2002.
47. Fujimoto S, Yamaguchi K, Gunjikake K: Mouth breathing: objective and subjective estimation. Presented at Second Meeting of Kyushu Orthodontic Society, 2007.
48. Harvold EP, Vargervik K, Chierici G: Primate experiments on oral sensation and dental malocclusions, *Am J Orthod* 63:494-508, 1973.
49. Tomer BS, Harvold EP: Primate experiments on mandibular growth direction, *Am J Orthod* 82:114-119, 1982.
50. McNamara JA: Influence of respiratory pattern on craniofacial growth, *Angle Orthod* 51:269-300, 1981.
51. Harvold EP, Tomer BS, Vargervik K, Chierici G: Primate experiments on oral respiration, *Am J Orthod* 79:359-372, 1981.
52. Yamaguchi K: Effects of experimental mouth breathing on dento-facial growth, *Nippon Kyosei Shika Gakkai Zasshi* 39:24-45, 1980.
53. Tomiyama N, Ichida T, Yamaguchi K: Electromyographic activity of lower lip muscles during chewing with the lips in contact and apart, *Angle Orthod* 74:31-36, 2004.
54. Throckmorton GS, Buschang PH, Hayasaki H, Pinto AS: Changes in the masticatory cycle following treatment of posterior unilateral crossbite in children, *Am J Orthod Dentofacial Orthop* 120:521-529, 2001.
55. Miyawaki S, Yasuda Y, Yashiro K, Takada K: Changes in masticatory jaw movement and muscle activity following surgical orthodontic treatment of adult skeletal Class III case, *Clin Orthod Res* 4:119-123, 2001.
56. Sohn BW, Miyawaki S, Noguchi H, Takada K: Changes in jaw movement and muscle activity after orthodontic correction of incisor crossbite, *Am J Orthod Dentofacial Orthop* 112:403-409, 1997.
57. Matsuka Y, Kitada Y, Mitoh Y, et al: Effect of a bite-raising splint on the duration of the chewing cycle and the EMG activities of masticatory muscles during chewing in freely moving rabbits, *J Oral Rehabil* 25:159-165, 1998.
58. Karkazis HC, Kossioni AE: Re-examination of surface EMG activity of the masseter muscle in young adults during chewing of two test foods, *J Oral Rehabil* 24:216-223, 1997.
59. Papargyriou G, Kjellberg H, Kiliaridis S: Changes in masticatory mandibular movements in growing individuals: a six-year follow-up, *Acta Odontol Scand* 58:129-134, 2000.

CHAPTER 15

Efficient Mechanics and Appliances to Correct Vertical Excess and Open Bite

■ *Flavio Andres Uribe and Ravindra Nanda*

In the past century of orthodontic history, diagnosis and treatment planning have focused primarily on the anteroposterior (AP) skeletofacial dimension. Not surprisingly, the current classification system of malocclusions remains as described by Edward Angle, which in essence does not provide any information regarding the vertical or transverse dimension.

It took decades before the importance of the vertical facial dimension was highlighted. Sassouni and S. Nanda[1] were among the first to describe the vertical proportions of the face and the skeletal characteristics associated with open bites and deep bites. Nanda[2] later found that the vertical facial pattern was established early in life and maintained through growth. Therefore, this finding implied that in order to affect the vertical growth pattern, a therapeutic intervention was necessary.

Although the vertical dimension lends itself to mechanical control, alteration of the vertical facial pattern is difficult, and instability with treatment may be expected.[1,3,4] Many have contended that adequate control of the vertical dimension is crucial for a successful AP correction.[5-8] A clear reciprocity exists between the dimensions.

There are two extremes in the vertical facial pattern: (1) excessive vertical growth and (2) deficient vertical facial height. Many terms have been used to describe excessive facial height, including hyperdivergency, high angle, dolichofacial pattern, and leptoprosopic pattern. Likewise, terms used to describe reduced facial height have included hypodivergency, low angle, brachyfacial pattern, and euryprosopic pattern. The dolichofacial pattern is often associated with an open-bite malocclusion and the brachyfacial pattern with a deep-bite malocclusion.

It is important to be aware that the occlusal relationship does not always follow the facial pattern because dental compensations are usually found at both extremes.[9] Additionally, there are ranges of vertical excess, and some patients may not present with an extreme type of vertical pattern, but rather with a slight or moderate tendency toward one of the two extremes.

The purpose of this chapter is to describe the characteristics of excessive vertical skeletofacial pattern and outline different mechanics for its correction. Also, the soft tissue, skeletal, and dental characteristics of a vertical skeletofacial pattern are discussed, as well as their influence on the outcome of the vertical facial form. Different treatment alternatives are presented, each addressing the problem from a different perspective. Furthermore, the importance of timing is emphasized because treatment decisions differ significantly between growing and nongrowing patients.

ETIOLOGY OF DOLICHOFACIAL PATTERN

The dolichofacial pattern can be attributed primarily to genetic factors, although environmental factors are also considered important in establishing this pattern.[10,11] The heritability of the facial heights has been studied in monozygotic and dizygotic twins, in whom the lower facial height appears to be under strong genetic influence.[12] Research studies evaluating the environmental causes of the dolichofacial pattern have attributed abnormal function such as mouth breathing, abnormal swallowing, and tongue posture as primary etiologic factors.[10,11,13] However, the concept of environmental causes as the sole etiology responsible for establishment of the dolichofacial pattern is strongly debated.[14,15]

The influence of the soft tissues is evident in the dolichofacial pattern via the muscle architecture. Indeed, it has been suggested the masticatory muscles in individuals with a vertical excess exert a diminished occlusal force compared to individuals with a normofacial or brachyfacial pattern.[16] Boyd et al.[17] described the masseter muscles in these individuals as having a higher percentage of type II (fast) fiber muscles. On the contrary, Rowlerson[17a] found greater percentages of type II fibers in the brachyfacial sample. Korfage et al.[18] noted that the discrepancy in these findings may be caused by the large intraindividual and interindividual variability. Analyzing and identifying the type of muscle fiber may ultimately be important in the treatment of these patients, but it may also have connotations in the long-term stability of treatment.

CHARACTERISTICS OF VERTICAL EXCESS

Vertical excess has specific skeletal, dental, and soft tissue characteristics. The soft tissue characteristics can be evaluated clinically, anthropometrically, and cephalometrically. The analysis of the vertical dimension is possible from a frontal and a profile view. The absolute length measurements in the vertical distances between anatomic landmarks are not as important as the *proportions* of the face. To evaluate these proportions, the face is initially divided into equal thirds, with the middle and lower third being the most important because they contain the majority of facial structures. More specifically, the lower third is of utmost importance because is it is the facial area that can be significantly altered with orthodontic treatment.[6]

The lower third of the face can be further divided into thirds: the inferior two thirds from stomium to menton and the superior one third from subnasale to stomion. Existing disproportions can be evaluated though the analysis of these measurements, but clinically one of the most important characteristics of the vertical facial excess is found in the lower facial third: a large "interlabial gap" at rest. The presence of a large interlabial gap can be further confirmed when the patient closes the lips lightly and mentalis muscle strain is noticed.[6] Another clinical characteristic associated with a large interlabial gap in patients with vertical facial excess is an excessive gingival display on smile. Keep in mind that the large interlabial gap and excessive gingival display may not result exclusively from vertical facial excess, but rather may be caused partially or totally by a short upper lip.[19] Comparison of a patient's lip length to normative data can help determine any deficiencies.

The lateral cephalometric radiograph is the most common means used to evaluate, quantify, and classify a patient with vertical facial excess. These radiographic findings can be correlated with the clinical and anthropometric analysis. Other useful skeletofacial measurements and ratios may be obtained by a lateral cephalogram; for example, upper and lower hard tissue facial heights can be determined. Ideally, the face should be divided anteriorly into two halves, with the upper half slightly smaller than the lower half (45:55). Using the lateral cephalogram, the relationship between the anterior and posterior facial height may also be evaluated. On average, the posterior facial height measured from sella to gonion should be approximately 60% of the anterior facial height.[20]

One of the most common cephalometric measurements used to classify a patient as "hyperdivergent" is the inclination of the mandibular plane. An angle measurement above 36 degrees to the sella-nasion plane is usually an important indicator of vertical facial excess. Other characteristics suggestive of this pattern, as described by Björk,[21] are growth indicators that anticipate the development of extreme facial excess. He believed that these features serve as predictive characteristics of what has been described as "backward growth," which ultimately develops into a dolichofacial pattern.

Finally, in the lateral cephalogram, vertical dental characteristics can be measured and compared to normative data. Of these, the dentoalveolar heights in the maxilla and the mandible are measured to the palatal plane and the mandibular plane, respectively. The occlusal table of the first molar to these reference lines usually is excessive in these patients, especially the maxillary molar to the palatal plane. Anteriorly, the distance from this reference plane may also be excessive, that is, palatal plane to the maxillary central incisor. In this case, although a vertical facial pattern is evident, an open bite would not be seen anteriorly because the incisors may have supraerupted, compensating for the posterior vertical excess. It is important to note that although a patient may have a dolichofacial pattern, only a small percentage of these patients have a corresponding anterior open bite.[9,15]

The differentiation between a skeletal and a dental open bite has been controversial.[15,22] As just described, the major characteristics of a skeletal open bite are determined through cephalometric measurements. Usually a dental open bite is related to a habit that inhibited the vertical development of the incisors.[22] The open bite can also be initiated or perpetuated by a tongue thrust. Diverging occlusal planes anterior to the premolars is a feature that may be indicative of a dentoalveolar open bite. This clinical and cephalometric feature is usually caused by a finger habit. On the contrary, skeletal open bites generally display two occlusal planes that start diverging more posteriorly than the first premolar, usually from the second premolar or first molar (Fig. 15-1).

A clear distinction between the two types is generally not obvious, and often some individuals with vertical facial excess may have a habit (e.g., thumb sucking) and thus features of both skeletal and dental open bite (Fig. 15-2).

VERTICAL EXCESS AND SMILE ESTHETICS

Smile esthetics has always been a common goal among all the disciplines in dentistry. In the past, orthodontics emphasized the attainment of good occlusion as the primary goal, and alignment of the dental arches was the most important factor in achieving esthetics.

Recently, more characteristics have been defined to describe the esthetic smile.[23] One of these characteristics related to the vertical dimension is the *incisor display* or *gingival tissue display* at rest and smile. This characteristic can be categorized as excessive, normal, or deficient. The excessive display may be caused by excessive vertical height of the maxilla, supraeruption of the upper incisors, short upper lip, or a combination of all these factors.[19] The clinical diagnosis of the vertical excess is evaluated in the posed smile; therefore a differential diagnosis is necessary through the evaluation of lip mobility. A hypermobile lip will give the appearance of vertical maxillary excess because a significant amount of gingival tissue will be displayed at smile, even though the amount of incisor display at rest may be normal. Thus a patient may have excessive gingival display at smile without vertical facial excess (Fig. 15-3).

When evaluating the gingival display at smile, another differential diagnosis of vertical maxillary excess is *altered passive eruption.* In this situation the crowns of the incisors appear to be short in height because of inadequate apical migration of the dentogingival complex, resulting in more apparent gingival tissue on smiling. Again, the clinical analysis of the smile must be correlated with the cephalometric and anthropometric data to obtain a complete diagnosis.

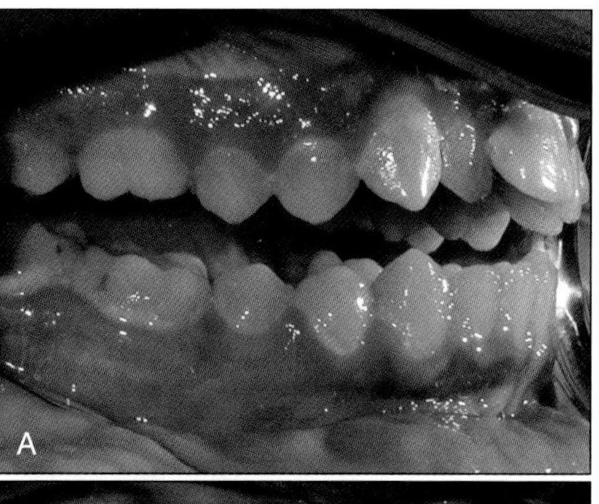

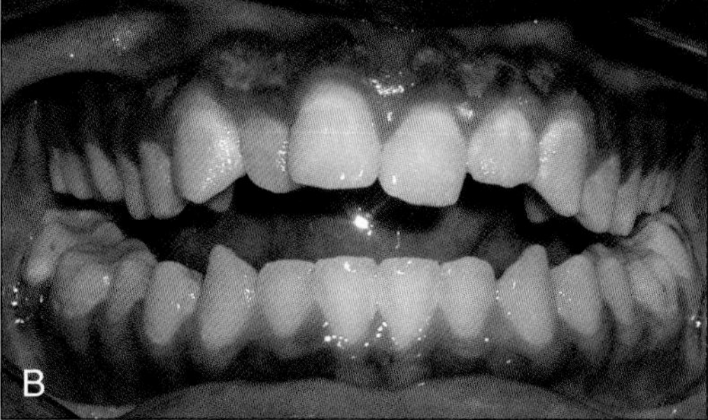

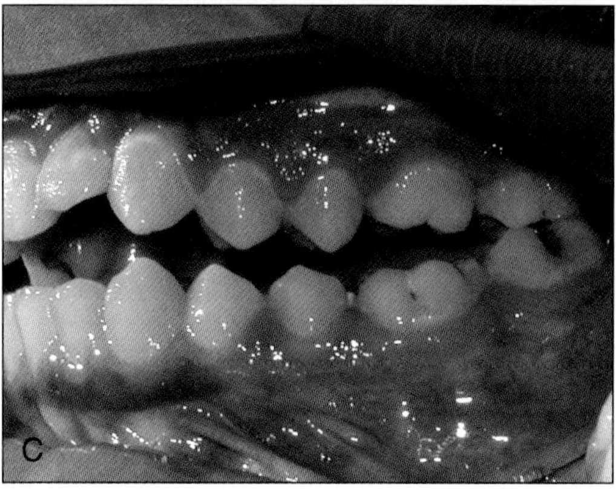

Fig. 15-1 **A** to **C**, Significant anterior open bite with occlusal planes that diverge anteriorly from the second and third molars. Generally, this clinical feature suggests a skeletal rather than a dental open bite.

TREATMENT STRATEGIES

After reviewing all the multiple etiologies for the hyperdivergent facial profile, treatment strategies need to include soft tissue, dental, and skeletal evaluations. The vertical dimension can readily be altered by controlling the posterior teeth.[6,24] In these patients the ultimate goal is either to intrude or to maintain the vertical position of the molars.[15]

The methods available to achieve the vertical control of the molars vary depending on the age of the patient. The specific aim of treatment in the growing patient is to hold the vertical position of the molars while normal vertical maxillary and mandibular growth is occurring. Generally, the different orthodontic appliances for the vertical control are targeted to the maxillary molars, although vertical control of the mandibular molars has also been described.[5,6]

Appliances

Different appliances have been used to restrict the vertical maxillary growth and inferior displacement of the molars. These appliances apply the force directly or indirectly to the first molars. Headgear is the classic example of an appliance that delivers a force directly to the molar in an intrusive direction. Occipital and vertical-pull headgears have been recommended because both types have a vertical component to the force. Although the occipital type does not provide a purely vertical force, the distally directed component of the force may be indicated in patients with vertical maxillary excess and a convex profile. To deliver this type of force vector, the pulling force of the headgear should approximate the center of resistance of the maxillary molar. This is obtained by adjusting the height and the length of the outer bow. *Key ridge* serves as an anatomical landmark to estimate the center of resistance of the maxillary molar. Any vector of the force that does not go through the center of resistance of the molar will generate a clockwise or counterclockwise rotation of the molar (Fig. 15-4). This tipping movement of the molar can be used favorably in certain sagittal occlusal relationships (i.e., Class II molar).

Another appliance that aids in controlling the vertical dimension has been proposed by Pearson[5] and involves the application of mandibular headgear. This design controls the eruption of the lower molar, especially when using Class II elastics.[5,25] By inhibiting the lower molar eruption, the vertical dimension is, in theory, more readily controlled. Reportedly, lower alveolar height increases more than the maxillary molar height during orthodontic treatment, in which case mandibular headgear becomes particularly

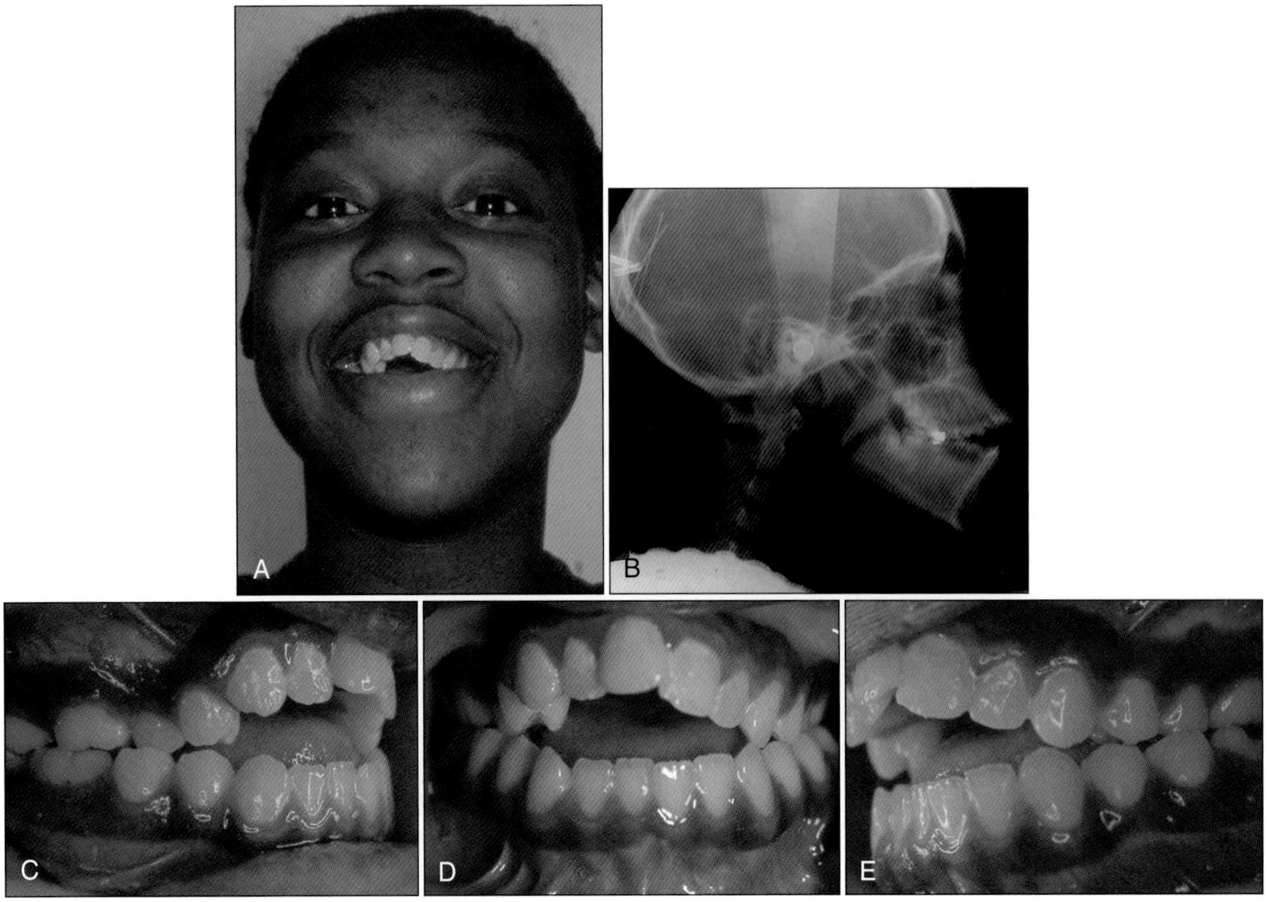

Fig. 15-2 Patient with history of thumb-sucking habit showing combined features of a skeletal and dental open bite. **A,** Patient showing a reverse smile with an anterior open bite. **B,** Lateral cephalogram shows numerous characteristics of a skeletal open bite. **C** to **E,** Occlusal planes diverge anteriorly from the first premolars, which is usually associated with a dental open bite caused by a finger habit.

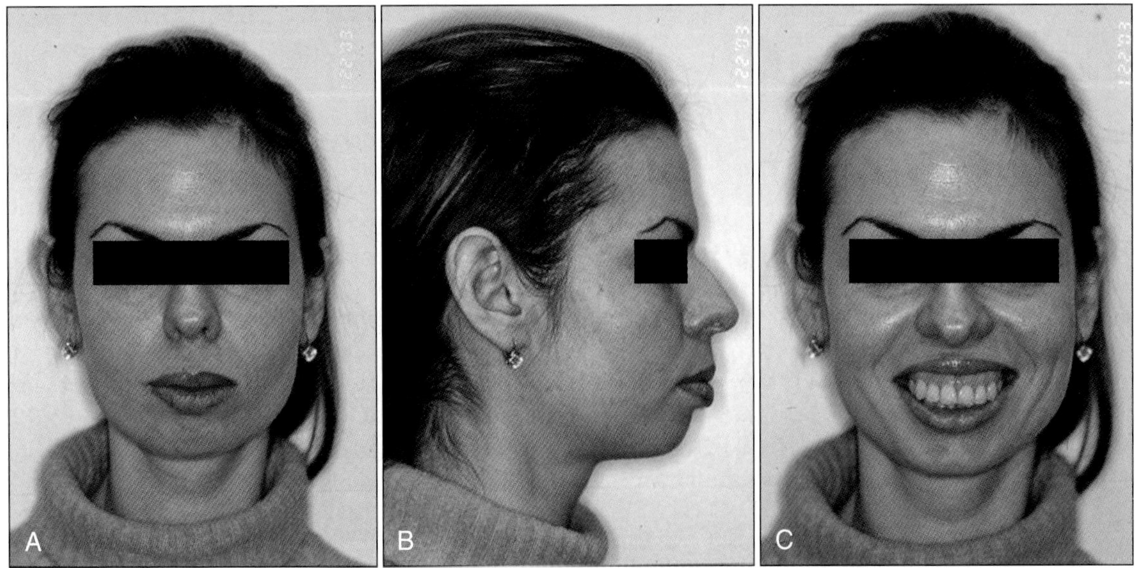

Fig. 15-3 **A** and **B,** Brachyfacial pattern with an uncharacteristic excessive gingival display on smile (**C**). Differential diagnosis is needed: maxillary excess, short upper lip, hypermobile lip, or supraerupted maxillary incisors. Surgical correction of the excessive gingival display on smile through maxillary impaction in a patient with this vertical facial pattern may be detrimental to vertical facial proportions, because the lower facial height would most likely be further reduced.

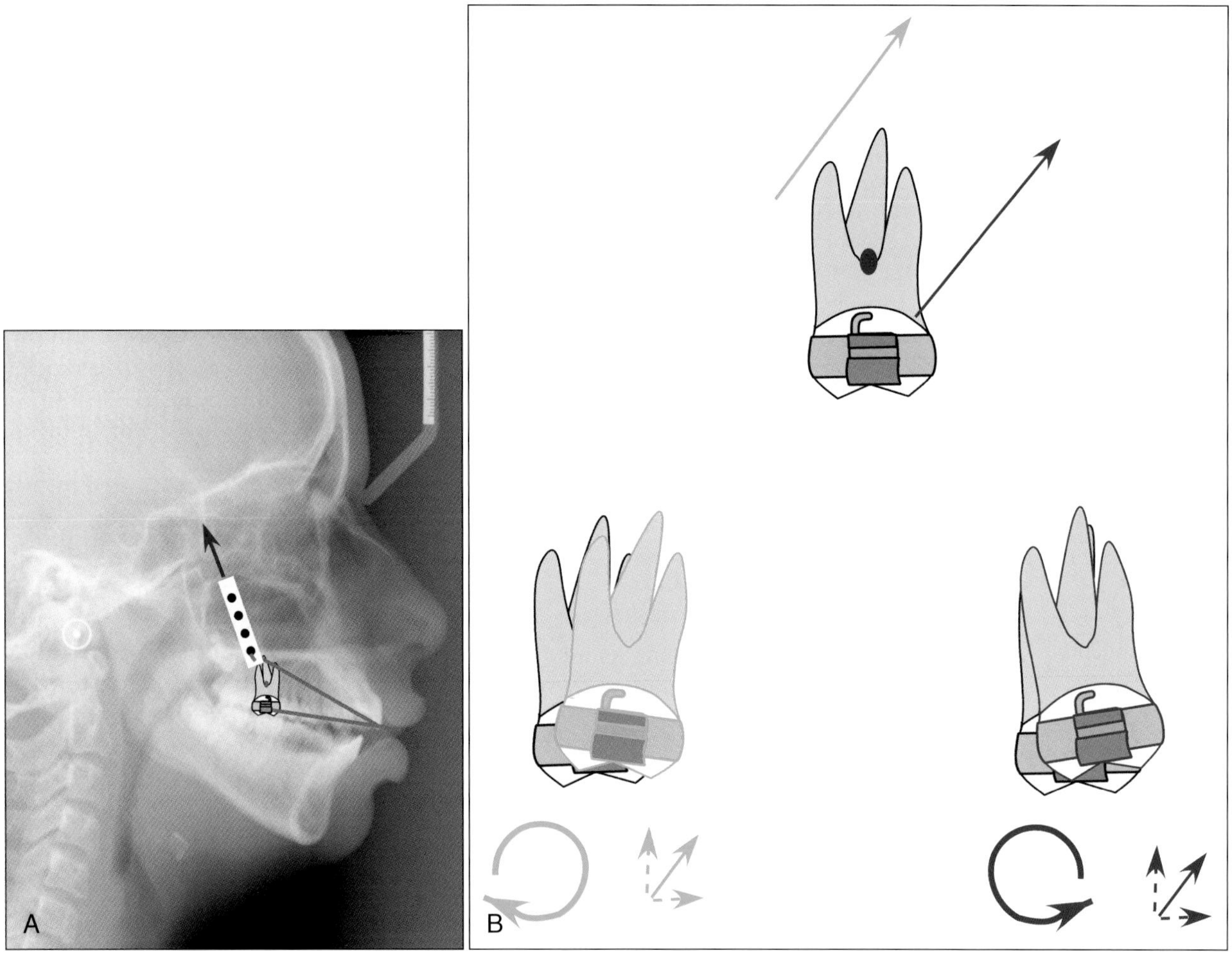

A B

Fig. 15-4 **A,** The *vector* of the headgear force is defined by the strap connecting the head cap to the outer bow. The relationship of this force vector to the molar defines the type of tooth movement. Key ridge is a good anatomical landmark to estimate the center of resistance of the maxillary first molar. **B,** The green force vector will generate an intrusive and distal molar displacement in conjunction with counterclockwise rotation. The blue force vector will generate an intrusive and distal movement with a clockwise rotation of the molar.

attractive.[5] The only disadvantage of this appliance is that a purely vertical force cannot be delivered; a distal component of the force is always present. This distal component of the force can be decreased by lengthening the outer bow (Fig. 15-5). However, this adjustment would also tend to increase the distal tipping effect on the molar because of the moment of the force. Mandibular headgear could certainly be a treatment option for vertical control, but it is not a popular modality.

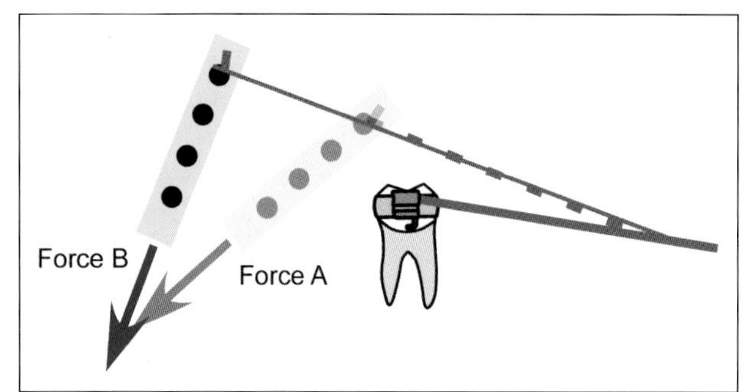

Fig. 15-5 The longer the outer bow is in mandibular headgear, the more vertical the component of the force that is achieved. However, the distal tipping moment of the force is also increased.

Indirect Delivery of Force

The maxillary and mandibular molars can also be controlled vertically in the growing patient though indirect delivery of the force. This can be accomplished through the different muscles during normal function. The two primary muscle groups involved in these indirect forms of force delivery are the masticatory muscles and the muscles of the tongue.

During normal function, *masticatory muscles* transfer their contractile forces to the occlusal surface of the posterior teeth. Although present under normal conditions, these forces do not predictably inhibit vertical molar eruption. Muscle activity needs to be concentrated and redirected to achieve an inhibitory effect. It has been proposed that isometric masticatory muscle exercises can accomplish this. After performing specific muscle exercises, vertical eruption of the molars can be inhibited.[24] For example, vertical dimension control has been achieved with some degree of success in growing children when they are taught to clench their teeth at regular intervals daily.[26]

Masticatory muscle tone can be enhanced by impinging in the "free-way space" by means of a bite block (approximately 3-4 mm in thickness) placed between the posterior teeth. The effect on the molars is produced through a constant force at rest and in function. Muscle exercises can also be prescribed with a bite block to achieve a synergistic effect. Moreover, the inhibitory effect can be enhanced through forces in equal and opposite direction delivered through intermaxillary magnets on the occlusal surface of the bite blocks.[27-29] Woods and Nanda[30] showed positive vertical effects on growing nonhuman primates.[30] Although positive vertical control has been reported in growing children, problems have been encountered in two ways: (1) the gingival tissue above the erupting second molars prevented any significant reduction in the vertical dimension, and (2) the uncontrolled delivery of the magnet forces generated crossbites in some children.[27,31]

The indirect effect of the masticatory pull can also be enhanced in another manner. A *vertical-pull chin cup* (VPCC) has been described that inhibits vertical facial growth.[25] This effect is achieved predominantly during postural muscle activity and typically is used with an intermaxillary bite block.[32,33]

The *tongue* contains the other group of muscles that can indirectly affect the vertical position of the molars. The tongue posture can be affected in a similar manner as described for the masticatory muscles, by impinging in the postural space and by regular swallowing and mastication. Normally the tongue rests against the roof of the palate. By placing a bar away from the palate, the postural and functional forces of the tongue are translated to the maxillary molars. This effect was reported in a clinical study in which a palatal arch was placed at different distances from the roof of the palate.[34] The results showed that a transpalatal arch 6 mm from the roof of the palate delivered on average about 200 g/cm^2 of force to the second molars, and this force was significantly higher than that obtained from a bar placed 2 mm away from the palate. In a variation of this design, the "vertical holding appliance," a thick acrylic button placed on the roof of the palate produced less than 1-mm inhibition of maxillary molar vertical development during a 2-year period.[35]

Wedge Effect

The vertical dimension also can be altered by the "wedge effect," which shows the interrelationship of the vertical and anteroposterior dimensions. In essence the "wedge," or narrow tip of the triangle bordered by the posterior maxillary and mandibular molars, is decreased by means of extraction of the first molars. The result is a corresponding decrease in the vertical dimension. The wedge is removed by extracting first molars and translating the second molars anteriorly. First molars are chosen because, as shown clinically, no reduction in vertical dimension is accomplished with first premolar extraction.[36] However, both second premolar and first molar extractions have shown a reduction in the mandibular plane angle.[37]

Treatment for the Growing Patient

The treatment modalities used to control the vertical position of the molars in a growing patient can be employed separately or in tandem. As mentioned, for example, a bite block is often used in combination with a VPCC or vertical-pull headgear[32,33,38] (Fig. 15-6). In a retrospective two-phase study, Schulz et al.[38] compared the efficiency of VPCC and bonded *rapid palatal expander* (RPE). A bonded RPE was given to patients with increased vertical dimension. These patients also underwent a second phase of treatment with fixed appliances. A second group underwent the same procedures, but in addition, a VPCC was prescribed throughout the two phases of treatment. The VPCC group had a slightly reduced increase in vertical skeletal measurements. Curiously, this reduction was more apparent during the first phase than in the second phase of treatment. However, this study was limited by the absence of a control group. Thus prospective randomized clinical trials are needed to measure the efficiency of different combinations of these appliances in vertical dimension control.[39,40]

Treatment for the Nongrowing (Adult) Patient

For nongrowing patients, all these treatment modalities can be used for vertical control of the molars. However, the goal in the fully grown patient is to intrude the molars instead of holding them against growth. Although extraoral appliances can be used to achieve this effect, adult patients often are not receptive to this treatment option. Unfortunately, the alternatives (e.g., intraoral appliances) have limitations as well. They often act as a speech impediment and are unesthetic. Of these, the least visible is the *palatal button;* however, this appliance used alone would probably have minimal intrusive effect on the maxillary molar.

Therefore in an adult patient the best option is directly delivering an intrusive force to the molars to correct the vertical dimension. The magnitude of this force to achieve significant intrusion has been reported to be about 200 g.[41,42] To deliver this force orthodontically, temporary anchorage devices (TADs) offer a good solution capable of delivering

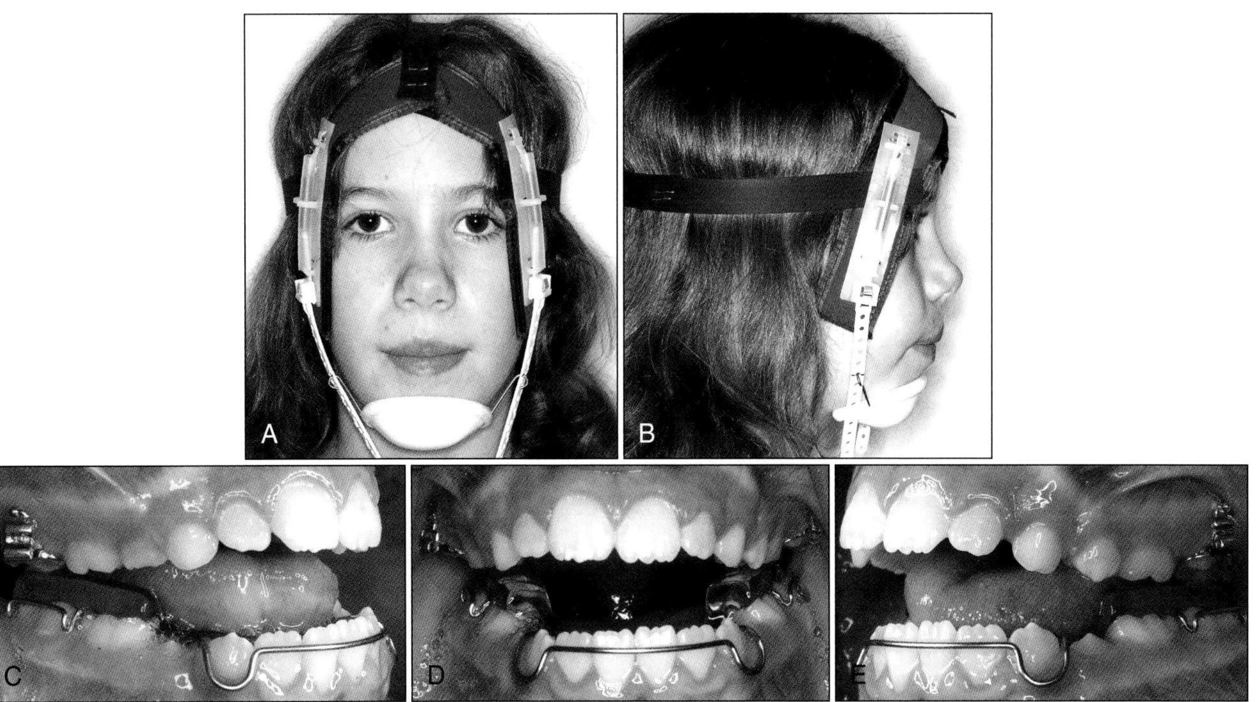

Fig. 15-6 **A** and **B,** Patient wearing a vertical-pull chin cup in conjunction with a bite plate (**C-E**) to control the eruption of the buccal segments and inhibit molar eruption. A synergistic effect is obtained using these two appliances together.

this force magnitude directly to the molars in the adult (nongrowing patient) without the need for bulky, unesthetic appliances. Understandably, the popularity of these appliances has risen significantly in the past few years. Before their availability, the only treatment alternative for these patients was surgery if significant intrusive displacement was needed.[43]

Mechanically, molar intrusion using skeletal anchorage has been accomplished with all the different TAD types. The selection should be determined from a biomechanical standpoint. Before selecting the type of TAD to be used, the line of force needed to produce molar intrusion should be defined. Thus TADs are planned from a biomechanical analysis and not based on the anatomical availability of alveolar bone. Only when the desired line of force is defined can the anatomical area for TAD placement be identified.

The simplest TAD to place is the *miniscrew.* Its use has been widespread because of the ease of placement and cost. The major disadvantage to this system is that it fits tightly between the roots of adjacent teeth and therefore limits the direction and amount of tooth movement possible. To offset this constraint, some clinicians have proposed the miniscrew be placed in the infrazygomatic crest of the maxillary bone[44] or in a palatal position near the midpalatal raphe away from the roots of the maxillary teeth.[41]

The other options of skeletal anchorage, such as *miniplates* and *palatal implants,* ensure placement away from the tooth structures and allow greater latitude of movement. Both rely on an arm that can be extended from the fixed

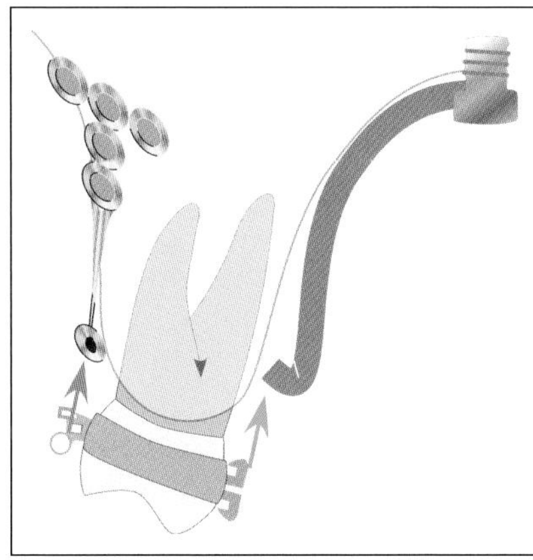

Fig. 15-7 Mini-implants and miniplates allow free dental movement in the three planes of space. To deliver the force from these temporary anchorage devices, long arms are extended to an area near the gingival third of the teeth.

location of the plate or implant, allowing for any desired line of force, depending on the prescribed direction of the extension arm (Fig. 15-7). In general, although versatile, miniplates are limited to the facial aspect of the maxillary and mandibular bones, whereas the palatal implant is generally placed in the palate.

Figure 15-8 shows an interesting approach to reduce the vertical dimension using skeletal anchorage and the concept of a "wedge effect." In this patient, skeletal anchorage was used to intrude the lower second molars responsible for the

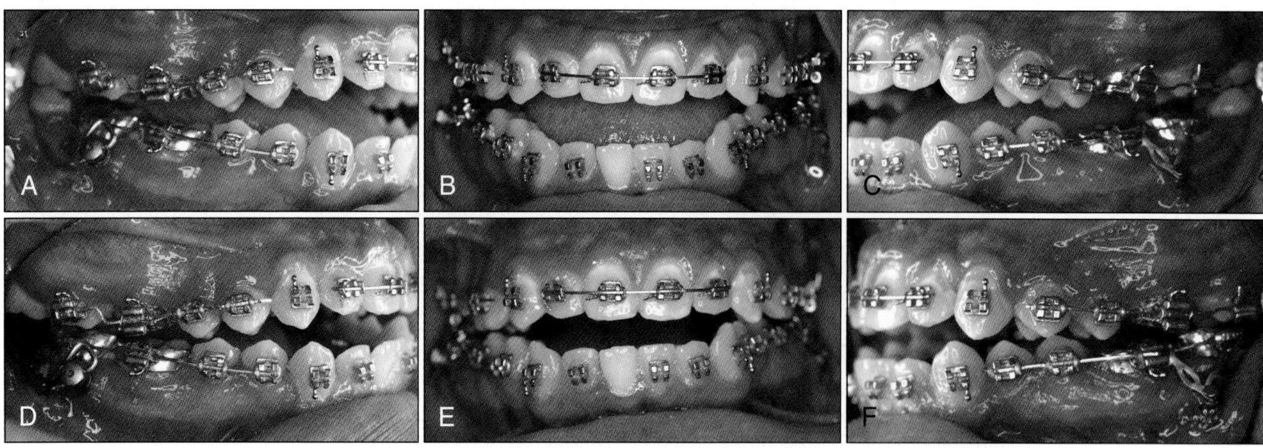

Fig. 15-8 Patient with significant open bite (initial intraoral photos, see Fig. 15-1). Miniscrew and miniplate were placed to intrude the mandibular second molars. **A** to **C,** Third molars were only contacting after initial mandibular second molar intrusion. **D** to **F,** Mandibular third molars were extracted, removing the wedge. Approximately 3 mm of anterior open-bite closure was immediately achieved.

posterior wedge and significant open bite. The third molars also contributed to the wedge. After approximately 2 mm of intrusion of the lower second molars, the lower third molars were extracted. Because the third molars were the only teeth maintaining the vertical dimension, an immediate reduction in the open bite was observed. The magnitude of the open bite was greatly reduced in conjunction with the vertical dimension. The full correction of the open bite can be achieved from this point through mild extrusion of the incisors and continuation of the intrusion in the buccal mandibular segments.

One important aspect to consider is the alleged "compensatory eruption" of the antagonizing molars with molar intrusion.[45] As molars are intruded, space is created between the arches. Supraeruption of the opposing dentition into the newly established space can be expected. To offset this tendency, the opposing occlusion should be held in check. Although more evidence is needed to support this view, placing skeletal anchorage devices in all quadrants while actively intruding the maxillary or mandibular molars should thwart this tendency and allow for a net gain in the vertical dimension.[46]

With skeletal anchorage to correct vertical excess, Erverdi et al.[47] proposed the use of three components working in conjunction to reduce vertical excess: titanium (Ti) plates, a cemented bite block, and a low transpalatal arch (TPA).[47] From the Ti plates a direct anchorage force can be applied to the posterior segment, which is then splinted to an acrylic bite block, which in turn increases the intrusive forces on the maxillary molars through occlusion. Finally, a low TPA transfers vertical intrusive forces to the buccal segments by exploiting the forces produced by the tongue.

A final option for the adult patient to reduce vertical excess is the surgical approach. A LeFort I impaction is the most common procedure used to achieve reduction of the vertical facial excess.[43] In these patients the maxilla can be impacted evenly (anteriorly and posteriorly) or unevenly, depending on the overbite and the amount of desired final incisor display. If the patient's incisor position is to be maintained vertically, while the occlusal plane diverges anteriorly from the first molar or premolars, a three-piece maxillary impaction may be indicated. This procedure would involve superior movement of the maxillary posterior segments, thereby autorotating the mandible. In this manner, the desired simultaneous reduction in the facial height and mandibular plane angle would be achieved; if necessary, the vertical excess can be reduced further by performing a sliding genioplasty. This additional procedure is indicated when a convex soft tissue profile is also present; as the chin slides up, the vertical height is reduced, and more anterior projection of the chin is obtained.

ANTERIOR OPEN BITE AND THE VERTICAL DIMENSION

Complicating the treatment of vertical excess, about one sixth of vertical excess patients also present with a significant anterior open bite.[15] As mentioned, the correction of the vertical excess depends on vertical control of the molars. By addressing the vertical control of the molars and reducing the vertical excess, a concomitant reduction in the open bite may be achieved.

In these patients the open bite needs to be treated separately in specific clinical situations (Fig. 15-9). In such cases, incisor extrusion is often necessary with diligent maintenance (not reduction) of the vertical dimension of the molars. For example, incisor extrusion is a viable option in patients with an anterior open bite and a lack of incisor display. In these patients the etiology is often a previous habit. Although a vertical excess pattern may also be present,

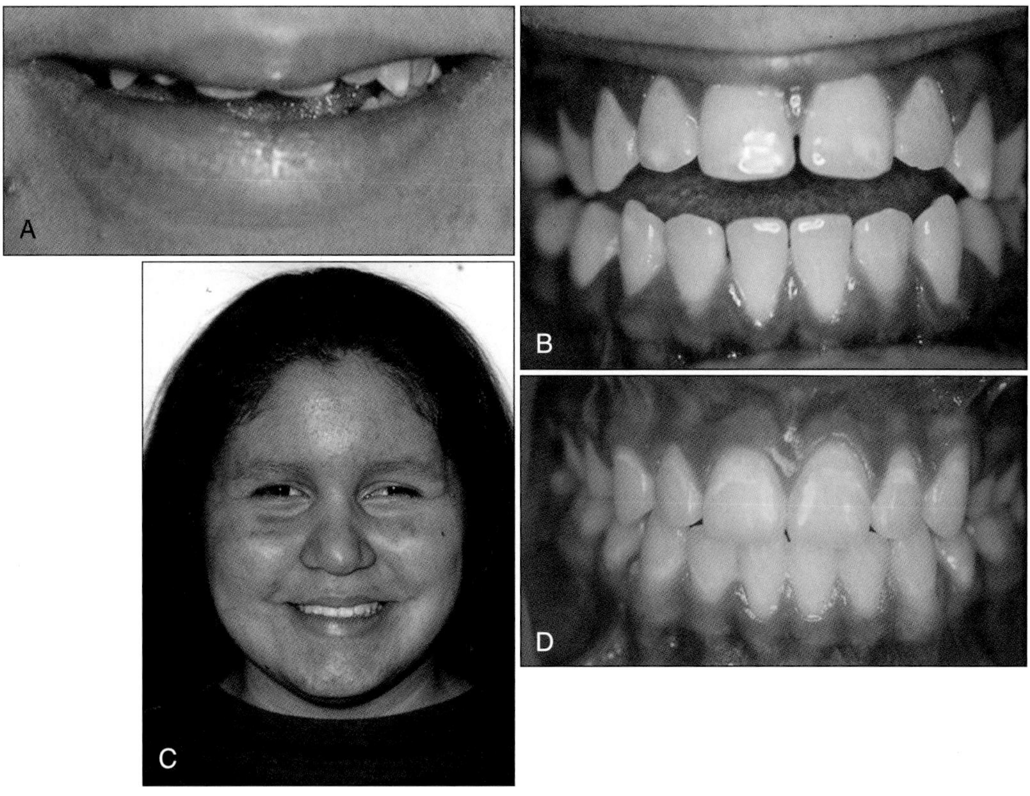

Fig. 15-9 **A** and **B**, Patient with anterior open bite and deficient incisor display on smile. **C** and **D**, Extrusion of the incisors with orthodontic treatment significantly enhanced the smile esthetics and solved the occlusal problem.

the malocclusion and the esthetics require closure of the open bite by extrusion of the incisors. Depending on the severity of the open bite, some of the closure can be accomplished by a combination of molar intrusion and incisor extrusion. However, vertical molar control may be easier to accomplish in a growing patient. In the adult patient the molar intrusion component can be achieved only with skeletal anchorage or surgery. Finally, an important factor to consider when correcting an anterior open bite is the stability of the correction. This area is more controversial and is discussed later.

A technique that has gained some acceptance for the correction of open bite is the *multiloop edgewise archwire* (MEAW) technique. Initial reports suggest that during treatment the maxillary occlusal plane rotates in a clockwise direction while the mandibular occlusal plane rotates counterclockwise.[48] The reports imply that molar intrusion is involved in the correction. However, published data have shown that the correction is primarily obtained through eruption of the incisors.[49] Rotation of the occlusal plane may contribute to a better stability; however no data are available to support this claim.

Skeletal anchorage can facilitate the rotation of the occlusal plane and can be accomplished in different ways. For example, one method is to place a rigid sectional wire in the posterior segment of the maxilla and then place a force distal to the center of resistance of that segment. Another method is to place a segment of a wire between a skeletal anchorage system and a rigid buccal segment. This design encourages rotation of the occlusal plane by a couple, which will rotate the segment around the center of resistance (Fig. 15-10).

A similar concept is used to rotate occlusal planes, but without skeletal anchorage. The patient in Figure 15-11 has third molars that were to be extracted at the end of treatment. The third molars are used as anchorage units to obtain the desired movement. The force system included a moment and an extrusive force placed between the canine and the premolar (Fig. 15-12). The moment is in a clockwise direction, thus closing the bite. The ancillary extrusive force helped to correct the divergent occlusal planes. Although using skeletal anchorage devices would be an option in such patients with fully erupted third molars, adding TADs would clearly be redundant and unnecessary because the existing anchorage using the third molars is sufficient.

Extraction therapy is another treatment modality that allows for closure of the anterior open bite. As mentioned, in cases involving vertical excess, the vertical dimension is reduced by first molar or second premolar extraction. This theory is applicable to open-bite cases as well. After second premolar extraction therapy, the molar will move anteriorly, reducing the open bite through a wedge effect. The remaining portion of the extraction space is closed through incisor

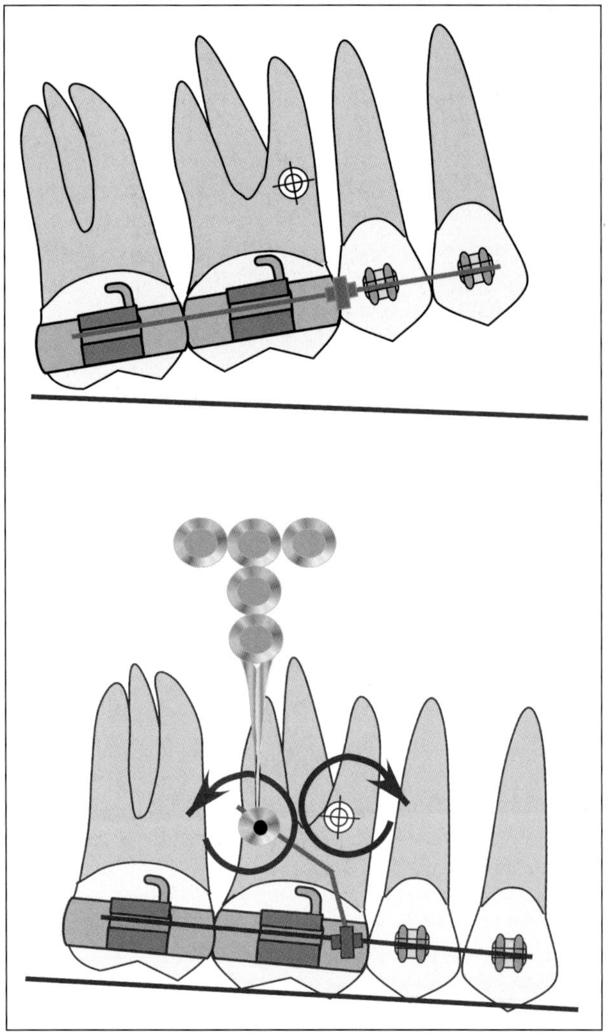

Fig. 15-10 Occlusal plane rotation achieved through a two-couple system from a miniplate. Equal and opposite moments generate the clockwise rotation of the maxillary occlusal plane.

retraction. As the incisors are retracted, the bite deepens because the retraction force is applied to the crown, resulting in extrusion of the incisal end caused by the moment of the force (Fig. 15-13). The incisor retraction also has a positive effect on soft tissue conformation; the lips close in response to incisor retraction. The lips not only move back but also inferiorly, thereby reducing the interlabial gap.

Finally, if a habit is responsible for the development of an anterior open bite, the first objective is to find a method of convincing the patient to stop. Usually this involves administering a habit-inhibiting appliance. Habit appliances influence mostly the incisors, so once the habit ceases, the correction is achieved through natural incisor extrusion. In other words, most habits such as thumb sucking impose a force on the incisors that inhibit natural extrusion. Once the habit is eliminated, the incisors respond naturally by moving into the space they would otherwise have occupied.

It is important to evaluate the etiology of the open bite. Some patients may have not only an anterior open bite caused by a habit, but also a vertical skeletal excess. Indeed, the side effects of the habit may mask an underlying skeletal excess. The maxillary incisors may be in an adequate vertical position, as reflected by an appropriate incisor display, but once the habit is removed, a clear vertical excess will be expressed (Fig. 15-14). In this patient, although the habit must stop, molar vertical control is crucial to level the occlusal planes through relative intrusion of the molars.

STABILITY

The stability of any type of corrective treatment relies primarily on the elimination of the etiology. In the patient with vertical excess it can be assumed that the main etiology is genetic; secondary environmental influences such as mouth breathing caused by nasal obstruction may contribute to the facial pattern. As described previously, the correction of the vertical excess in these individuals relies primarily on the molar intrusion. Because the treatment varies in growing versus nongrowing patients, stability must be described separately for these groups.

The clinical studies involving growing patients and control of the vertical molar position have shown promise, particularly in the short term using the appliances described earlier.[50] However, long-term studies are needed to verify that these short-term changes are maintained. Only long-term verification will justify the need for early treatment of these patients.

Follow-up surgical records for nongrowing patients regarding long-term stability of reduced vertical excess indicate adequate stability. Data from the University of North Carolina (UNC) reveal that the long-term stability of vertical excess reduction is relatively successful with maxillary impaction.[51] A double-jaw surgery is also stable as long as the counterclockwise rotation of the mandible is not done at the expense of increasing the pterygomasseteric sling. This UNC conclusion contradicts findings of an earlier study that found a fairly high amount of skeletal relapse with vertical correction.[52] The discrepancy between these two studies could be partially attributed to the type of skeletal fixation devices used.

As outlined, the other alternative for molar control in the adult patient is skeletal anchorage. Since the TAD era is still dawning, long-term reports are scant. Molar intrusion with orthodontic appliances is still in its infancy, but short-term findings have shown approximately 30% relapse in the vertical molar position.[46] More long-term data are needed to assess the stability of the correction in the molar position and the vertical skeletal pattern by means of TADs.

Anterior open-bite stability is difficult to evaluate; the criteria used to define a stable correction in anterior open bites is somewhat vague. Studies evaluating open-bite stability have used different criteria and reference planes.[53] Overall, the evidence indicates that surgical correction and a nonsurgical approach result in a similar amount of relapse. Evaluating outcome is difficult because the studies had different targets for achieving correction. Before skeletal anchorage,

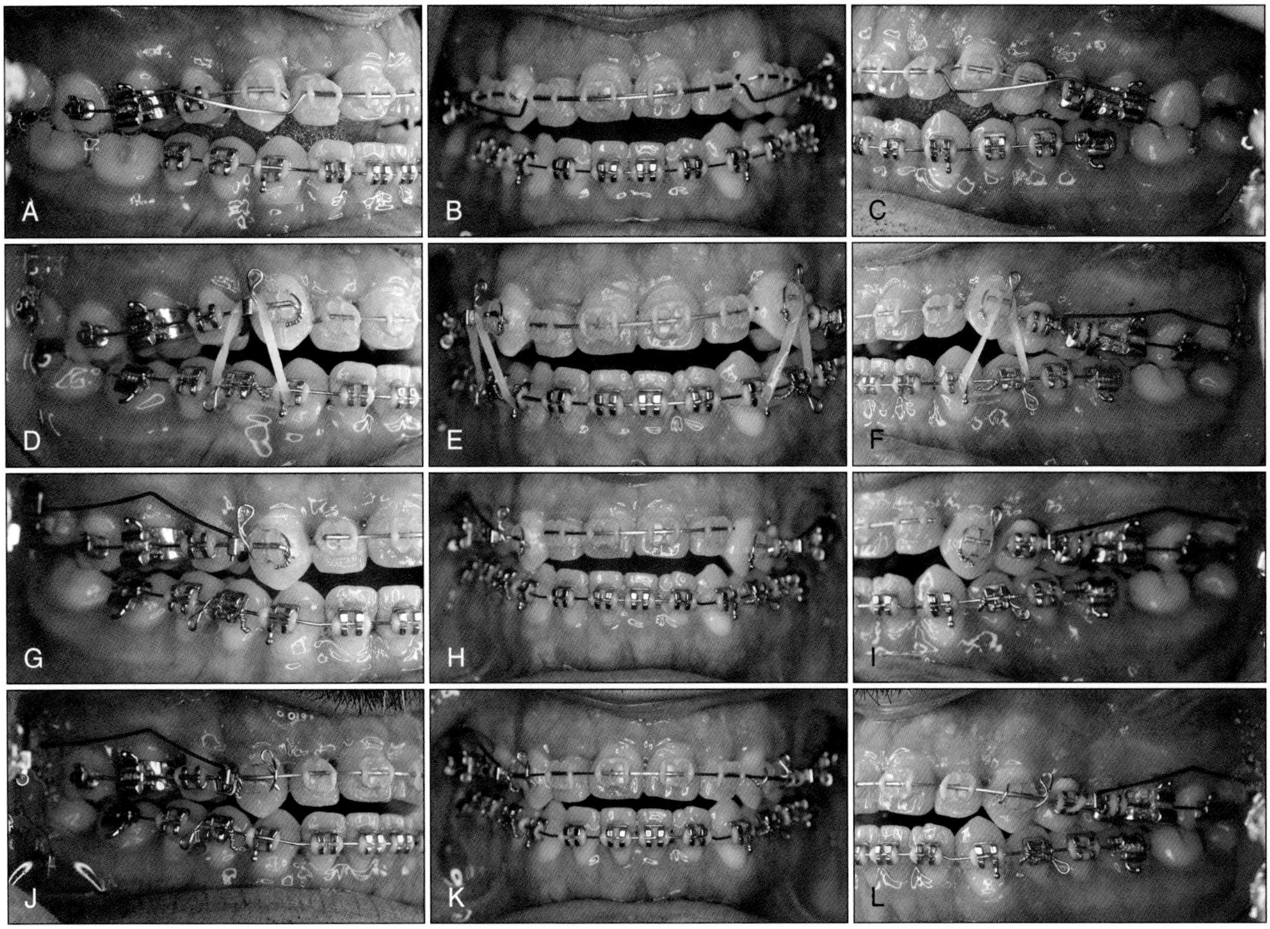

Fig. 15-11 A to C, Similar concept applied for occlusal plane rotation as in Fig. 15-10. In this patient, instead of a temporary anchorage device (TAD), maxillary third molars were used as anchor units to deliver the desired force system. An extrusion arch is placed from the maxillary molars to the incisors using segmental mechanics. **D** to **F,** Intermaxillary seating elastics are used to control for the side effect on the buccal segments of the extrusion arch. **G** to **I,** Sectional wire with an off-centered V-bend is placed from the maxillary third molars to the buccal segments to create a favorable clockwise rotation of the latter to correct the posterior open bite. The side effects on the third molar are not relevant because these teeth will be extracted at the end of orthodontic treatment. The mechanics are reinforced by intermaxillary seating elastics. **J** to **L,** Results of this mechanical approach on the maxillary buccal segments.

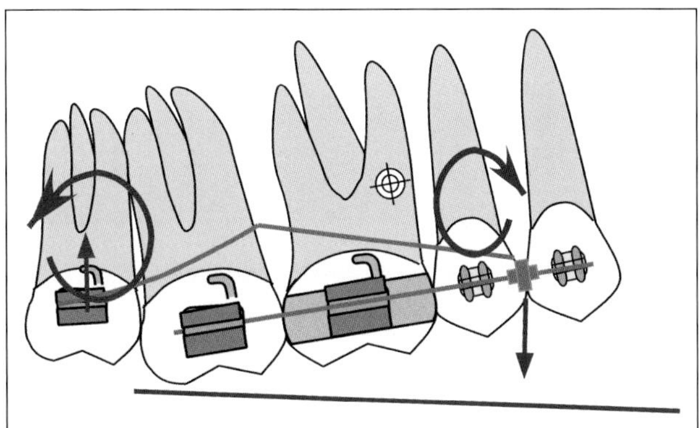

Fig. 15-12 Description of the force system used in the patient in Fig. 15-11. A two-couple system was used to achieve clockwise rotation of the maxillary buccal segments. An extrusive force in the anterior segment is also generated with this Class V geometry V-bend. The side effects on the maxillary third molars are distal tipping and slight intrusion.

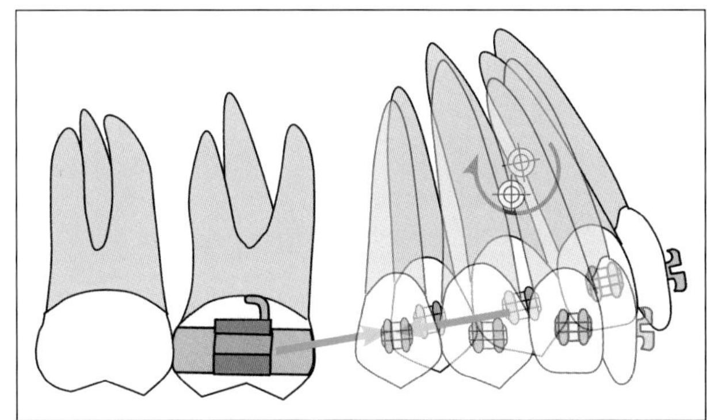

Fig. 15-13 The distal component of the force applied to the anterior teeth during space closure, after extraction of the second premolar, aids in the closure of the anterior open bite. Extraction of second premolars in patients with anterior open bite may also aid in the correction of this malocclusion through the "wedge effect."

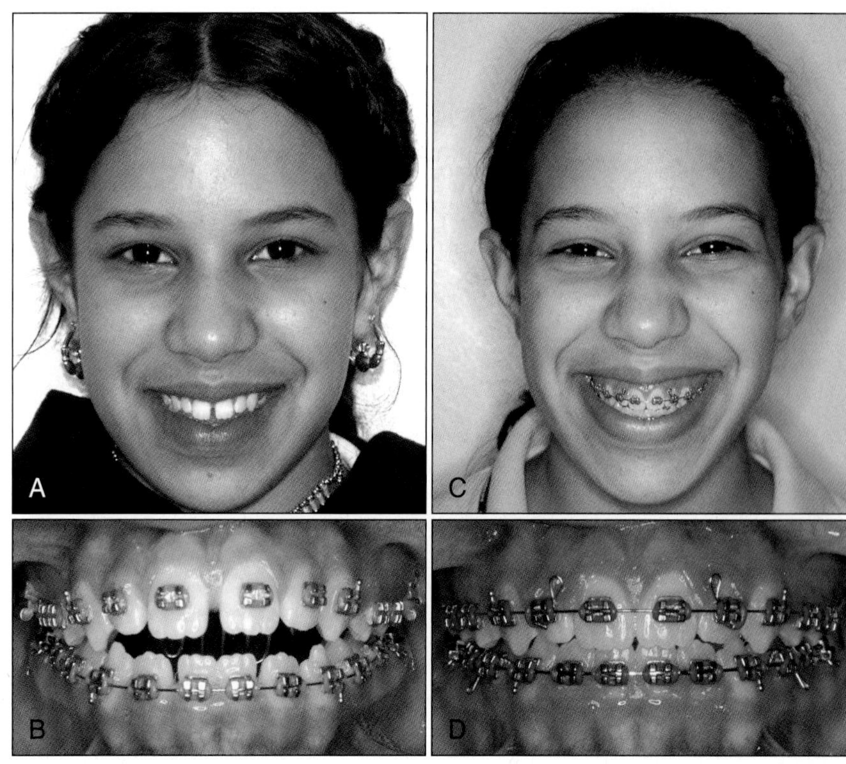

Fig. 15-14 **A,** Patient with an anterior open bite and adequate incisor display on smile. **B,** A habit appliance was used to correct the open bite. **C** and **D,** The resulting incisor extrusion leveled the maxillary occlusal plane at the expense of more anterior gingival display.

orthodontic open-bite correction relied primarily on extrusion of the incisors, whereas surgical correction mainly addressed the molar superior reposition through maxillary impaction. Regardless of the means used to achieve correction, inherent instability appears to be present in open-bite cases. Presumably the soft tissues, including the tongue, may be important contributors to the relapse tendencies in some patients.

Only when etiology is more precisely diagnosed will corresponding treatment be implemented, and then stability may improve. Unfortunately, hard tissues are subject to the dynamic soft tissue environment; until these soft tissue influences can be predictably altered, improvement in long-term stability of open-bite correction will remain a challenge.

Overall, retention of the vertical correction in the dolichofacial patient depends on molar control. However, retention of the occlusal relationship in a patient with an open-bite malocclusion depends on maintenance of not only the vertical control of the molars, but also the vertical control of the incisors. Controlling the vertical dimension clearly requires interarch communication, and few appliances have this ability. Therefore the instability of open-bite correction may be related to a deficiency in the efficacy of retention appliances.

One solution suggested during the retention phase is use of positioners. This treatment involves the application of isometric pressure to the molars through intermittent chewing exercises daily.[54,55] A similar approach involves chewing gum consistently and with aggressive vertical force.[56] Another alternate method is continuous wearing of the active appliances to control molar position during retention. In other words, the continuous use of headgear during the retention period, a clearly unrealistic option.

On the other hand, with skeletal anchorage, retention stability can be accomplished in two ways. First, the vertical molar correction can be achieved earlier in treatment and maintained by means of ligature wires attached to the TADs during the finishing phase to allow periodontal fiber remodeling. Second, after appliance removal, the TADs can be maintained to control any relapse tendencies, should they occur, by means of sectional mechanics.

The vertical position of the incisors can be maintained by using Essix retainers with small, bonded attachments. Figure 15-15 shows a patient who required treatment for vertical relapse and had new appliances placed to close the bite again. The vertical relationship was maintained after re-treatment with a Vacu-form retainer, and the correction has been maintained.

CONCLUSION

Excess in the vertical dimension is a ubiquitous problem seen in various forms in the orthodontic office. If an esthetic profile and functional occlusion are major goals in orthodontics, vertical issues must be corrected. Patients with vertical excess and open bite are certainly a group who require orthodontic treatment because of the clear negative influences on facial proportions. The etiology is multifactorial but with a strong genetic influence. Vertical molar control

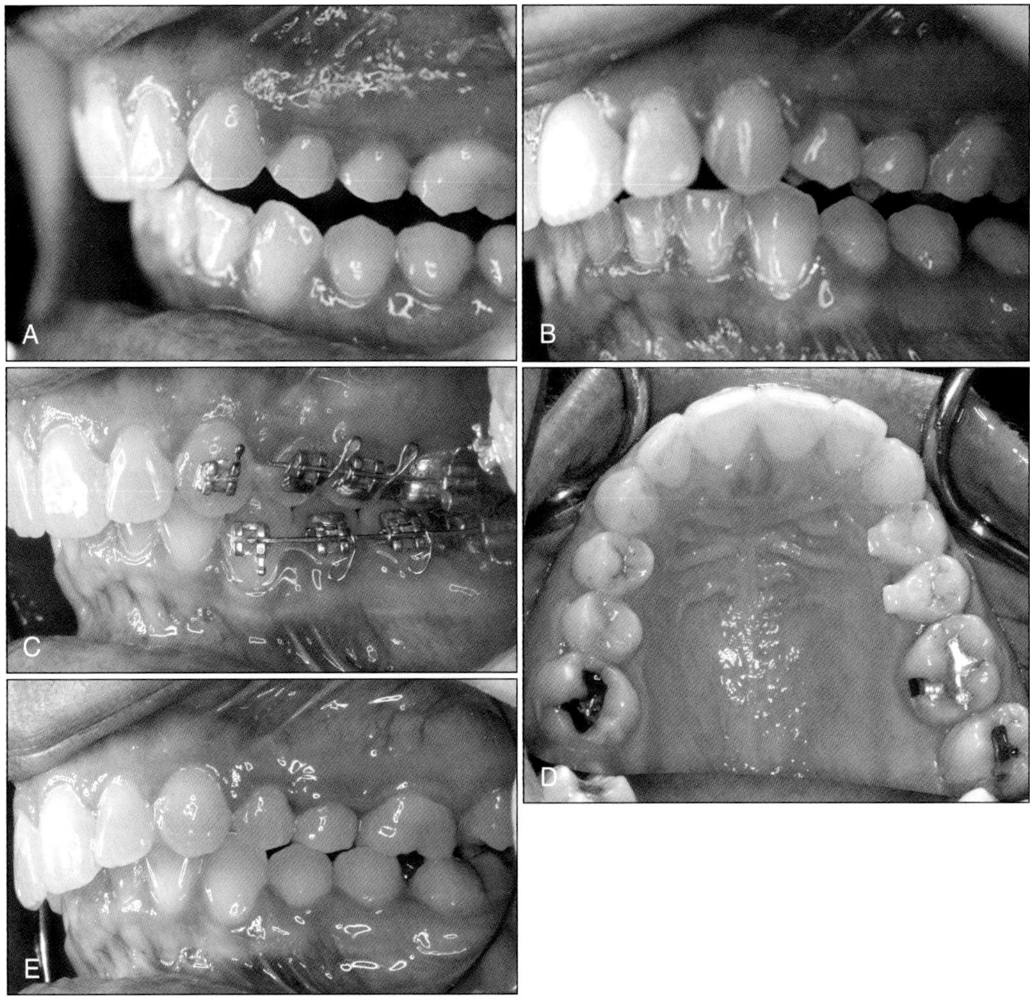

Fig. 15-15 **A** and **B,** Patient was initially treated for a lateral open bite that recurred. **C** and **D,** Patient was re-treated, and vertical retention of the left buccal segment was maintained with Vacu-form retainer that engaged vertical stops on the lingual aspect of the canine and premolars. **E,** Vertical correction has been maintained.

is the critical factor in the correction of the dolichofacial pattern. Headgear, bite blocks, and vertical-pull chin cups have been used somewhat successfully to hold the vertical position of the molars during growth. In the nongrowing patient the vertical dentoalveolar excess has been corrected primarily through surgery.

Recently, skeletal anchorage has become a promising therapeutic adjunct to orthodontic correction of this facial pattern. However, only a transitory change results, with minimal long-term stability expected in most patients. Stability is the perennial issue, particularly with open-bite patients, in whom the key to success is not alterability of the vertical pattern but rather maintenance of the correction. Some treatment alternatives are innovative and promising, but the ability to establish true stability remains unclear. Future studies using these new devices will reveal this truth.

ACKNOWLEDGMENT

Special thanks to Dr. Brett Holliday for her contribution in the preparation of this manuscript.

References

1. Sassouni V, Nanda SK: Analysis of dentofacial vertical proportions, *Am J Orthod* 50:801-823, 1964.
2. Nanda SK: Patterns of vertical growth in the face, *Am J Orthod Dentofacial Orthop* 93:103-116, 1988.
3. Nemeth RB, Isaacson RJ: Vertical anterior relapse, *Am J Orthod* 65:565-585, 1974.
4. Engel G, Cornforth G, Damerell JM, et al: Treatment of deepbite cases, *Am J Orthod* 77:1-13, 1980.
5. Pearson LE: Vertical control through use of mandibular posterior intrusive forces, *Angle Orthod* 43:194-200, 1973.

6. Kuhn RJ: Control of anterior vertical dimension and proper selection of extraoral anchorage, *Angle Orthod* 38:340-349, 1968.
7. Schudy F: Vertical growth versus anteroposterior growth as related to function and treatment, *Angle Orthod* 34:75-93, 1964.
8. Fotis V, Melsen B, Williams S, Droschl H: Vertical control as an important ingredient in the treatment of severe sagittal discrepancies, *Am J Orthod* 86:224-232, 1984.
9. Dung DJ, Smith RJ: Cephalometric and clinical diagnoses of open bite tendency, *Am J Orthod Dentofacial Orthop* 94:484-490, 1988.
10. Trask GM, Shapiro GG, Shapiro PA: The effects of perennial allergic rhinitis on dental and skeletal development: a comparison of sibling pairs, *Am J Orthod Dentofacial Orthop* 92:286-293, 1987.
11. Linder-Aronson S: Adenoids: their effect on mode of breathing and nasal airflow and their relationship to characteristics of the facial skeleton and the dentition—a biometric, rhino-manometric and cephalometro-radiographic study on children with and without adenoids, *Acta Otolaryngol Suppl* 265:1-132, 1970.
12. Hartsfield JK: Development of the vertical dimension: nature and nurture, *Semin Orthod* 8:113-119, 2002.
13. Harvold EP, Tomer BS, Vargervik K, Chierici G: Primate experiments on oral respiration, *Am J Orthod* 79:359-372, 1981.
14. Vig KW: Nasal obstruction and facial growth: the strength of evidence for clinical assumptions, *Am J Orthod Dentofacial Orthop* 113:603-611, 1998.
15. Proffit WR, White RP, Sarver DM: Long face problems. In Proffit WR, White RP, Sarver DM, editors: *Contemporary treatment of dentofacial deformity,* St Louis, 2003, Mosby, pp 464-506.
16. Ingervall B, Thilander B: Relation between facial morphology and activity of the masticatory muscles, *J Oral Rehabil* 1:131-147, 1974.
17. Boyd SB, Gonyea WJ, Finn RA, et al: Histochemical study of the masseter muscle in patients with vertical maxillary excess, *J Oral Maxillofac Surg* 42:75-83, 1984.
17a. Rowlerson A, Raoul G, Daniel Y, et al: Fiber-type differences in masseter muscle associated with different facial morphologies, *Am J Orthod Dentofacial Orthop* 127:37-46, 2005.
18. Korfage JA, Koolstra JH, Langenbach GE, van Eijden TM: Fiber-type composition of the human jaw muscles. Part 2. Role of hybrid fibers and factors responsible for inter-individual variation, *J Dent Res* 84:784-793, 2005.
19. Sarver DM: Facial analysis and the facial esthetic problem list. In Sarver DM, editor: *Esthetic orthodontics and orthognathic surgery,* St Louis, 1998, Mosby, pp 2-55.
20. Siriwat PP, Jarabak JR: Malocclusion and facial morphology: is there a relationship? An epidemiologic study, *Angle Orthod* 55:127-138, 1985.
21. Björk A: Prediction of mandibular growth rotation, *Am J Orthod* 55:585-599, 1969.
22. Cangialosi TJ: Skeletal morphologic features of anterior open bite, *Am J Orthod* 85:28-36, 1984.
23. Sarver DM, Ackerman MB: Dynamic smile visualization and quantification. Part 2. Smile analysis and treatment strategies, *Am J Orthod Dentofacial Orthop* 124:116-127, 2003.
24. English JD: Early treatment of skeletal open bite malocclusions, *Am J Orthod Dentofacial Orthop* 121:563-565, 2002.
25. Pearson LE: Vertical control in treatment of patients having backward-rotational growth tendencies, *Angle Orthod* 48:132-140, 1978.
26. Ingervall B, Bitsanis E: A pilot study of the effect of masticatory muscle training on facial growth in long-face children, *Eur J Orthod* 9:15-23, 1987.
27. Kalra V, Burstone CJ, Nanda R: Effects of a fixed magnetic appliance on the dentofacial complex, *Am J Orthod Dentofacial Orthop* 95:467-478, 1989.
28. Kuster R, Ingervall B: The effect of treatment of skeletal open bite with two types of bite-blocks, *Eur J Orthod* 14:489-499, 1992.
29. Dellinger EL, Dellinger EL: Active vertical corrector treatment: long-term follow-up of anterior open bite treated by the intrusion of posterior teeth, *Am J Orthod Dentofacial Orthop* 110:145-154, 1996.
30. Woods MG, Nanda RS: Intrusion of posterior teeth with magnets: an experiment in growing baboons, *Angle Orthod* 58:136-150, 1988.
31. Kiliaridis S, Egermark I, Thilander B: Anterior open bite treatment with magnets, *Eur J Orthod* 12:447-457, 1990.
32. Iscan HN, Akkaya S, Koralp E: The effects of the spring-loaded posterior bite-block on the maxillo-facial morphology, *Eur J Orthod* 14:54-60, 1992.
33. Sankey WL, Buschang PH, English J, Owen AH 3rd: Early treatment of vertical skeletal dysplasia: the hyperdivergent phenotype, *Am J Orthod Dentofacial Orthop* 118:317-327, 2000.
34. Chiba Y, Motoyoshi M, Namura S: Tongue pressure on loop of transpalatal arch during deglutition, *Am J Orthod Dentofacial Orthop* 123:29-34, 2003.
35. Deberardinis M, Stretesky T, Sinha P, Nanda RS: Evaluation of the vertical holding appliance in treatment of high-angle patients, *Am J Orthod Dentofacial Orthop* 117:700-705, 2000.
36. Staggers JA: Vertical changes following first premolar extractions, *Am J Orthod Dentofacial Orthop* 105:19-24, 1994.
37. Aras A: Vertical changes following orthodontic extraction treatment in skeletal open bite subjects, *Eur J Orthod* 24:407-416, 2002.
38. Schulz SO, McNamara JA Jr, Baccetti T, Franchi L: Treatment effects of bonded RME and vertical-pull chincup followed by fixed appliance in patients with increased vertical dimension, *Am J Orthod Dentofacial Orthop* 128:326-336, 2005.
39. Torres F, Almeida RR, de Almeida MR, et al: Anterior open bite treated with a palatal crib and high-pull chin cup therapy: a prospective randomized study, *Eur J Orthod* 28:610-617, 2006.
40. Pedrin F, Almeida MR, Almeida RR, et al: A prospective study of the treatment effects of a removable appliance with palatal crib combined with high-pull chincup therapy in anterior open-bite patients, *Am J Orthod Dentofacial Orthop* 129:418-423, 2006.
41. Lee JS, Kim DH, Park YC, et al: The efficient use of midpalatal miniscrew implants, *Angle Orthod* 74:711-714, 2004.
42. Yao CC, Wu CB, Wu HY, et al: Intrusion of the overerupted upper left first and second molars by mini-implants with partial-fixed orthodontic appliances: a case report, *Angle Orthod* 74:550-557, 2004.
43. Bailey LJ, Proffit WR, Blakey GH, Sarver DM: Surgical modification of long-face problems, *Semin Orthod* 8:173-183, 2002.
44. Liou EJ, Chen PH, Wang YC, Lin JC: A computed tomographic image study on the thickness of the infrazygomatic crest of the

maxilla and its clinical implications for miniscrew insertion, *Am J Orthod Dentofacial Orthop* 131:352-356, 2007.

45. Kuroda S, Katayama A, Takano-Yamamoto T: Severe anterior open-bite case treated using titanium screw anchorage, *Angle Orthod* 74:558-567, 2004.
46. Sugawara J, Baik UB, Umemori M, et al: Treatment and post-treatment dentoalveolar changes following intrusion of mandibular molars with application of a skeletal anchorage system (SAS) for open bite correction, *Int J Adult Orthod Orthog Surg* 17:243-253, 2002.
47. Erverdi N, Usumez S, Solak A: New generation open-bite treatment with zygomatic anchorage, *Angle Orthod* 76:519-526, 2006.
48. Kim YH: Anterior openbite and its treatment with multiloop edgewise archwire, *Angle Orthod* 57:290-321, 1987.
49. Kim YH, Han UK, Lim DD, Serraon ML: Stability of anterior openbite correction with multiloop edgewise archwire therapy: a cephalometric follow-up study, *Am J Orthod Dentofacial Orthop* 118:43-54, 2000.
50. Cozza P, Mucedero M, Baccetti T, Franchi L: Early orthodontic treatment of skeletal open-bite malocclusion: a systematic review, *Angle Orthod* 75:707-713, 2005.
51. Proffit WR, Bailey LJ, Phillips C, Turvey TA: Long-term stability of surgical open-bite correction by Le Fort I osteotomy, *Angle Orthod* 70:112-117, 2000.
52. Denison TF, Kokich VG, Shapiro PA: Stability of maxillary surgery in openbite versus nonopenbite malocclusions, *Angle Orthod* 59:5-10, 1989.
53. Huang GJ: Long-term stability of anterior open-bite therapy: a review, *Semin Orthod* 8:162-172, 2002.
54. Nolan PJ, West KS: Finishing and retention. In McNamara JA Jr, editor: *Orthodontics and dentofacial orthopedics,* Ann Arbor, Mich, 2002, Needham Press, pp 453-474.
55. Proffit WR: The third stage of comprehensive treatment: finishing. In Proffit WR, editor: *Contemporary orthodontics,* St Louis, 1993, Mosby, pp 516-533.
56. Kondo E, Aoba TJ: Nonsurgical and nonextraction treatment of skeletal Class III open bite: its long-term stability, *Am J Orthod Dentofacial Orthop* 117:267-287, 2000.

CHAPTER 16

ETIOLOGY, DIAGNOSIS, AND TREATMENT OF DEEP OVERBITE

■ *Madhur Upadhyay and Ravindra Nanda*

Deep overbite is perhaps one of the most common malocclusion and the most difficult to treat successfully. The amount of incisor overlap varies greatly and is primarily a manifestation of dental malocclusion.[1] Understanding the concept of overbite is imperative to any discussion of deep-bite malocclusion. In 1950, Strang[2] defined overbite as "the overlapping of the upper anterior teeth over the lowers in the vertical plane." However, the crown length of the upper and lower incisors varies significantly in individuals. Therefore a definition of overbite that includes "percentage" is more descriptive and useful: hence it would be more appropriate to redefine overbite as "the amount *and percentage* of overlap of the lower incisors by the upper incisors."

The ideal overbite in a normal occlusion may range from 2 to 4 mm, or more appropriately, 5% to 25% (overlap of mandibular incisors by maxillary incisors) (Fig. 16-1). According to Nanda,[3] a range of 25% to 40% without associated functional problems during various movements of the temporomandibular joint (TMJ) may be considered "normal." However, overlap greater than 40% should be considered "excessive" (deep bite) because of the potential for deleterious effects on the overall health of the surrounding periodontal structures and the TMJ. At 5 to 6 years of age the percentage of overbite varies between 36.5% and 39.2%.[4] From 9 to 12 years of age the overbite usually increases, whereas it decreases at 12 years to adulthood.[5] Thereafter, overbite remains largely unchanged, varying between 37.9% and 40.7%, unless affected by other factors, such as abrasion or loss of teeth, which can potentially reduce vertical dimension.

A severe expression of excessive overbite is the *cover bite*[6] (Fig. 16-2, *A-C*). Cover bite is associated primarily with the Class II, Division 2 malocclusion. This condition was first recorded in 1912 in the German literature as *Deckbiss*.[7] Cover bite is characterized by complete covering (concealment) of the mandibular incisor crowns resulting from excessive overbite and retroclination of the maxillary incisors. Another term used to denote a severe form of deep bite is *closed bite*[8] (Fig. 16-2, *D-F*). Closed bite is mainly seen in adults and rarely in young children and is characterized by excessive overbite resulting from loss of posterior teeth.

ETIOLOGY

Developmentally, a skeletal or dental overbite is caused by genetic or environmental factors, or a combination of both. *Skeletal* deep bites usually have a horizontal growth pattern and are characterized by (1) growth discrepancy of the maxillary and mandibular jawbones, (2) convergent rotation of the jaw bases, and/or (3) deficient mandibular ramus height. In these patients the anterior facial height is often short, particularly the lower facial third. On the other hand, *dental* deep bites show supraocclusion (overeruption) of the incisors,[2,9] infraocclusion (undereruption) of the molars,[2,5,9,10] or a combination. Other factors that can affect deep bite are alterations in tooth morphology, premature loss of permanent teeth resulting in lingual collapse of the maxillary or mandibular anterior teeth, mesiodistal width of anterior teeth, and natural, age-related deepening of the bite.

Deep bites that are primarily caused by environmental factors can also be classified as *acquired* deep bites. It is well known that a dynamic equilibrium exists between the structures around the teeth (tongue; buccinator, mentalis, and orbicularis oris muscles) and the occlusal forces, which assist in the balanced development and maintenance of the occlusion. Any environmental condition that disrupts this

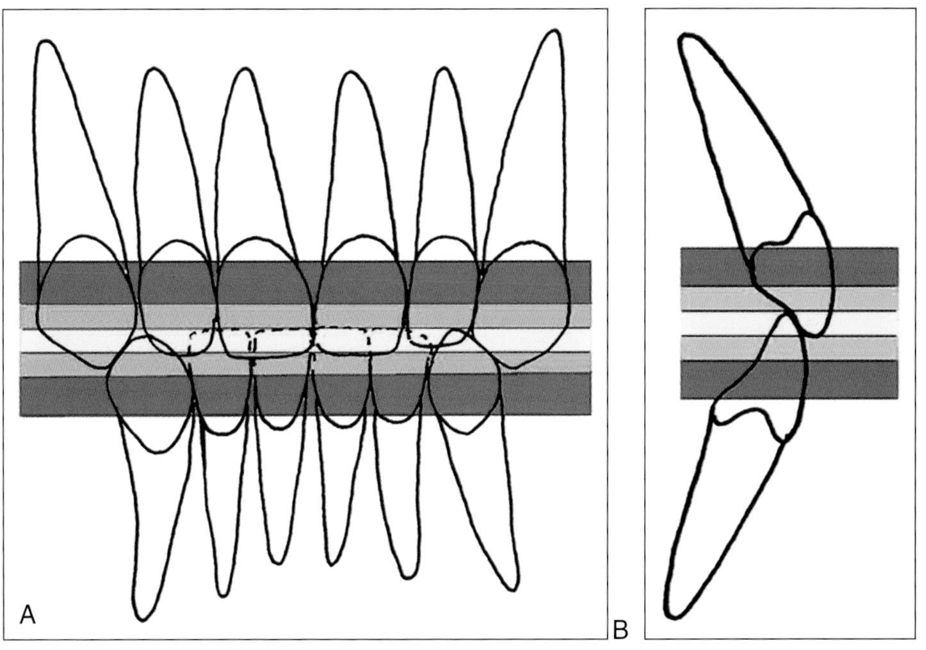

Fig. 16-1 Zones of overbite. From 5% to 25% is normal *(yellow)*, 25% to 40% is increased overbite *(orange)*, and greater than 40% is excessive (deep) overbite *(red)*. **A**, frontal view, **B**, Lateral view.

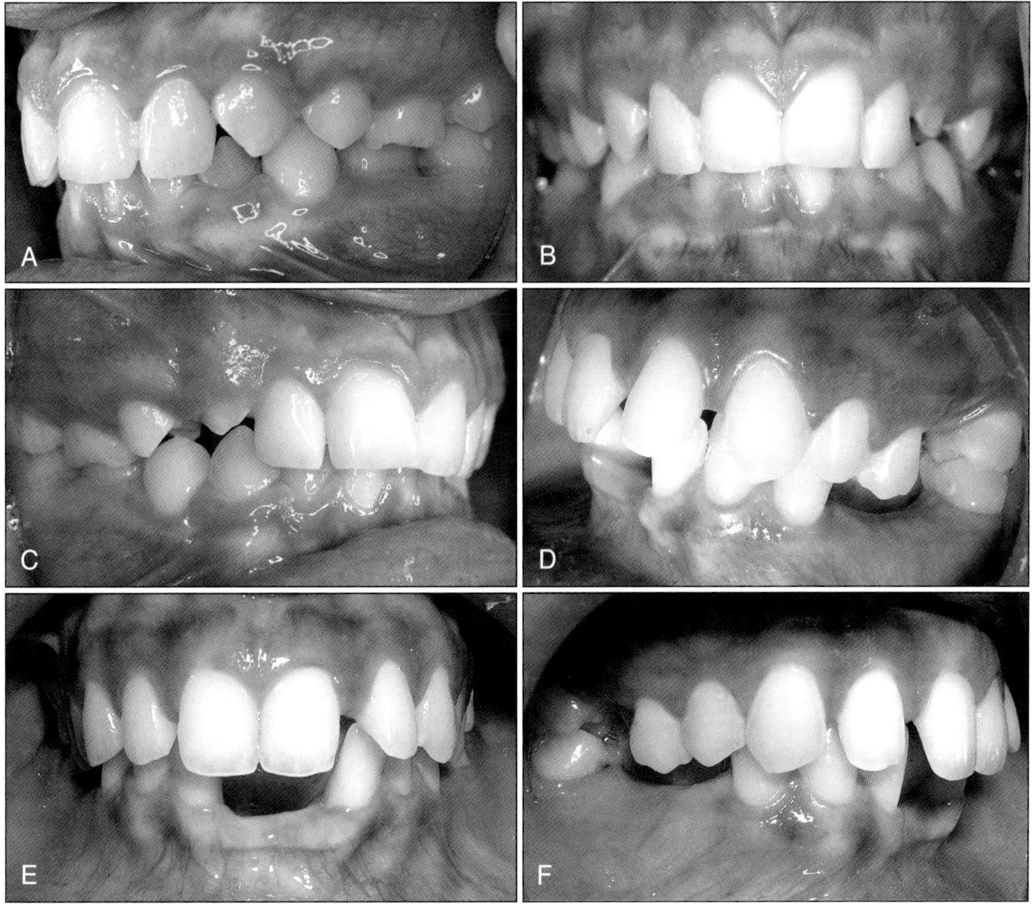

Fig. 16-2 **A** to **C,** Example of cover-bite malocclusion. Note how the lower incisors are completely concealed by the upper incisors. **D** to **F,** Example of closed-bite malocclusion.

dynamic harmony can lead to a malocclusion, such as the following:

- A lateral tongue thrust or abnormal tongue posture causing infraocclusion of the posterior teeth
- Wearing away of the occlusal surface or tooth abrasion
- Anterior tipping of the posterior teeth into extraction sites
- Prolonged thumb sucking

Deep-bite etiology must be considered in detail to formulate a comprehensive diagnosis and treatment plan for each patient so that optimal skeletal, dental, and esthetic results can be attained.

DIAGNOSIS

A deep overbite can be corrected by extrusion of posterior teeth or by inhibition and genuine intrusion of anterior teeth, or by a combination (Fig. 16-3). The choice of treatment is based in part on the etiology of deep bite, the amount of growth anticipated, the vertical dimension, relationship of the teeth with the adjoining soft tissue structures, and the desired position of the occlusal plane.

Growth Considerations

It is widely accepted that correction of deep bite is both easier to accomplish and more stable when performed on growing patients than when attempted on those with no appreciable growth remaining.[11,12] Because growth tends to increase the vertical distance between maxilla and mandible, it is probably useful to treat such patients during a period of active mandibular growth. During the growth period, tooth eruption can be stimulated in posterior segments and inhibited in anterior segments because condylar growth allows for dentoalveolar growth.

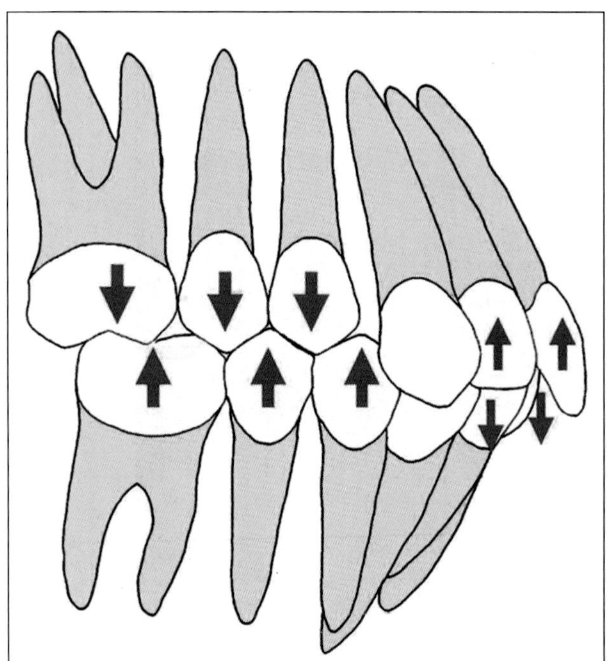

Fig. 16-3 Deep-bite malocclusion can be treated by either intrusion of incisors or extrusion of posterior teeth.

In adults, however, such a movement is counteracted by the posterior occlusion, especially in those with a hypodivergent skeletal pattern. The stability of such tooth movement, if performed, is highly questionable because it leads to alterations in muscle physiology, increasing the risk of relapse. In these malocclusions and others in which growth stimulation is no longer possible, fixed or removable mechanical appliances are needed to achieve optimal treatment results. Some patients might require a surgical procedure. For example, in patients with vertical maxillary excess, a LeFort I osteotomy with maxillary impaction might be required to achieve optimum dentofacial esthetics. A detailed discussion on this subject is beyond the scope of this chapter and can be found elsewhere.[13]

Assessment of the Vertical Dimension

Schudy[14] advocated correction of deep bite with eruption of premolars and molars as the treatment of choice, whereas others have preferred intrusion of incisors for treating most of their patients.[3,15] In addition to the above information, which is primarily anecdotal, it is important to carefully consider the influence of extrusive or intrusive mechanics on the vertical facial height of a patient, which in turn may affect the anteroposterior relationship of the maxilla and mandible.

In general, eruptive mechanics should not encroach on the "free-way space,"[8] or *interocclusal space,* defined as the distance between the occlusal or incisal surfaces of the maxillary and mandibular teeth when the mandible is in the physiological rest position. The average interocclusal space is 2 to 4 mm. It is less for the posterior teeth and more for the anterior. When there is a larger-than-normal "free space," greater opportunities exist for correction by guiding vertical alveolar development. For example, in a Class II, Division 2 patient with a hypodivergent facial pattern, redundant lips, and a flat mandibular plane angle, the deep bite can be corrected and facial esthetics improved by increasing the lower facial height or facial convexity. In most other Class II malocclusions, however, it is not always desirable to increase the vertical dimension, because it would tend to accentuate the point A–point B discrepancy and also increase an abnormally large lower face.

Soft Tissue Evaluation

Soft tissue relationships form an important diagnostic tool for deep-bite correction. The clinician should always consider the maxillary incisor position relative to the lip position to determine whether to maintain, intrude, or extrude the maxillary incisors relative to the upper lip. With the increased emphasis on smile esthetics and smile design, the use of "dynamic smile analysis" is supplementing static photographs in diagnosing malocclusions and formulating the appropriate treatment plan.[16]

Incisal exposure should be considered in three different clinical situations during initial examination: in relaxed-lip position, while smiling, and during speech. In a relaxed-lip position, 2 to 4 mm of incisor exposure, which includes the incisal edges, is considered acceptable. When smiling, the average incisor exposure is almost two thirds of the upper incisor, according to Maulik and Nanda.[16] They also report that in most "pleasing" smiles, the upper lip in men does not show gingiva, whereas women can have 1 to 2 mm of gingival exposure. If this condition is met and a deep bite is still present, the treatment plan should focus either on posterior extrusion (if the vertical parameters permit) or lower incisor intrusion (Fig. 16-4). In contrast, an occlusal plane "significantly" below the ideal might show excessive gingiva and

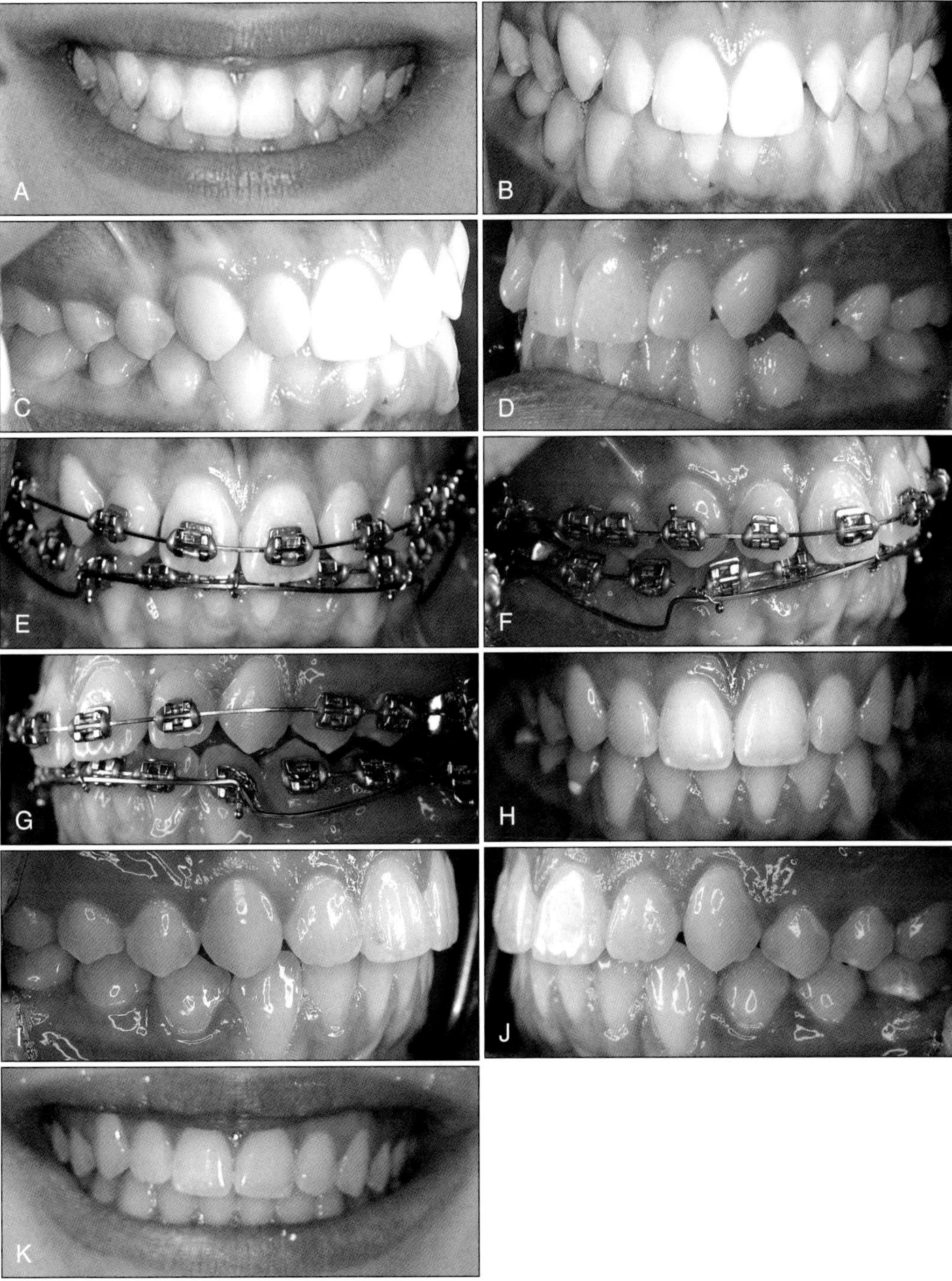

Fig. 16-4 **A** to **D,** The chief complaint of this adolescent female patient was excessive overbite. Careful analysis revealed that her upper incisor exposure was adequate both at rest and during smiling. **E** to **G,** The treatment decision was to intrude the lower incisors only, so that the deep-bite malocclusion could be resolved without significantly affecting the patient's smile esthetics. Segmental intrusion of the lower incisors was performed with an overlay intrusion arch. **H** to **K,** Final treatment results showing considerable improvement in the overbite.

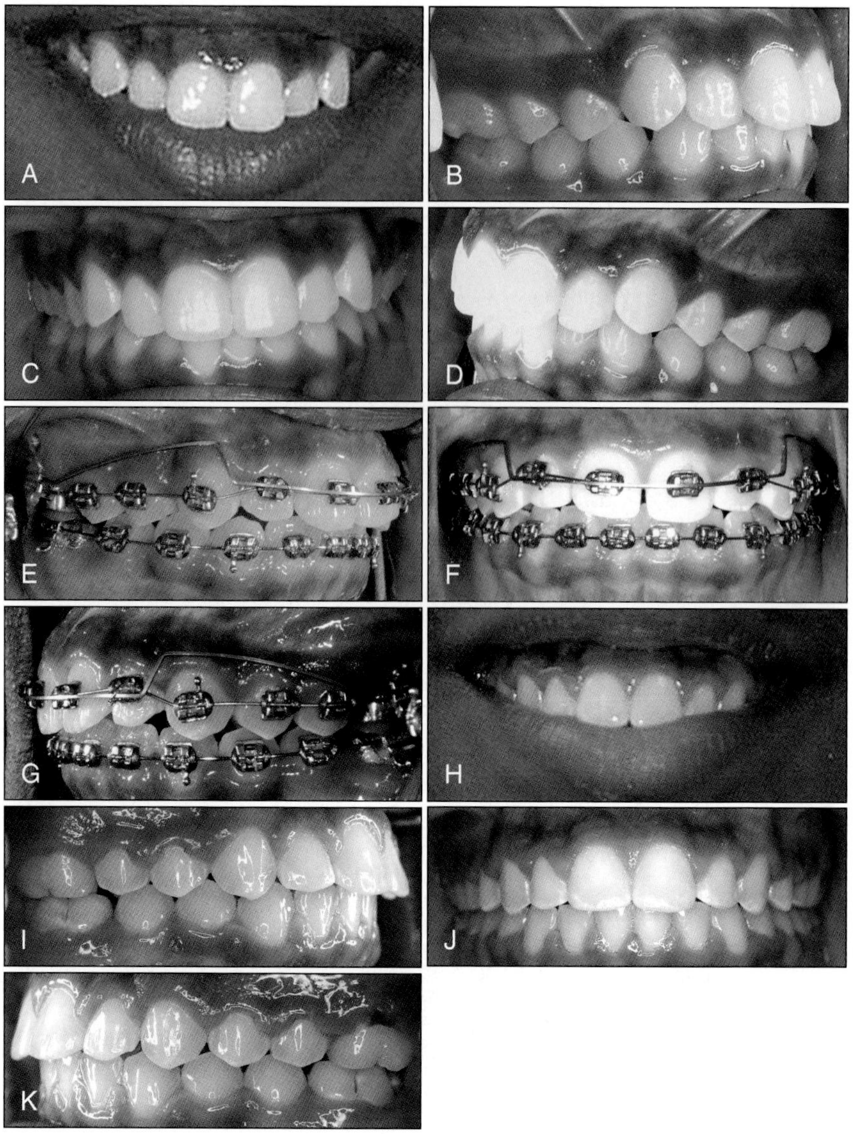

Fig. 16-5 **A** to **D**, Patient with excessive gingiva and deep overbite. **E** to **G**, Extremely light forces delivered through a CTA (Connecticut intrusion archwire) were used selectively to intrude only the upper central incisors. **H** to **K**, Treatment results show a significant improvement in the gingival exposure and the smile together with the correction of the deep overbite.

then require selective intrusion of the upper incisors (Fig. 16-5). Incisor exposure during speech may also give additional information because different facial muscles are involved.

Another important factor to consider is the *interlabial gap*. In patients exhibiting large interlabial gap, performing posterior extrusive mechanics may be contraindicated because this could further worsen esthetics by increasing the interlabial gap. In fact, an increase in the interlabial gap may cause several other problems, such as inability to close the lips without strain and associated functional problems. However, in individuals with redundant upper and lower lips, or no interlabial gap, but who show excessive overbite, posterior extrusive mechanics may be indicated.

Flaring (proclining) the incisors is another option, which, however, primarily camouflages deep bites. Nonetheless it is useful in patients presenting with retroclined incisors (e.g., Class II, Division 2 cases) at the initial visit. However, rapid labial tipping of mandibular incisors must be avoided to minimize risk of root resorption, gingival recession, and bone dehiscence, especially on a narrow symphysis with questionable labiolingual width of the alveolar bone.[17] Another contraindication may be undesirable facial esthetics.

TREATMENT

Treatment mechanics for deep-bite correction depends not only on the associated etiological variables but also on the treatment plan formulated for the malocclusion. Nevertheless, as mentioned, there are three ways to treat deep-bite malocclusions. These are as follows:

1. Intrusion of upper/lower incisors
2. Extrusion of upper/lower posterior teeth
3. A combination of intrusion/extrusion

Intrusion of Upper/Lower Incisors

Incisor intrusion is generally indicated in a patient with a vertical maxillary excess, a large interlabial gap, a long lower facial height, or a steep mandibular plane. The primary goal of the appliances is to achieve "true incisor intrusion."[18]

Intrusion arch

An intrusion arch (Ortho Organizers) can be made of .016 × .022–inch or .017 × .025–inch CNA archwires. Alternatively, preformed intrusion archwires can also be used; the Connecticut intrusion arch (CTA; Ultimate Wireforms, Bristol, Conn.), fabricated from nickel-titanium alloy, provides the advantage of shape memory, spring back, and light, continuous force distribution[19] (Fig. 16-6, *A*). The appliance setup includes two passive posterior (stabilizing) units and one active anterior unit (the intrusion arch). The passive units consist of stiff or rigid segmented wires (.017 × .025–inch or greater stainless steel wires) in the molars and premolars bilaterally. Inclusion of as many teeth as possible in the posterior segment minimizes side effects. The anterior segment, which includes either two or four incisors, is constructed with similar wires. Remember, the greater the dimension of the stainless steel wires, more predictable is the tooth movement.

The intrusion arch is activated by placing a 30-degree gingival bend 2 to 3 mm mesial to the molar tubes so that the wire lies passively in the vestibular sulcus. Activation is accomplished by bringing the intrusion arch occlusally and tying it to the anterior segment so that only a point contact is made versus placing it directly into the bracket slots, as done with the utility arch.[20,21] The intrusion arch utilizes a one-couple force system, which makes the appliance "statically determinant"; that is, the various forces and moments in this setup can be quantified to an appreciable degree of accuracy. The intrusion arch can also be tied back or cinched to prevent flaring of the incisors if the intrusive force is being applied anterior to the *center of resistance* (Cres) of the incisors. The reciprocal action of the intrusion arch on the molars or the buccal segments is the extrusion and distal tip-back of the crowns and mesial movement of the roots (Fig. 16-6, *B*). This can be very helpful in a Class II, Division 1 patient requiring correction of the molar relationship to a Class I. In such patients a buccal segment is often not needed because it may prevent distal tip-back of molars. In Class I malocclusions with deep bite, however, a tip-back may cause steepening of the occlusal plane. Increasing the number of teeth in the anchor unit is one way of minimizing such side effects. Another method is to use relatively low forces of about 40 g for the upper four incisors and 30 g for the lower incisors.

As a general guideline, 10 to 15 g of force per incisor is acceptable to prevent posterior side effects. Recent evidence has shown that the intrusive forces can be made so light that reactive forces on the anchor teeth remain well below the force levels needed for extrusion and tipping.[22] Therefore the use of a headgear to prevent side effects is completely avoidable. Also, low forces help in minimizing root resorption. On average, after the initial activation period of 3 to 4 weeks, the base arch should intrude 0.4 to 0.6 mm per month.[23]

Another useful clinical application of the intrusion arch is preventing the side effects from canine retraction. A popular method of canine retraction is "frictional mechanics" employing a continuous arch system. The advantages of this system (over frictionless mechanics) are reduced risk of unintended canine movement (e.g., rotation, flaring, extrusion) and minimal wire bending. However, when an archwire with a low load-deflection rate is used, it tends to deform, leading to undesirable side effects on the anterior teeth, including extrusion of the incisors and deepening of the bite.[24] This type of deep bite can also be termed *iatrogenic* deep bite, which in this context means deep bite induced inadvertently by the clinician (Fig. 16-7). With larger or more rigid archwires, the system might develop excessive friction, leading to delayed tooth movement, anchorage loss, or even cessation of canine retraction. Therefore the use of a .016 × .022–inch CTA as an overlay archwire is recommended, to optimize the biomechanical system for canine

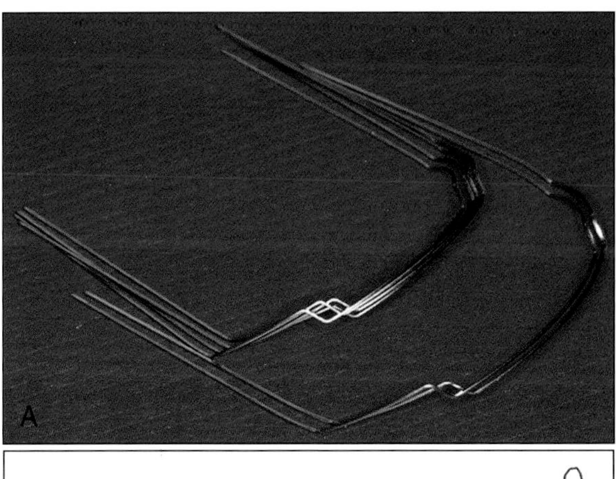

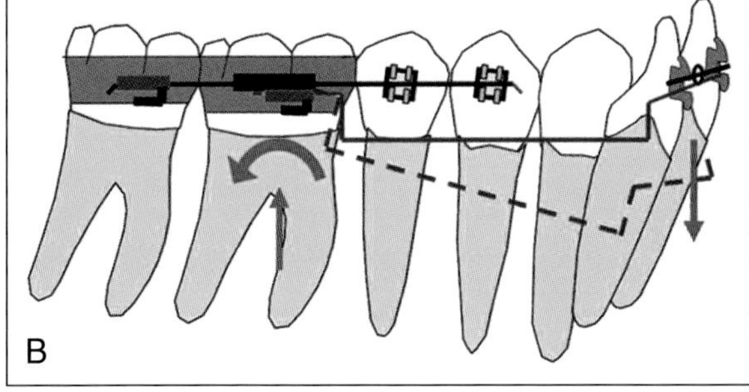

Fig. 16-6 **A,** Preformed upper and lower CTA made from nickel-titanium alloy. **B,** Biomechanical design of lower incisor intrusion with the CTA.

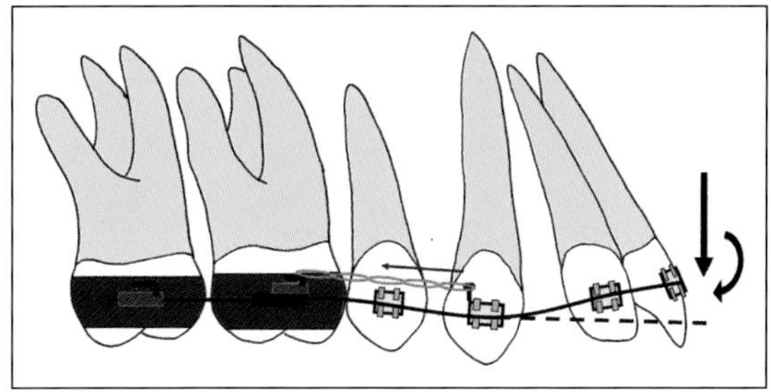

Fig. 16-7 Development of deep bite (iatrogenic) during canine retraction (sliding mechanics) from occlusal deflection of the archwire.

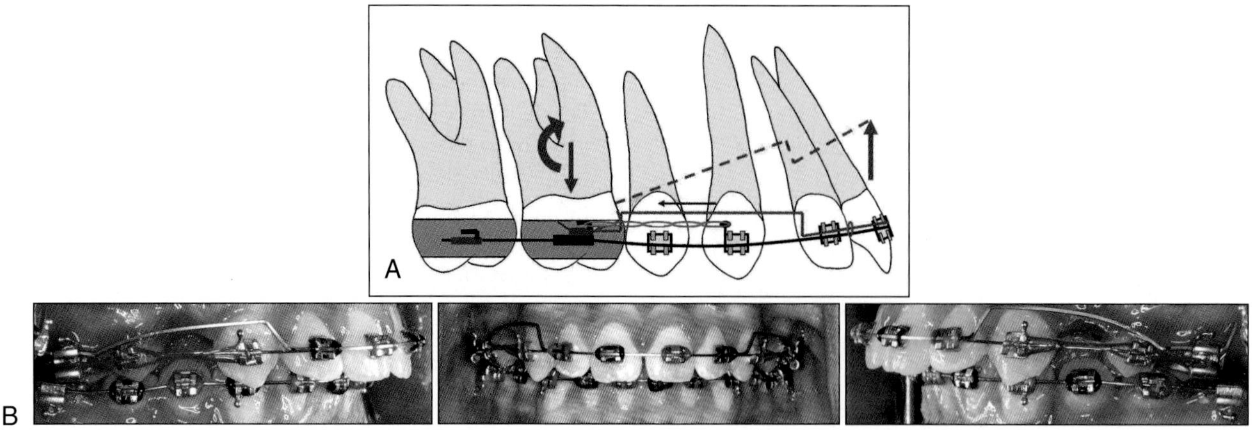

Fig. 16-8 Application of CTA to prevent deepening of the bite and simultaneously to augment anchorage during canine retraction. **A,** Biomechanical force system involved. **B,** Clinical pictures.

retraction (Fig. 16-8). The anticlockwise moment (if tied anterior to Cres of anterior teeth) and the intrusive force on the incisors ensure the stability of the incisors by counteracting the iatrogenic forces generated by canine retraction. Also, molar anchorage is reinforced because of a tip-back moment on the posterior segment.

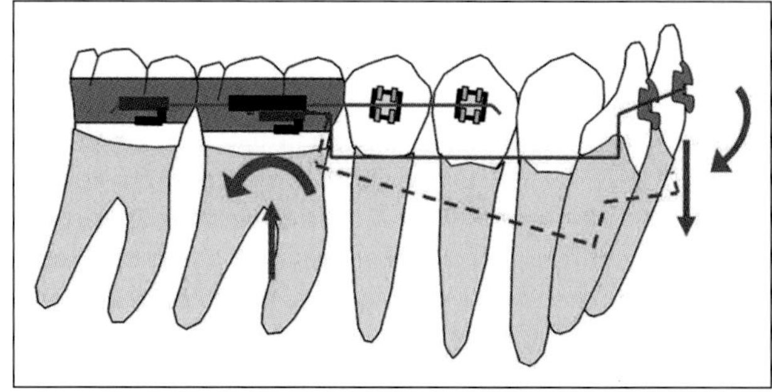

Fig. 16-9 Biomechanical design of lower incisor intrusion with Rickett's utility arch.

Utility arch

The utility arch is similar in design to the CTA. It is stepped down at the molars, passes through the buccal vestibule, and is stepped up at the incisors to avoid distortion from occlusal forces (Fig. 16-9). The difference from CTA is that for intrusion, the utility arch is tied into the incisor brackets, which creates a two-couple force system, the moment of which tends to tip the incisor crowns facially and the molar distally. Although the facial tipping of incisors can be avoided by cinching or tying back the intrusion utility arch, any force that tends to bring the anchor teeth mesially is undesirable. Incorporating a "twist" or "torque bend" in the incisor segment is another way of controlling this tendency of the teeth to tip facially; however, this will increase the intrusive force on the incisor segment and the extrusive force on the molar. It is well known that heavier forces do not increase the amount or rate of intrusion.[25,26] Another problem is that, unlike the CTA, the utility arch is a two-couple system and thus it is impossible to accurately determine the magnitude of the reactive forces ("statically indeterminant"), which in turn makes it impossible to adjust the archwire to prevent side effects.

Therefore in their clinical practice, the authors routinely choose the CTA. Also, considerable chair time is saved because the CTA involves no wire bending and needs minimal adjustment.

Three-piece intrusion arch

Labial tipping of incisors gives the clinical impression of deep-bite correction because it influences the vertical incisal edge position. Similarly, during extensive retraction of incisors, development of a deep bite (iatrogenic) is common because of uprighting of the incisors (Fig. 16-10). It is therefore important to control the labiolingual inclination of the anterior teeth as they are intruded and retracted, especially if they are initially flared.

A three-piece intrusion arch[27] uses segmental mechanics to intrude and retract incisor teeth simultaneously in a highly predictive manner. With some modifications, the passive units are constructed in the same way as described for the intrusion arch (Fig. 16-11). The active units consist of two segmented springs made from .016 × .022–inch or .017 × .025–inch CNA, with wires activated by placing a 30-degree gingival bend 2 to 3 mm mesial to the molar tubes. The gingival bend can be increased or decreased based on the desired amount of intrusive force. The units are hooked to the distal extensions on the anterior segmented wire at a point close to the estimated Cres of the incisors. Application of a light, distal force delivered by a Class I elastic or a power chain to the anterior segment helps to alter the direction of the intrusive force on the anterior segment, so that the forces are directed in an upward and backward direction through the Cres of the anterior teeth, or as required in a particular patient (Fig. 16-12).

Extrusion of Upper/Lower Posterior Teeth

Bite planes

Currently, bite planes are the most popular appliances for deep bite correction (Fig. 16-13). These appliances load the incisors for an intrusive effect but leave the posterior teeth free to erupt, thereby leveling the curve of Spee primarily by posterior extrusion. Studying the vertical changes of molars and incisors with bite-plane treatment, Sleichter[28] found that alveolar height in the molar region increased, with minimal change in the incisal area. The intrusive effect on the incisors is, at best, minimal.

Two types of bite planes can be used; removable or fixed. *Removable* bite planes consist of an acrylic platform anchored to the maxillary dentition with arrowhead, Adams, ball-end, or crib clasps. Anteriorly, a labial bow helps to stabilize the bite plate and contact the teeth at the incisal one third. By acting as a premature incisal stop, usually within the confines of the interocclusal space, the block forces the posterior teeth from occlusal contact and allows them to erupt. It is advisable not to disocclude the posterior teeth by more than 2 mm; this allows close supervision of the follow-up and treatment progress and prevents any sudden TMJ or myofunctional change.

Fixed, or bonded, bite planes are blocks of composite or glass ionomer cement that can be bonded on the lingual surface of maxillary incisors to disocclude the posterior teeth. The advantages over removable bite planes are integration with fixed-appliance mechanotherapy, no patient compliance issue, and less bulky appliance.

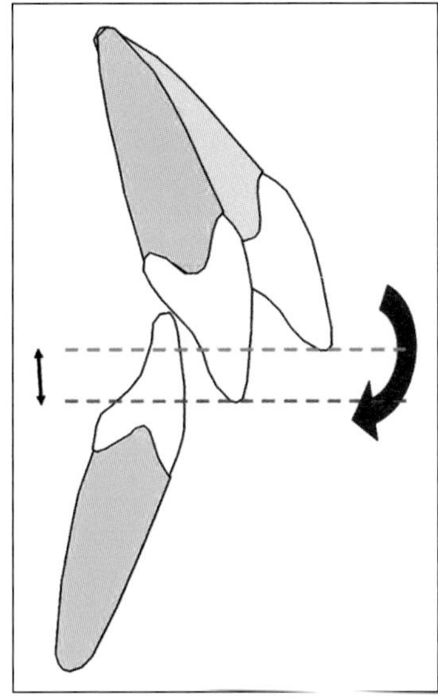

Fig. 16-10 Uprighting (or retraction) of proclined incisors during orthodontic treatment might lead to development of deep bite (iatrogenic).

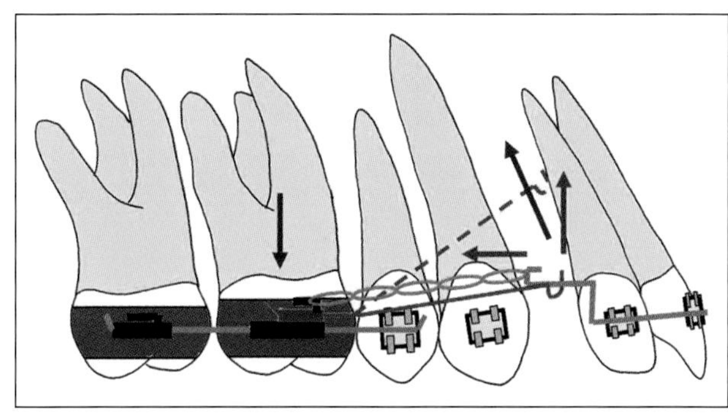

Fig. 16-11 Biomechanics involved when using three-piece intrusion arch for simultaneous intrusion and retraction of maxillary incisors.

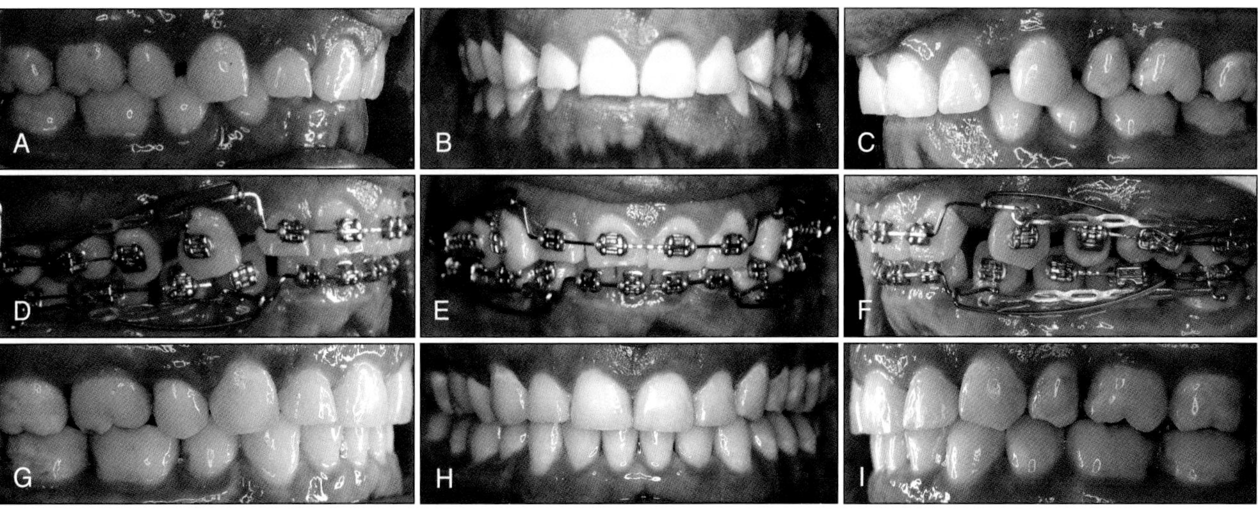

Fig. 16-12 **A** to **C,** Adult patient with severe deep bite caused by supraeruption of incisors. **D** to **F,** Three-piece intrusion arches were placed in the upper and lower arches for deep-bite correction. **G** to **I,** Optimum overbite and overjet were established at the end of treatment.

Functional appliances

Functional appliances can also be used to achieve posterior extrusion to correct deep bites, especially in low-angle Class II malocclusions. Functional appliances help in positioning the lower jaw forward to an edge-to-edge relationship, thereby disoccluding the posterior teeth, which are then free to erupt. Eruption can be augmented by using elastics during fixed-appliance mechanotherapy. For treatment to succeed, however, the appliance must be worn almost full-time. Unfortunately, a significant number of patients do not fully comply, and appliances are often worn only part-time or may be lost or broken while out of the mouth. Many of these problems can be overcome by using fixed functional appliances, such as the Twin Force (Fig. 16-14).

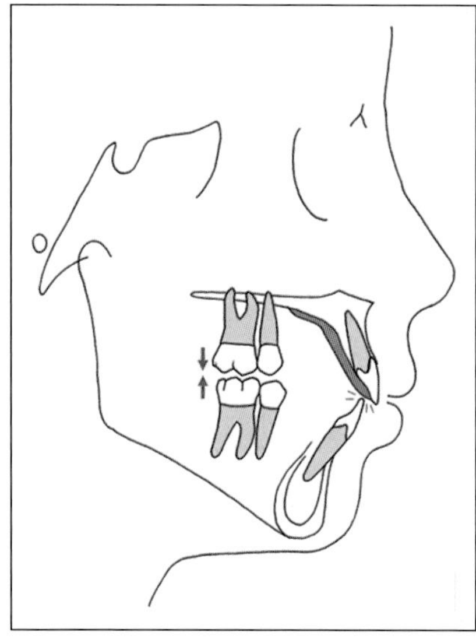

Fig. 16-13 Mechanism of action for anterior bite plane.

Combination of Intrusion and Extrusion

By positioning anterior brackets occlusally and posterior brackets gingivally, or by using reverse-curve archwires, simultaneous intrusion of anterior teeth and extrusion of posterior teeth can be achieved (Fig. 16-15). However, there is no definitive control over such mechanics. Drawbacks that need to be addressed include changes in the axial inclination of the buccal teeth and flaring of incisors caused by an intrusive force anterior to the Cres. Also, because extrusion is more easily accomplished than intrusion, a reverse "curve of Spee" wire will extrude posterior teeth while obtaining minimal, if any, anterior intrusion.[29]

IMPLANTS FOR DEEP-BITE CORRECTION

Anchorage control, especially in the vertical dimension, is paramount if bite opening needs to be achieved by genuine intrusion of the anterior teeth. Also, if instead of only four incisors, intrusion of all six anterior teeth (including the canines) is desired, as in a cover-bite malocclusion, extraoral appliances become a prerequisite to withstand the additional burden of anchorage. According to Burstone,[15] it is not possible to intrude all six anterior teeth at one time without producing undesirable axial inclination in the posterior segment. An additional 20 to 30 g of force would be required on each side to intrude the canine, taking into account the root size and the dense surrounding bone. Although effi-

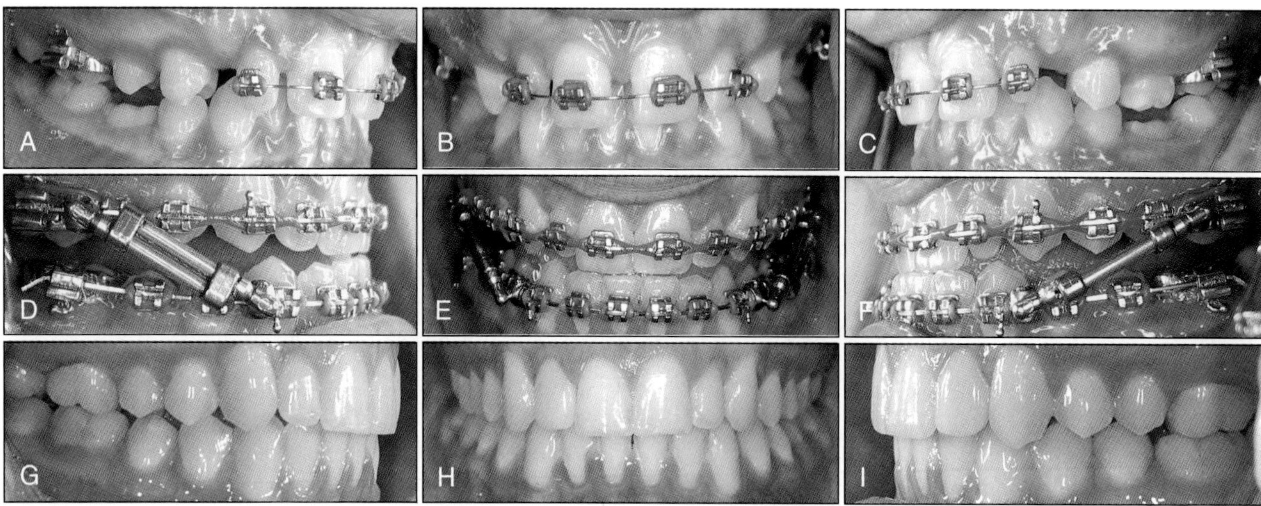

Fig. 16-14 **A** to **C**, Clinical photographs of Class II, Division 1 patient with severe deep bite. **D** to **F**, The patient was treated with the Twin Force bite corrector (fixed functional appliance). Note how the anterior positioning of the mandibular teeth in an edge-to-edge relationship with the maxillary incisors disoccludes the posterior teeth, which are then free to erupt. Alternatively, elastics can also be used to augment their eruption. **G** to **I**, Final treatment results showing Class I molar and canine relation with normal overbite.

cient, extraoral appliances require extensive patient compliance. A recent study also shows that the chances of root resorption increase with these appliances, possibly from the "jiggling effect."[30] Esthetics and social issues may be concerns as well.

In the past decade, skeletal anchorage systems such as miniplates, palatal implants, mini-implants, and miniscrews have revolutionized orthodontic anchorage and biomechanics by making anchorage more stable.[31-35] Mini-implants can be effectively used for en masse intrusion of anterior teeth[36] (Fig 16-16).

Factors to consider when placing mini-implants for intrusion of anterior teeth include availability of sufficient interdental bone, less soft tissue irritation, and a larger anterior segment (if all six anterior teeth are included), which requires greater control. In the authors' experience the interdental bone between the roots of the canine and lateral incisors (bilaterally) is an appropriate location for placement of mini-implants. The selection of the point of application of the intrusive force with respect to the Cres of the anterior segment is also important in the placement of the implants, so that the tooth movement can be predicted more accurately. The Cres of the six anterior teeth has been estimated to be halfway between the Cres of the four incisors and canines.[36] True intrusion without axial inclination change can be obtained only by directing the intrusive force through the Cres of the anterior teeth. In the patient described in Fig. 16-16, a light distal force was delivered by an elastic chain to the anterior segment to alter the direction of the intrusive force, so that true intrusion of the anterior teeth could be achieved on their long axes (Fig. 16-17). The distal force used was of very low magnitude, primarily to redirect the line action of the intrusive force.

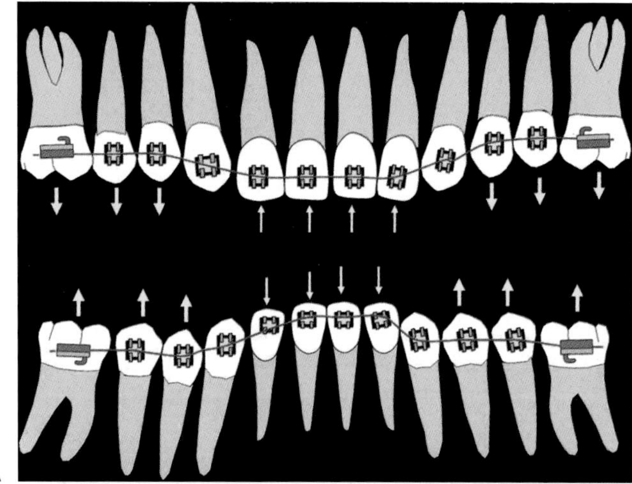

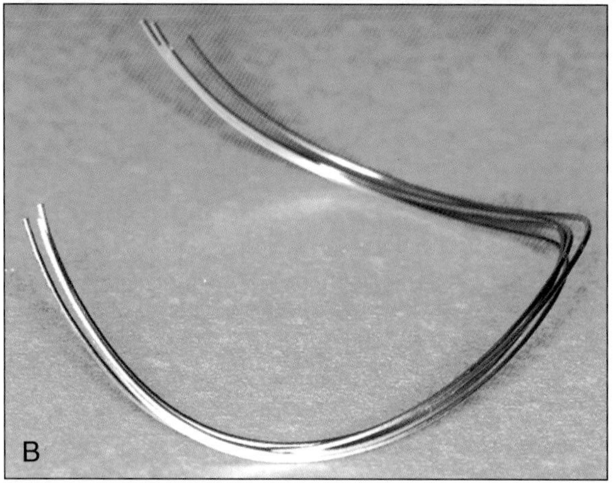

Fig. 16-15 **A,** Simultaneous intrusion of anterior teeth and extrusion of posterior teeth can be accomplished by occlusal positioning of anterior brackets relative to posterior brackets. **B,** Using reverse-curve archwires produces a similar effect.

RETENTION AND STABILITY

As previously discussed, correction of deep-bite malocclusion can be achieved by a variety of methods with fairly predictable results. The real challenge, however, is maintaining the overbite over time. The results of most studies on the stability of overbite correction suggest a decrease in overbite during treatment, followed by an increase in the overbite after appliance removal, although clinically this might not be significant.[37] Factors to consider when planning retention for deep-overbite correction include age of the patient, facial type, molar extrusion/incisor intrusion, and interincisal angle.

Age

Deep-bite correction is usually achieved by the simultaneous intrusion of incisors and extrusion of the posterior teeth. Growing patients benefit the most with this approach because active vertical growth during deep-bite correction ensures greater stability. Because growth tends to increase the vertical distance between the jaw bases, performing treatment during this period is most advantageous.

Facial Type

Certain facial types have a greater potential for permanent correction than other types. Hyperdivergent facial types usually exhibit a more favorable reaction to overbite correction than hypodivergent types. This can be attributed to the growth rate in the vertical direction, which is the highest and lasts the longest in high-angle patients.

Molar Extrusion/Incisor Intrusion

Molar extrusion in growing patients is a fairly stable procedure if the interocclusal space is not violated. Any eruptive movement beyond the interocclusal space might not be stable because of strong posterior occlusion or muscle stretching, especially in low-angle individuals. For the same reason in adults, incisor intrusion is regarded as more stable. Other factors that can lead to relapse of incisor intrusion are continued lower incisor eruption, canting of the occlusal plane, incomplete leveling of the curve of Spee, and forward rotation of the mandible.

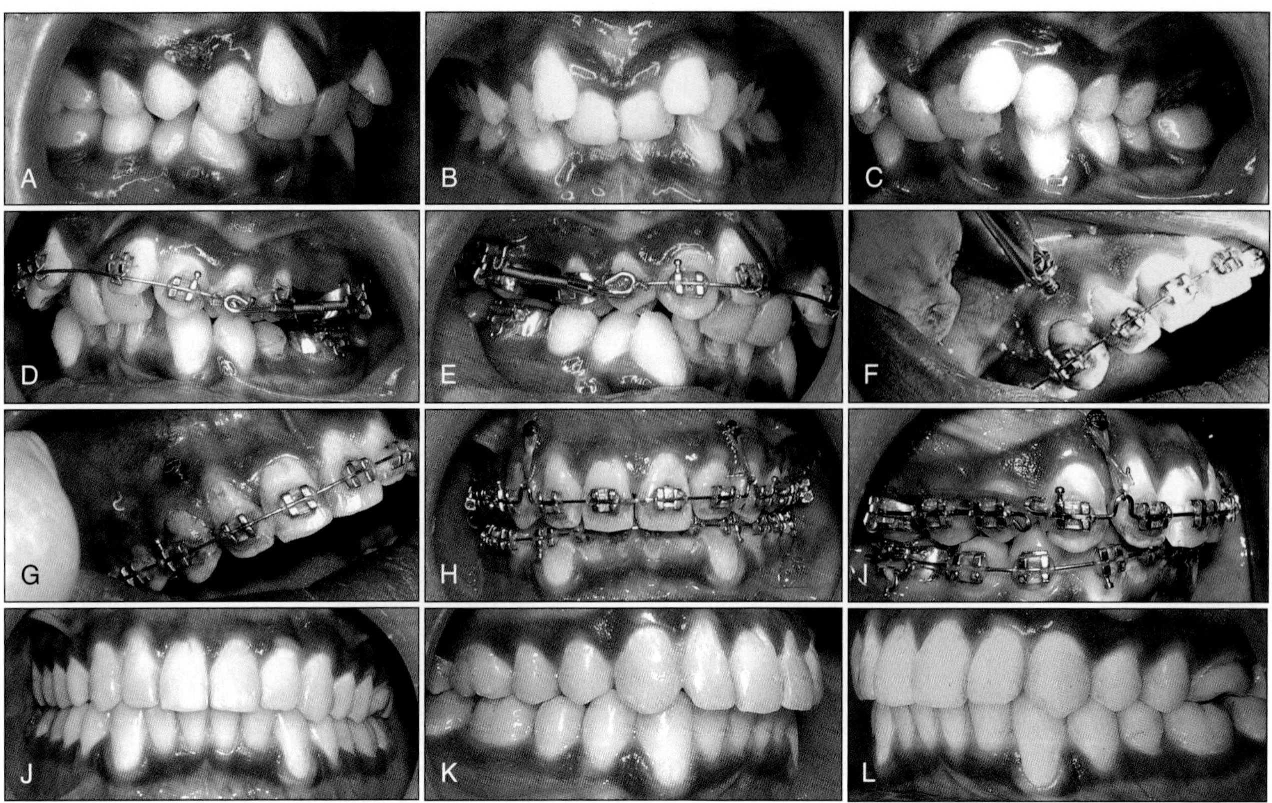

Fig. 16-16 **A** to **C,** Postpubertal 16-year-old male patient with severe Class II, Division 2 malocclusion with 100% deep bite. **D** and **E,** First phase of treatment. "Jones Jig" appliance was used to distalize the maxillary molars by more than 6 mm, to achieve a Class I molar relationship. **F** to **I,** Second phase of treatment. Mini-implants were inserted between the roots of the maxillary lateral incisor and canine (**F** and **G**) to intrude all the maxillary anterior teeth en masse in a single step. More than 4 mm of intrusion was achieved without any posterior teeth extrusion. The implants remained stable throughout treatment. In the mandibular arch the incisors were proclined to alleviate the severe crowding. **J** to **L,** Good overjet and overbite were achieved after completion of active orthodontic treatment.

Interincisal Angle

Reidel[38] suggested that a large interincisal angle at the end of treatment is associated with relapse of deep overbite, possibly because a large interincisal angle tends to force the crowns of the mandibular incisors lingually and the apex of the maxillary incisors labially.[12] Burzin and Nanda[37]showed that the axial inclination of the incisors did not change significantly during a 2-year posttreatment observation period. They suggested that ideal axial inclination of the incisors at the end of treatment could be a factor in overbite stability. Therefore, maintaining optimum interincisal angle, incisal stops, and guidance between the maxillary and mandibular incisors is essential for maintaining overbite correction. The interincisal angle can be greater for dolichofacial patterns and less for brachyfacial patterns. In general, however, an angle of 125 to 135 degrees ensures good stability for deep-bite correction.

CONCLUSION

Deep overbite is a common component of malocclusion in adults and children. The importance of accurate diagnosis, which entails precise identification of the etiological factors, cannot be overemphasized because effective treatment of deep bite and long-term retention depend on it. Additionally, esthetic considerations, including maxillary incisor–to-lip relationship and the gingival exposure on smiling, are also important diagnostic features that must be considered in the treatment plan.

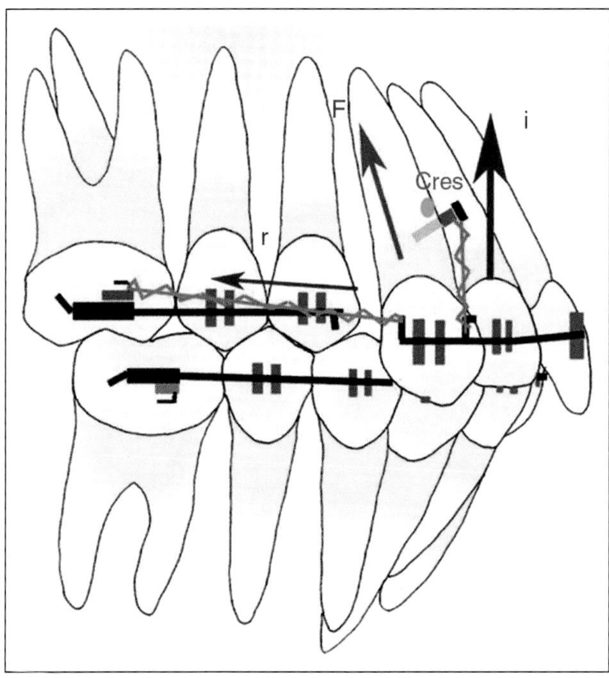

Fig. 16-17 Biomechanical design for the en masse intrusion of the maxillary anterior teeth: *i,* intrusive force; *r,* distal force; *F,* resultant force; *Cres,* center of resistance of anterior teeth.

References

1. Goldstein MS, Stanton FL: Various types of occlusion and amounts of overbite in normal and abnormal occlusion between two and twelve years, *Int J Orthod Oral Surg* 22:549-569, 1936.
2. Strang RHW: *A textbook of orthodontia*, Philadelphia, 1950, Lea & Febiger.
3. Nanda R: The differential diagnosis and treatment of excessive overbite, *Dent Clin North Am* 25:69-84, 1981.
4. Dermaut LR, Pauw GD: Biomechanical aspects of Class II mechanics with special emphasis on deep bite correction as a part of the treatment goal. In Nanda R, editor: *Biomechanics in clinical orthodontics,* Philadelphia, 1997, Saunders, pp 86-98.
5. Flemming HB: Investigation of the vertical overbite during the eruption of the permanent dentition, *Angle Orthod* 31:53-62, 1961.
6. Peck S, Peck L, Kataja M: Class II Division 2 malocclusion: a heritable pattern of small teeth in well-developed jaws, *Angle Orthod* 68:9-17, 1998.
7. Mayrhofer B: *Lehrbuch der Zahnkrankheiten*, Jena, Germany, 1912, G Fischer, pp 60-62.
8. Moyers RE: *Handbook of orthodontics*, ed 4, Chicago, 1988, Year Book Medical Publishers, pp 422-424.
9. Prakash P, Margolis HI: Dento-cranofacial relations in varying degrees of overbite, *Am J Orthod* 38:657-673, 1952.
10. Wylie WL: The relationship between ramus height, dental height and overbite, *Am J Orthod Oral Surg* 32:57-67, 1946.
11. Bell W, Jacobs J, Legan H: Treatment of Class II deep bite by orthodontic and surgical means, *Am J Orthod* 85:1-19, 1984.
12. Simons M, Joondeph D: Change in overbite: a ten-year post-retention study, *Am J Orthod* 64:349-367, 1973.
13. Proffit WR, White RP, Sarver DM: Long face problems. In Proffit WR, White RP Jr, Sarver DM, editors: *Contemporary treatment of dentofacial deformity,* St Louis, 2003, Mosby, pp 464-506.
14. Schudy FF: The control of vertical overbite in clinical orthodontics, *Angle Orthod* 38:19-38, 1968.
15. Burstone CR: Deep overbite correction by intrusion, *Am J Orthod* 72:1-22, 1977.
16. Maulik C, Nanda R: Dynamic smile analysis in young adults, *Am J Orthod Dentofacial Orthop* 132:307-315, 2007.
17. Wehrbein H, Bauer W, Diedrich P: Mandibular incisors, alveolar bone, and symphysis after orthodontic treatment: a retrospective study, *Am J Orthod Dentofacial Orthop* 110:239-246, 1996.
18. Ng J, Major PW, Heo G, Flore-Mir C: True incisor intrusion attained during orthodontic treatment: a systematic review and meta-analysis, *Am J Orthod Dentofacial Orthop* 128:212-219, 2005.
19. Nanda R, Marzban R, Kulhberg A: The Connecticut intrusion arch, *J Clin Orthod* 32:708-715, 1998.
20. Ricketts RM: Bioprogressive therapy as an answer to orthodontic needs. Part I, *Am J Orthod* 70:241-248, 1976.
21. Ricketts RM: Bioprogressive therapy as an answer to orthodontic needs. Part II, *Am J Orthod* 70:359-397, 1976.
22. Steevenbergen EV, Burstone CJ, Prahl-Andersen B, Aartman IHA: The influence of force magnitude on intrusion of the maxillary segment, *Angle Orthod* 75:723-729, 2005.
23. Faber ZT: The relationship of tooth movement to measured force systems: a prospective analysis of the treatment effects of orthodontic intrusion arches, 1994, Division of Orthodontics, University of Connecticut (master's thesis).
24. Nanda RS, Ghosh J: Biomechanical considerations ion sliding mechanics. In Nanda R, editor: *Biomechanics in clinical ortho dontics,* Philadelphia, 1997, Saunders, pp 188-217.
25. Dellinger EL: A histologic and cephalometric investigation of premolar intrusion in the *Macaca speciosa* monkey, *Am J Orthod* 53:325-355, 1967.
26. Reitan K: Initial tissue behavior during apical root resorption, *Angle Orthod* 44:68-82, 1974.
27. Shroff B, Nanda R: Biomechanics of class II correction. In Nanda R, editor: *Biomechanics in clinical orthodontics,* Philadelphia, 1997, Saunders, pp 143-155.
28. Sleichter CG: Effects of maxillary bite plane therapy in orthodontics, *Am J Orthod* 40:850-870, 1954.
29. Woods MG: The mechanics of lower incisor intrusion: experiments in non-growing baboons, *Am J Orthod* 93:186-195, 1988.
30. Deguchi T, Murakami T, Kuroda S, et al: Comparison of the intrusion effects on the maxillary incisors between implant anchorage and J-hook headgear, *Am J Orthod Dentofacial Orthop* 133:654-660, 2008.
31. Nanda R, Uribe FA: *Temporary anchorage devices in orthodontics*, St Louis, 2008, Mosby-Elsevier.
32. Upadhyay M, Yadav S, Nagaraj K, Patil S: Treatment effects of mini-implants for en-masse retraction of anterior teeth in bialveolar dental protrusion patients: a randomized controlled trial, *Am J Orthod Dentofacial Orthop* 134:18-29, 2008.
33. Nagaraj K, Upadhyay M, Yadav S: Mini-implant anchorage for a skeletal Class II malocclusion with missing mandibular incisors: a case report, *World J Orthod* 9:155-166, 2008.

34. Upadhyay M, Yadav S: Mini-implants for retraction, intrusion and protraction in a Class II Division 1 patient, *J Orthod* 34:158-167, 2007.
35. Upadhyay M, Nagaraj K, Yadav S, Saxena R: Mini-implants for en masse intrusion of maxillary anterior teeth in a severe Class II Division 2 malocclusion, *J Orthod* 35:79-89, 2008.
36. Melsen B, Fotish V, Burstone CJ: Vertical force considerations in differential space closure, *J Clin Orthod* 24:678-683, 1990.
37. Burzin J, Nanda R: The stability of deep overbite correction. In Nanda R, Burstone CJ, editors: *Retention and stability in orthodontics,* Philadelphia, 1993, Saunders, pp 61-79.
38. Riedel RA: A review of the retention problem, *Angle Orthod* 30:179-194, 1960.

PART III

Management of Adult and Complex Cases

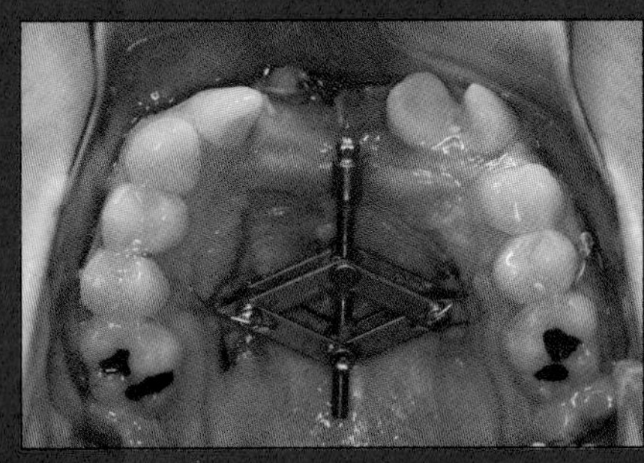

CHAPTER 17

Orthodontic Treatment in Adult Patients with Reduced Periodontal Attachment

Julia Harfin

Esthetics and the conservation of youthful traits are important to most people. Orthodontics plays an essential role not only in maintaining teeth but also in improving the patient's smile. This is one of the primary reasons why adult patients seek orthodontic treatment: to improve their smile despite their age. This trend has increased over time, and now there is general acceptance of the beneficial effects of adult orthodontics.

SPECIAL CONSIDERATIONS IN ADULT PATIENTS

Before discussing adult treatment further, it is necessary to consider the important differences between the treatment of children and adults:

- In children the amount and direction of growth determines the treatment plan. In adults there is no residual growth to take advantage of, and the sutures are more closely intertwined.
- Adults normally start treatment with fewer teeth than adolescents, especially in the posterior region, and therefore anchorage considerations become more important.
- Gingivitis is normally present in children, whereas different degrees of periodontitis are present in adults.[1-5]
- Frequently, adults are more concerned with esthetics and are more demanding than children and adolescents.
- Some adults have temporomandibular syndromes that make treatment objectives more difficult to achieve.

It is impossible to treat all patients with a similar approach, especially when dealing with periodontal attachment loss. This issue is often more critical than the chronological age.[6-10] It is important to remember that the *center of resistance* is related to the amount of periodontal attachment and indicates the amount and direction of the force that must be applied.

Another factor to consider with adult patients is their past medical treatments, especially those who are or have been taking different medications. This can have a significant effect on the bone turnover, especially in women during menopause. In treating middle-aged women, it is important to consider whether they are menopausal and if they are taking hormonal replacement drugs or being treated with bisphosphonates. Antidepressant or antihypertensive drugs may cause side effects such as dryness of the mucosa and ulceration. These patients require the use of dull-surfaced appliances to avoid lesions affecting the mucosa.[11]

The activation period should be longer and less frequent (6-8 weeks) to allow the patient's bone time to recover. Loss of 2 mm of root length in a patient with 80% to 90% of periodontal attachment is not the same as in a patient with only 20% attachment. For example, in the patient shown in Fig. 17-8, the longevity of the tooth would be compromised.[12]

New medical advances have reduced the risks of treating malocclusions in patients with acquired immunodeficiency syndrome (AIDS), osteoporosis, or endocrine disturbances, as well as in long-term users of corticosteroids or immunosuppressants.[13-19]

TREATMENT USING MINISCREWS

In certain cases, prosthodontists need to upright or intrude molars to normalize the curve of Spee and the occlusal plane. Miniscrews are frequently used in orthodontic treatment as a device for skeletal anchorage when needed.

Figure 17-1 shows a 39-year-old patient who sought treatment to correct the position of the left lower second molar. It was decided to use a miniscrew to help in correcting its position, and this case is a good example of how to upright a molar with the use of microimplant anchorage.[5]

A miniscrew also can be effectively used with the over-eruption of maxillary molars caused by loss of the opposing teeth, which could create occlusal interferences. Its correction is an essential step before initiating prosthodontic procedures. The intrusion of upper molars is a challenging situation for the prosthodontist. Although a prosthodontic reduction with an endodontic procedure and a crown restoration is an option, the author prefers to solve the problem with microimplants, as shown in Fig. 17-2.[20] After treatment, pulpal vitality was maintained and periodontal health improved. The occlusal plane discrepancy was corrected without surgical procedures. At the end of the treatment the occlusal space was sufficient to rebuild the posterior occlusion by using an implant prosthesis.[21]

In certain situations the orthodontist must work as a "tissue engineer," moving teeth to create bone for future implants.

TREATMENT OF DIASTEMAS

One of the most common clinical problems seen in adult patients involves closing upper and lower diastemas. For many years, total recovery of the dental papillae after closing the anterior diastema was considered only a chance result. In 1992, however, Tarnow et al.[22] showed that the recovery of the papillae is determined by the distance between the

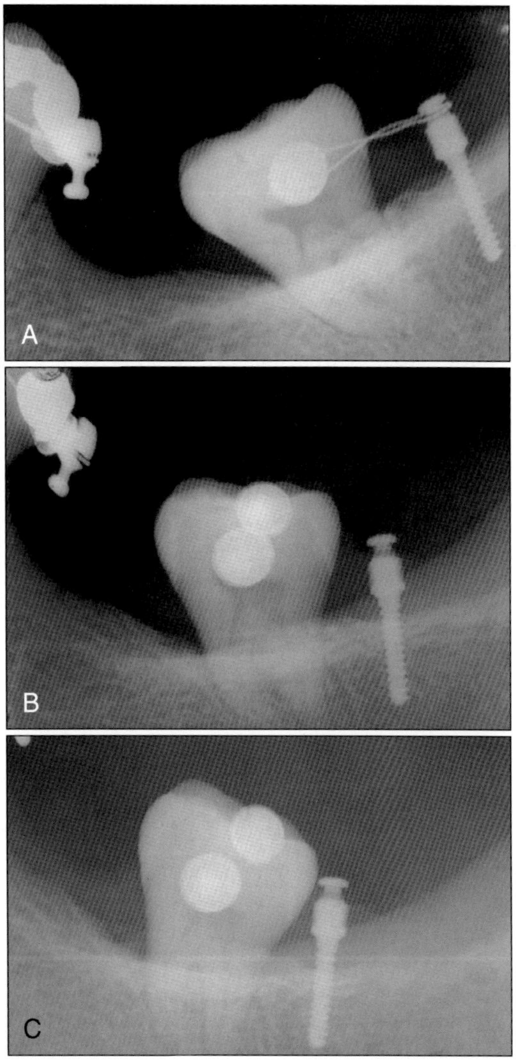

Fig. 17-1 Radiographs of mesially inclined second molar in 39-year-old patient. **A** and **B,** After 9-mm miniscrew was placed 5 mm distally, a ligature wire was placed 20 days later between a labio-lingual button and the miniscrew and activated every 20 days. **C,** Results after 5 months of treatment. The molar is totally uprighted.

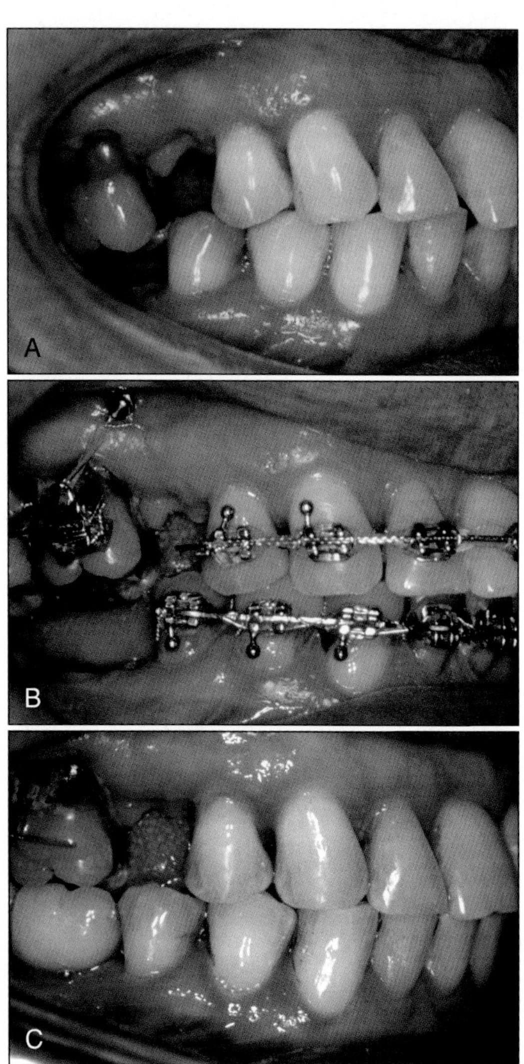

Fig. 17-2 **A,** Significant extrusion of first upper-right molar in 43-old-patient. **B,** A 9-mm microimplant is placed mesially to the first molar and activated every 20 days through a ligature wire. **C,** Results after 8 months of treatment. The intrusion of the first molar is clearly visible.

incisor contact point and the crestal bone height. Orthodontists can predictably move the dental contact point to achieve the desired results.

However, to accomplish this, it is necessary first to determine the cause of the diastema. Eliminating the underlying etiology along with closure of the diastema ensures greater stability and less chance of relapse. The malocclusions in which diastemas may be seen can be divided into the following four main groups:

1. Occlusal disturbances caused by premature contacts in the posterior region, which might induce the mandible to move forward during the closing pathway. As a consequence, changes in the normal contact points at the anterior region produce eccentric forces, resulting in diastemas.
2. Loss of teeth in the posterior region, causing anterior teeth to drift distally.
3. Lack of leveling of the occlusal plane.
4. Periodontal problems.

It is crucial to know the true cause creating or increasing the diastema. Otherwise, relapse is highly probable. Additionally, periodontal therapy before, during, and after orthodontic treatment is essential to achieve good and stable results. It is impossible to retain the closure of the diastema when an active periodontal problem is present.[23-25]

It is well known that similar results can be obtained when the teeth are endodontically treated. Endodontically treated teeth may be less susceptible to apical resorption than vital teeth. In both cases, good recovery of the papillae is obtained. The normalization of the occlusal plane, overjet, and overbite with a normal cuspid and incisor guide is an important prerequisite to achieve long-term stability. Figure 17-3 shows the closure of a large diastema when one of the teeth has been endodontically treated.

Diastemas Resulting from Tongue Thrusting

The presence of the diastema in the anterior region has often been associated with tongue thrusting. It is difficult to determine whether the anterior position of the tongue is responsible for the diastema, a consequence of it, or a combination of both. Nevertheless, when the diastema has been successfully closed, the patient must be sent to a speech therapist to normalize lingual function.[26-28]

Figure 17-4 shows a 49-year-old man who wanted a second opinion regarding the presence of a diastema between

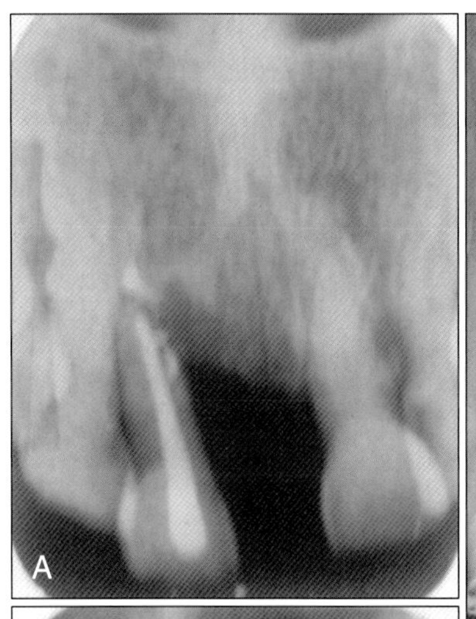

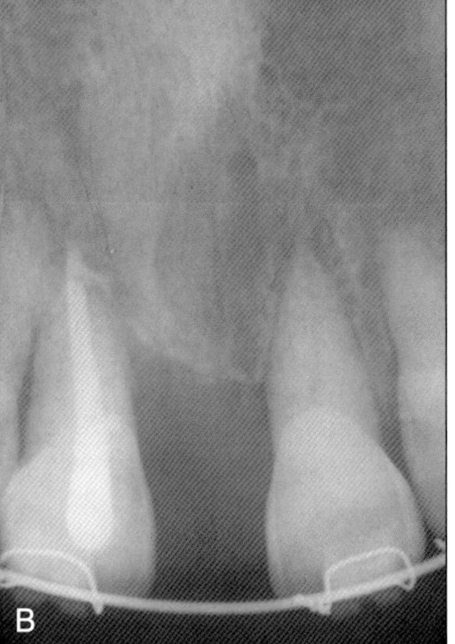

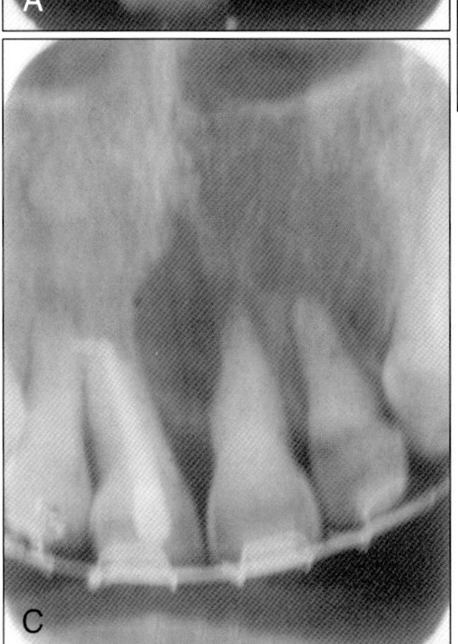

Fig. 17-3 Radiographs of significant diastema in 73-year-old patient. **A,** Right upper central incisor shows endodontic treatment and only 20% periodontal attachment. **B,** Esthetic brackets were placed in conjunction with .014-inch stainless steel arch. After alignment was completed, the space was closed with ligature wires and activated every 4 weeks. **C,** Results after 14 months of treatment. The diastema is totally closed, and an important osseous repair is achieved.

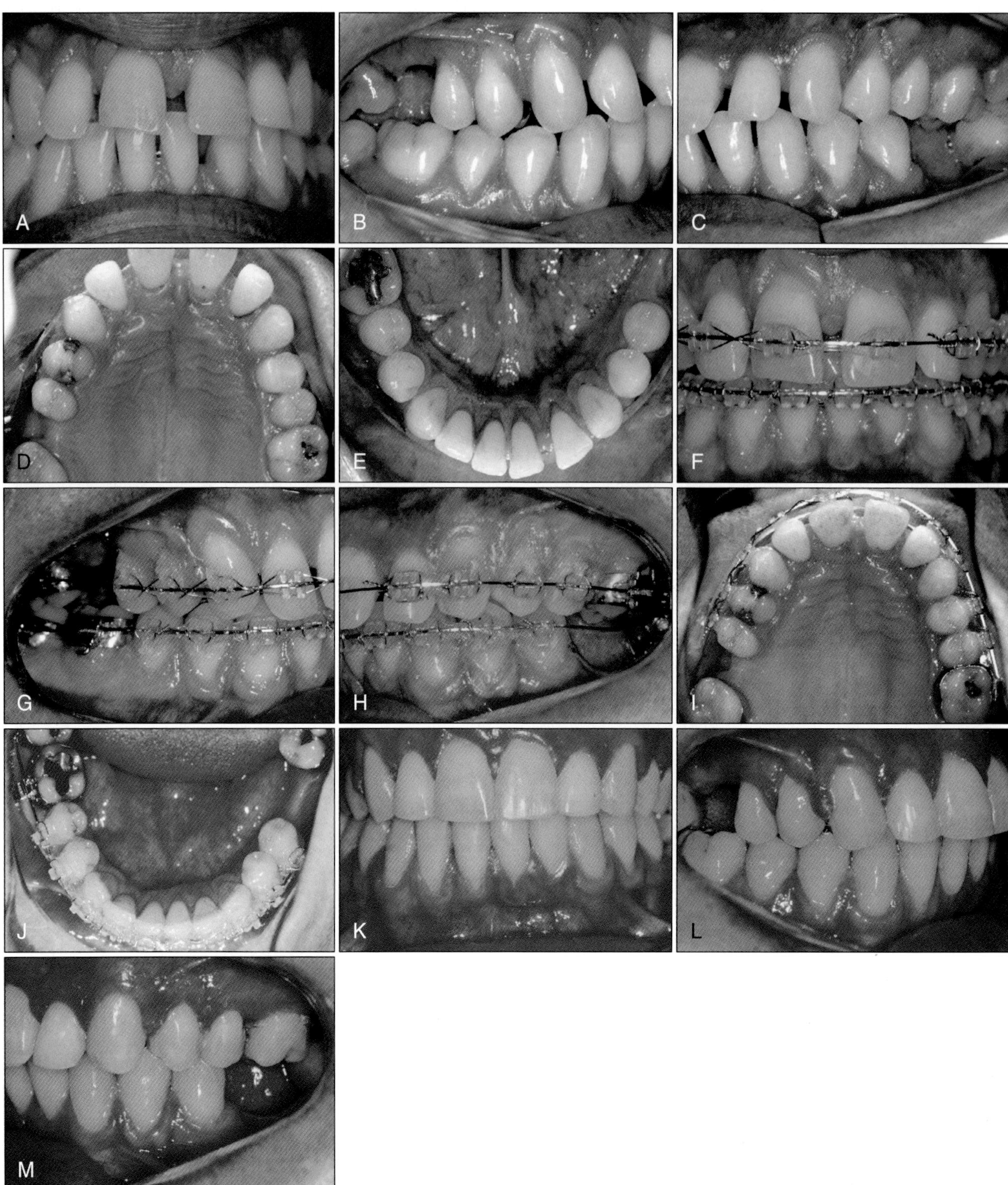

Fig. 17-4 **A,** Upper and lower diastemas and lack of interdental papillae in 49-year-old man. **B** and **C,** Extrusion and inclination of upper and lower incisors noticeable in lateral views; first upper-right molar and first lower-left molar absent. **D** and **E,** Photographs of upper and lower arches confirmed the diastemas and lack of papillae. **F** to **H,** Esthetic brackets with metal slots were recommended. After completion of the leveling and alignment of the arches, the diastemas were closed, with monthly activation of ligature wires. **I** and **J,** Upper and lower arches at completion of first phase of treatment. **K,** Final results. All the diastemas are closed and the papillae totally recovered. **L** and **M,** Right and left Class I canines are achieved. Some gingivitis is present, more evident on the right side.

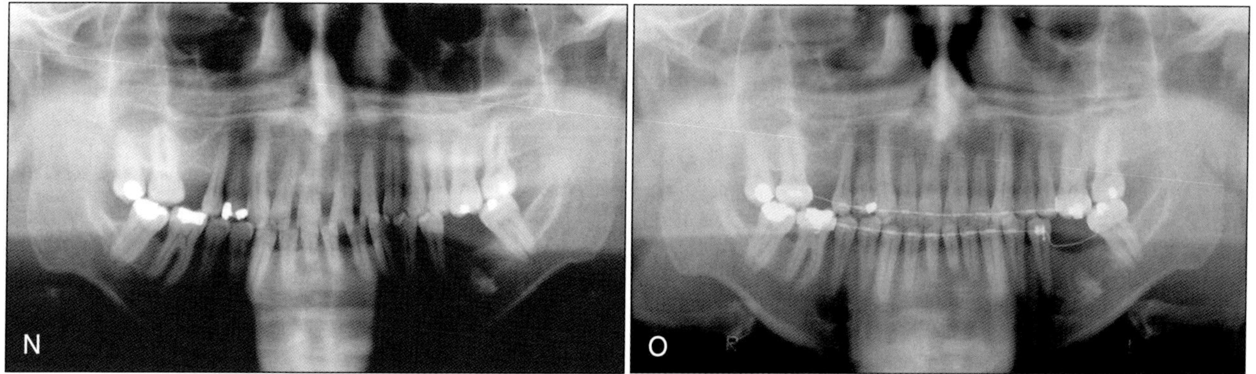

Fig. 17-4, cont'd **N,** Pretreatment, and **O,** posttreatment, panoramic radiographs.

the upper central incisors. His dentist suggested larger central incisor crowns to close the diastema. His dental history indicated that the upper and lower diastemas had improved significantly during the last 2 years, after the extraction of the upper and lower left molars. The lack of interdental papillae was his main concern, as evident from the frontal photograph (Fig. 17-4, *A*).

The extrusion and an increase in the inclination of the anterior incisors were evident and had been worsened by a tongue-thrust habit. As with every treatment plan, periodontal treatment was the first step. It is impossible to move teeth in the presence of bacterial plaque or with active periodontal pockets. In such cases, periodontal monitoring every 2 to 3 months is highly recommended.[29,30]

Esthetic brackets with a metallic slot were used to diminish friction. It is advisable to begin with low-load deflection archwires (stainless steel .012 × .014–inch Ni-Ti-Cu) to achieve alignment and level the arches (Fig. 17-4, *F-J*). The spaces in the lower arch should be closed first, so as to have the necessary space to close the diastema in the upper arch. To achieve a good result, it is recommended to activate the ligature wires every 4 weeks. It is important to remember that the arch form of each patient requires specific bends. For example, the same arch form used in a severely dolichofacial 12-year-old patient can never be used in a 60-year-old patient with a severe brachyfacial biotype and few teeth. The differences are too great from one patient to another to have preformed archwires for every patient.

Diastemas were closed in the upper and lower arch (Fig. 17-4, *K-M*). The interdental papillae recovered to their normal shape and size. The midline was coincident, and Class I molar and canine relationships were achieved. The occlusal plane was also normalized. The immediate replacement of the missing molars was highly recommended.

Permanent retention with fixed retainers was advised for both upper and lower arches. A Hawley's plate is not advisable because the palatal acrylic reduces the space for the tongue, which makes it move forward, causing the anterior spaces to reopen. As mentioned previously, treatment by a speech therapist is also required to normalize the position of the tongue. The total recovery of the papillae is only achieved when the gingivoperiodontal tissues are normalized.

Figure 17-5 shows that similar results can also be obtained by using lingual brackets. Pretreatment photographs show a 32-year-old patient with severe diastemas in the upper and lower arches (Fig. 17-5, *A-E*). As evident from the photos, the interdental papillae are absent. Lingual brackets were placed (G7 from Ormco, Orange, Calif.) with a .016-inch titanium molybdenum archwire (TMA). The diastemas were closed with ligature wires (Fig. 17-5, *F* and *G*). Vertical elastics with lingual brackets were used to improve occlusion (Fig. 17-5, *H*). After 15 months of treatment, the upper and lower diastemas were closed, and the papillae totally recovered (Fig. 17-5, *I-K*). A lower and upper fixed retainer was recommended for avoiding any form of relapse.[31,32]

TREATMENT OF PATIENTS WITH SIGNIFICANT PERIODONTAL PROBLEMS

Loss of Maxillary Incisor

Figure 17-6 shows a 39-year-old female patient whose upper-left lateral incisor was lost because of periodontal problems a few months earlier. She came to the author's office for a second opinion, referred by the Department of Periodontology at Maimonides University. Her chief complaint was replacement of the upper-left lateral incisor. Her medical history was unremarkable.[9,33-38] The pretreatment clinical photographs clearly showed her periodontal problems, especially in and around the incisor region (Fig. 17-6, *A-E*). Significant pathological migration of the anterior teeth was present. Periapical radiographs of the upper and lower incisors confirmed the loss of periodontal attachment (Fig. 17-6, *F* and *G*).

The patient's lower incisors were splinted with composite to diminish their mobility. The following questions arose before the final treatment plan could be determined:

- Is there any specific bracket prescription that can be used to treat this patient?

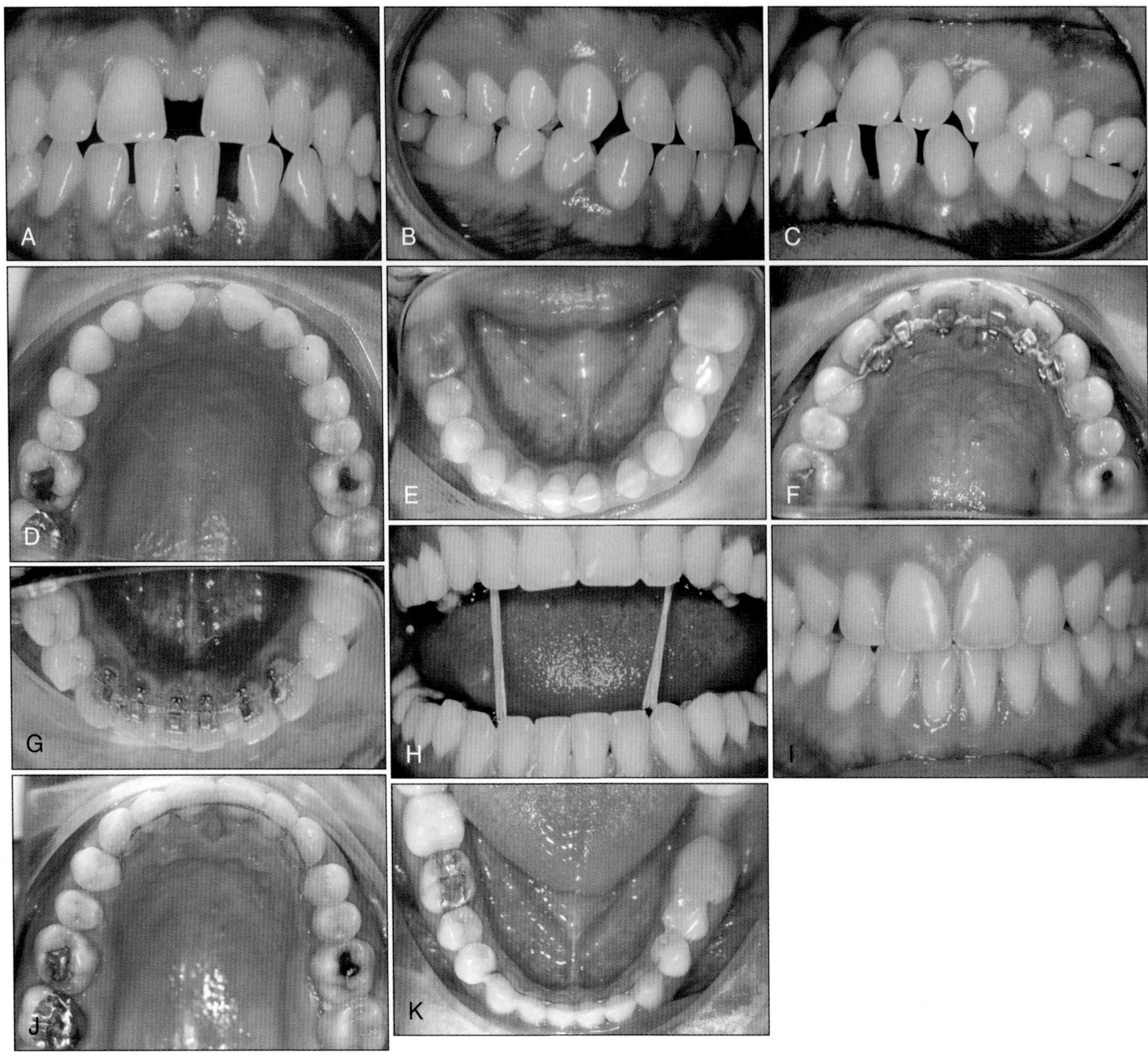

Fig. 17-5 **A,** Multiple diastemas in 32-year-old patient; no papillae present. **B** and **C,** Lower incisors more labially inclined than upper incisors; Class I right and left molars present. **D** and **E,** Photographs of upper and lower arches confirmed the diastemas. **F** and **G,** All the diastemas were closed using lingual brackets and TMA .016-inch wire. **H,** Vertical elastics were used to improve overjet and overbite. **I,** Results at completion of treatment. All the diastemas are closed, and the midline is normalized. Overjet and overbite are almost normal. **J** and **K,** Upper and lower fixed retention wires were recommended for 5 to 7 years.

- Should the upper-left lateral incisor's space be maintained for a future implant, or should it be closed?
- What would be the best decision regarding the upper-right lateral incisor and the lower incisors?

After analyzing the case with the periodontologist, the following treatment plan was determined:

1. Periodontal treatment
2. Three-month periodontal evaluation
3. Alignment and leveling of the arches
4. Closure of the space of the upper-left lateral incisor
5. Extraction of the central lower-right incisor
6. Periodontal monitoring every 4 to 8 weeks during treatment
7. Establishment of normal overbite and overjet
8. Application of fixed upper and lower retainer wires

Preprogrammed brackets were used (Fig. 17-6, *H-L*). After 7 months of treatment the space of the upper-left lateral incisor was closed. The central lower-right incisor space was closed with stainless steel ligature wire and

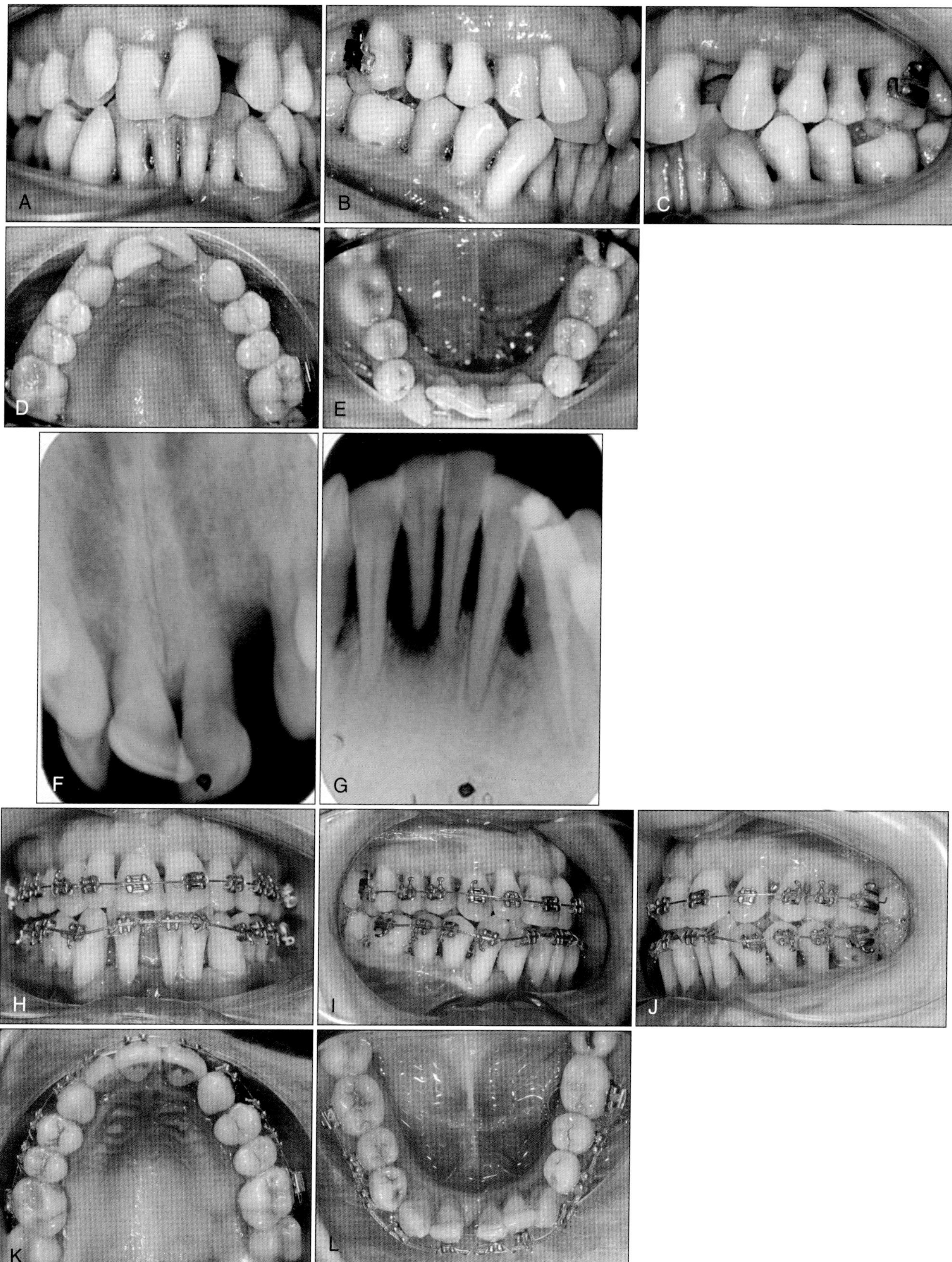

Fig. 17-6 **A,** Frontal view of 39-year-old woman with severe periodontal problems. Upper and lower anterior teeth were in worse condition than posterior teeth. **B** and **C,** Lateral photographic views confirmed absence of lateral incisors. Right lateral incisor was totally displaced labially. **D** and **E,** Photographs of upper and lowers arches confirmed presence of severe crowding. **F,** Upper, and **G,** lower, radiographs clearly show significant loss of the periodontal attachment. Right lower incisor was completely lost. **H,** Preprogrammed .022-inch metal brackets were used. Central lower-right incisor was extracted. Turbo-wire (.017 × .025 inch) was recommended to align and level the arches. **I** and **J,** With a periodontal patient, it is preferable to use tubes instead of bands at the first molars. The space of the upper-left lateral incisor was closed. **K** and **L,** Upper and lower arches at this stage of treatment.

Continued

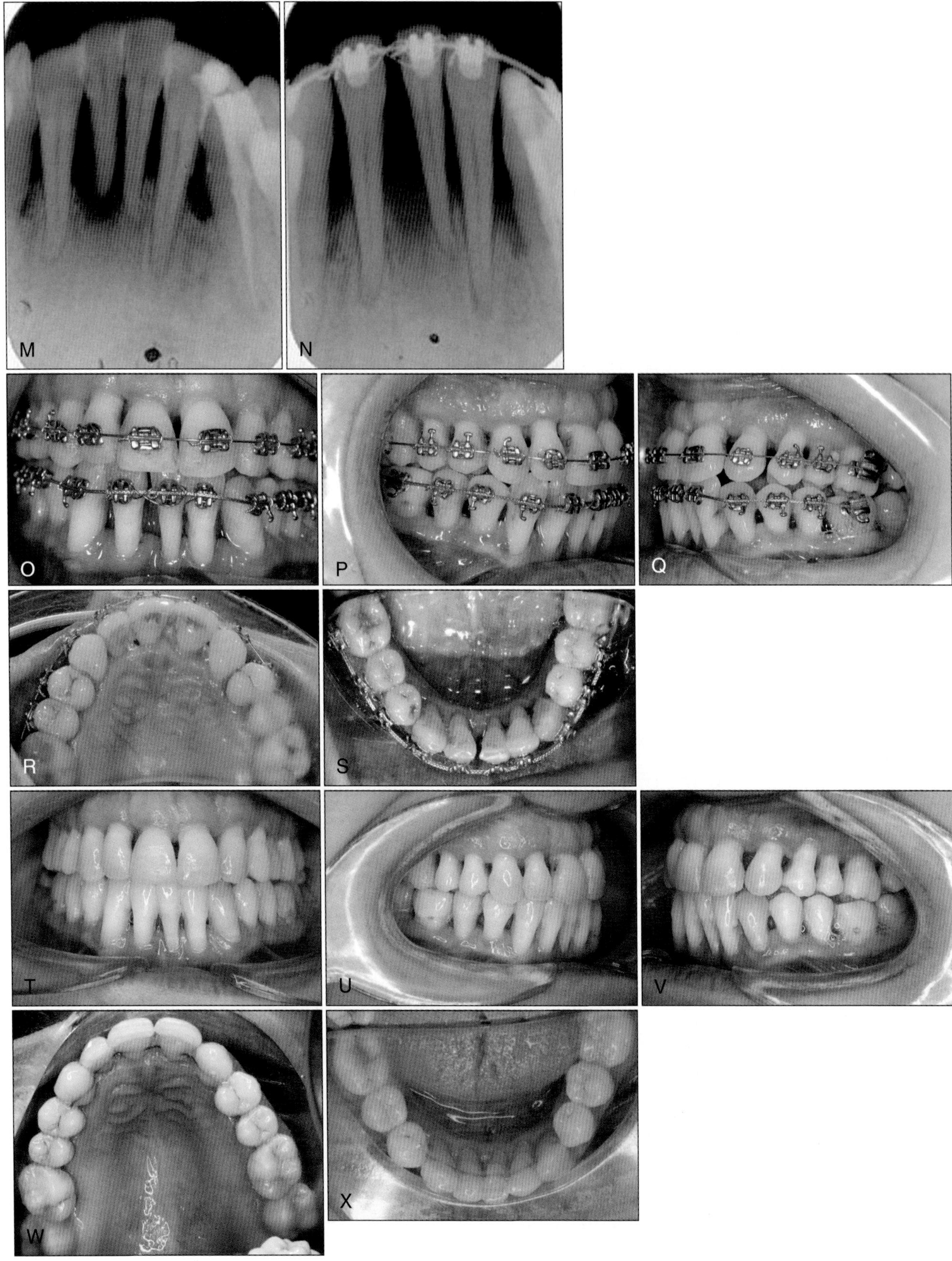

Fig. 17-6, cont'd **M,** Pretreatment, and **N,** 1-year posttreatment, radiographs show that the lower incisor could be moved with very low periodontal attachment. **O,** Treatment at 6 months shows that almost all the spaces were closed. Because of patient's severe periodontal problems, TMA wire was recommended in upper arch and Turbo-wire in lower arch. **P** and **Q,** Normalization of occlusal plane and gingival line is achieved. **R** and **S,** Upper and lower arches at this stage of treatment. **T,** Final results. All the spaces of the missing incisors are closed. **U** and **V,** Lateral photographic views at completion of treatment. **W** and **X,** Upper and lower arches showing final treatment results.

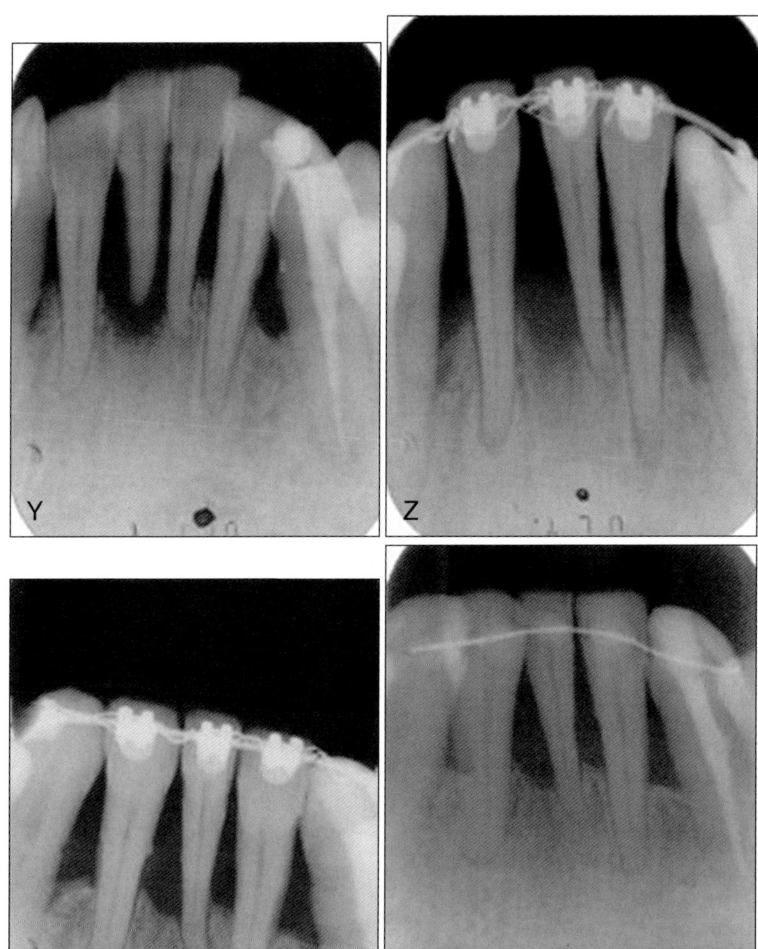

Fig. 17-6, cont'd **Y,** Pretreatment; **Z** and **AA,** treatment; and **BB,** posttreatment; radiographic views.

activated every 6 to 8 weeks to control the parallelism of the roots.[35,36,39-42]

Figure 17-6, *M* and *N,* compare the lower incisors before treatment and after 12 months of treatment. No progression of the periodontal problem occurred during the orthodontic movement. The space is almost closed, and the overjet and overbite had improved (Fig. 17-6, *O-S*).

At the end of treatment the anticipated results were achieved (Fig. 17-6, *T-X*). The upper-right lateral incisor occupied its correct place, the space of the upper-left lateral incisor was closed, the crowding of the lower incisors was corrected, and the gingivoperiodontal tissues clearly had improved. The comparison of the periapical radiographs before (Fig. 17-6, *Y*), during (*Z* and *AA*), and after *(BB)* treatment confirmed the hypothesis that it is possible to move teeth with reduced periodontal attachment when the periodontal disease is under control. The improvement with the osseous repair is evident.[43-50]

Loss of Mandibular Incisor

Figure 17-7, *A,* shows a 59-year-old patient examined after the spontaneous loss of the mandibular left central incisor. Changes were seen in the gingivoperiodontal tissues of the surrounding area. Some mobility of the lower incisors was also present.

After oral hygiene instructions and scaling and root planing at the lower anterior area, the orthodontic treatment began. Esthetic edgewise brackets were used to treat the patient. The space was closed using a round, stainless steel wire with steel ligature that was activated every 6 weeks (Fig. 17-7, *B*). It is important to avoid elastomeric rings for better plaque control in such patients.

At the end of the treatment the space of the mandibular central lower incisor was completely closed (Fig. 17-7, *C*). The gingivoperiodontal tissues were healthy. Periodontal maintenance at regular intervals (6-8 weeks) was carried out during the first 2 years and then every 3 months.[51,52] Figure 17-7, *D,* shows the control 9 years after treatment. The gingivoperiodontal tissues appear much better than expected.[38,53-57] It is interesting to note the extensive bone destruction at the beginning of treatment (Fig. 17-7, *E*) versus the osseous repair at the end of treatment *(F)* and 9 years after treatment *(G)*. Significant improvement in oral hygiene during and after the orthodontic treatment played an important role.

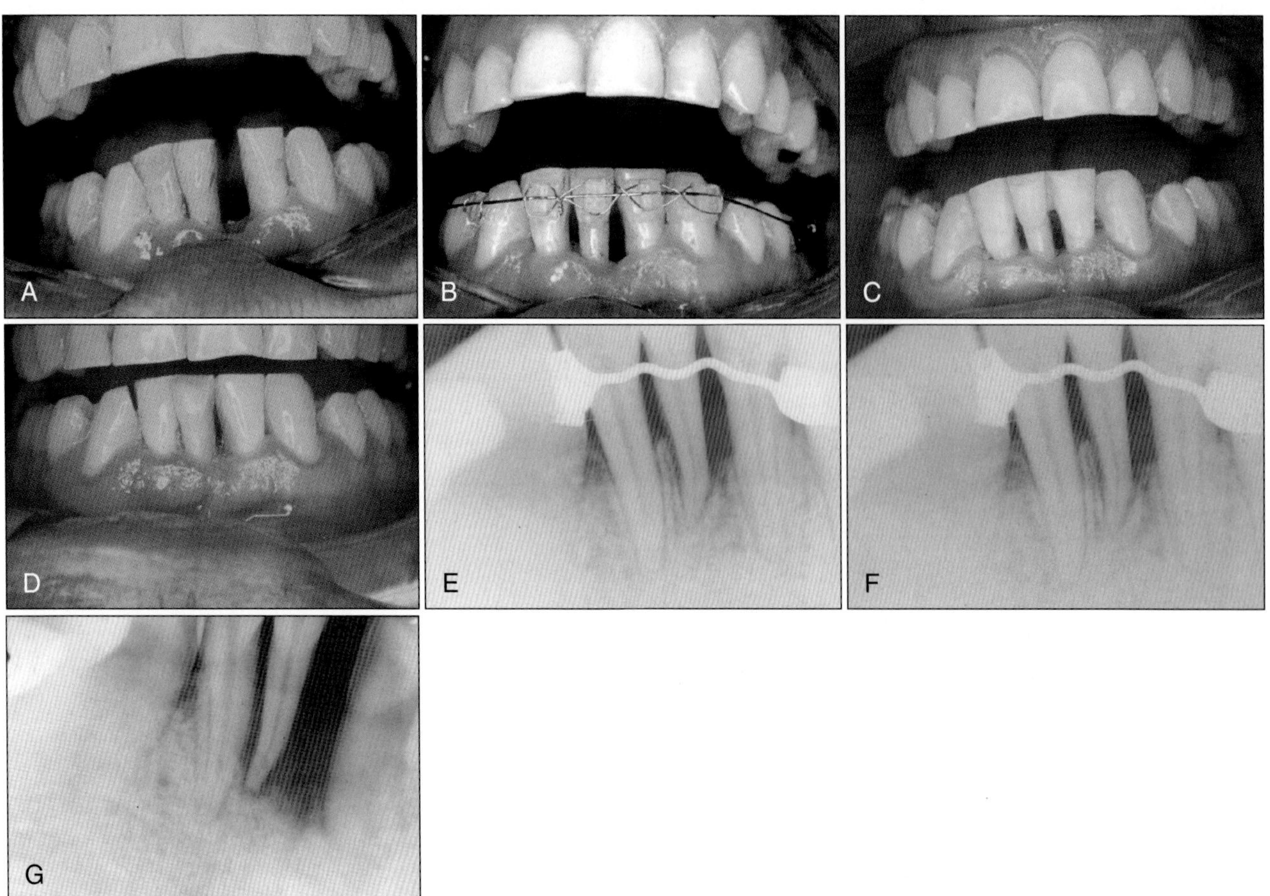

Fig. 17-7 Spontaneous loss of mandibular left central incisor in 59-year-old patient. **A,** Pretreatment photograph. **B,** Esthetic .018-inch brackets were used with .014-inch stainless steel arch. **C,** Posttreatment, and **D,** 9-year posttreatment, photographic views. **E,** Pretreatment; **F,** posttreatment; and **G,** 9-year posttreatment; radiographic views.

A clear understanding of the biological process is necessary to achieve a positive result. Active pockets must be eliminated before the orthodontic movement is initiated, to prevent further bone destruction during the treatment.[58-62] Figure 17-7 is a good example of the important role of orthodontics in the treatment of such challenging patients. The bone recovery has been maintained after 9 years of treatment. The key in achieving such significant osseous repair is the combination of continuous periodontal control, very low forces, and long-term retention. It is important to remember that orthodontic patients with moderate or advanced periodontal disease require an individualized treatment and retention plan.[26,28,63,64]

Crowding, Mobility, and Periodontal Breakdown

Figure 17-8, *A,* shows an 83-year-old woman who was referred for treatment by her daughter (a colleague of the author) after the daughter attended an odontogeriatric lecture. Remarkably, no teeth were missing despite the patient's advanced age. She had significant crowding in the upper and lower arches, and periodontal breakdown was present at the posterior regions of both the arches[57,65-69] (Fig. 17-8, *B-D*). This caused significant problems for the patient and was the reason for the consultation. Previously, another dentist had tried to fix the central lower incisors with wire to reduce their mobility (Fig. 17-8, *E*), but they were totally lost.

The following questions arose when determining the treatment plan for this patient:

- Is it possible to move the lower lateral incisors to close the space in an 83-year-old patient with such significant osseous defects?
- If the answer is "yes," what would be the best biomechanical procedure?

After discussing the patient's case with her family dentist and the periodontologist, the following individualized treatment plan was devised, taking into account her age and the severe periodontal problem[23,24,34,70]:

1. Periodontal treatment
2. Extraction of the central lower incisors
3. Closure of the space
4. Periodontal monitoring every month during treatment
5. Application of fixed retention

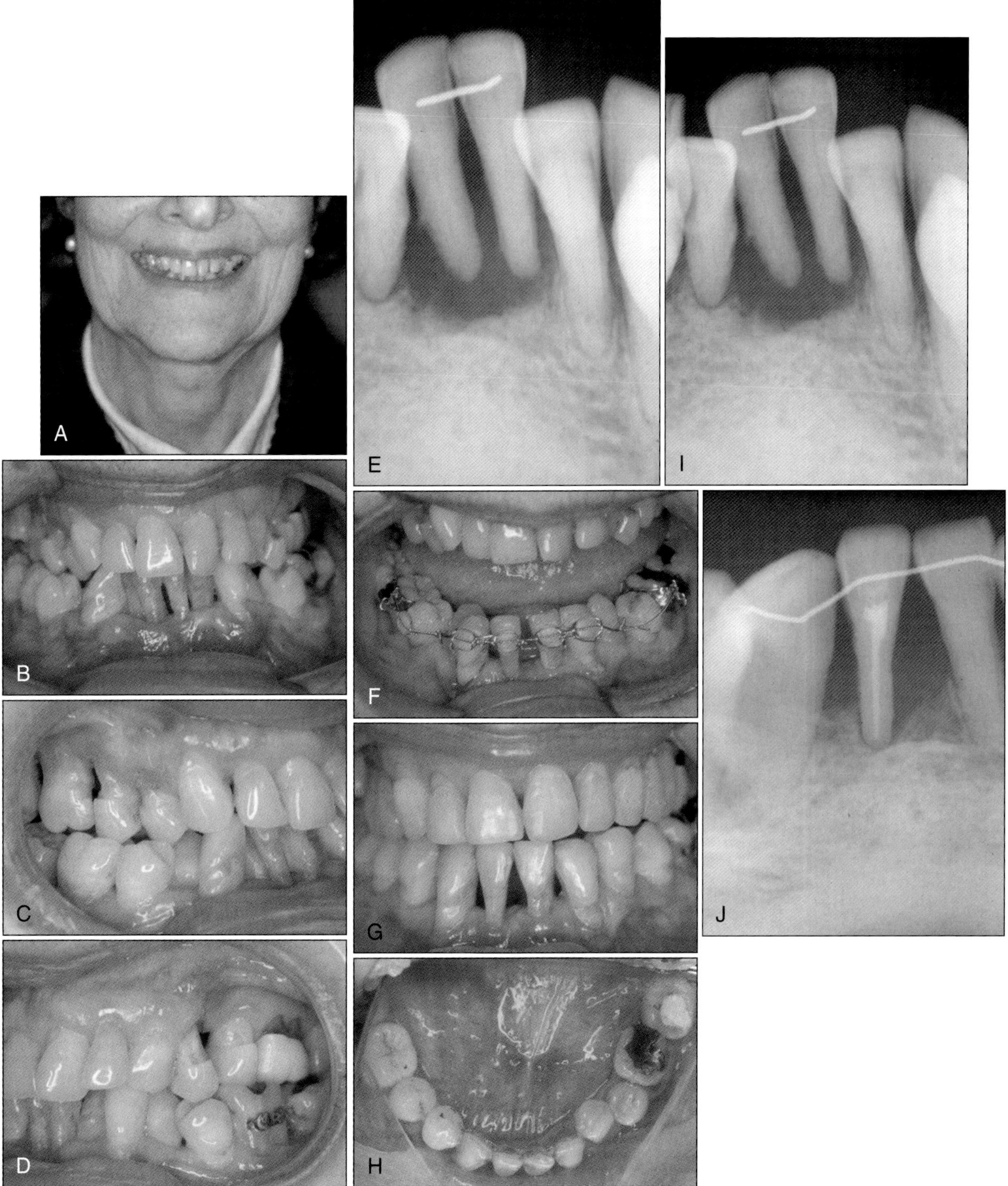

Fig. 17-8 **A** and **B,** Pretreatment facial and intraoral photographs of 83-year-old woman showing significant crowding. **C** and **D,** Lateral photographic views showing severe periodontal problems. **E,** Lower central incisors completely lost. **F,** Esthetic .022-inch brackets were placed. The spaces were closed with ligature wire. **G** and **H,** Final results. Long-term fixed retention was recommended. **I,** Pretreatment, and **J,** posttreatment, radiographs. An important osseous repair is achieved.

After periodontal treatment, brackets were placed in the lower arch to close the space and unravel the crowding (Fig. 17-8, *F*). The initial archwire was a .014-inch stainless steel wire used for leveling and aligning the lower teeth. The space was closed with a ligature wire activated every 6 to 8 weeks. It is recommended that a controlled force be used according to the amount of periodontal attachment present. Some gingivitis was present at this time, so the patient was seen by the periodontist every 2 weeks.

Figure 17-8, *G* and *H,* show the results at the end of 18 months of treatment. The gingivoperiodontal tissues were normalized, making it easier for the patient to maintain good oral hygiene.[22,71-73] The treatment objectives were achieved, and the periodontal condition remained under control. A permanent fixed retention was recommended at the end of treatment.

An endodontic treatment had been performed months earlier for the lower-right lateral incisor, and the results were significantly better than expected. An important osseous repair was present (Fig. 17-8, *I* and *J*), as demonstrated earlier.[74-76]

These results confirmed the experimental studies, which have shown that with adequate periodontal treatment and exhaustive periodontal maintenance therapy, teeth with reduced but healthy periodontal attachment may not experience further loss of bone support during orthodontic movement. Unfortunately, no one prescription exists for all patients. The best method for tooth movement must be determined for each patient according to the amount of periodontal attachment present.[68,77,78]

CONCLUSION

Orthodontic treatment in adult patients with reduced but healthy periodontium should be performed by an interdisciplinary team whose combined efforts may transform patients with unattractive dentition into persons with an esthetically pleasing smile. No cephalometric norms work for all patients, and no specific guidelines fit all patients.[10,31,32,77,79-81]

The periodontal condition must be a primary consideration before initiating orthodontic treatment and must be constantly monitored during the treatment and retention periods. Patients with unhealthy periodontal tissues may experience further breakdown and tooth loss during orthodontic treatment. Careful treatment protocol and regular periodontal monitoring are essential for obtaining good results. In some patients, osseous repair can also be obtained, thereby improving the overall prognosis of the dentition in the long term.

Orthodontic treatment in patients with large periodontal destruction is a challenge for dentists. However, when all the biological bases of tooth movement and their limitations are taken into account, excellent esthetic and functional results can be achieved. Without specific and individualized treatment goals, treatment success cannot be measured or achieved. Specific goals are the only way orthodontic and periorestorative treatment can be planned with the end result in mind. A long or rather permanent retention period is always advisable and strongly recommended.[10,80-86]

REFERENCES

1. Axelsson P, Lindhe J, Nystom B: On the prevention of caries and periodontal disease: results of a 15-year longitudinal study in adults, *J Clin Periodontol* 4:278-293, 1977.
2. Axelsoon P, Lindhe J: Effect of controlled oral hygiene procedures on caries and periodontal disease in adults: results after 6 years, *J Clin Periodontol* 5:133-151, 1978.
3. Bolin A, Eklund G, Frithiof L, Lavstedt S: The effect of changed smoking habits on marginal alveolar bone loss: a longitudinal study, *Swed Dent J* 17:211-216, 1993.
4. Boyd RL: Mucogingival considerations and their relationship to orthodontics, *J Periodontol* 49:67-76, 1978.
5. Brown S: The effect of orthodontic therapy on certain types of periodontal defects, *J Periodontol* 44:742, 1973.
6. Artun J, Urbye KS: The effect of the orthodontic treatment on periodontal bone support in patients with advanced loss of marginal periodontium, *Am J Orthod Dentofacial Orthop* 93:143-148, 1988.
7. Atherthon JD: The gingival response to orthodontic tooth movement, *Am J Orthod* 58:179-186, 1979.
8. Axelsoon P, Lindhe J: The significance of maintenance care in the treatment of periodontal disease, *J Clin Periodontol* 8:281-294, 1981.
9. Bakdash B: Oral hygiene and compliance as risk factors in periodontitis, *J Periodontol* 65:539-544, 1994.
10. Zachrisson BU: The bonded lingual retainer, *J Clin Orthod* 17:838-884, 1983.
11. Grossi SG, Skrepinsky FB, DeCaro T, et al: Response to periodontal therapy in diabetics and smokers, *J Periodontol* 67:1094-1102, 1996.
12. Musich DR, Crossetti H: Assessment and description of the treatment need of adult patients for orthodontic therapy. III. Characteristics of the multiple provider group, *Int J Adult Orthod Orthog Surg* 1:251-274, 1986.
13. Darveau RP, Tanner A, Page RC: The microbial challenge in periodontitis, *Periodont 2000* 14:12-32, 1997.
14. Dennison DK, Gottsegen R, Rose LF: Diabetes and periodontal diseases, *J Periodontol* 67:166-176, 1996.
15. Emrich LJ, Schlossman M, Genco RJ: Periodontal disease in non-insulin-dependent diabetes mellitus, *J Periodontol* 62:123-131, 1991.
16. Genco R, Zambon J, Christersson L: The origin of periodontal infections, *Adv Dent Res* 2:245-259, 1988.
17. Grossi S, Genco R, Machtei E, et al: Assessment of risk of periodontal disease: risk indicators for attachment loss, *J Periodontol* 65:23-29, 1994.
18. Jenkins WM, Kinane DF: The "high risk" group in periodontitis, *Br Dent J* 167:168-171, 1989.
19. Oliver RC, Tervonen T: Periodontitis and tooth loss: comparing diabetes with general population, *J Am Dent Assoc* 124:71-76, 1993.
20. Yao CC, Wu CB, Wu HY, et al: Intrusion of the overerupted upper left first and second molars by mini-implants with partial-fixed orthodontic appliances: a case report, *Angle Orthod* 74:550-557, 2004.

21. Page R: Frontiers in periodontics, *Pac Coast Soc Orthod Bull* 63:39-41, 1991.
22. Tarnow DP, Magner AW, Fletcher P: The effect of the distance from the contact point to the crest of the bone on the presence or absence of the interproximal dental papillae, *J Periodontol* 63:119-125, 1992.
23. Brown LJ, Loe H: Prevalence, extent, severity and progression of periodontal disease, *Periodont 2000* 2:57-71, 1993.
24. Caffese RG, Sweeney PL, Smith BA: Scaling and root planing with and without periodontal flap surgery, *J Clin Periodontol* 13:205-210, 1986.
25. Chasens A: Periodontal disease, pathologic tooth migration and adult orthodontics, *N Y J Dent* 49:40-43, 1979.
26. Kokich VG: Enhancing restorative, esthetic and periodontal results with orthodontic therapy. In Schlunger S, Youdelis R, Page R, Johnson R, editors: *Periodontal therapy,* Philadelphia, 1990, Lea & Febiger, pp 433-460.
27. Kokich VG: Anterior dental esthetics: an orthodontic perspective, *J Esthet Dent* 5:174-178, 1993.
28. Kokich VG: The role of orthodontics as an adjunct to periodontal therapy. In Newman MG, Carranza FA, Takei H, editors: *Carranza's clinical periodontology,* ed 9, Philadelphia, 2002, Saunders, pp 423-452.
29. Geiger AM: Mucogingival problems and the movement of the mandibular incisors: a clinical review, *Am J Orthod* 78:511-527, 1980.
30. Kessler M: Interrelatioships between orthodontics and periodontics, *Am J Orthod* 70:154-172, 1976.
31. Zachrisson BU, Alnaes L: Periodontal condition in orthodontically treated and untreated individuals. II. Alveolar bone loss: radiographic findings, *Angle Orthod* 43:402-411, 1974.
32. Zachrisson BU: Periodontal changes during orthodontic treatment. In McNamara JA Jr, Ribbens KA, editors: *Orthodontic treatment and the periodontium,* Monograph 15, Craniofacial Growth Series, Center for Human Growth and Development, Ann Arbor, 1984, University of Michigan, pp 43-62,
33. Beck J: Methods of assessing risk for periodontitis and developing multifactorial models, *J Periodontol* 65:468-478, 1994.
34. Boyd RL, Leggott PJ, Quinn RS, et al: Periodontal implications of orthodontic treatment in adults with reduced or normal periodontal tissues versus those in adolescents, *Am J Orthod Dentofacial Orthop* 96:191-199, 1989.
35. Eliasson LA, Hugoson A, Kurol J, et al: The effects of orthodontic treatment on periodontal tissues in patients with reduced periodontal support, *Eur J Orthod* 4:1-9, 1982.
36. Gazit E, Lieberman M: Occlusal and orthodontic considerations in the periodontally involved dentition, *Angle Orthod* 50:346-349, 1980.
37. Kokich VG, Spear F: Guidelines for managing the orthodontic-restorative patient, *Semin Orthod* 3:3-20, 1997.
38. Kokich VG: Esthetics: the orthodontic-periodontic-restorative connection, *Semin Orthod* 2:21-30, 1996.
39. Ericsson I, Thilander B, Lindhe J, et al: The effect of orthodontic tilting movements on the periodontal tissue on infected and non-infected dentitions in the dog, *J Clin Periodontol* 4:115-127, 1977.
40. Ericsson I, Thilander B, Lindhe J: Periodontal condition after orthodontic tooth movement in the dog, *Angle Orthod* 48:210-218, 1978.
41. Ericsson J, Lindhe J: Effect of longstanding jiggling on experimental marginal periodontitis in the beagle dog, *J Clin Periodontol* 9:497-503, 1982.
42. Lindhe J, Ericsson J: The influence of trauma from occlusion on reduced but healthy periodontal tissues in dogs, *J Clin Periodontol* 3:110-122, 1976.
43. Sjolien T, Zachrisson BU: Periodontal bone support and tooth length in orthodontically treated and untreated persons, *Am J Orthod* 64:28-37, 1973.
44. Socransky SS, Haffajee AD, Goodson JM, et al: New concepts of destructive periodontal disease, *J Clin Periodontol* 11:21-32, 1984.
45. Socransky SS, Hafjee AD: The bacterial etiology of destructive periodontal diagnosis, *J Clin Periodontol* 13:175-181, 1986.
46. Thilander B, Nyman S, Karring T, Magnusson I: Bone regeneration in alveolar bone dehiscences related to orthodontic tooth movements, *Eur J Orthod* 5:105-114, 1983.
47. Wagenberg BD, Eskow J: Orthodontics: a solution for the advanced periodontal or restorative problem: the interim tooth movement into infrabony defects, *J Periodontol* 55:197-202, 1984.
48. Wennstrom J, Lindskog-Stokand B, Nyman S, et al: Periodontal tissue response to orthodontic movement of teeth with infrabony pockets, *Am J Orthod Dentofacial Orthop* 103:313-319, 1993.
49. Wehrbein H, Furhamann RAW, Diedrich PR: Periodontal conditions after facial root tipping and palatal root torque of incisors, *Am J Orthod Dentofacial Orthop* 106:455-462, 1994.
50. Wilson TG Jr: Supportive periodontal treatment introduction: definition, extent of need, therapeutic objectives, frequency and efficacy, *Periodontol 2000* 12:11-15, 1996.
51. Polson AM, Meitner SW, Zander HA: Trauma and progression of marginal periodontitis in squirrel monkeys. III. Adaptation of interproximal alveolar bone to repetitive injury, *J Periodontol Res* 11:279-289, 1976.
52. Polson A, Caton J, Polson AP, et al: Periodontal response after tooth movement into infrabony defects, *J Periodontol* 55:197-202, 1984.
53. Kurth J, Kokich VG: Open gingival embrasures after orthodontic treatment in adults: prevalence and etiology, *Am J Orthod Dentofacial Orthop* 120:116-123, 2001.
54. Lindhe J, Haffajee AD, Socransky SS: Progression of periodontal disease in adult subjects in the absence of periodontal therapy, *J Clin Periodontol* 10:433-442, 1983.
55. Lindhe J, Nyman S: Long term maintenance of patients treated for advanced periodontal disease, *J Clin Periodontol* 11:504-505, 1984.
56. Lindhe J, Nyman S: Scaling and granulation tissue removal in periodontal therapy, *J Clin Periodontol* 12:374-388, 1985.
57. Loe H, Theilade E, Jensen S: Experimental gingivitis in man, *J Periodontol* 36:177-187, 1965.
58. Machtei E, Dunford R, Haussman E, et al: Longitudinal study of prognostic factors in established periodontitis patients, *J Clin Periodontol* 24:102-109, 1997.
59. Marks M, Corn H: Periodontics and orthodontics: coordinating the disciplines for optimal treatment planning, *Alpha Omega* 76, Fall 1983.
60. Martinez-Canut P, Lorca A, Magan R: Smoking and periodontal disease severity, *J Clin Periodontol* 22:743-749, 1996.
61. Melsen B: Limitations in adult orthodontics. In Melsen B, editor: *Current controversies in orthodontics,* Chicago, 1991, Quintessence, pp 147-180.
62. Melsen B, Agerbark N, Markenstam G: Intrusion of incisors in adult patients with marginal bone loss, *Am J Orthod Dentofacial Orthop* 96:232-241, 1989.

63. Karring T, Nyman S, Thilander B, Magnusson B: Bone regeneration in orthodontically alveolar bone dehiscences, *J Periodont Res* 17:309-315, 1982.
64. Krampf J: Multidisciplinary treatment: ortho-perio-restorative dentistry, *Dent Clin North Am,* July 1972.
65. Lang NP, Loe H: The relationship between the width of the attached gingiva and gingival health, *J Periodontol* 43:623, 1972.
66. Levitt H: Orthodontic treatment for the adult periodontal patient, *J Can Dent Assoc* 57:787-789, 1991.
67. Lindhe J, Okamoto H, Yoneyama T, et al: Periodontal loser sites in untreated adult subjects, *J Clin Periodontol* 16:671-678, 1989.
68. Musich DR: Assessment and description of the treatment need of adult patients for orthodontic therapy. II. Characteristics of the dual provider group, *Int J Adult Orthod Orthog Surg* 1:101-117, 1986.
69. Park YC, Lee SY, Kim DH, et al: Intrusion of posterior teeth using mini screw implants, *Am J Orthod Dentofacial Orthop* 123:690-694, 2003.
70. Goldman MJ, Ross IF, Goteiner D: Effect of periodontal therapy on patients maintained for 15 years or longer, *J Periodontol* 57:347-353, 1986.
71. Salama M, Salama H: An interdisciplinary approach to the management of the adult mutilated dentition: a case report, *Compend Contin Educ Dent* 13:328-338, 1992.
72. Sadowsky C, BeGole EA: Long tem effects on orthodontic treatment on periodontal health, *Am J Orthod* 80:156-172, 1981.
73. Sherman PR, Hutchens LH Jr, Jewson LG: The effectiveness of subgingival scaling and root planing. II. Clinical responses related to residual calculus, *J Periodontol* 61:9-15, 1990.
74. Musich DR: Assessment and description of the treatment need of adult patients for orthodontic therapy. I. Characteristics of the solo provider group, *Int J Adult Orthod Orthog Surg* 1:55-67, 1986.
75. Newman GU, Wagenberg BD: Treatment of compromised teeth: a multidisciplinary approach, *Am J Orthod* 76:530-537, 1979.
76. Pihlstrom BL, Anderson KA, Aeppli D, et al: Association between signs of trauma from occlusion and periodontitis, *J Periodontol* 57:1-6, 1986.
77. Harfin J: *Tratamiento ortodóntico en el adulto,* ed 2, Buenos Aires, 2005, Editorial Médica Panamericana.
78. Moore PA, Weyant RJ, Mongelluzzo MB, et al: Type I diabetes mellitus and oral health: assessment of periodontal disease, *J Periodontol* 70:409-417, 1999.
79. Harfin J: *Tratamiento ortodóntico en el adulto,* Buenos Aires, 1999, Editorial Médica Panamericana.
80. Wilson TG Jr: Compliance and its role in periodontal therapy, *Periodontol 2000* 12:16-23, 1996.
81. Zachrisson BU: A histological study of experimental gingivitis in man, *J Periodont Res* 3:293-298, 1968.
82. Tonetti MS: Cigarette smoking and periodontal diseases: etiology and management of disease, *Ann Periodontol* 3:88-101, 1998.
83. Vanarsdall RL: Complications of orthodontic treatment, *Curr Opin Dent* 1:622-633, 1991.
84. Vanarsdall RL: Correction of periodontal problems through orthodontic treatment. In Hosl E, Zachisson BU, Baldauf A: *Orthodontics and periodontics,* Chicago, 1985, Quintessence, pp 127-167.
85. Zachrisson BU: Adult retention: a new approach. In Graber LW, editor: *Orthodontics: state of art, essence of the science,* St Louis, 1986, Mosby, pp 310-327.
86. Zachrisson BU: Clinical implications of recent ortho-perio research findings, *Semin Orthod* 2:4-12, 1996.

CHAPTER 18

Diastemas: Is Permanent Retention Really Necessary?

Thomas F. Mulligan

Instability following orthodontic tooth movement has been a recurring problem for the practicing orthodontist and the profession. Many dental professionals who see such patients later assume incompetence on the part of the treating orthodontist.

Treatment of diastemas is common after space closure[1-3] (Fig. 18-1). Many orthodontists view permanent retention as the only realistic approach to maintaining closure (Fig. 18-2). Removable appliances used for retention create back-and-forth movement as a result of being worn "on and off" (Fig. 18-3). Although many orthodontists resort to frenectomies and circumferential fibrotomies,[4] the outcome in these cases is often frustrating because undesirable side-effects still occur.[5] Thus, even with surgical procedures,[6] some form of retention is frequently required.

ARCHWIRE REMOVAL AND CLINICIAN CONCERNS

This chapter addresses an approach used by the author for many years in which all archwires are removed during treatment as a mandatory phase of orthodontic tooth movement.[7] This approach has a better than 90% success rate. Such wires are removed for at least 6 weeks, but often longer as situations demand (e.g., summer vacation). This does not mean, however, that archwires must be removed for every type of instability,[8] such as crossbites, open bites, overbites, and rotations. These different areas may be checked for stability versus instability at the same time. Common sense prevails in this regard; treatment time should not be extended because of archwire removal.

The typical orthodontist resists removing archwires during orthodontic treatment because of possibly losing some of the movement achieved. It is for this very reason, however, that archwires are removed. Teeth "rebound" for several reasons,[5] but in any case will attempt to put themselves into equilibrium with muscles and function. Cephalometrics may encourage the placement of teeth in certain anteroposterior as well as transverse positions. However, the numbers and angles involved do not apply to each patient treated, but rather to a collection of such patients.

Averages can be misleading when individualizing tooth movement for the patient. If a clothing store carried only trousers with the average size for men, theoretically there might not be a single pair of trousers that fits any of them. Although unlikely, this illustrates that the best "fit" for the patient is one that has been "tailor-made" for the individual in question. This means recognizing that tooth position is determined by muscles, function, and habits, along with duration and related factors.

But how can all this be achieved? There must be a better way than the traditional approach, associated with such a high degree of failure in the absence of permanent retention.

All orthodontists are aware of cause-and-effect relationships. However, not all orthodontists necessarily ask, "Why?" when observing undesirable outcomes, and instead frequently resort to some type of appliance, laboratory or otherwise, to resolve the problem. In other words, treatment often involves treating the "effect" rather than the cause.

"GEDANKEN" EXPERIMENT

In attempting to solve the problem of stabilizing diastema closure without permanent retention, the author decided to use the same approach that Einstein used so successfully when arriving at a number of still-valid scientific facts. Einstein was often criticized for creating experiments in his mind without actually performing them; he became famous for his *Gedanken* ("thought") experiments.[9] This frustrated his fellow scientists, who believed that validating results required actual experiments.

In using a "gedanken experiment" to try and resolve the diastema problem, the author first needed to ask the following question: "Do we know of any other situations in orthodontic tooth movement that result in the creation of space following space closure?" One answer would be the space opening orthodontists frequently witness after space closure in a four first-bicuspid extraction case for adults (Fig. 18-4). As a "thought" experiment only, one can visually ask, if the space readily reopened after paralleling of the roots, what might happen if the crowns were severely tipped toward each other, instead of paralleling the roots? Obviously, this would create serious periodontal problems and would not be considered a solution, but only a mental experiment. However, one could still conclude (without actually doing it) that the greater the tipping, the greater the probability of increased stability following space closure. The logical question would then be, "Why?"

As can be seen in Fig. 18-5, the occlusal forces acting on the cuspid and bicuspid would take place through a greater perpendicular distance from the centers of resistance in these teeth, thus creating so-called functional moments. Also, if the central incisors were observed with the same angular displacement as shown with the cuspid and bicuspid, the incisal forces would produce the same increased "functional moments," for the same reason. Although with the central incisors the angular displacement would require primarily root displacement, it is the increased separation of the centers of resistance that results in these functional moments.

Although diverging the roots to this extent would never be considered, in this gedanken experiment one can reasonably conclude that stability lies somewhere between these two extremes. This mental experiment provides the knowledge that "somewhere" there is stability when the centers of resistance have been sufficiently displaced during such exaggerated tooth inclination. It now remains to be discovered whether such change in inclination remains within acceptable limits for the patient.

In the case of a diastema, the central incisor crowns can only move together until contact is made, at which time the remaining movement consists of only distal movement of the central incisor roots. Any time a moment is applied to teeth—whenever crown movement is prevented in one direction—root movement occurs in the opposite direction. This is demonstrated many times as this experiment progresses.

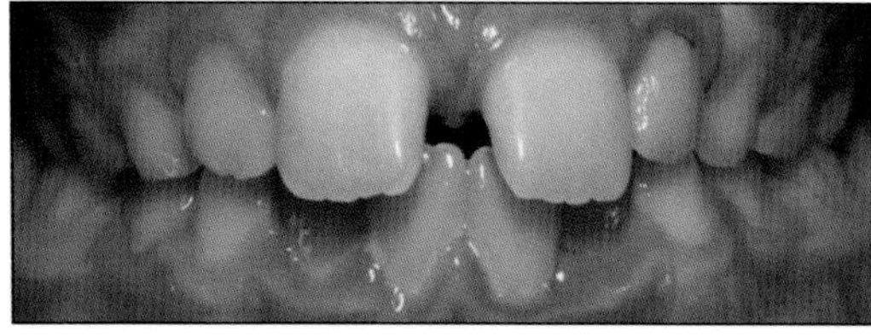

Fig. 18-1 Intraoral view of a diastema.

STABILITY CONSIDERATIONS

How long will it take for the required movements to occur in order to reach stability? The answer lies with the individual patient and can only be determined by archwire removal.

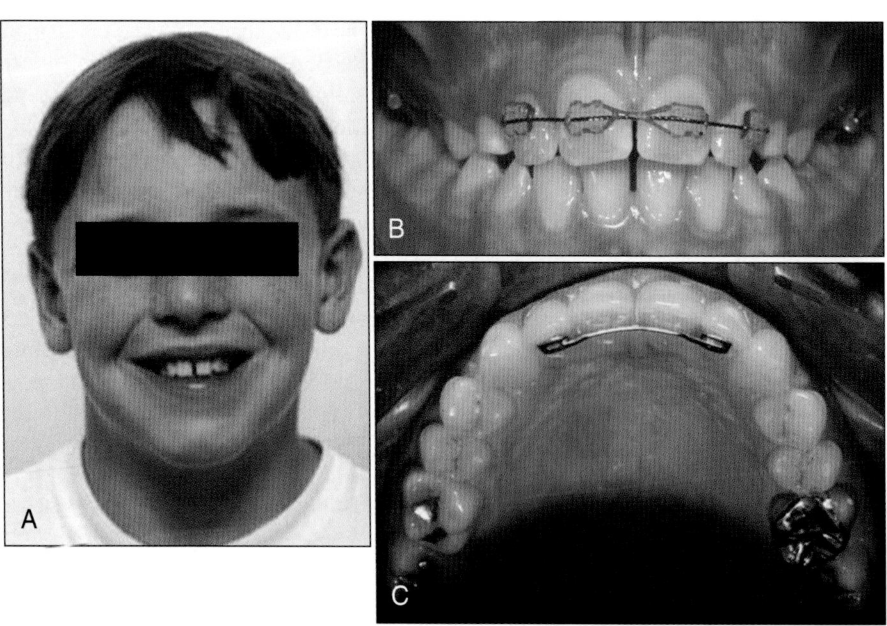

Fig. 18-2 Use of permanent retention to treat a diastema. **A,** Pretreatment facial photograph. **B** and **C,** Permanent retainer in place.

The following factors are involved in the time for stability in each patient after diastema closure:

1. The parallel relationship between the incisor crowns and roots
2. The amount of crown divergency and apical convergency

Although a factor, patient age is not crucial to this discussion.

After space closure, if the patient is presented with converging apices (Fig. 18-6, *A*), more movement will be

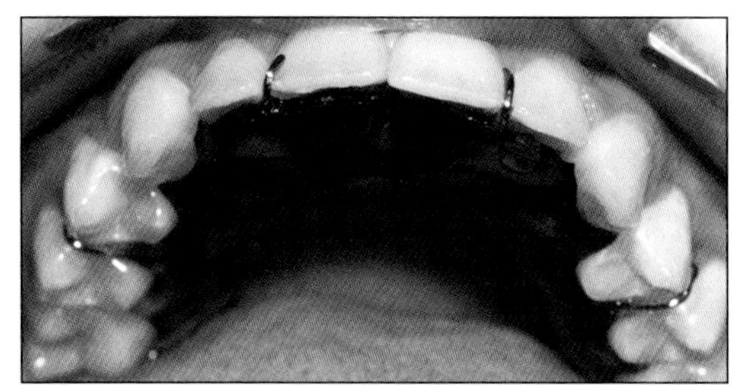

Fig. 18-3 Removable retainer.

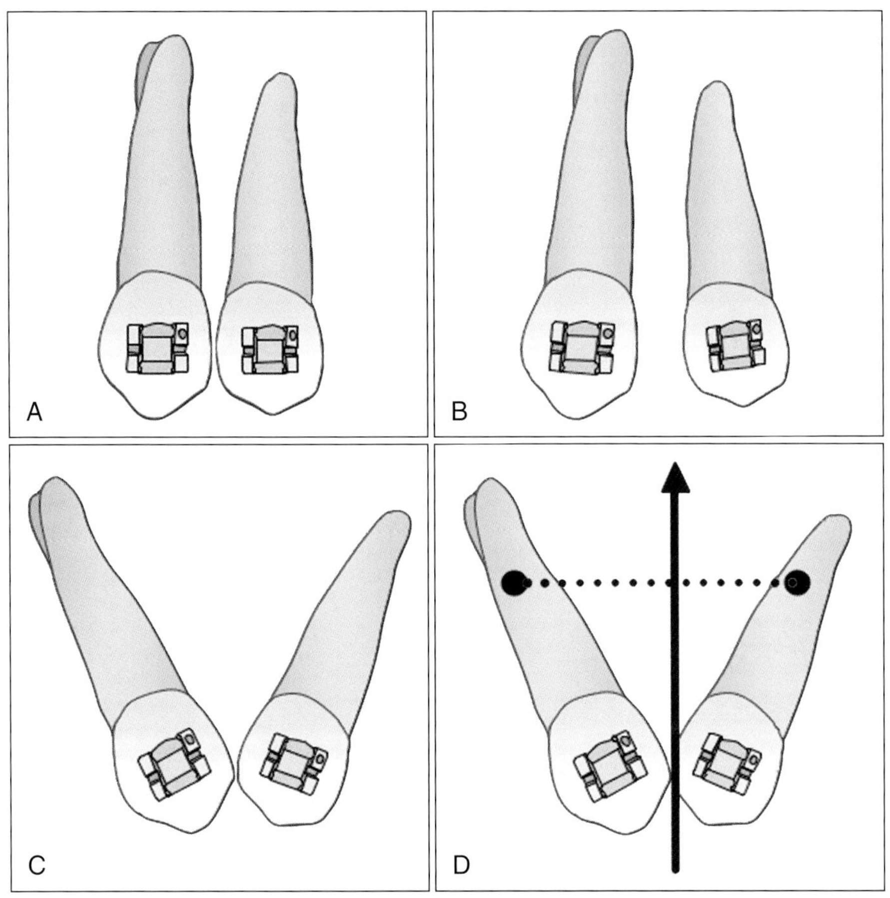

Fig. 18-4 Use of a "gedanken" (thought) experiment to resolve diastema problem. Space opening seen after space closure. **A,** Roots are parallel. **B,** Space has reopened after paralleling of roots. **C,** Crowns are severely tipped toward each other, which can cause periodontal problems. **D,** Greater tipping results in greater probability of increased stability following space closure.

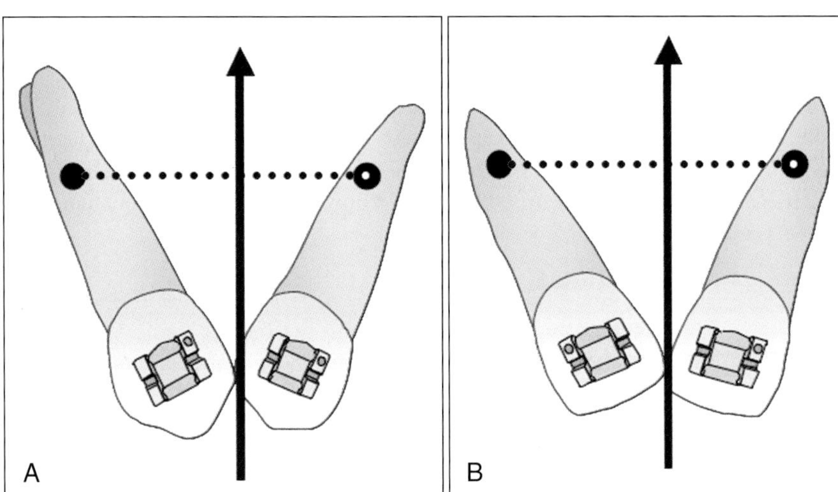

Fig. 18-5 Comparison of occlusal forces acting on **A,** cuspid, and **B,** bicuspid.

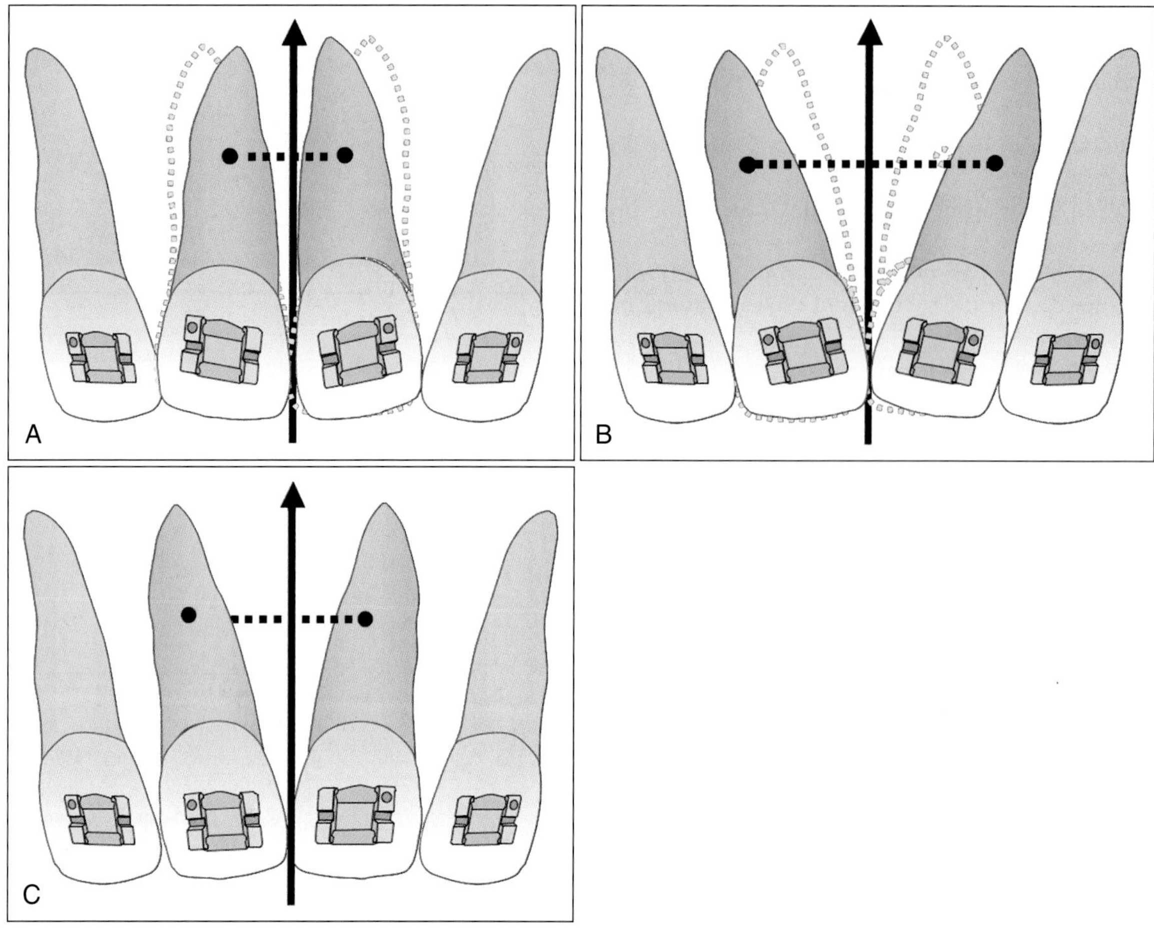

Fig. 18-6 **A,** Converging apices. **B,** Diverging apices. **C,** Normal relationship of roots following space closure.

required and therefore additional time. In Figure 18-6, *B*, the diverging apices will result in less time for movement because the roots already have a "head start." Figure 18-6, *C*, shows the more typical relationship of the roots to each other after space closure.

When checking these movements for stability, do not discard the wire used; it may again be inserted into the brackets for additional movement if there is evidence of space opening. If final stability is achieved, angulated brackets will now be present as a result of the change in tooth inclination. Only then should the wire be removed and the incisal edges, now canted, be reshaped with a diamond disk (Fig. 18-7). The brackets may be removed and rebonded with proper alignment for continued treatment, if necessary.

ROOT DIVERGENCY

In Figure 18-8, if crown widths are normal and proportionate to other teeth in the anterior segment, the divergence of roots will result in some overjet. After closure of the diastema, the overjet produced can be used effectively to solve other potential problems, such as the following:

- Diastemas
- Small lateral incisors
- The "dark triangle"
- Generalized spacing resulting from small lateral incisors
- Anterior "end-on" relationships
- Slight Class III anterior teeth

Treatment may involve the use of continuous arches, anterior segments with a center bend, or a bypass segment consisting of two off-center bends (Fig. 18-9). The latter two are frequently used in combination.

Clinical Examples

Figures 18-10 and 18-11 feature two sisters who were treated simultaneously. Although both would appear to have identical problems, one required removal of the archwire several times, whereas her sister required removal only once. Clearly, there is no predictable number of times for archwire removal to achieve stability. Experience will show, however, that the

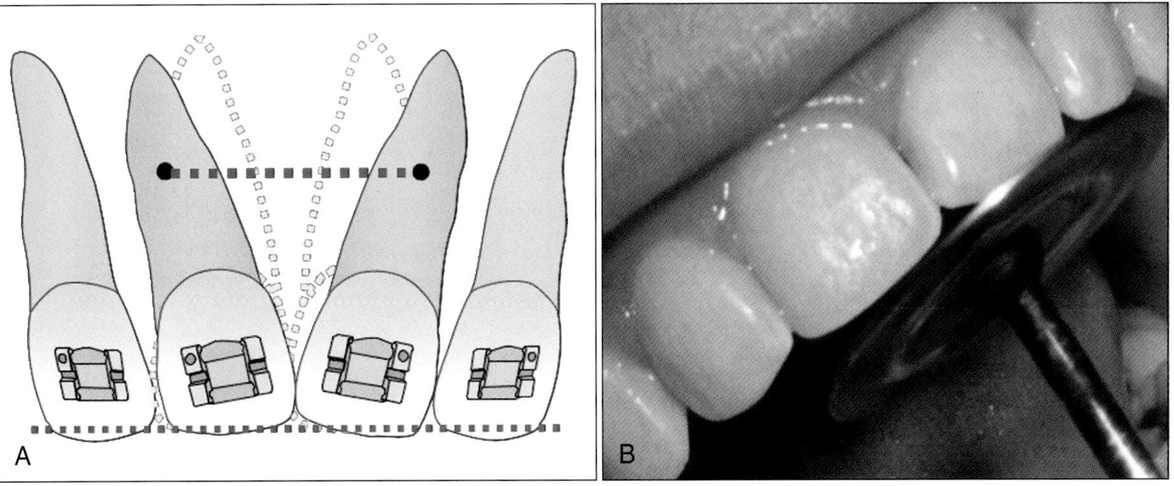

Fig. 18-7 **A,** When final stability is achieved, angulated brackets are present because of the change in tooth inclination. Only then should the wire be removed. **B,** The now-canted incisal edges are reshaped with a diamond disk.

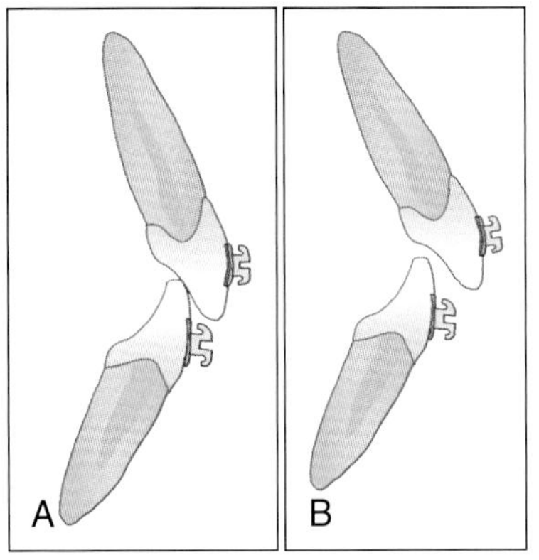

Fig. 18-8 **A,** Result of diverging incisor roots, showing **B,** increase in overjet that can result.

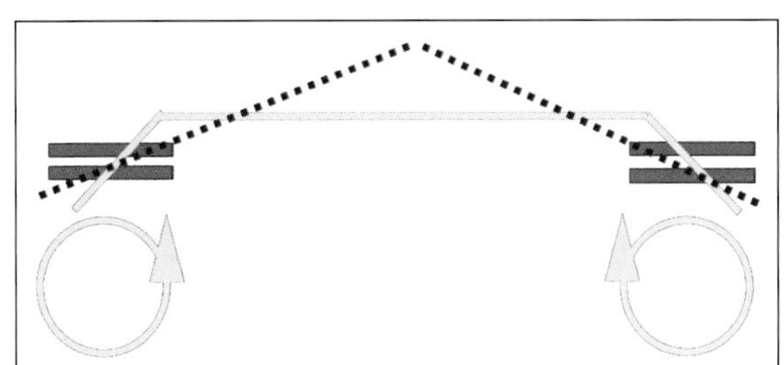

Fig. 18-9 In this arch the two off-center bends are the same as a center bend.

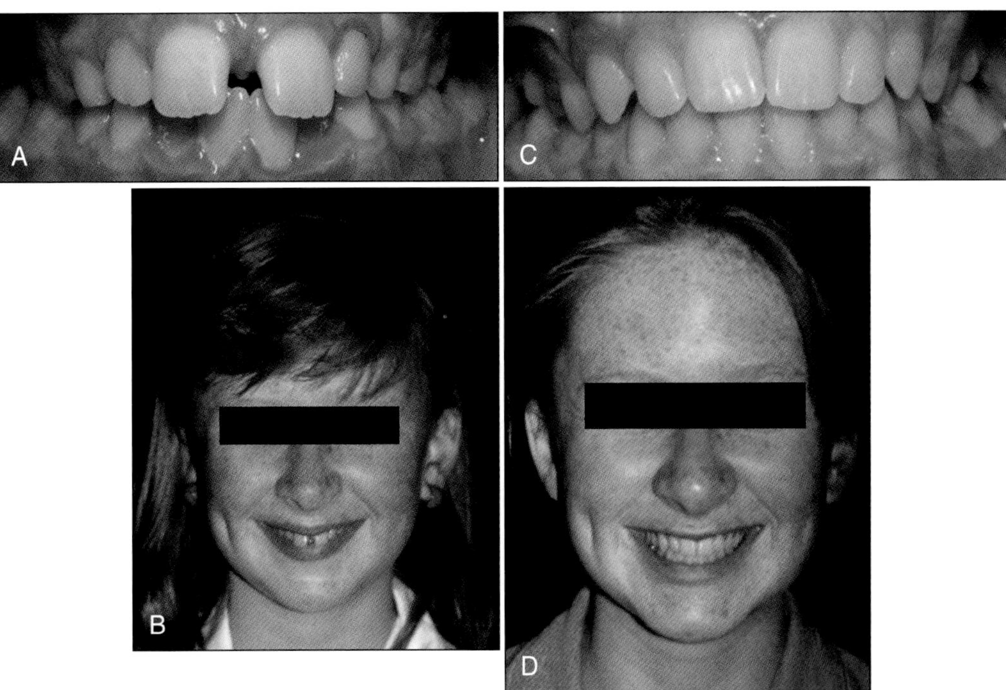

Fig. 18-10 **A** and **B**, Pretreatment intraoral and facial photographs. **C** and **D**, Intraoral and facial photographs 4 years after treatment. No retention was utilized. Patient's archwire was removed four times.

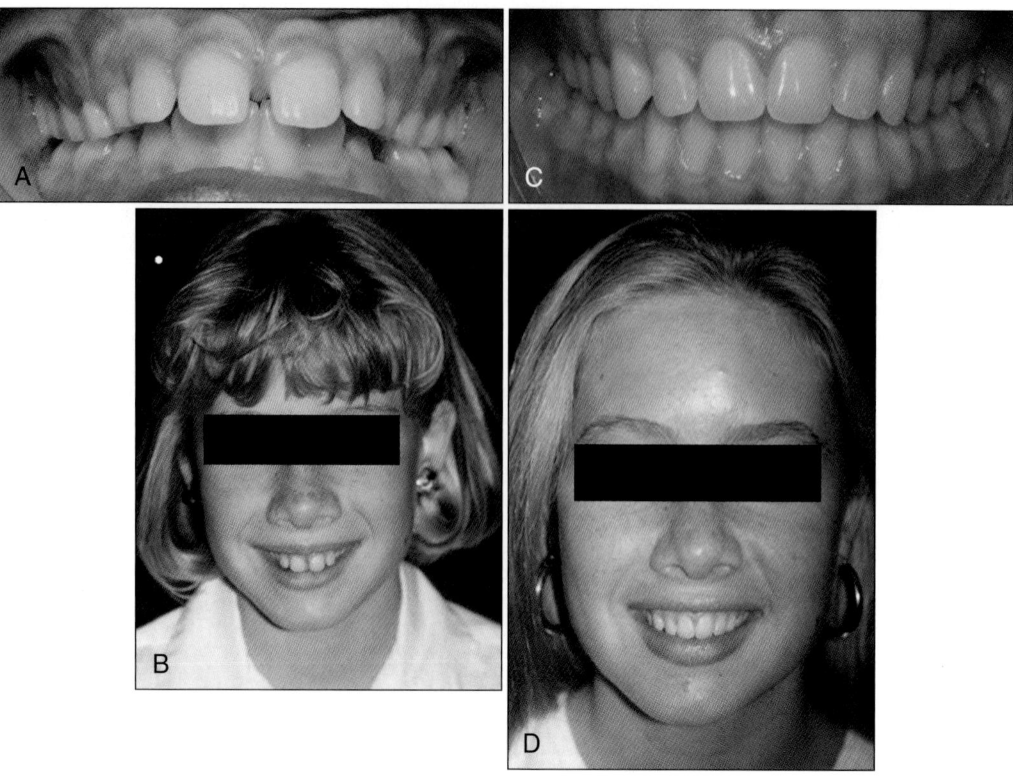

Fig. 18-11 Sister of patient in Fig. 18-10. **A** and **B,** Pretreatment intraoral and facial photographs. **C** and **D,** Intraoral and facial photographs 4 years after treatment. No retention was utilized. Patient's archwire was removed only once.

range usually is one to three times and varies with each patient. The first sister (see Fig. 18-10) was treated with only four incisor brackets and a wire segment,[7] which was removed four times (early in learning process). No retention was used, and the patient is shown 4 years later. Her sister (see Fig. 18-11) was treated in exactly the same manner and is shown 4 years later with no form of retention.

The patient in Figure 18-12 demonstrates an obvious convergency of the roots. Because of the delayed cuspid eruption, this was an excellent opportunity to observe stability without depending on interproximal contact with fully erupted cuspids for support. A continuous wire was used because treatment involved more than closure of the diastema. Figure 18-12, *D* to *F,* shows that there is no opening of the anterior space during the several months the cuspids erupted into position.

Figure 18-13 shows a patient whose roots are parallel following the original convergency (*A* and *B*). Movement continues following the parallel relationship *(C)*. At some point the orthodontist must remove the archwire when roots are divergent; experience will dictate a reasonable time. The appliance has been removed, with complete stability present *(D)*.

Figure 18-14 features a patient in whom convergency and rotation are present with the diastema *(A)*. The rotated incisor has been overcorrected and the incisor roots diverged (*B* and *C*). Two years after treatment, complete stability is present *(D)*.

Roots are diverged for several reasons. The patient in Figure 18-15 had contacts running the full length of the crown after space closure. A slight divergency permits the contact point to be moved slightly toward the incisal edges, improving the esthetics for the patient.

GENERALIZED SPACING

Within limits, the space resulting from narrow lateral incisors can be eliminated and esthetic restoratives avoided by diverging the lateral roots in addition to those involving the central incisors. Examination of the mesiodistal widths involved in an anterior segment of teeth (Fig. 18-16, *A*) shows the increased requirements that arise when such roots are diverged (Fig. 18-16, *B*). This requires special mechanics because a continuous wire will not produce the four equal moments required for these teeth.[7] When sufficient divergency is obtained and spaces are closed, the brackets will be canted as a result of this movement (Fig. 18-16, *C*). The incisal edges can now be reshaped (Fig. 18-16, *D*), and the brackets then rebonded and properly positioned for additional treatment, if needed.

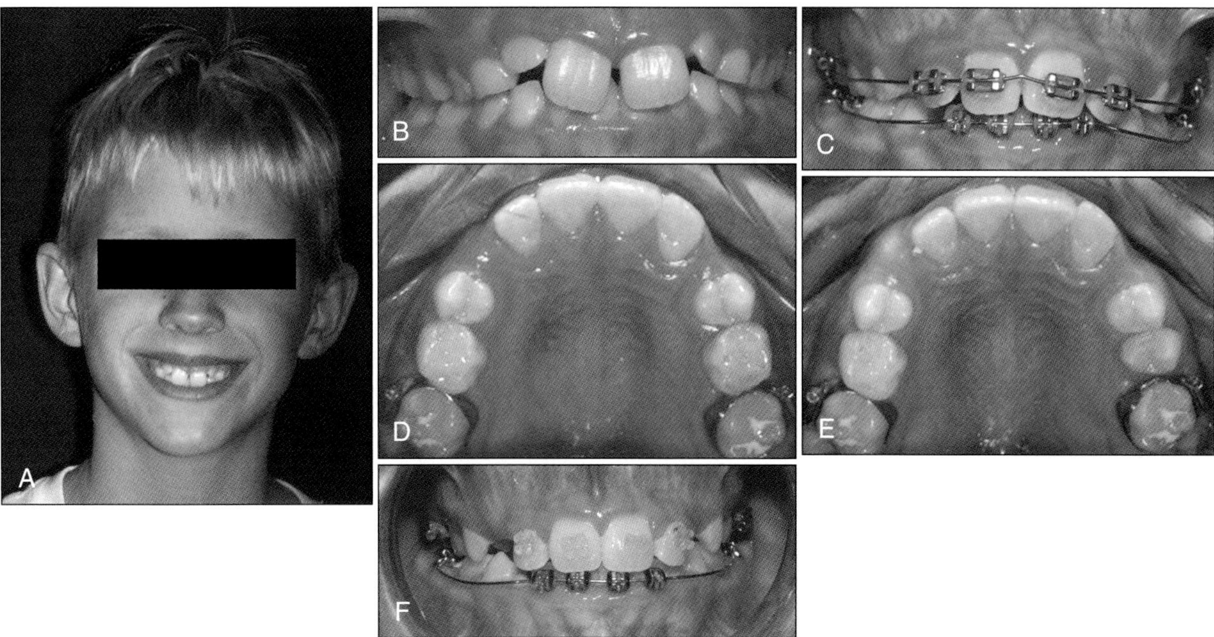

Fig. 18-12 Patient with obvious convergency of the roots. Smaller diastemas may require greater time when the roots are convergent because more movement is required for stability. **A** and **B,** Facial and intraoral photographs before treatment. **C,** Center band was placed after the roots were parallel. **D** to **F,** No opening of the anterior space was present during the time the cuspids erupted into position.

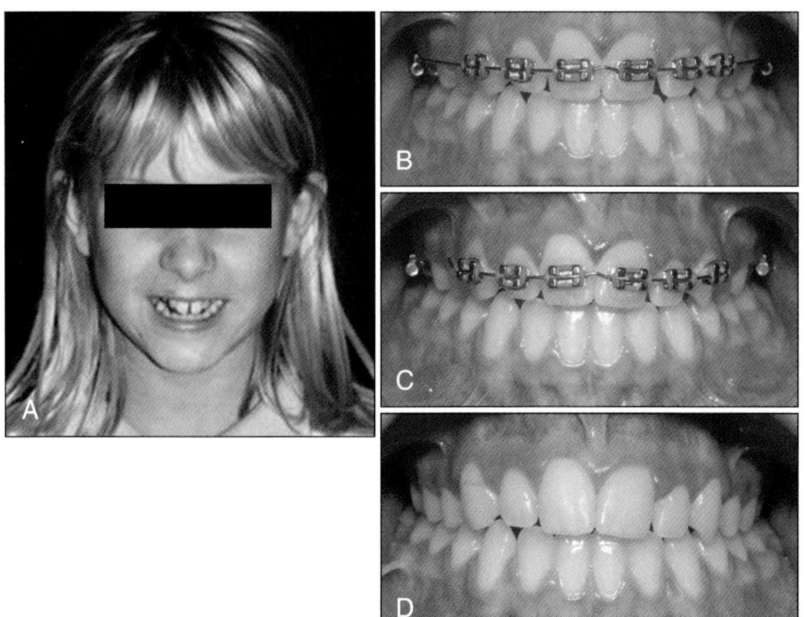

Fig. 18-13 Patient in whom the roots were parallel after original convergency. **A,** Pretreatment facial photograph. **B,** Center band was placed after the roots became parallel. **C,** When it became apparent the roots were divergent, the archwire was removed and the closure checked for stability. **D,** The root divergency proved to be sufficient for stability. This determination could be made only with removal of the archwire.

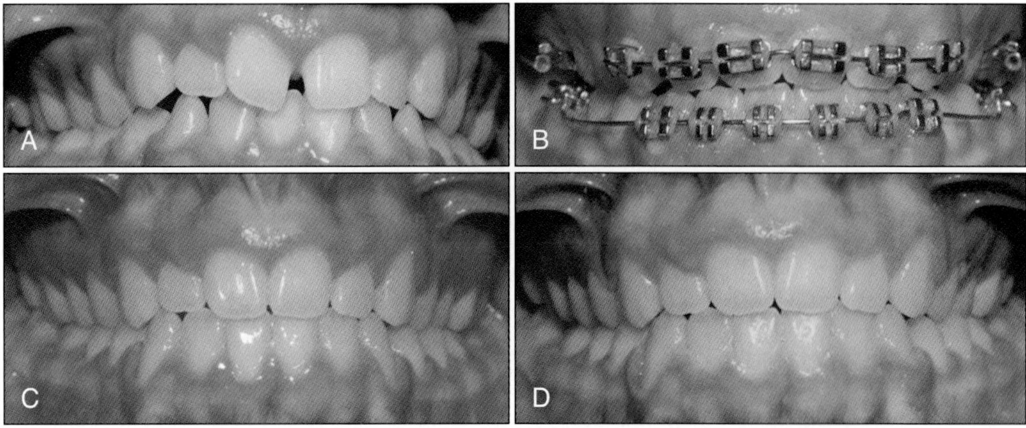

Fig. 18-14 Patient in whom convergency and rotation were present with a diastema. **A,** Pretreatment intraoral photograph. **B,** Overrotation and root divergency should be checked at archwire removal. **C,** Intraoral photo after appliance removal. **D,** Intraoral photo 2 years after treatment.

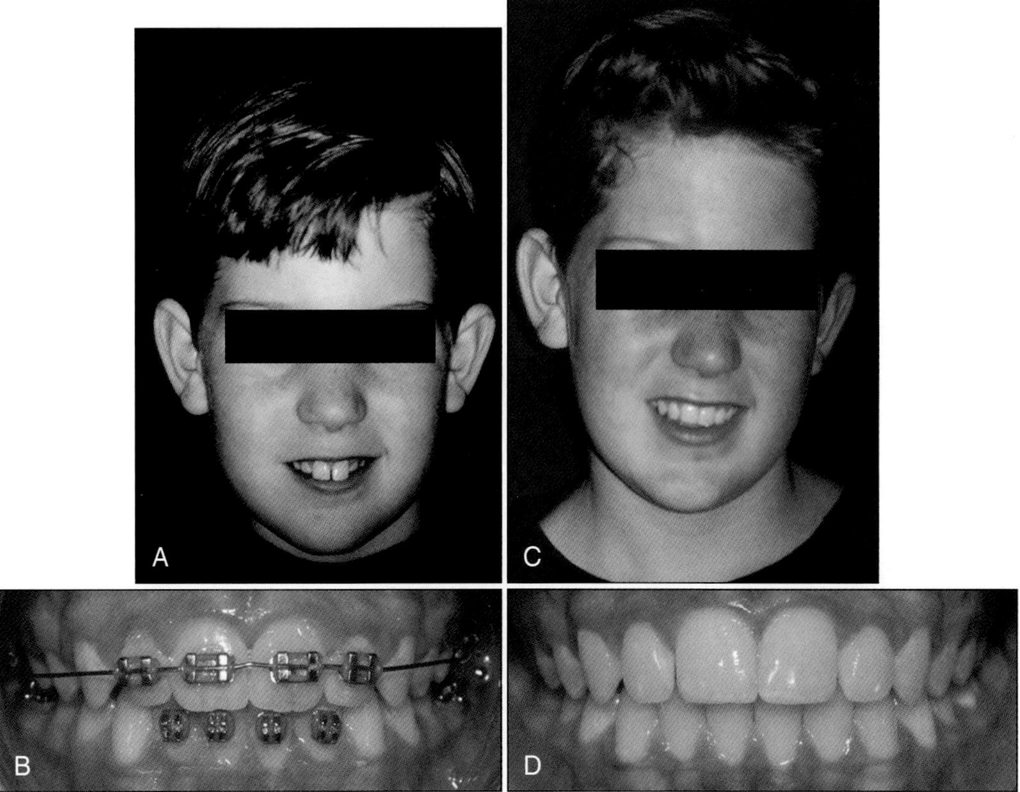

Fig. 18-15 Patient with contacts running full length of the crown after space closure. **A,** Pretreatment facial photograph. **B,** Slight divergency permits the contact point to be moved slightly toward the incisal edges. **C** and **D,** Esthetics are improved.

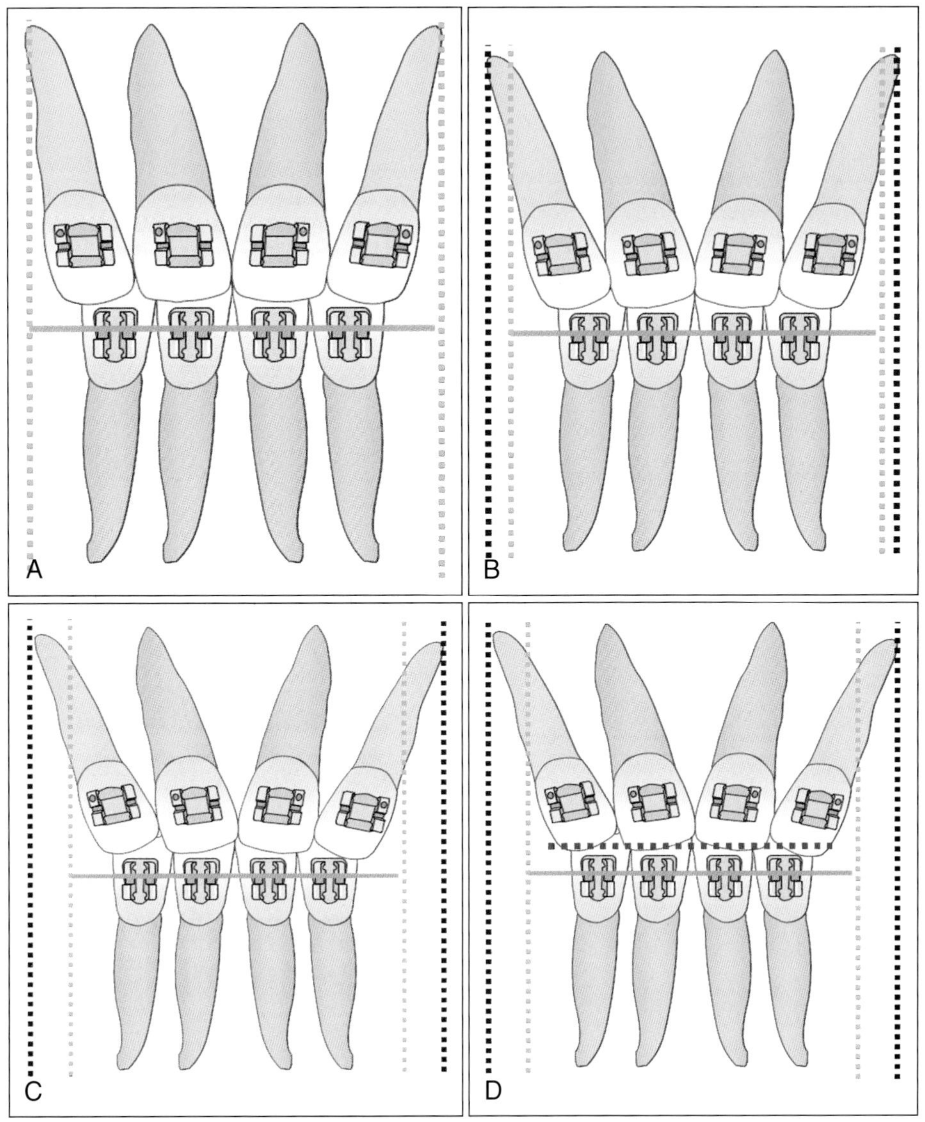

Fig. 18-16 Conservative approach to solving the problem of generalized spacing (e.g., narrow incisors). **A,** Root divergency can help in patients with generalized spacing. **B,** Mesiodistal width is increased. **C,** Increasing the mesiodistal width results in canted incisal edges. **D,** Incisal edges can now be contoured.

MODIFIED MECHANICS

Because a continuous arch engaged into all brackets cannot produce pure moments on the four incisor brackets, two individual segments can be used instead. One segment is referred to as a *center bend* and produces equal and opposite moments. The other segment involves two *off-center bends* and performs exactly the same function as the center bend. This permits the divergence of roots on all incisors at the same time (Fig. 18-17).

As in the previous cases, after archwire removal and verification of stability, the incisal edges may be contoured and the brackets repositioned for any continuation of treatment (Fig. 18-18).

Figure 18-19 shows a patient 8 years after elimination of a diastema. No retention was ever used. He was part of an original experimental group treated before cuspid eruption. All such patients were chosen with parental permission. Some had missing lateral incisors; none had erupted cuspids. Early treatment was done with the knowledge that stability produced at such an age would be further enhanced with the eruption of additional teeth. Radiographs were carefully studied to ensure no danger to the roots of developing incisors. This caution is not necessary for usual orthodontic work, however, because such patients would not be treated in this manner while root development was incomplete.

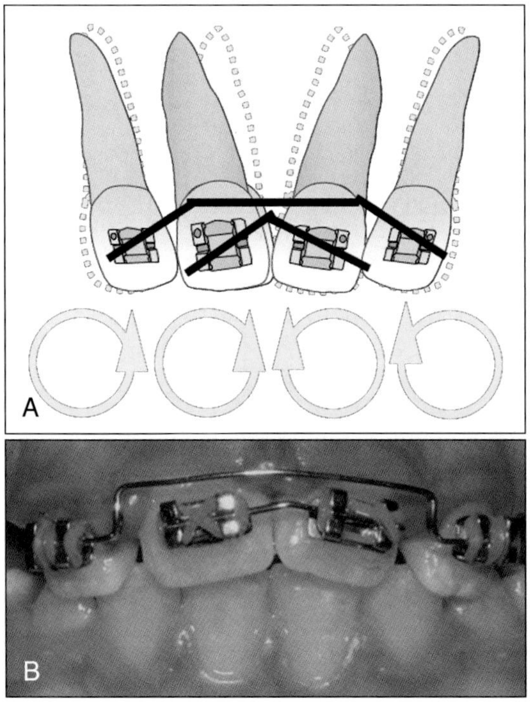

Fig. 18-17 Center bend with a round wire and bypass segment with .019 × .025–inch rectangular wire.

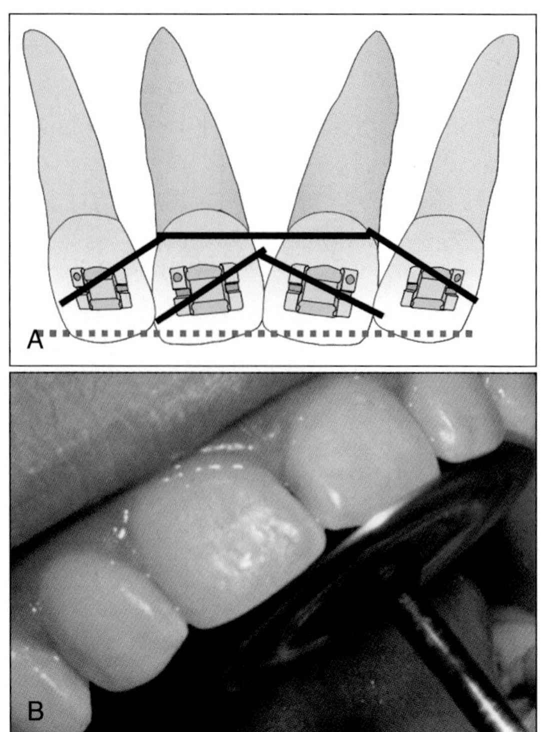

Fig. 18-18 After archwire removal and verification of stability, the brackets can be repositioned for any continuation of treatment, and the incisal edges may be contoured.

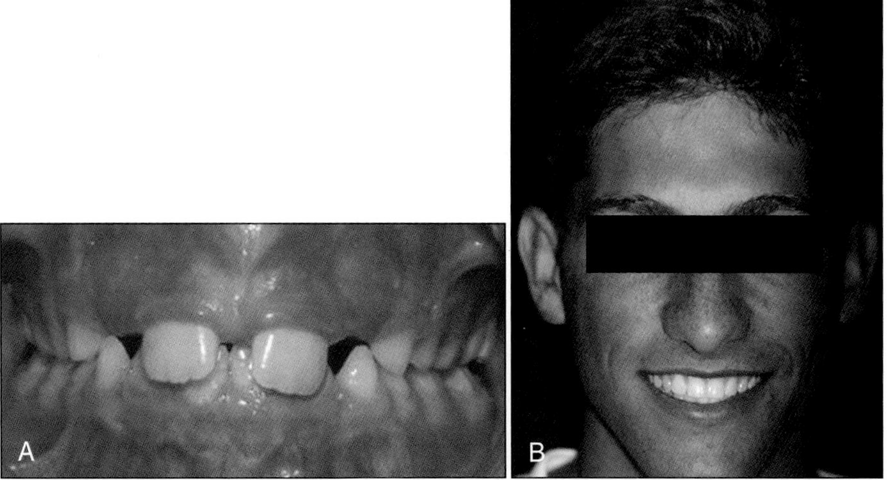

Fig. 18-19 Patient who was part of experimental group treated prior to cuspid eruption. **A,** Pretreatment intraoral photograph. **B,** Facial photograph 8 years after treatment to eliminate the diastema.

DARK TRIANGLE

All clinicians are familiar with the "dark triangle." As explained earlier, diverging incisor roots result in some degree of overjet if teeth are normal in their mesiodistal dimensions. Also, whatever prevents crown movement in one direction also results in root movement in the opposite direction. Therefore interproximal reduction of the central incisors must be accomplished before complete closure of the diastema, to prevent distal root movement instead of mesial crown movement.

In the cases cited earlier, interproximal reduction was accomplished after divergency, and the incisor segments retracted into normal overjet. However, with the dark triangle, such interproximal reduction must be accomplished before complete closure so as to permit the incisor crowns to move mesially a greater distance than demonstrated in the prior cases. In other words, in treating the dark triangle, there will be greater mesial movement of the incisor crowns and less distal movement of the roots, although the change in inclination will remain the same.

In Figure 18-20, *A*, overjet is created following root divergency. The amount of overlap that would occur without interproximal reduction is shown in Figure 18-20, *B*, simply to illustrate how much "stripping" can be achieved. Finally, after archwire removal to verify stability, brackets are rebonded for proper positioning (Fig. 18-20, *C*).

CONCLUSION

Before the author's treatment of diastemas as discussed in this chapter, a despondent young woman visited his office, stating that her family dentist thought she would be better off living with her problem than having it treated by an orthodontist (Fig. 18-21, *A-F*).

Space closure for this patient was accomplished with four anterior brackets and a power-chain elastic. The space was never eliminated, but simply divided into two halves, each located distal to the lateral incisors. Clearly, root divergency was not present (Fig. 18-21, *G-I*). She was given a removable appliance and was thrilled with the outcome (Fig. 18-21, *J* and *K*).

However, does this patient still have her retainer? Has she lost it? Has the space recurred? Has she lost hope in orthodontic treatment? If I could re-treat this young woman today, I would place four bonded brackets, using the two anterior segments previously discussed: a center bend and two off-center bends.

This type of treatment is so simple and rewarding to the patient and orthodontist that it seems archwire removal should become a mandatory procedure in orthodontics. I

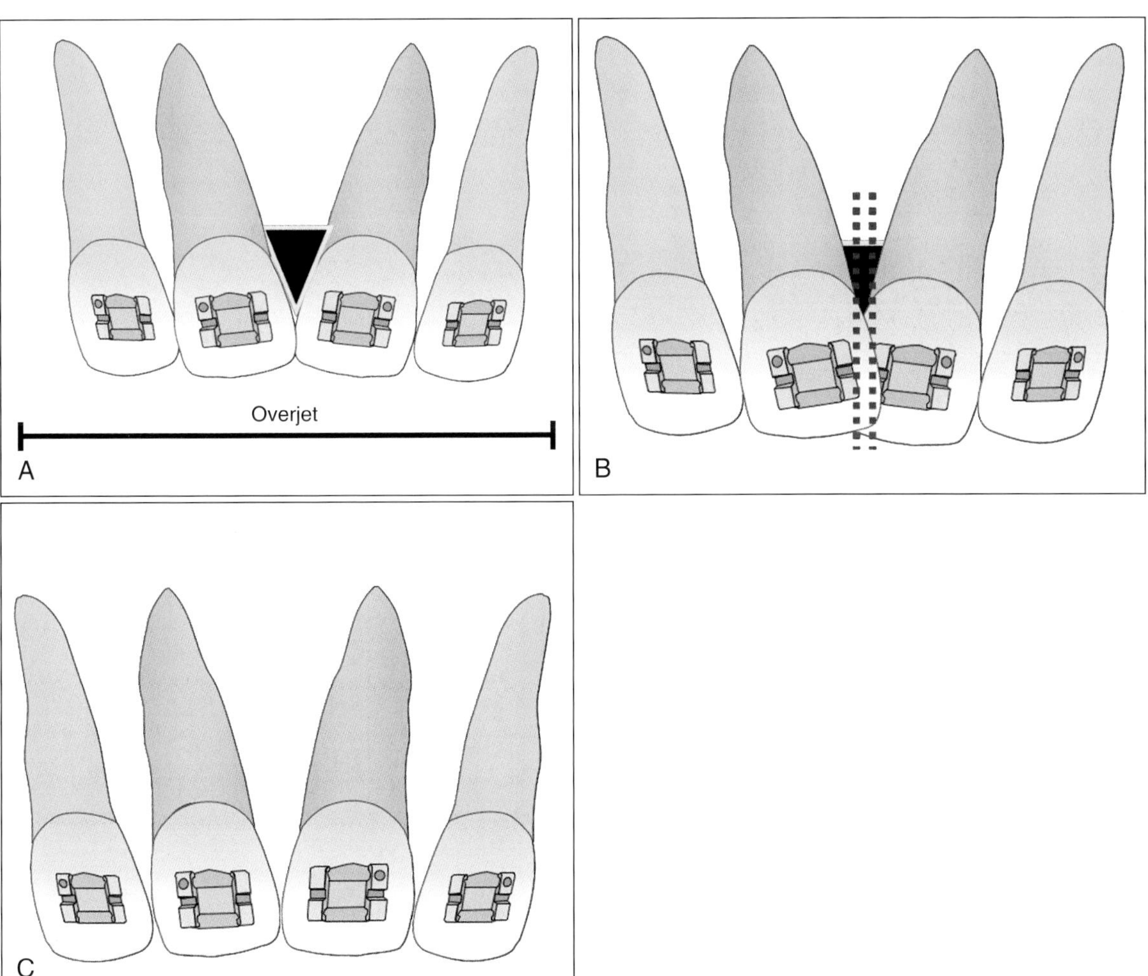

Fig. 18-20 **A,** Overjet created following root divergency. **B,** Amount of interproximal reduction with .003-inch disk. **C,** Brackets are ready to be rebounded for alignment.

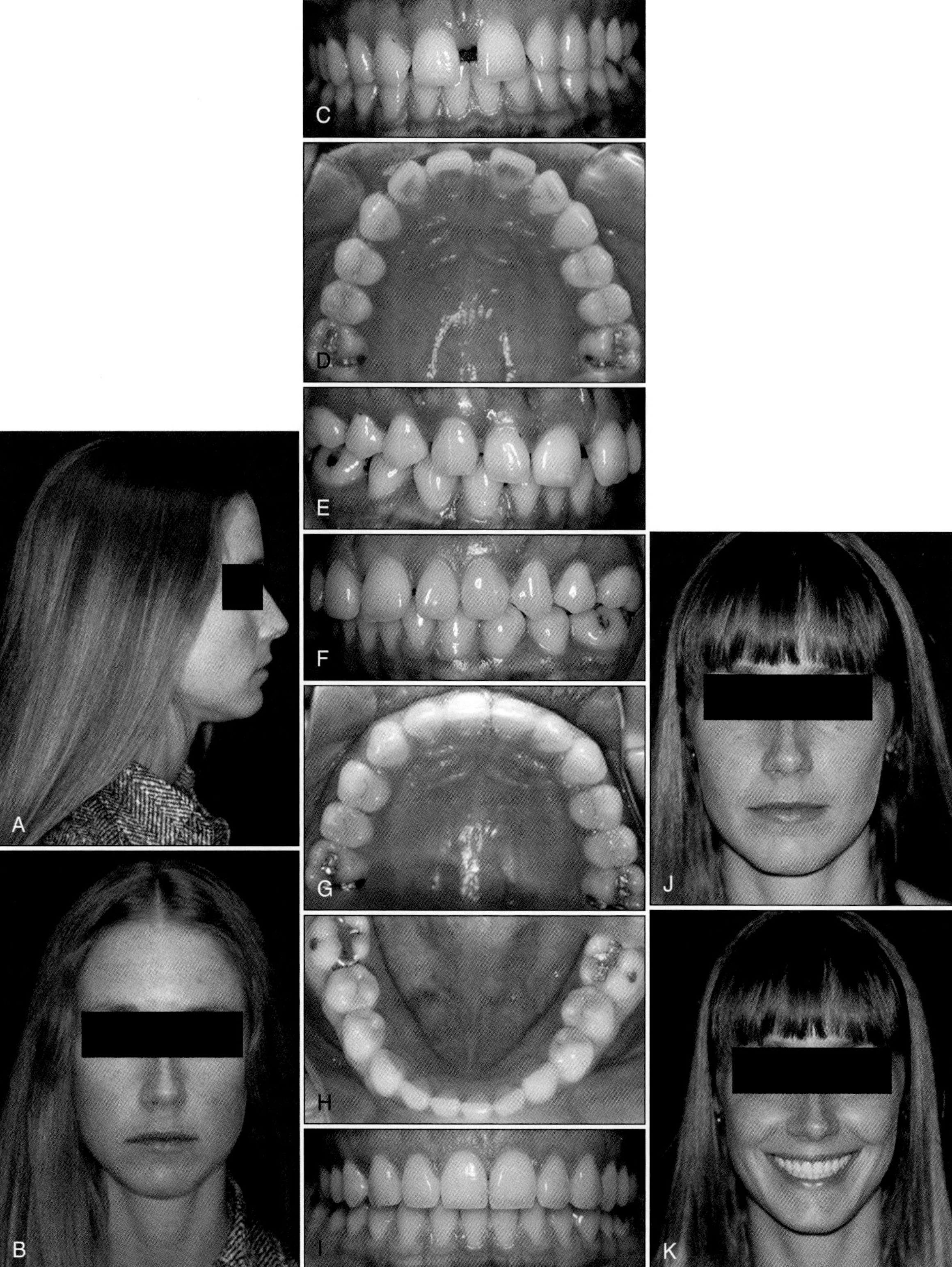

Fig. 18-21 Patient treated prior to the author adopting the treatment method discussed. **A** and **B,** Facial, and **C** and **D,** intraoral, photographs before treatment. **E** and **F,** The space was not eliminated but divided into two halves, each located distal to lateral incisors. **G** to **I,** Root divergency is not present. **J** and **K,** Facial photographs after treatment. Esthetics have improved, but were they maintained?

predict that in the future, all orthodontists seeking stability instead of permanent retention will begin removing archwires during treatment.

REFERENCES

1. West EE: Diastema, a cause for concern, *Dent Clin North Am* 8:86-95, 1968.
2. Baum AT: The midline diastema, *J Oral Med* 21:30-39, 1966.
3. Bishara SE: Management of diastemas in orthodontics, *Am J Orthod* 61:55-63, 1972.
4. Edwards JG: The diastema, the frenum, the frenectomy: a clinical study, *Am J Orthod* 71:489-507, 1977.
5. Edwards JG: Diastema relapse, *Dent Clin North Am* 37:212-225, 1993.
6. Bell WH: Surgical-orthodontic treatment of interincisal diastemas, *Am J Orthod* 57:158-163, 1970.
7. Mulligan TF: *Common sense mechanics in everyday orthodontics,* Phoenix, Ariz, 1998, CSM, pp 106, 171, 254.
8. Campbell PM, Moore JW, Matthew JL: Orthodontically corrected midline diastemas, *Am J Orthod* 67:139-158, 1975.
9. Hey T, Walters P: *Einstein's mirror,* Cambridge, England, 1997, Cambridge University Press, p 271.

CHAPTER 19

Optimizing Biomechanics in Complex and Compromised Cases

Sunil Kapila and R. Scott Conley

Every orthodontic patient presents with a unique set of dental, occlusal, and skeletal discrepancies that require individualized treatment approaches as well as specific biomechanics to place teeth in the most ideal and stable position. Although distinctly different biomechanical approaches can be used to accomplish tooth movement, some methods are more effective and efficient at delivering the forces and placing the teeth and roots closest to the desired location while minimizing undesirable side effects. A firm foundation in sound biomechanical principles provides the orthodontist with the knowledge to make creative and efficient biomechanics plans and to design appropriate appliances that, contrary to popular belief, can be both patient friendly *and* staff friendly.

To date, *continuous archwire mechanics* remains the most often used and popular form of mechanics. Although this mechanical approach has several advantages, including ease of use, patient comfort, short chair-side doctor time, and ability to delegate to the staff, it also has several limitations. Thus, in some clinical situations, continuous archwire mechanics may be inappropriate or inefficient to deliver the type of tooth movement desired.

In contrast, segmenting the arch enables the implementation of many novel and efficient force systems designed to enhance patient care and treatment results. *Segmented archwire mechanics* has several disadvantages, however, including potential difficulty in designing custom-spring applications, careful activation to obtain controlled tooth movement, some level of patient discomfort, and the decreased ability to delegate to staff. Alternatively, many clinical situations are optimally suited to enable the orthodontist to combine the advantages of both continuous archwire mechanics and segmented arch mechanics in an approach called *hybrid sectional mechanics.*

This chapter provides an overview of continuous and segmented mechanics, introduces the concept of hybrid sectional mechanics, and uses biomechanical principles to discuss the pros and cons of each of these approaches. This chapter also describes the selective use of continuous, segmented, and hybrid sectional mechanics for individual cases and arches to achieve optimal and efficient treatment results, particularly in complex and compromised cases.

RECOGNIZING COMPLEXITIES TO AVOID PITFALLS

Before implementing treatment, the orthodontist must make an accurate and appropriate diagnosis, derive the treatment objectives, critically assess the various treatment options, and select an optimal treatment plan for the patient. The full principles of orthodontic diagnosis and treatment planning are beyond the scope of this chapter and therefore are not discussed here. However, within the context of treatment planning, it is important to realize that in addition to making important decisions about the overall treatment approach, such as whether or not to extract, which teeth to extract, and whether to incorporate surgery, the clinician must be equally diligent in planning the biomechanics, appliances, and wire sequences. In other words, the comprehensive treatment plan incorporates decisions on extractions and surgery, as well as optimal and customized biomechanics.

One of the more challenging components of designing the patient's individualized biomechanical treatment plan is determining or predicting potential difficulties or adverse tooth movements that might occur during treatment. In general, it is more efficient to recognize these mechanical or treatment complexities before initiating treatment. Early recognition of potential problems enables the orthodontist to plan strategies to avoid difficulties or adverse tooth movements during treatment. Additional benefits of such a proactive approach to biomechanical planning include better treatment outcomes (as discussed later) and greater efficiency, resulting in increased orthodontic practice productivity and profitability with reduced stress.

CONTINUOUS ARCHWIRE MECHANICS

Indications

To enhance practice flow, orthodontists often use standardized treatment approaches that incorporate continuous archwire mechanics with the same or similar sequences of wires, retraction and space consolidation, detailing, and finishing for all patients. Although these "autopilot mechanics" have the benefits of the staff understanding and anticipating the next wire size or the next treatment stage, of possibly limiting clinician and staff time, and likely enhancing efficiency and productivity in most routine cases, the advantages of this approach may not apply to many complex and dentally or periodontally compromised cases. Indeed, the complications introduced by the use of routine mechanics in these cases will likely lead to increased treatment time, decreased productivity, and compromised esthetic and or functional results. Therefore, as a general rule, standard continuous archwire mechanics can be best used in most simple nonextraction cases, cases with spacing, extraction cases in which there is likely to be minimal round-tripping of teeth, or when decompensating in surgical cases.

Table 19-1 provides a listing of specific indications for continuous archwire mechanics and serves as a guide for clinical situations where alternate biomechanical approaches such as segmented archwire and hybrid sectional mechanics can be beneficial. Depending on the practice profile, approximately 40% to 70% of patients in a given practice would likely meet the criteria for use of routine continuous archwire mechanics to deliver the force systems necessary to produce the desired outcomes.

Although primarily indicated for relatively routine cases, continuous archwire mechanics can be beneficial even in a select number of cases that are quite complex in which none of the contraindications listed in Table 19-1 are present, as in the following case.

Deformed dentoalveolar structures and generalized spacing

Figure 19-1 shows a patient who had recently recovered from a 6-month coma during which he had oral intubation. He presented with wide dental arches, deformed dentoalveolar structures, severely proclined upper and lower incisors, overerupted maxillary molars, and generalized spacing (Fig. 19-1, *A-H*). The generalized spacing resulted from the intubation, multiple missing teeth, macroglossia, and partial tongue paralysis. Both the proclined incisors and the buccally inclined molars had compromised periodontal health.

Periodontal evaluation, treatment, and maintenance therapy were performed before initiating orthodontic care. In addition, an orthognathic surgery consultation for evaluation of the underlying skeletal discrepancy and a reduction glossectomy were performed. The comprehensive treatment plan included periodontal management and reduction glossectomy, followed by orthodontic treatment with continuous archwire mechanics to consolidate and redistribute spaces and remove compensations as best as possible. As space consolidation and redistribution progressed, a final determination of space needs for restorations and obtaining optimal occlusal results was made in consultation with a prosthodontist. The final treatment stage required orthog-

TABLE 19-1

Indications for Continuous Archwire, Segmented Archwire, and Hybrid Sectional Mechanics

	Continuous Archwire	Segmented Archwire	Hybrid Sectional
Generalized spacing	+++		
Mild crowding (nonextraction)	+++		
Crowding (extraction treatment; minimal round tripping anticipated)	+++		
Decompensations desired	+++		
Moderate to severe crowding (extraction treatment; round tripping anticipated)	—	+++	+++
Differential anchorage desired	—	+++	++
Severe canine/premolar root angulations	—	+++*	+
Asymmetric cases	—	+++	+
Multiple missing teeth	—	++	+++
Compromised periodontal health	—	++	+++
Preservation of dental compensations	—	+*	+++
Desire to perform multiple stages of treatment concurrently	—	+	+++

Degree of indication: +++, strong; ++, moderate; +, weak; no symbol indicates segmented or hybrid sectional mechanics can be used but are not necessary; —, contraindication.

*Initiate with segmented, and follow up with hybrid sectional mechanics if needed.

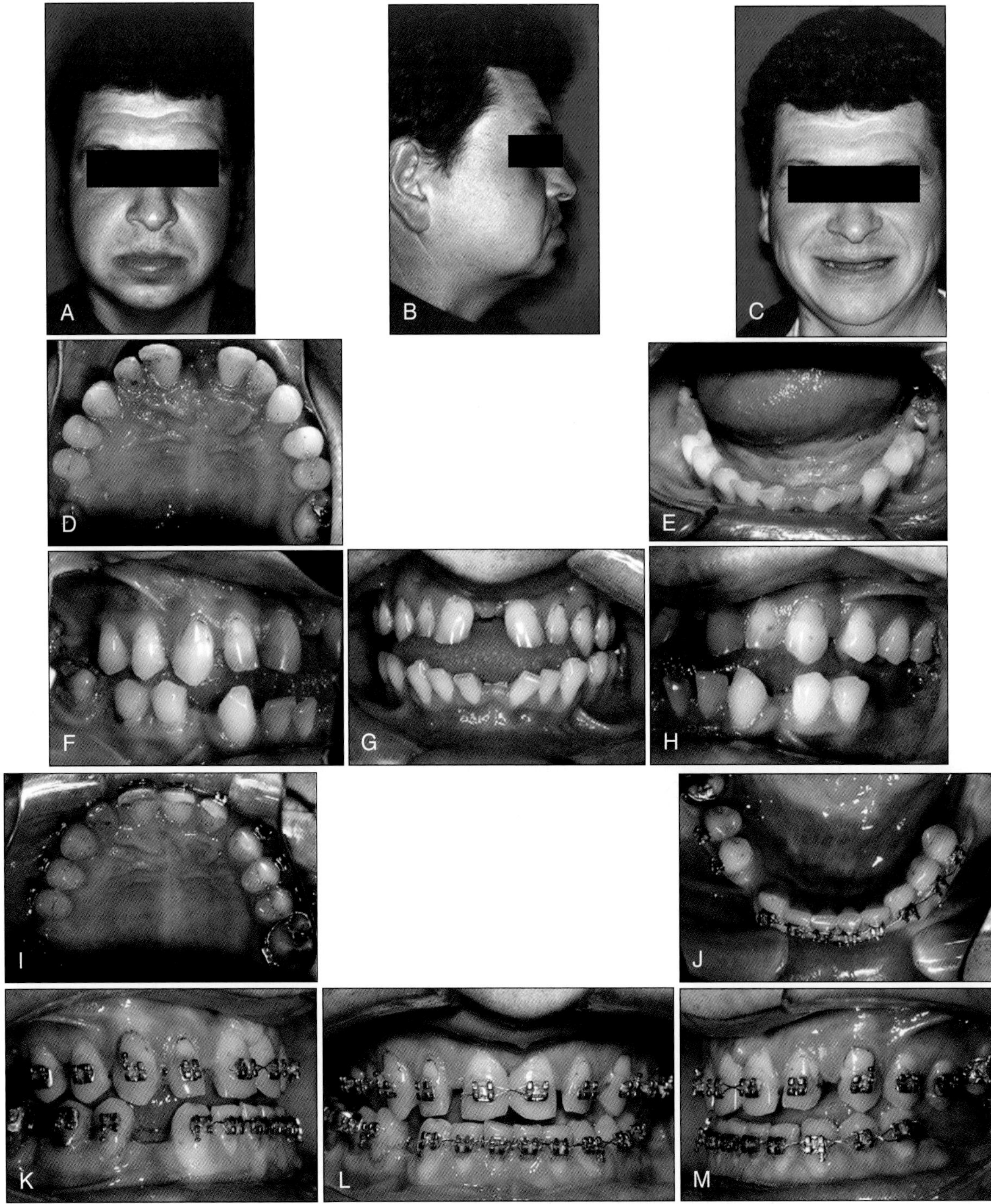

Fig. 19-1 **A** to **H,** Pretreatment facial and intraoral photographs of a patient with generalized spacing and distorted dentoalveolar structures. Because of the lack of round tripping and minimal adverse tooth movements anticipated with continuous archwire mechanics, this mechanics can be used in this patient. **I** to **M,** Presurgical photographs showing arch coordination, as well as incisor retraction and space redistribution after the reduction glossectomy and presurgical orthodontics. The spaces will be refined further postsurgically.

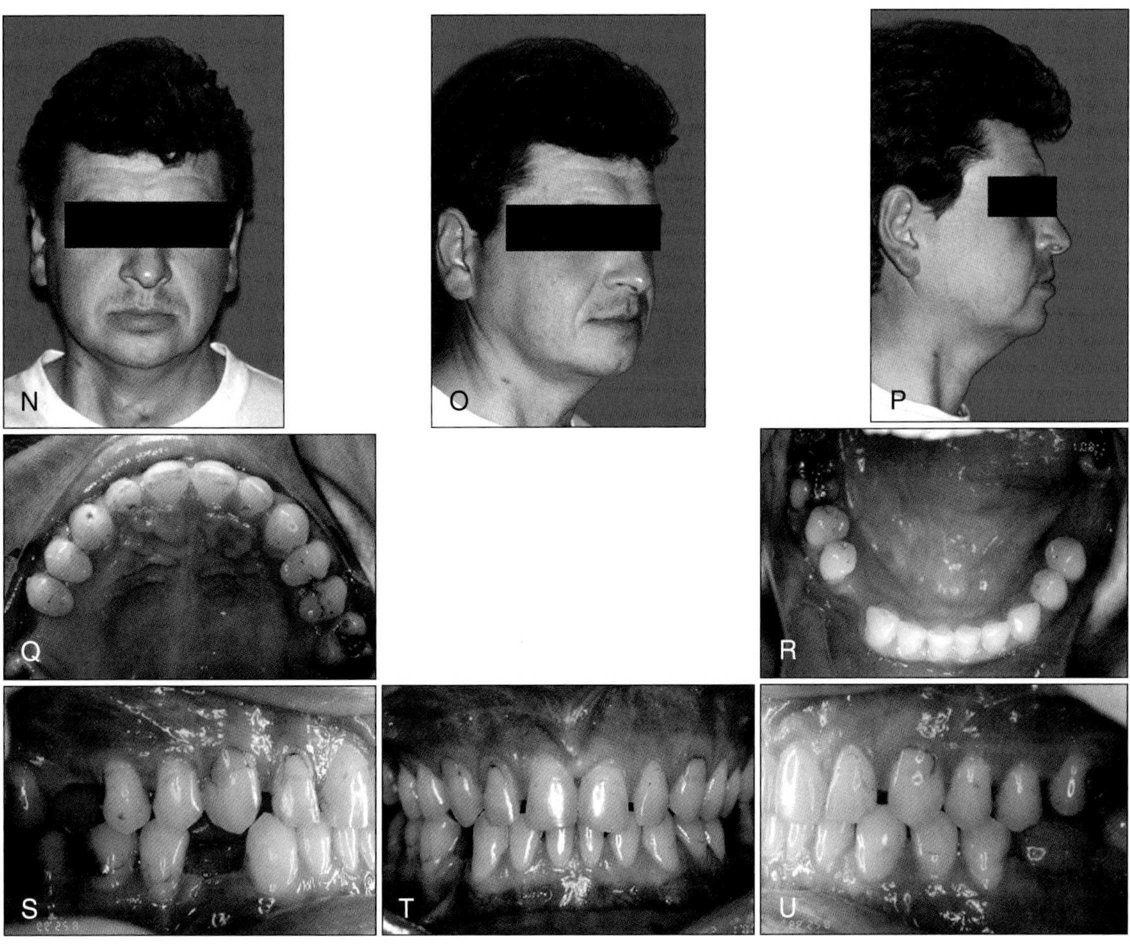

Fig. 19-1, cont'd **N** to **U**, An excellent finish was obtained using continuous archwire mechanics. Facial balance (**N-P**) and a stable occlusion (**Q-U**) have been established.

nathic surgery to achieve the best possible occlusal and esthetic results. Once orthodontic treatment was completed, the missing teeth would be replaced with a combination of implants and removable partial dentures.

Before orthodontic care began, the patient underwent a reduction glossectomy to enable retraction of the dentition. A decision was made to wait several months to allow for any self-correction of incisors resulting from the reduced tongue volume and pressure, which could alter the equilibrium on the teeth[1] and possibly cause them to move lingually. After 1 year, however, only minimal incisor uprighting was observed. Treatment was then initiated with continuous archwire mechanics because of spacing and the expectation that minimal adverse tooth movements, including round tripping, would result from these mechanics. A routine archwire sequence, including nickel-titanium (Ni-Ti) wires for alignment and stainless steel wires with elastomeric power chains for space consolidation were used. A low-hanging transpalatal arch (TPA) was also placed to intrude or prevent the extrusion of the upper molars.[2]

This patient was treated before the introduction of temporary anchorage devices (TADs). Had TADs been available, they would have been used to intrude the maxillary molars and maintain their anteroposterior position during space consolidation.

The decision on optimal space distribution and restorations were finalized as spaces were being closed. Presurgical records demonstrate the space consolidation and the significant amount of incisor retraction in both arches (Fig. 19-1, *I-M*). Small spaces were preserved in the maxillary anterior region because of an underlying maxillary Bolton deficiency. After surgery, the spaces were refined to enable the prosthodontist to fabricate appropriately sized central and lateral incisor restorations. The postorthodontic and postsurgical and prerestorative results demonstrate that in some complex cases, high-quality results are possible with conventional continuous archwire mechanics (Fig. 19-1, *N-U*).

Contraindications

Unlike the complex case in Fig. 19-1, other cases may present with occlusal discrepancies that are not well suited for continuous archwire mechanics. Such cases include patients with multiple missing teeth, compromised periodontal health, asymmetric malocclusions, and moderately to severely crowded arches where round tripping is

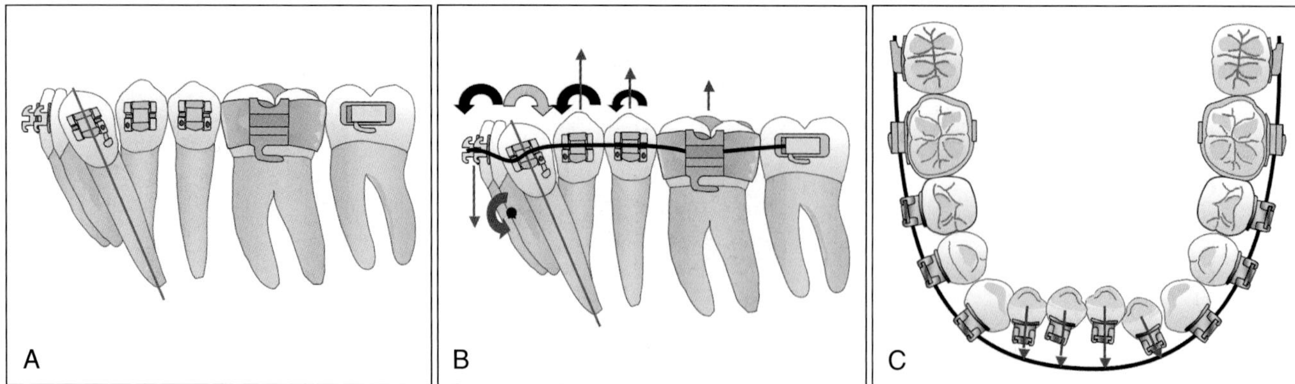

Fig. 19-2 **A,** Correction of severely tipped canines with continuous archwire mechanics will contribute to many adverse tooth movements. **B,** Placing a continuous archwire in a mesial crown/distal root, tipped mandibular canine generates the desirable moment on the canine *(yellow arrow)* but intrusive forces on the mandibular incisors, which produces incisor flaring, because the intrusive force is labial to the incisor center of resistance. The wire exiting distal to the severely inclined canine also produces extrusion of the lower posterior teeth. In addition to the undesirable intrusive and extrusive forces, moments are also generated on the teeth adjacent to the canine *(black arrows)*. These moments can result in the undesirable tipping of the "anchor" teeth and ultimately cant the entire occlusal plane. **C,** The flaring of the incisors can be exacerbated in situations where the canines are positioned more facially than the incisors.

undesirable, as well as those where dental compensations must be maintained (see Table 19-1).

Additional examples of such cases include those patients who present with severe angulations of the canine, which occurs more frequently than realized, particularly in the mandibular arch (Fig. 19-2, *A*). If the canine presents with a severe mesial crown/distal root angulation, a continuous archwire will generate significant protrusive and intrusive forces on the incisors. Intrusion may be desirable, but because the intrusive forces are applied labial to the lower incisor center of resistance, additional proclination or flaring of the anterior teeth can occur[3-5] (Fig. 19-2, *B*). Finally, because such a canine crown is often more labial than the incisors, it will tend to move the incisors labially (Fig. 19-2, *C*).

Of equal concern is the force system on the posterior portion of the arch resulting from the continuous archwire. As the continuous archwire exits the distal aspect of the canine bracket, it generates an extrusive force on the first and second premolars, as well as the first and second molars (Fig. 19-2, *B*). Large, multirooted teeth might be assumed to have enough anchorage to resist these extrusive forces, but this is not always the case.[6] Extrusive forces to the posterior dentition, particularly in patients with long faces and weaker facial musculature, can result in undesired eruption leading to the iatrogenic development of an anterior open bite.[7,8] In addition to these undesirable forces generated by the archwire, the teeth neighboring the canine also experience moments that cause the teeth to tip adversely (Fig. 19-2, *B*).

The consequences of such moments and forces in contributing to adverse and undesirable tooth movements are evident in the following case, which is followed by a description of the authors' method of choice for distalizing crowns or roots of severely angulated teeth.

Severe dental angulations

A 12-year-old girl presented with bimaxillary protrusion, incompetent lips from increased maxillary vertical excess and short upper lip, increased gingival display on smiling, and a Class I molar relationship with severe mandibular crowding (Fig. 19-3, *A-H*). Multiple viable treatment options ranging from orthognathic surgery to a variety of different extraction protocols could be used in this case. Because of the parent's desire not to undergo surgery and because patient compliance was considered questionable, the orthodontist planned the shortest treatment approach possible. This included extraction of the upper first premolars and lower canines, combined with routine continuous archwire mechanics.

Unfortunately, in choosing these biomechanics, no serious consideration was given to the negative effects that would result from placing the wire into the bracket on the severely mesial crown/distal root angulated lower left premolar (Fig. 19-3, *I*). Placement of the initial series of Ni-Ti continuous archwires for alignment generated the desired moment to upright the premolar, but this also introduced force systems to intrude and flare the mandibular incisors, extrude the left posterior teeth, and produce rotational moments on the incisors and premolars (Fig. 19-3, *J* and *K*). These adverse movements largely occur asymmetrically on the side with the mesially inclined premolar, resulting in canting of the anterior and posterior occlusal planes, an asymmetric left anterior and lateral open bite, and an increase in vertical face height caused by the posterior extrusion.

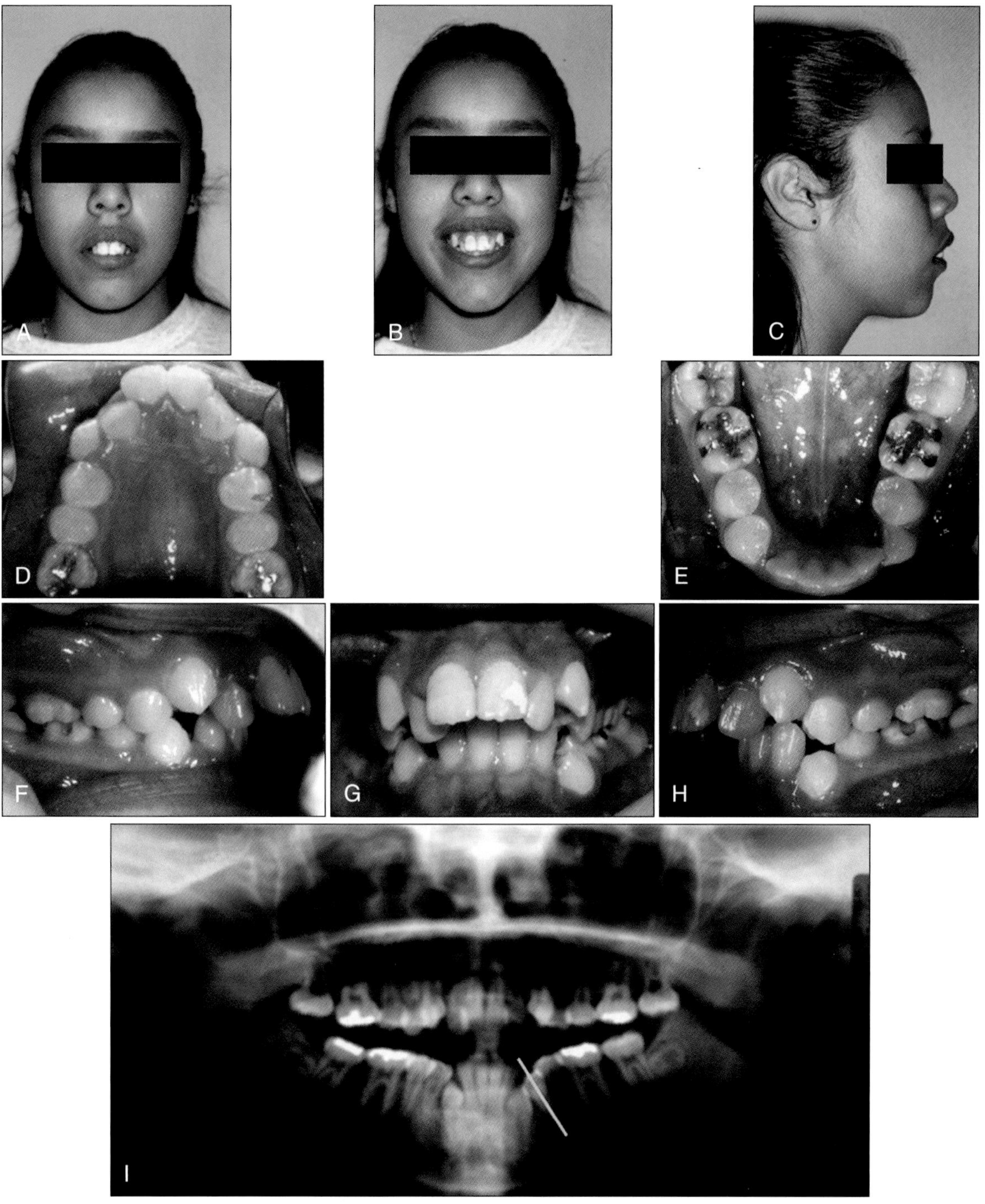

Fig. 19-3 **A** to **H,** Pretreatment facial and intraoral photographs of a patient with bimaxillary protrusion, excessive incisor and gingival display, severe crowding, severe mesial inclination of mandibular left first premolar, and blocked-out lower canines. **I,** Panoramic radiograph showing the severe mesial inclination of the mandibular left first premolar and impacted lower canines.

Continued

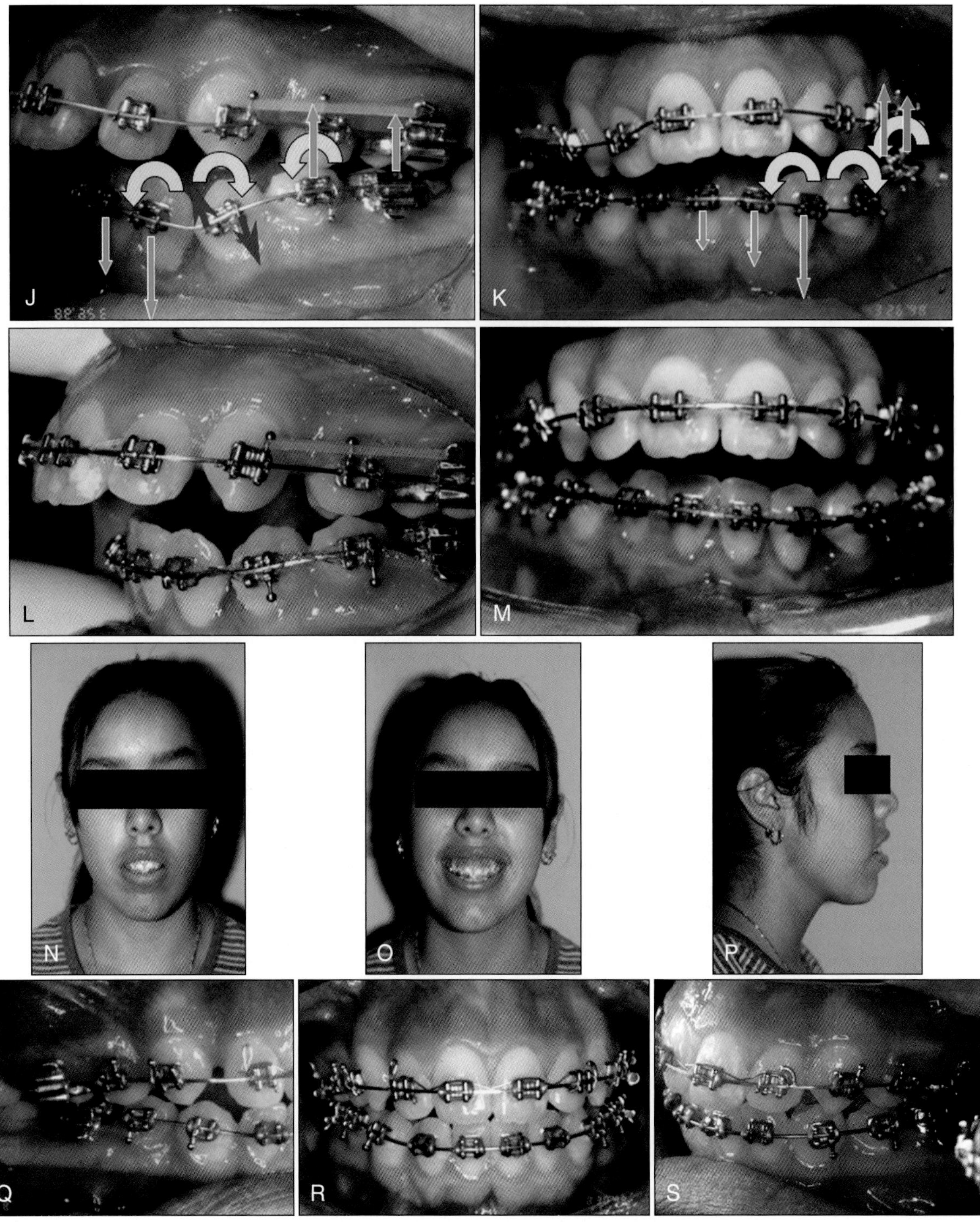

Fig. 19-3, cont'd **J** and **K,** The complex force systems resulting from the severely angulated mandibular left first premolar, even with a light Ni-Ti continuous archwire, is demonstrated clinically by the adverse changes in tooth positions. These movements result from the same intrusive/extrusive force system and associated moments described in Fig. 19-2. **L** and **M,** Lateral open bite and canted occlusal plane are maintained in a heavier stainless steel continuous archwire because of its delivery of adverse moments and forces to the teeth adjacent to the mandibular left first premolar. **N** to **S,** After correction of the lateral open bite and canted occlusal plane with interarch elastics, a reasonable occlusion has been established. Unfortunately, compared with the potential outcomes of using the appropriate mechanics, the substantially increased gingival display results in poorer esthetics, and the increased treatment time contributes to diminished clinical efficiency.

As stiffer, stainless steel wires were inserted and left to work until passive, they produced the clinical findings depicted in Figure 19-3, *L* and *M*, which displays the results that could have been predicted from a detailed pretreatment mechanical analysis. Because of the undesirable and iatrogenic eruption of the posterior teeth and the creation of an asymmetric lateral and anterior open bite, additional treatment time and complexity have been added to the case, which now requires complicated mechanics to resolve. Although not an optimal method for resolving these undesirable consequences, significant anterior elastic wear was used to compensate for the open bite. The pre-debond occlusion, although not optimal, is acceptable compared with the very poor occlusion during treatment (Fig. 19-3, *N-S*). However, the extrusion of the anterior teeth due to the extensive use of vertical elastics has resulted in substantially diminished esthetics due to excessive gingival display, not only when smiling but also in repose.

The poor choice of initial mechanics resulted in negative facial changes and substantially increased her treatment time to 4 years. These consequences are highly undesirable from both a patient and practice management perspective.

This case represents several occlusal discrepancies that contraindicate the use of continuous archwire mechanics (see Table 19-1). These include the severe angulation of the premolar and the asymmetry between left and right premolar angulations (Fig.19-3, *A-I*) that, when corrected with continuous archwire mechanics, is transferred to other parts of the arch (Fig. 19-3, *J-M*).

An alternative and optimal approach to correct this malocclusion would strategically focus first on correcting the premolar angulation with a segmented mechanical approach, as depicted in Fig. 19-4. Any type of segmental spring that introduces a moment that moves the premolar root mesially can be designed and engaged in the premolar and molar brackets. Using the principles of biomechanics, it is clear that the desired clockwise moment on the premolar generated by this spring results in an undesired extrusive force on the molar (Fig. 19-4, *A*). The extrusion of the molar resulting from this extrusive force can be minimized by enhancing anchorage on this tooth by (1) incorporating a sectional wire on the second premolar and the two molars, (2) adding a lower lingual arch between the molars, and (3) if necessary, further reinforcing the anchorage on the contralateral molar by placing an archwire segment that engages the right quadrant up to the left lateral incisor (Fig. 19-4, *A* and *B*). Alternatively, these additional features for enhancing anchorage may be replaced by a TAD placed gingival and distal to the left molar and simply tied to the molar to prevent adverse vertical and mesial movements of the molar (Fig. 19-4, *C*). Once the premolar has been fully uprighted, the case could be routinely finished through continuous archwire mechanics.

Round Tripping

Another clinical problem that can be difficult to avoid with continuous archwire mechanics is "round tripping." When initial alignment is performed in a crowded arch using a continuous archwire, the clinician is attempting to align crowded teeth by increasing the overall length of the arch, which generally translates into expansion at the incisors, commonly referred to as "proclination." This will occur in crowded arches even if teeth have already been extracted (Fig. 19-5, *A* and *B*). Subsequently, after canine retraction the incisors are also retracted (Fig. 19-5, *C*). The initial proclination of the incisors followed by their retraction is often referred to as "round tripping" (Fig. 19-5, *D*).

The final position of the teeth after "retraction" might not be significantly different from the start position, but the path traveled by the teeth is extensive. Also, if the incisors are overly proclined during initial alignment in a patient with thin alveolar bone support, it may be accompanied by tissue destruction such as gingival stripping or loss of crestal bone height,[9-11] as depicted in Figure 19-6. Another potentially

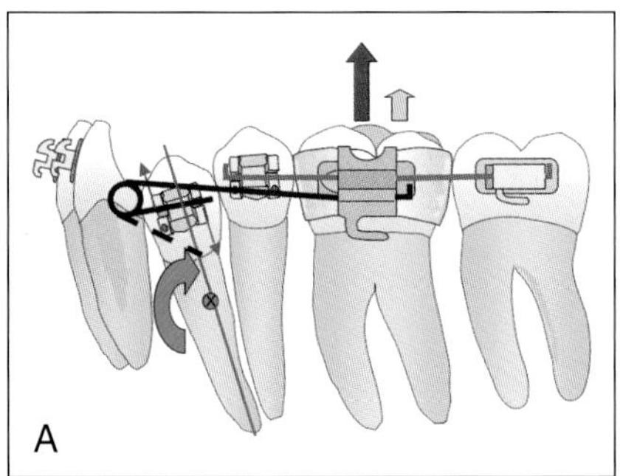

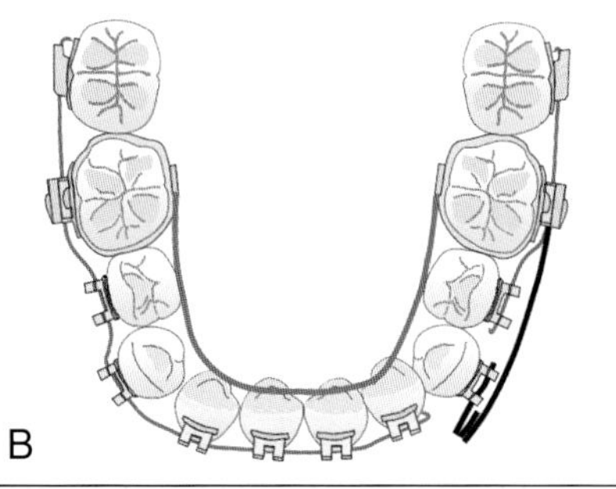

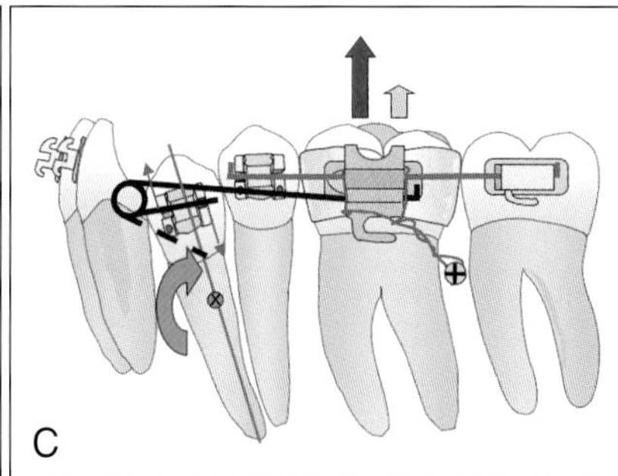

Fig. 19-4 **A,** Segmental uprighting spring to correct premolar angulation can be fabricated to minimize adverse effects on anterior portion of the arch. Resultant effects of extrusive forces on the molar can be minimized by reinforcing anchorage with a wire segment on the second premolar and molars. **B,** This can be further combined with a lower lingual arch with or without a segmented arch extending from the contralateral molars to the lower left incisor. **C,** Alternatively, a temporary anchorage device (TAD) can be placed and ligated to the first molar to minimize its extrusion and mesial movement. The red and yellow extrusive arrows on the molar represent the magnitude of extrusion without and with reinforced anchorage, respectively.

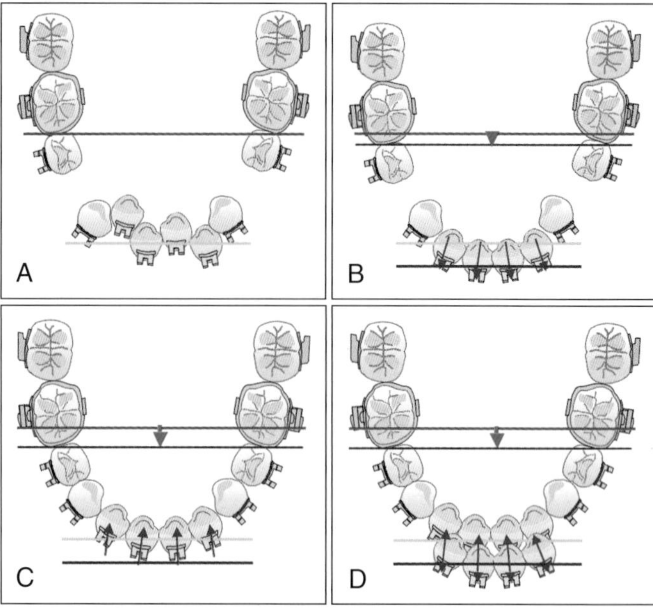

Fig. 19-5 "Round tripping" of crowded incisors with continuous archwire mechanics. Placing a continuous archwire in arches with moderate to severe incisor crowding (**A**) results in increased arch circumference (**B**) caused by proclination of the incisors *(red arrows)* even when extractions have been performed. This may cause some anchorage loss *(green arrowhead)* and contribute to tissue damage. **C,** After canine and incisor retraction, the incisors are positioned close to their original starting position *(yellow line)*. The retraction of the canines and also the incisors from their proclined position results in additional anchorage loss *(green arrow)*. **D,** Composite of incisor proclination and retraction demonstrating round tripping *(red arrows)* and molar anchorage loss *(green arrow)* in a moderate incisor crowding case treated with continuous archwire mechanics.

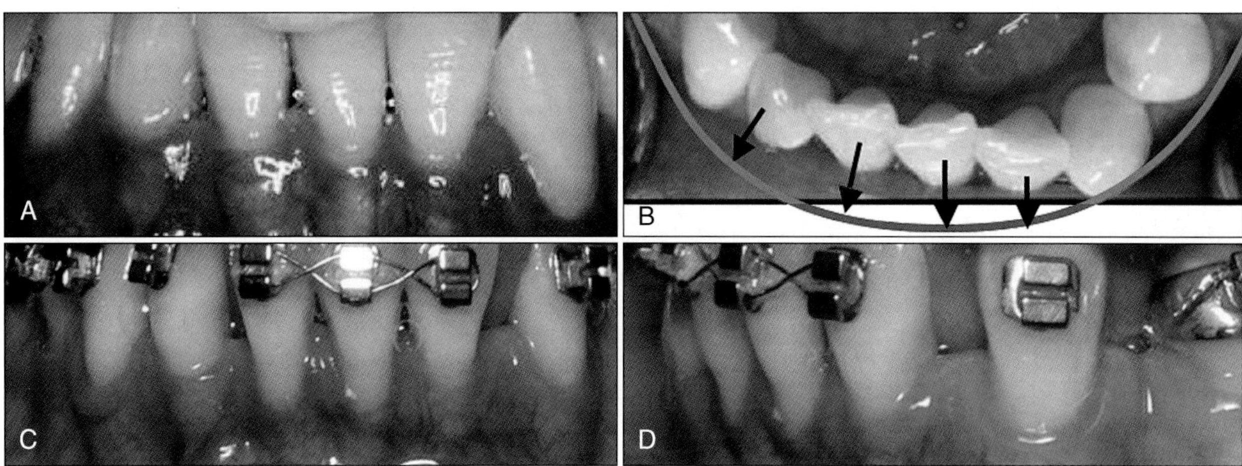

Fig. 19-6 **A** and **B,** Pretreatment intraoral frontal and lower occlusal photographs demonstrating crowding and thin attached gingiva on lower incisors. Placing a continuous archwire would result in labial forces on the incisors and their resultant proclination (**B**). **C** and **D,** In patients with thin alveolar housing and minimal attached gingiva, such mechanics could result in gingival recession.

negative consequence of round tripping may be root resorption resulting from unnecessarily proclining the incisors and placing their roots in contact with the lingual or palatal cortical plate[12] or from the increased magnitude of tooth movement[13] and time in treatment.[14]

An additional potential adverse effect of round tripping is increased anchorage loss and its negative consequences on final incisor position and lip prominence. The anchorage loss occurs not only during initial alignment (i.e., posterior teeth drift forward as incisors procline) but also during retraction of the incisors from a more anterior position than at the start of treatment (see Fig. 19-5, *B-D*). This results in less extraction space for retraction. If the goal of treatment is to perform significant retraction of incisors to improve incisor position and lip esthetics and competency, the desired facial goals may not be achieved.

Examination of the patient's pretreatment records, particularly the casts and the lateral cephalogram, can help identify situations where incisor round tripping may have negative consequences. In this regard, situations that have incisor crowding or incisor flaring are of particular concern because placement of a continuous archwire will lead to their further proclination. Patients who also exhibit thin periodontal biotypes are at further increased risk of adverse changes. Thin biotypes are identified when the periodontal probe inserted into the gingival sulcus is visible through the patient's translucent tissues,[15] and by observing prominent roots on the labial aspect of the alveolus.

Another diagnostic aid for assessing the ability of periodontal supporting structures to adapt to proclination or round tripping of incisors is the thickness of the alveolar bone, which can be readily observed in lateral cephalograms,[16,17] as demonstrated later. In some patients in whom the alveolar process around the incisor roots is relatively thin, significant labial or even lingual movement may contribute to tissue damage and loss in periodontal support. In the future, three-dimensional cone-beam computed tomography (CBCT) will likely provide additional diagnostic information that will be important in assessing the limits to which round tripping or proclination of incisors can be performed while maintaining integrity of bony structures housing the incisors.

Anchorage Considerations

An additional caveat of continuous archwire mechanics is that it poses a challenge in adequately controlling the anchorage at its extremes. The two extremes of anchorage are commonly described as *maximum* anchorage (or "A" anchorage) and *minimum* anchorage (or "C" anchorage).[18] Symmetrically activated closing loops, coil springs, and elastomeric power chains all produce reciprocal space closure because these mechanics are unable to produce differential moment/force ratios in the anterior and posterior regions.[19] Differential space closure with these mechanics is often achieved through intermaxillary elastics, which can provide some assistance to differential space closure but with drawbacks. Class II elastics will extrude the mandibular posterior dentition and extrude and retrocline the maxillary anterior teeth and potentially result in greater incisal display. The mandibular posterior extrusion will contribute to posterior occlusal plane anomalies, increase the vertical face height, and result in occlusal interferences. Class III elastics have similar effects but in opposing directions.

Orthodontists also attempt to use other anchorage devices to aid in cases with high anchorage needs, but sometimes these approaches are "sprinkled in" haphazardly or implemented once trouble is observed. Two such approaches are use of a Nance holding arch and use of a TPA. The Nance appliance, originally proposed by Hayes Nance in 1947, utilizes a stainless steel .036-inch wire bent along the contours of the maxillary arch to connect the maxillary first molars. Once contoured and soldered to the maxillary molars, cold-cured acrylic is applied to the anterior portion of the wire to establish a rest on the palatal mucosa. It is hoped that the pressure exerted by continuous space closure mechanics onto the palatal mucosa and underlying palatal bone will be sufficient to resist anchorage loss. Unfortunately, according to some reports, this and other forms of anchorage may have less anchorage value than previously thought.

The TPA has also been used as an anchorage auxiliary. Controversy exists regarding the anchorage value of the traditional TPA, with a recent report suggesting similar levels of anchorage loss with or without a passive TPA.[20] Orthodontists who use the TPA for anchorage suggest that part of the anchorage resistance results from using an active rather than a passive TPA.

Another approach to enhancing anchorage includes the use of headgear. This can include Klöhn-type headgear in high-pull, cervical-pull, or straight-pull directions. Other treatment disciplines recommend "J hook" headgear directly to the canines or the anterior portion of the maxillary and mandibular arches. The biggest limitation of headgear is the need for patient compliance.

The introduction of TADs is likely to diminish the need for many of these approaches for anchorage preservation. However, as with other aspects of orthodontic treatment, TADs should be used rationally and with careful attention to detail in planning and optimizing the biomechanics to be used.

INDIVIDUALIZING TREATMENT OBJECTIVES AND BIOMECHANICS

As stated previously, each patient presents to the orthodontic office with his or her unique set of treatment needs. This requires that an optimal treatment plan and treatment objectives be developed for each patient. Besides the universally accepted treatment objectives that are generically applicable to most patients (e.g., achieving good facial esthetics with balanced facial proportions, positioning the dentition upright over basal bone, developing a functional and stable occlusion, and preserving the health of the teeth and the periodontium), patient-specific treatment objectives must also be defined. These generic and specific treatment objectives together are essential to derive the optimal biomechanical plan for each patient and arch. However, although the literature is replete with individualized treatment objectives, it often lacks individualized mechanical analysis and the biomechanical plan necessary to achieve the stated objectives.

To meet patient-specific objectives and adequately prepare the biomechanics plan, it is helpful to determine both the magnitude and the direction of tooth movement needed to achieve each of these objectives. Helpful tools to establish patient-specific treatment objectives include the practitioner's cephalometric, arch length, and facial analyses of choice. Another tool is the occlusogram, which enables the practitioner to perform treatment on an acetate tracing first to determine the feasibility of the proposed treatment.[21-23] Recent advances have enabled three-dimensional (3D) computerized occlusograms to be performed.[24] Because treatment objectives and mechanics should ideally be planned concurrently in all three planes of space to adequately and completely treat the malocclusion, the 3D occlusogram and other 3D imaging aids are likely to become increasingly important tools in diagnosis and treatment planning.

Once the specific or individualized treatment goals, including the anchorage requirements and precise numbers of millimeters and degrees of correction required, have been established, the practitioner can determine the biomechanics and the biomechanical sequencing necessary to achieve the established treatment objectives. By establishing case-specific treatment objectives before initiating treatment, the orthodontist must evaluate the case more critically, then define the individualized biomechanics plan. In this way the orthodontist can evaluate potential adverse tooth movements and implement strategies to prevent their occurrence and better plan and sequence the overall treatment for enhanced treatment efficiency. Strategies to prevent adverse tooth movements include the use of anchorage auxiliaries (e.g., Nance appliance, TPA, headgear, TADs) that should be planned and implemented proactively, rather than haphazardly sprinkling these anchorage aids during treatment or after adverse tooth movements are observed.

Because of the shortcomings of continuous archwire mechanics in specific cases where its use is contraindicated (see Table 19-1), the use of alternative biomechanical approaches is not just an option but is highly recommended to achieve optimal results. Fortunately, the repertoire of biomechanics available to the clinician is broader than just continuous archwire mechanics that is traditionally used by most orthodontists. Two alternative approaches are segmented mechanics (and its various modifications) and hybrid sectional mechanics, which incorporates the advantages of segmented and continuous archwire mechanics. These alternative approaches are described below in greater detail and should be used in specific cases when indicated.

Segmented Mechanics

The most common alternative mechanical approach is segmented-arch mechanics as originally proposed by Dr. Charles Burstone, with its many subsequent modifications and iterations. The overall purpose of the original segmented approach was to break up the arch into three segments of teeth, or what may be regarded as three large, multirooted teeth. These consist of one anterior segment mesial to the canines and two posterior segments typically consisting of the second premolar through second molar. By only including three teeth in the posterior segment, a precise and resolvable force system is created. This simplifies the derivation of moments and forces generated by any given appliance in the individual segments, which enables the orthodontist to implement additional mechanical strategies to counteract undesirable tooth movements. In addition, specific operator-determined force systems can be created and implemented.[4,25,26]

This approach is in contrast with continuous archwire mechanics, in which the forces and moments generated are infinitely complex or indeterminate, and therefore strategies to counteract undesirable tooth movements are difficult or impossible to derive and implement. As such, in complex cases, continuous archwire mechanics are more likely to lead to negative occlusal changes and treatment results (see Figs. 19-3 and 19-6). Another important difference between segmented and continuous archwire mechanics is the sequence in which the treatment is performed. Thus, unlike the sequence of leveling and aligning in continuous archwire mechanics, followed by canine retraction and incisor retraction, segmented mechanics involves canine retraction first, followed by incisor retraction and then leveling and aligning (Table 19-2). The final stage in both continuous archwire and segmented mechanics is detailing and finishing.

Although segmented mechanics are highly desirable in most complex and compromised cases, there are specific disadvantages to these mechanics as compared with continuous archwire mechanics. These include the complexity of appliance design and activation, difficulty in arch coordination, potentially increased chair-side time particularly during appliance construction, decreased ability to delegate chair-side work to staff, patient discomfort from loops and springs, and potential difficulty in maintaining oral hygiene[27] (Table 19-3). However, many of these drawbacks are largely negated by the benefits of these mechanics. For example, the disadvantages of increased chair-side time during initial appliance design, placement, and subsequent activations is heavily outweighed by the chair-side time and increased length in treatment that would result from inappropriately using continuous archwire mechanics in a complex case for which it is contraindicated (see Fig. 19-3).

The difficulty in maintaining arch coordination in segmented mechanics remains a major limitation. This limitation is generally overcome by using a TPA, which also provides cross-arch stabilization.[28-30] Failure to understand the force systems involved in TPA activation can lead to rapid deterioration in arch coordination and iatrogenic malocclusion. With segmented mechanics, other than the TPA, few intersegmental connections are made. For example, during arch leveling the only connection between the two posterior segments and the anterior segment is the intrusive or extrusive base arch. This consists of two to four connections from the intrusive base arch to the anterior segment wire, where stainless steel ligatures tie the two together (Fig.

TABLE 19-2

Typical Treatment Sequencing in Continuous Archwire, Segmented, and Hybrid Sectional Mechanics

Step	Continuous Archwire	Segmented	Hybrid Sectional
1	Leveling and aligning	Canine retraction	Canine retraction, incisor aligning and leveling
2	Canine retraction	Incisor retraction (and intrusion if indicated)	Incisor retraction (and intrusion if needed)
3	Incisor retraction	Align (and level if indicated)	Coordination, detailing, and finishing
4	Coordination, detailing, and finishing	Coordination, detailing, and finishing	—

TABLE 19-3

Comparison of Pros and Cons of Continuous Archwire, Segmented, and Hybrid Sectional Mechanics

Continuous Archwire		Segmented		Hybrid Sectional	
Pros	**Cons**	**Pros**	**Cons**	**Pros**	**Cons**
Simple appliance	Indeterminate force system	Known force systems	Decreased ability to delegate	Simple appliance	Patient discomfort (loops)
Ease of arch coordination	Unable to avoid adverse tooth movements	Precise spring design	Difficulty in arch coordination	Ease of arch coordination	Uses small segments of expensive wires
Decreased chair-side time	Causes incisor proclination and round tripping	Minimizes adverse tooth movements	Increased chair-side time	Decreased chair-side time	
Increased ability to delegate			Patient discomfort (loops)	Ability to delegate	
Minimal or no loops			Difficulty with hygiene maintenance	Minimizes adverse tooth movements	
Ease of maintaining hygiene				Ease of maintaining hygiene	

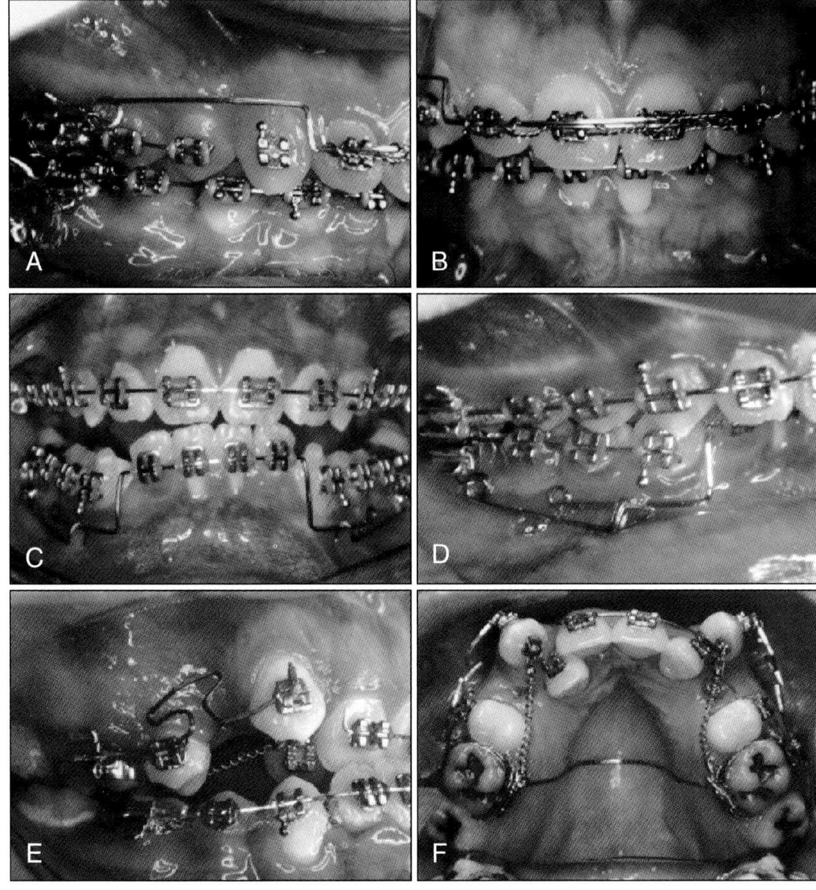

Fig. 19-7 Three clinical situations demonstrating aspects of segmented archwire mechanics. **A** and **B,** Intrusion of the upper incisors in which the intrusive arch is tied to the incisor segmental wire by two ligatures. Because the intrusive forces are anterior to the center of resistance of the incisors, these teeth will undergo some proclination during intrusion. **C** and **D,** Lower incisor intrusion using right and left intrusive cantilevers in which the intrusive forces are placed in the same plane as the center of resistance of the incisors and should result in pure intrusion. **E** and **F,** Space closure using a segmented titanium molybdenum alloy (TMA) closing loop. This mechanical approach requires cross-arch stabilization with a transpalatal arch (TPA).

19-7, *A* and *B*), or where the intrusive cantilever clips over the distal extension of the anterior segment wire (Fig. 19-7, *C* and *D*). During space closure, the anterior to posterior segment connection occurs only through the titanium molybdenum alloy (TMA) wire auxiliary closing loop, which connects the posterior segments from the first molar auxiliary tube to the canine that has a specialized bracket with a vertical or horizontal tube (Fig. 19-7, *E* and *F*).

If the TPA is not used or is used with imprecise or incorrect activation, arch form aberrations and poor segment alignment will result in various planes of space. Thus, for example, because the space closure forces are applied at a distance from the center of resistance of the posterior segments, these segments will undergo mesial rotation in the sagittal plane and palatal rotation in the transverse plane. The anterior segment does not undergo adverse movements because similar retraction forces are applied to both right and left sides of this segment.

Hybrid Sectional Mechanics

Hybrid sectional mechanics attempts to combine the simplicity and other advantages of continuous archwire mechanics with the precision and control of the segmented arch technique. This approach uses traditional twin brackets that are used in any practice and therefore offers the versatility to use either continuous archwire mechanics or hybrid sectional mechanics, or sequentially to use both mechanics, as required by the case and stage of treatment. The practitioner is also not required to have multiple bracket prescriptions or inventories of specialized brackets, easing difficulties in inventory control and minimizing staff and doctor confusion. Instead, it is the mechanics that are modified to address the needs of each patient.

As with segmented mechanics, if complexities or negative force systems are anticipated, hybrid sectional mechanics should be incorporated from the beginning as the individualized mechanics of choice for the patient. This enhances treatment efficiency by not moving teeth into adverse positions before moving the teeth to the desired position. In other cases, should problems arise during treatment with continuous archwire mechanics, hybrid sectional mechanics can be implemented without changing any brackets.

The underlying principle of hybrid sectional mechanics includes simplifying treatment by "segmenting" posterior and anterior regions of the arch. However, rather than employing true segments, a single continuous wire is placed in brackets from second molar up to the canines but bypassing the incisors (Fig. 19-8, *A* and *B*). The primary reason for this segmentation is that it eliminates the early engagement and round tripping of the incisors, potentially eliminating or minimizing its adverse consequences (see Figs. 19-3 and 19-6). Also, because anterior teeth are more often poorly aligned while the posterior teeth are more reasonably positioned, not engaging the incisor segments and having a long span of unengaged wire in the anterior region allows treatment to be initiated in heavier wires, permitting retraction of the canines very early in treatment.

The hybrid sectional mechanics technique is also compatible with different wire sizes and materials in different segments of the arch, as a variation of Burstone's principle of "variable-modulus orthodontics."[31] This strategic combination of wires and mechanics enables different types of tooth movement, such as canine retraction, incisor alignment, and incisor intrusion, to be performed concurrently, as summarized in Table 19-4, thereby reducing the patient's overall treatment time, relative to continuous archwire mechanics

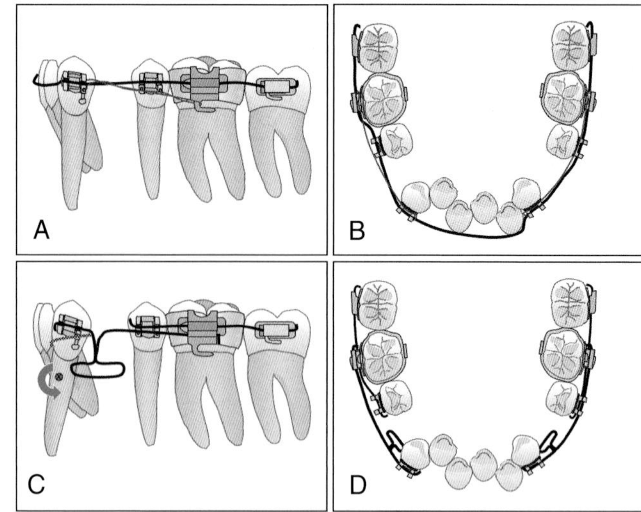

Fig. 19-8 Step 1 of hybrid sectional mechanics is performed if the canines or posterior teeth are not well aligned. **A** and **B,** Use of a .018 × .018 or .018 × .025–inch continuous Ni-Ti archwire in the posterior teeth and canine brackets that bypasses the incisors. **C** and **D,** Use of segmented .017 × .025–inch TMA retraction or uprighting spring combined with Ni-Ti segmented wires in the brackets on the posterior teeth.

(Table 19-5). The sequence of treatment with hybrid sectional mechanics is similar to that of segmented mechanics, except that aligning and leveling are performed concurrently with canine and incisor retraction, such that as soon as these stages are completed, detailing and finishing can be implemented.

Hybrid sectional mechanics is strongly indicated in patients with moderate to severe incisor crowding in whom extractions will be performed and where round tripping of teeth is undesirable (see Table 19-1). The sequence of mechanics and wires with this approach is summarized in Table 19-4. After extraction of the premolars, the first and second molars are banded or bonded, and the premolars and canines are bonded. If the posterior dentition is poorly aligned, initial alignment is performed usually using .018 × .018–inch or .018 × .025–inch Ni-Ti wire in a .022-inch slot, or smaller wires in a .018-inch slot (Fig. 19-8, *A* and *B*).

In patients in whom the canine root has moderate or severe mesial inclination, a .017 × .025–inch TMA T-loop segmented retraction spring should be used to distalize the root into adequate alignment to avoid the adverse consequences of correcting with a continuous archwire, as discussed previously (Fig. 19-8, *C* and *D*). The T-loop is engaged in the auxiliary tube of molar and canine bracket and activated approximately 30 to 40 degrees (alpha leg) to provide an uprighting moment to the canine. The segment is then cinched both anteriorly and posteriorly to provide a constraining force so that distal canine root movement rather than mesial canine crown movement occurs. The effects of the resultant extrusive forces on molars can be minimized by engaging a sectional wire in the premolar and molar

TABLE 19-4

Sequence of Procedures and Wires in Classic Hybrid Sectional Mechanics*

Step	Stage	Clinical Presentation	Materials and Mechanics
1	Initial canine/posterior teeth alignment	Mesially inclined canine roots Poor alignment of posterior teeth	Distal root tip with .017 × .025–inch TMA T-loop. .018 × .018 or 0.018 × 0.025–inch Ni-Ti wire bypassing incisors.
2A	Canine retraction and incisor unraveling	Canines corrected in step 1 or minimally malaligned canines	.016 × .022 or .018 × .025–inch SS anterior stepdown archwire; retract canines with Ni-Ti springs or power chains.
2B	Canine retraction and incisor alignment	Incisors unraveled	Continue canine retraction as above. Bond 2-2 and place Ni-Ti wire; increase up to .016 × .022 or .018 × .025–inch SS wire.
2C	Canine retraction and incisor intrusion	Incisors aligned	Continue canine retraction as above. Intrude incisors when necessary by piggyback of incisor segment on stepdown wire.
3	Incisor retraction	Minimal <2 mm	Place .018 × .025–inch SS continuous archwire and consolidate with Ni-Ti springs or power chains.
		Moderate >2 mm	Use .019 × .025–inch TMA T-closing loop.
4	Detailing and finishing	Minimal detailing	.019 × .025 or .021 × .025–inch SS archwire depending on desired torque expression.
		Substantial detailing	.019 × .025 or .021 × .025–inch TMA archwire depending on desired torque expression.

*Using .022-inch bracket slot. The wire sizes can be adjusted down in size when using .018-inch bracket slot.
Ni-Ti, Nickel-titanium; *SS,* stainless steel; *TMA,* titanium molybdenum alloy.

TABLE 19-5

Approximate Treatment Time: Continuous Archwire vs. Hybrid Sectional

Continuous Archwire		Hybrid Sectional	
Step	**Duration**	**Step**	**Duration**
Leveling and aligning	3-5 mo	Canine retraction, incisor aligning and leveling	0-3 mo *or* 5-7 mo
Canine retraction	5-7 mo	Incisor retraction and, if necessary, leveling	3-5 mo
Incisor retraction	4-6 mo	Coordination, detailing, and finishing	3-5 mo
Coordination, detailing, and finishing	3-5 mo	—	
Total	15-23 mo	Total	11-20 mo

brackets, as described earlier (see Fig. 19-4). Once the second-order canine correction has been obtained, the loop and the canine tip-back can be reactivated to continue translational canine retraction, or the case can be converted to hybrid sectional mechanics.

Continuous archwire mechanics is also contraindicated in cases where the canine has moderate to severe distal root or mesial crown tip, as previously described (see Fig. 19-3). Although mild mesial canine crown angulations can be managed through hybrid sectional mechanics with the canine bracket tied back, canines with moderate or severe angulation require segmental uprighting springs with auxiliaries incorporated into the system to prevent undesirable tooth movements (see Fig. 19-4 and Fig. 19-8, *C* and *D*).

Once initial alignment is achieved, the patient is then ready to begin the next step of canine retraction using methods similar to those used for cases in which the canines and posterior teeth are initially well aligned. In these latter cases, the first step involving posterior segment alignment or canine correction can be skipped. Instead, a moderate-stiffness .016 × 0.022–inch or 0.018 × 0.025–inch stainless steel wire with an anterior stepdown bend about 5 mm in height can be used for mild alignment and to start retracting the canines (Fig. 19-9, *A* and *B*). To prevent mesial canine crown movement in situations where the canine root is mildly mesially inclined, the canine should be tied back to the molar with a stainless steel ligature tie. For patient comfort, plastic tubing should be placed around the anterior region of the initial Ni-Ti wire (if used in the first stage) or the stainless steel wire in the area that bypasses the incisors. Because of multiple long, interbracket wire spans, the clinician should cinch back these initial wires to prevent them from dislodging from the molar tubes and causing patient discomfort.

Canine retraction is performed with either elastomeric power chain or Ni-Ti coil springs. This results in the incisors unraveling and aligning as space develops during canine

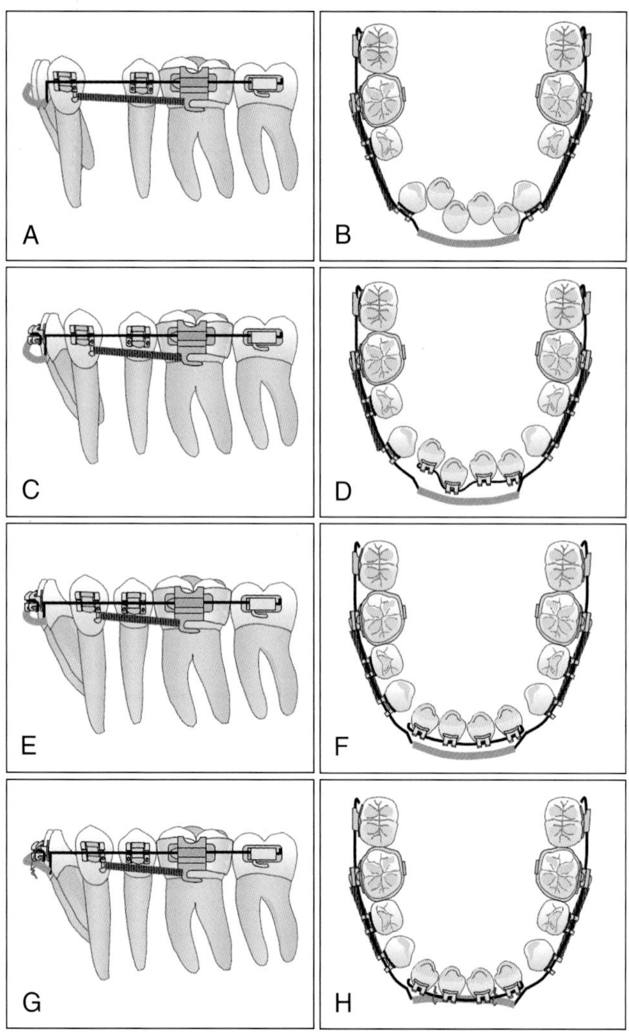

Fig. 19-9 Step 2 of hybrid sectional mechanics. **A** and **B,** If the canines and posterior teeth are relatively well aligned or have undergone initial alignment (as described in Fig. 19-8), .016 × .022 or .018 × .025–inch stainless steel archwires are placed with a 5-mm gingival step anteriorly, and canine retraction is started. **C** and **D,** When the incisors have unraveled and sufficient space for their alignment is evident, the incisors are bonded and aligned with Ni-Ti wire while canine retraction continues. **E** and **F,** After incisor alignment, .016 × .022 or .018 × .025–inch stainless steel segment is placed on these teeth. **G** and **H,** If any incisor intrusion is indicated, the anterior segment is tightly ligated to the gingival step in the main archwire while canine retraction proceeds.

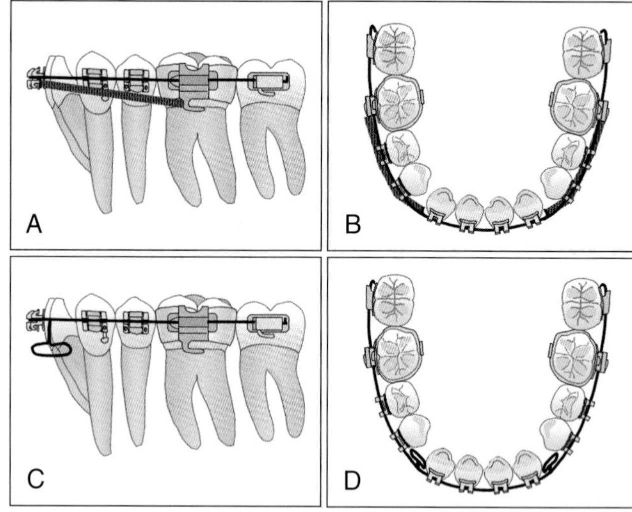

Fig. 19-10 Step 3 of hybrid sectional mechanics. **A** and **B,** Small residual spaces (<2 mm) can be closed with Ni-Ti springs placed on a hook on the wire or elastomeric chain tied to the distal wing of the lateral incisors, with all incisors ligated together. **C** and **D,** Consolidation of larger spaces (>2 mm) can be performed with .019 × .025–inch TMA closing T-loops.

retraction. Once the incisors have unraveled adequately, where they have minimal or no overlap, they are bonded and aligned without flaring (Fig. 19-9, *C* and *D*). Initial alignment of the anterior segment can be accomplished with the anterior segment of a .016 or .018 × .018–inch Ni-Ti arch. A segment from the patient's archwire utilized in the first stage of initial posterior teeth and canine alignment can be reused in the anterior segment at this stage, thereby reducing material costs. When initial alignment of the anterior teeth has occurred, a stiffer stainless steel segment, usually .016 × .022 or .018 × .025–inch, is placed in the anterior portion of the arch (Fig. 19-9, *E* and *F*). If there is a deep bite and incisor intrusion is indicated, this wire segment is ligated to the gingival step down region of the main stainless steel archwire (Fig. 19-9, *G* and *H*). Although these intrusive forces lie facial to the center of resistance of the incisors and will contribute to some mild proclination of the incisors, these teeth are generally fairly upright at this stage in hybrid sectional mechanics, and their proclination is often desirable. Canine retraction can continue during the incisor alignment and incisor intrusion stages of treatment.

Once the canines are completely retracted and incisor alignment and leveling have occurred, the third stage of hybrid sectional mechanics involving residual space closure is initiated. Because in the previous stages of treatment the size and stiffness of the anterior segment wire have been increased to the same or similar stiffness as the main step-down archwire, the arches at this stage are often well aligned and leveled enough to place a relatively stiff continuous archwire. Thus, with few exceptions, as when tooth compensations need to be maintained, at this stage the case is ready to be switched to routine continuous archwire mechanics.

In cases of severe crowding, minimal residual space will likely be left to close following canine retraction and incisor unraveling. When 2 mm or less of residual space is present, space closure can be performed on a continuous arch stainless steel wire (usually .018 × .025–inch) in one of several ways. One particularly attractive method involves retracting the incisors with Ni-Ti closed-coil springs attached to the molar hook and to a hook on the archwire located distal to the incisors (Fig. 19-10, *A* and *B*). If incisor torque must be maintained, a curve can be swept into the archwire. Alternatively, standard edgewise techniques of placing anterior torque in the wire can be used to maintain incisor torque.

In less severely crowded cases, more space may exist at the end of the canine retraction and incisor alignment stage. When the amount of space closure exceeds 2 mm, incisor retraction is performed with a continuous 0.019 × 0.025–inch TMA T-loop (Fig. 19-10, *C* and *D*), using a mild reverse or accentuated curve to maintain incisor torque. If the clinician prefers to revert back to his or her continuous arch space closure mechanics of choice, including wires with alternative loop designs, he or she can do so at this treatment stage.

The final stage of treatment involves detailing the occlusion and finishing. Two key clinical considerations in selecting the archwire size and material for this stage are the desired degree of torque to be expressed and the magnitude of detailing required. Cases that require high torque expression are usually finished in .021 × .025–inch wires, whereas those that require lower torque expression are finished in .019 × .025–inch wires. Also, when greater detailing is required, TMA archwires are beneficial to allow larger activations without generating high force levels. If minimal detailing is required, stainless steel archwires can be used.

Examples of the use of hybrid sectional mechanics are presented in the following three cases.

Hybrid sectional mechanics in a moderately crowded case

An adult male patient presented for orthodontic treatment with a Class I molar relationship bilaterally, an end-on-end right canine relationship, and a retained primary left maxillary canine showing Class I relationship (Fig. 19-11, *A-H*). The maxillary right canine is positioned buccally with significant distal rotation, and the maxillary right first premolar is distally rotated. The maxillary left canine is palatally impacted. The maxillary right second premolar is extremely carious with only retained roots present. The mandibular arch has moderate to severe dental crowding with a buccally positioned and mesially rotated right canine.

Without the maxillary left canine impaction and the unsalvageable maxillary right second premolar, this case would commonly be treated with four first premolar extrac-

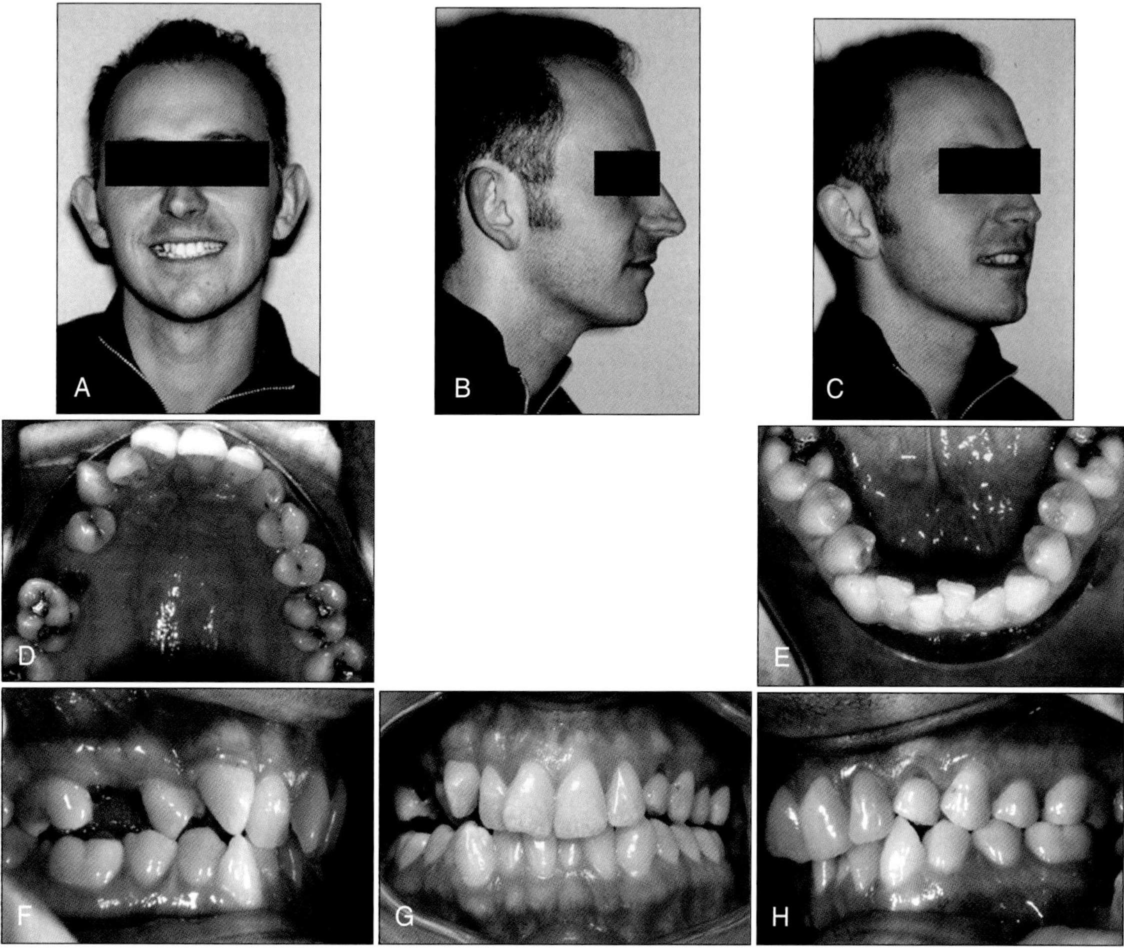

Fig. 19-11 **A** to **H,** Pretreatment facial and intraoral photographs of patient with nontraditional extraction pattern, asymmetric dental rotations, and moderate crowding. The maxillary left canine was palatally impacted, maxillary right second premolar was nonsalvageable, and the severely rotated maxillary right canine made the case ideal for hybrid sectional mechanics.

Continued

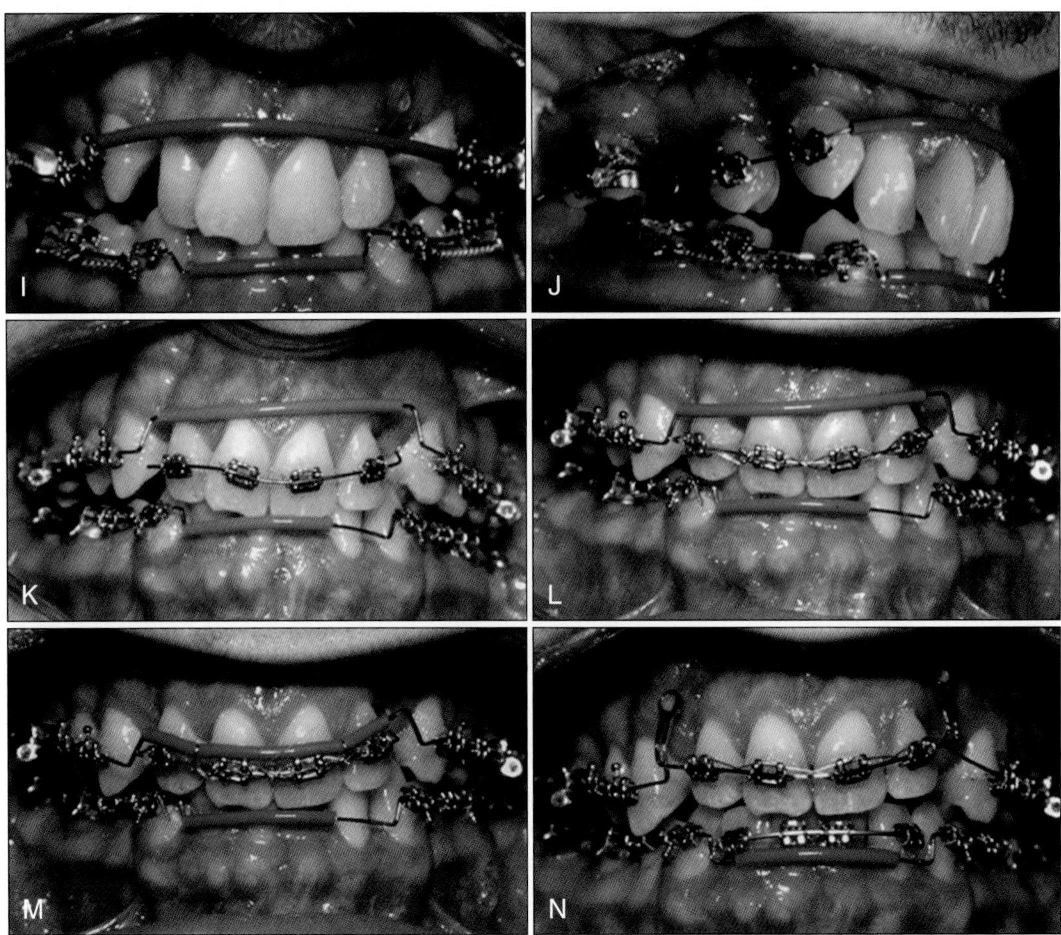

Fig. 19-11, cont'd **I** and **J,** Initial alignment in the upper arch was performed with a Ni-Ti archwire. Because the lower posterior teeth were relatively well aligned, treatment that included canine retraction with Ni-Ti springs was commenced in a stainless steel anterior stepdown archwire. **K,** As maxillary incisors unraveled, these teeth were initially aligned with a Ni-Ti wire segment. The lower incisors continued to unravel as the canines were retracted. **L** and **M,** Once the maxillary incisors were adequately aligned, a stainless steel segment was inserted and intrusive forces were applied by tying the segment to the anterior stepped archwire. The lower incisors continued to unravel, leaving minimal residual spaces to be closed. **N,** Finally, with the bite opened, a helical closing loop was fabricated to retract, torque, and intrude the maxillary anterior dentition. Final treatment would involve the use of continuous archwires to consolidate residual spaces and upper and lower arch detailing.

tions. However, because of the patient's desire to keep treatment as short as possible and the questionable prognosis of the impacted maxillary left canine, this tooth, the maxillary right second premolar roots, and lower first premolars were extracted to address the tooth size–arch length discrepancy. This resulted in the implementation of asymmetric treatment mechanics. Because of the crowding, the tissue constraints, and the anchorage needs, it was decided to treat this patient with hybrid sectional mechanics rather than continuous archwire mechanics.

To best illustrate the need for specialized mechanics in this patient, each quadrant is examined individually to compare the force system that would be generated by continuous archwire mechanics as opposed to the force system that can be created with hybrid sectional mechanics. Placing a continuous wire into all the teeth of the maxillary right quadrant would result in a significant flaring tendency of the maxillary incisors. This proclining force is produced in two ways: (1) the distal rotation of the maxillary right canine, which causes the wire to exit buccally from the mesial aspect of the canine bracket, and (2) the severe distal root tip of the canine, which would lead to intrusion and flaring of the incisors with a continuous archwire. Although cinching back on this wire would somewhat reduce the flaring forces, it would also lead to enhanced anchorage loss. The combined flaring and intrusion would likely result in an iatrogenic, unilateral anterior open bite as observed in a previous case (see Fig. 19-3).

On the surface, the maxillary left quadrant does not appear to have any potential pitfalls; however, changing the extraction pattern also changes the anchorage needs. Extracting farther forward in the maxillary left quadrant than in the mandibular left quadrant will result in different or asymmetric anchorage needs in the two arches. In addition, because the maxillary left first premolar needs to function as the canine and is currently in a Class III "canine" relationship, the anchorage must be carefully titrated in this quadrant. The mandibular left canine needs to move distally through the entire extraction space, or the maxillary left quadrant needs to shift forward, or some combination of both, to allow the first premolar to function in the canine position.

The 6 mm of crowding in the mandibular arch, in addition to the requirement to maintain a Class I molar relationship, dictates moderate to maximum anchorage requirements. If continuous archwire mechanics is used, it will be difficult to achieve these high-anchorage needs. In addition, placing a continuous lower archwire would result in proclination of the lower incisors, with potential adverse effects on periodontal tissue integrity and inefficient treatment resulting from round tripping.

The case was treated using hybrid sectional mechanics (Fig. 19-11, *I-N*). Alignment of the maxillary posterior segments was performed with a .018 × .025–inch cinched Ni-Ti archwire (*I*). The lower canines were aligned and retracted with Ni-Ti coil springs on a .016 × .022–inch stainless steel archwire with a small gingival step in the incisor region (*I* and *J*). Following alignment of the maxillary buccal segment, the upper canine retraction was performed on a .016 × .022–inch stainless steel anterior step down archwire using Ni-Ti springs. As canine retraction progressed, sufficient space was created in the maxillary anterior region to begin initial alignment with a segmented Ni-Ti wire *(K)*. The lower incisors were allowed to continue to unravel on their own because of the actions of the transseptal fibers as the canines were retracted. Next, the upper incisor segment was increased in stiffness to a .016 × .022–inch stainless steel wire *(L)*. A mild intrusive force was applied from the incisor segment to the gingivally stepped main archwire *(M)*. This resulted in the 5-mm overbite decreasing to 2 mm within 2 months (*M* and *N*). During this time the lower canines were retracted completely, and the lower incisors continued to unravel, leaving minimal residual space for closure. These incisors were bonded and aligned (*N*), and spaces were then consolidated with Ni-Ti springs on a continuous stainless steel archwire as described previously (see Fig. 19-10, *A* and *B*). A helical closing-loop continuous archwire was placed both to retract and to provide a labial crown/palatal root torque to the maxillary incisors *(N)*. After incisor retraction, the case was finished with continuous archwires as already discussed.

Maintaining compensations using hybrid sectional mechanics

A different clinical situation where hybrid sectional mechanics can also be beneficial is in the group of patients who present with dental compensations caused by an underlying skeletal discrepancy. As part of the patient consultation, the orthodontist must educate the patient regarding the cause(s) of the malocclusion and the treatment options. Some patients then choose to proceed with surgery, whereas others request a nonsurgical treatment approach when possible. With mild skeletal discrepancies, an orthodontics-only approach may be possible. Generally, when orthodontic camouflage treatment is performed in these patients, rather than removing the dental compensations, the pretreatment compensations need to be maintained or potentially even increased. Maintaining dental compensations with continuous archwire mechanics can be difficult, particularly when trying to minimize incisor flare in one or both arches. The use of hybrid sectional mechanics in a patient requiring maintenance of dental compensations is demonstrated in the following case.

A postadolescent female patient presented with a well-balanced, esthetic face and smile in the frontal view (Fig. 19-12, *A-H*). She exhibited a mildly concave profile, largely because of a mild decrease in midface projection, as well as a slightly increased mandibular projection with a Wits measurement of −6 mm. Intraorally, she had Class III molar and canine relationship, minimal overbite, slight midline discrepancy of approximately 1.5 mm, and anterior crossbite on four teeth. The lower canines were also positioned facially, such that placing a continuous archwire would have resulted in proclination of the incisors, thereby aggravating the anterior crossbite. Cephalometrically, the lower incisors were retroclined (Fig. 19-12, *I*).

After a conference with oral and maxillofacial surgeons, it was determined that both nonsurgical and surgical options were feasible. Because of the existing favorable profile and smile esthetics, not addressing the underlying Class III skeletal relationship provided a viable nonsurgical option. However, when correcting such a skeletal malocclusion with an orthodontics-only approach, it is important to consider the magnitude of orthodontic movement required to correct the malocclusion, and whether it will be feasible before initiating treatment. In this patient, because of the level of mandibular crowding, Class III molars, and dental compensations, it was determined that an orthodontics-only approach would be possible with lower premolar extractions, provided that the incisor compensations were maintained. After a presentation of the nonsurgical and surgical options to the patient, she opted to pursue the orthodontics-only option.

After extraction of the lower first premolars, hybrid sectional rather than continuous archwire mechanics was used in the lower arch to minimize the likelihood of removing the dental compensations, avoid round tripping and its accompanying potential for tissue damage, and enhance treatment efficiency. Besides the negative effects of round tripping on anchorage control, this patient presented with narrow alveolar structures (Fig. 19-12, *I*) around the lower incisor roots that would likely be accompanied by periodontal bone loss if the teeth were flared. To maintain the incisor compensations throughout treatment, hybrid mechanics was contin-

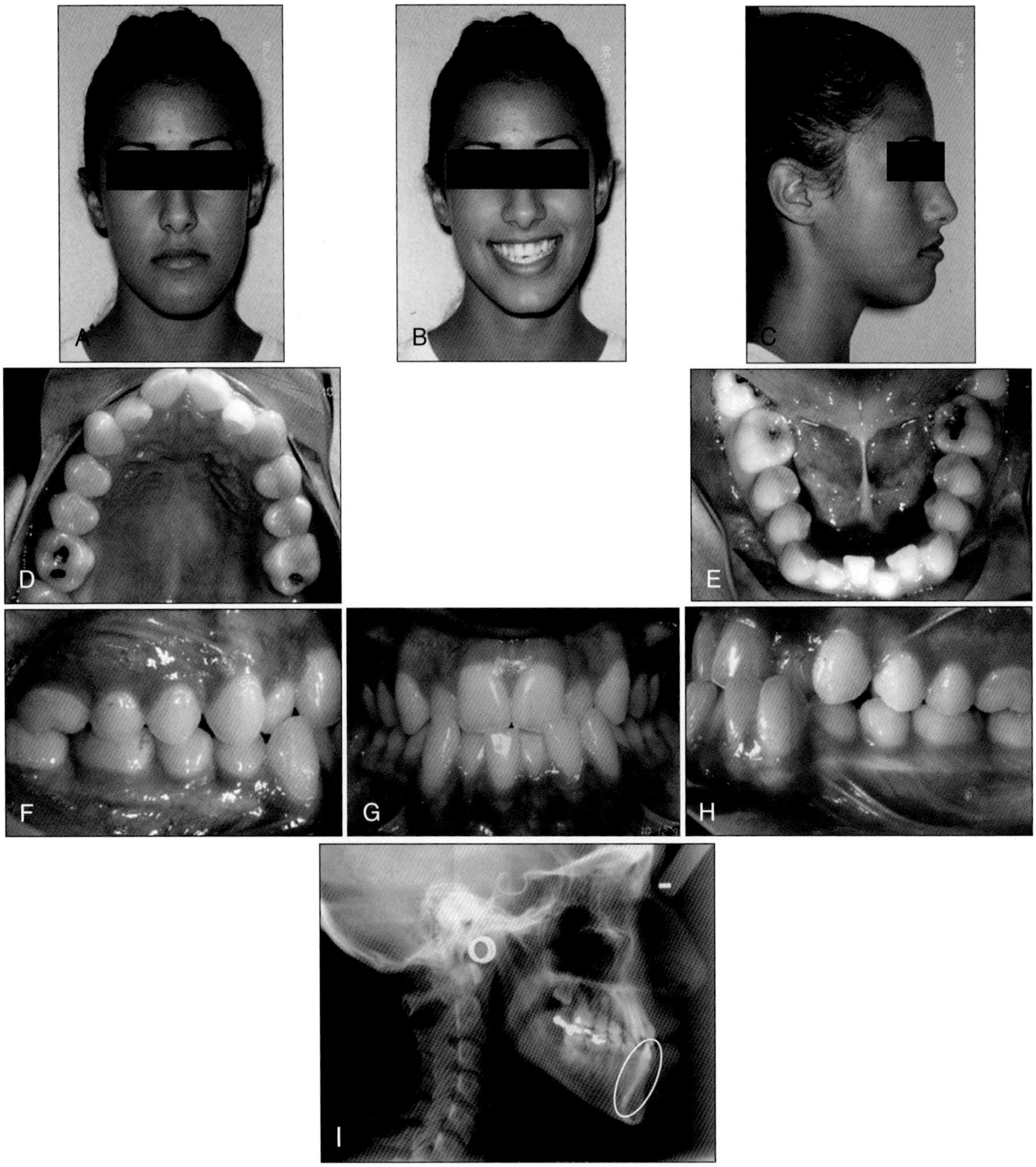

Fig. 19-12 **A** to **H,** Pretreatment facial and intraoral photographs of a patient with a mild skeletal and dental Class III malocclusion. An orthodontics-only treatment was performed because the skeletal malocclusion was mild and the patient preferred nonsurgical treatment. To aid in maintaining the incisor compensations and keep these teeth within the narrow alveolar housing (seen in **I**), hybrid sectional mechanics were used in the lower arch from start to finish of treatment. **I,** Pretreatment cephalogram showing retroclined lower incisors that are placed within a very narrow alveolar housing.

ued to the end of treatment. In the maxilla, because of minimal crowding and a desire for mild proclination of the maxillary incisors, continuous archwire mechanics was used.

The progress photographs show retraction of the lower canines and alignment of lower incisor segment while maintaining good anchorage and lower incisor compensations (Fig. 19-12, *J* and *K*). Had continuous archwire mechanics been used, even with extractions, the lower incisors would have first flared such that a complete anterior crossbite would have been established. This would also have increased the potential for anchorage loss in the lower arch into a greater than full-cusp Class III relationship. By pitting only the lower canines against the rest of the lower arch, anchorage was preserved. The use of hybrid sectional mechanics prevented incisor round tripping.

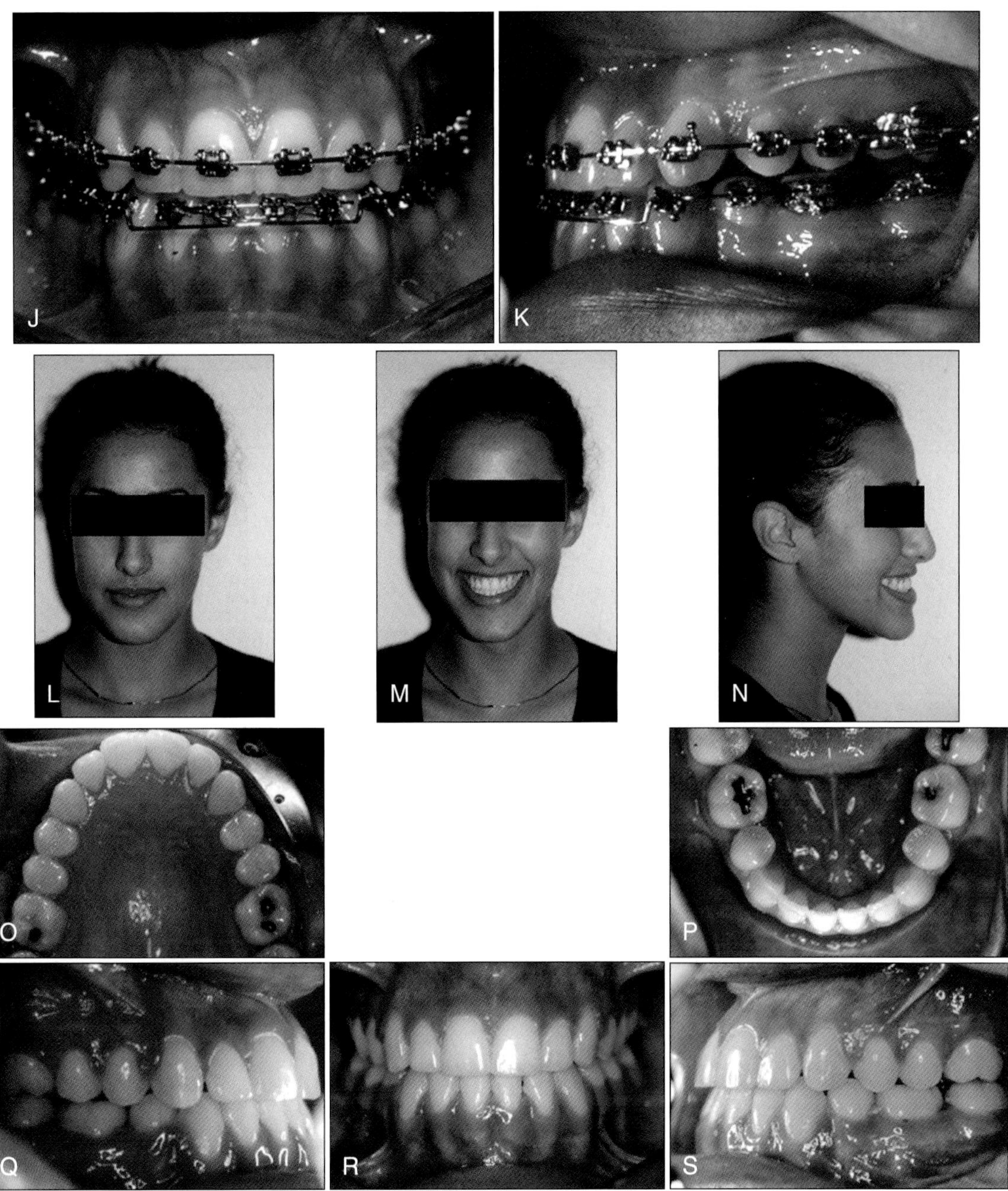

Fig. 19-12, cont'd **J** and **K,** Progress photographs demonstrate excellent maxillary and mandibular alignment and preservation of the mandibular incisor compensations resulting from use of lower hybrid sectional mechanics. **L** to **S,** Patient's treatment, which lasted only 18 months, was performed entirely with hybrid sectional mechanics in the mandibular arch to maintain lower incisor compensations. Posttreatment photographs show a well-interdigitated Class I canine relationship after lower first premolar extraction treatment.

The posttreatment results showed that the facial esthetics were maintained or even improved, dental compensations maintained, midlines corrected, and ideal overbite and overjet achieved in only 18 months (Fig. 19-12, *L-S*). Also important to note is the absence of tissue destruction.

Modifications to hybrid sectional mechanics

Hybrid sectional mechanics can also be used in other, nontraditional ways as demonstrated in the following case.

An adult male patient presented with a long, narrow face and mandibular asymmetry to the left (Fig. 19-13, *A-H*). Intraorally, he demonstrated a significant 5-mm anterior

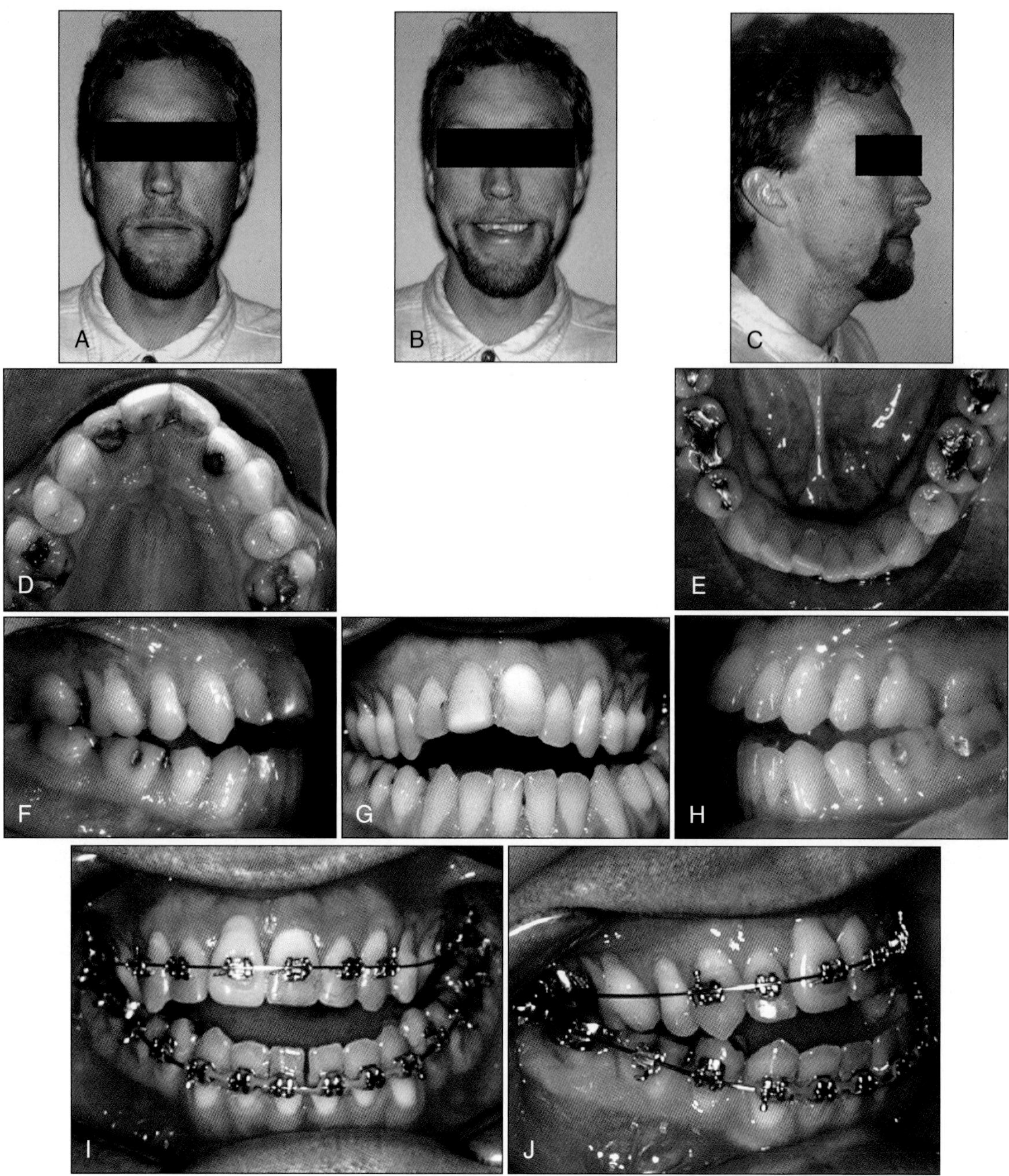

Fig. 19-13 **A** to **H,** Pretreatment facial and intraoral photographs of a patient previously treated with four first premolar extractions and maxillary expansion as an adolescent. Note complications resulting from the periodontal condition, missing maxillary incisor, and open bite. These complicating factors precluded the use of long-term traditional orthodontics. **I** and **J,** Presurgical photographs showing that the maxillary premolars and first molars were not bonded at the beginning of treatment, to avoid dental expansion and further periodontal bone loss. These teeth were bonded just before surgery, and a passive stainless steel archwire was placed to minimize undesirable orthodontic arch expansion.

open bite and a maxillary transverse deficiency with bilateral posterior crossbite, but a reasonably well-aligned mandibular arch. His previous orthodontic treatment as an adolescent included four first premolar extractions and maxillary expansion that had relapsed. In addition to the orthodontic problems, he had significant gingival recession and loss of alveolar bone support on the maxillary right and left first molars and second premolars. In addition, the maxillary incisors had moderate root resorption.

Before initiating care, the patient was referred for periodontal evaluation. A frank discussion of the potential consequences of further orthodontic treatment was necessary

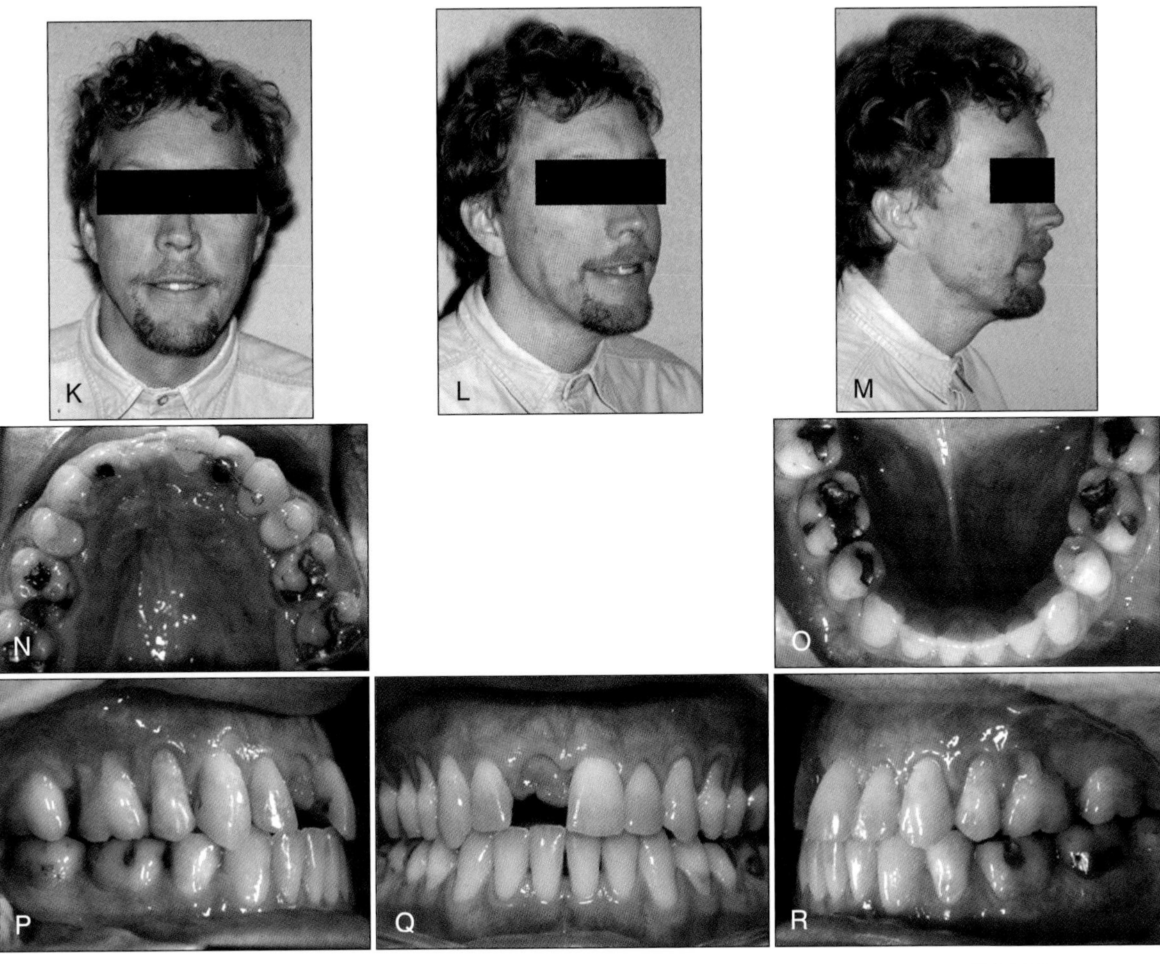

Fig. 19-13, cont'd K to R, By carefully planning the mechanics and performing most of the movements surgically in the maxilla, an excellent result was obtained in this patient, who traditionally would have been turned away from treatment.

because multiple teeth were at risk of being lost from root resorption or lack of periodontal support. After periodontal consultation and scaling, the plan included removing his maxillary incisor pontic and placing full orthodontic appliances in the mandibular arch and limited presurgical upper arch appliances to minimize dental expansion. His surgical treatment would include two-jaw orthognathic surgery to impact and expand the maxilla while simultaneously addressing the mandibular asymmetry.

The mandibular arch was treated with continuous archwire mechanics to realign and level the arch. The mandible was used as the template arch to determine the amount of segmental surgical maxillary expansion that would be required. In the maxillary arch, brackets were placed on all teeth except the maxillary second premolars and first molars so as to avoid any further orthodontic expansion and additional bone loss presurgically. This essentially resulted in segmented approach to treatment. Immediately before surgery (Fig. 19-13, *I* and *J*), brackets were placed on the maxillary teeth that were previously not bonded, and a continuous archwire was placed passively in all the brackets. During surgery the maxilla was segmented distal to the maxillary canines bilaterally. Through a combination of inferiorly positioning the maxillary anterior segment and superiorly positioning the right and left posterior segments, the maxilla was leveled and expanded simultaneously to fit the mandibular template arch. Additionally, a mandibular surgery was performed to correct that mandibular asymmetry.

After surgery, minimal orthodontic manipulation was required. A space was left for a maxillary right central incisor implant. Although this represents a nontraditional approach, an excellent result was obtained (Fig. 19-13, *K-R*). A modification of hybrid sectional mechanics with careful attention not to expand the maxillary posterior segments orthodontically allowed a severely compromised case to be treated with minimally increased risk to the dentition.

CONCLUSION

Continuous archwire mechanics has several advantages; it can be used in a relatively large number of cases and offers simplified and assistant-delegated treatment approach.

Unfortunately, continuous archwire mechanics also has several limitations. These include its limited ability to produce differential anchorage, optimal tooth movements, or control for adverse responses in complex cases, as well as its ability to cause round tripping of teeth, with potential adverse effects on anchorage and tissue integrity. With a sound foundation in biomechanical principles, a clinician can utilize alternate mechanics, including segmented and hybrid sectional mechanics, as viable and desired options in complex and compromised cases. Segmented mechanics provides excellent control but limited ability for chair-side delegation and potential difficulties in arch and segment coordination. Hybrid sectional mechanics strives to provide the ease of use similar to that of continuous archwire mechanics with the versatility and control of tooth movements associated with segmented mechanics.

To obtain optimal and efficient treatment, the clinician must select the ideal mechanical approach for the individual patient and arch. A well-considered proactive selection of optimal biomechanics, careful appliance design, and implementation of strategies to minimize adverse tooth movements are likely to produce the most desirable and efficient results in any orthodontic patient.

References

1. Proffit WR: Equilibrium theory revisited: factors influencing position of the teeth, *Angle Orthod* 48:175-186, 1978.
2. Deberardinis M, Stretesky T, Sinha P, Nanda RS: Evaluation of the vertical holding appliance in treatment of high-angle patients, *Am J Orthod Dentofacial Orthop* 117:700-705, 2000.
3. Christiansen RL, Burstone CJ: Centers of rotation within the periodontal space, *Am J Orthod* 55:353-369, 1969.
4. Burstone CJ, Koenig HA: Force systems from an ideal arch, *Am J Orthod* 65:270-289, 1974.
5. Koenig HA, Vanderby R, Solonche DJ, Burstone CJ: Force systems from orthodontic appliances: an analytical and experimental comparison, *J Biomech Eng* 102:294-300, 1980.
6. Ricketts RM, Bench RW, Gugino CF, et al: *Bioprogressive therapy,* Denver, 1979, Rocky Mountain Orthodontics.
7. Garcia-Morales P, Buschang PH, Throckmorton GS, English JD: Maximum bite force, muscle efficiency and mechanical advantage in children with vertical growth patterns, *Eur J Orthod* 25:265-272, 2003.
8. Throckmorton GS, Finn RA, Bell WH: Biomechanics of differences in lower facial height, *Am J Orthod* 77:410-420, 1980.
9. Alstad S, Zachrisson BU: Longitudinal study of periodontal condition associated with orthodontic treatment in adolescents, *Am J Orthod* 76:277-286, 1979.
10. Dorfman HS: Mucogingival changes resulting from mandibular incisor tooth movement, *Am J Orthod* 74:286-297, 1978.
11. Trentini CM, Moriarty JD, Phillips C, Tulloch JF: Evaluation of the use of orthodontic records to measure the width of keratinized tissue, *J Periodontol* 66:438-442, 1995.
12. Kaley J, Phillips C: Factors related to root resorption in edgewise practice, *Angle Orthod* 61:125-132, 1991.
13. Hollender L, Ronnerman A, Thilander B: Root resorption, marginal bone support and clinical crown length in orthodontically treated patients, *Eur J Orthod* 2:197-205, 1980.
14. Reitan K: Initial tissue behavior during apical root resorption, *Angle Orthod* 44:68-82, 1974.
15. Melsen B, Allais D: Factors of importance for the development of dehiscences during labial movement of mandibular incisors: a retrospective study of adult orthodontic patients, *Am J Orthod Dentofacial Orthop* 127:552-561, 2005.
16. Wehrbein H, Bauer W, Diedrich P: Mandibular incisors, alveolar bone, and symphysis after orthodontic treatment: a retrospective study, *Am J Orthod Dentofacial Orthop* 110:239-246, 1996.
17. Handelman CS: The anterior alveolus: its importance in limiting orthodontic treatment and its influence on the occurrence of iatrogenic sequelae, *Angle Orthod* 66:95-110, 1996.
18. Burstone CJ: The segmented arch approach to space closure, *Am J Orthod* 82:361-378, 1982.
19. Braun S, Sjursen RC Jr, Legan HL: On the management of extraction sites, *Am J Orthod Dentofacial Orthop* 112:645-655, 1997.
20. Zablocki HL, McNamara JA Jr, Franchi L, Baccetti T: Effect of the transpalatal arch during extraction treatment, *Am J Orthod Dentofacial Orthop* 133:852-860, 2008.
21. Faber RD: Occlusograms in orthodontic treatment planning, *J Clin Orthod* 26:396-401, 1992.
22. White LW: The clinical use of occlusograms, *J Clin Orthod* 16:92-103, 1982.
23. Marcotte MR: The use of the occlusogram in planning orthodontic treatment, *Am J Orthod* 69:655-667, 1976.
24. Fiorelli G, Melsen B: The "3-D occlusogram" software, *Am J Orthod Dentofacial Orthop* 116:363-368, 1999.
25. Burstone CJ: The mechanics of the segmented arch techniques, *Angle Orthod* 36:99-120, 1966.
26. Burstone CJ: Rationale of the segmented arch, *Am J Orthod* 48:805-822, 1962.
27. Marcotte MR: *Biomechanics in orthodontics,* St Louis, 1990, Mosby.
28. Burstone CJ: Precision lingual arches: active applications, *J Clin Orthod* 23:101-109, 1989.
29. Burstone CJ, Koenig HA: Precision adjustment of the transpalatal lingual arch: computer arch form predetermination, *Am J Orthod* 79:115-133, 1981.
30. Burstone CJ, Manhartsberger C: Precision lingual arches: passive applications, *J Clin Orthod* 22:444-451, 1988.
31. Burstone CJ: Variable-modulus orthodontics, *Am J Orthod* 80:1-16, 1981.

CHAPTER 20

Role of Orthodontics in Obstructive Sleep Apnea

■ *R. Scott Conley and Harry L. Legan*

Depending on the disease progression, chronic *obstructive sleep apnea* (OSA) can be a severely debilitating disorder. People of all ages can be affected, but middle-age adult men who are moderately to severely overweight have the highest prevalence of OSA.[1] Women can be affected, but to a lesser degree.[2] Recently, OSA is being increasingly seen in the pediatric and adolescent populations.[3] Some of these patients may be unaware of the condition and may not see their primary care physician routinely.[4]

With expertise in facial growth and development as well as craniofacial and dentofacial anomalies, orthodontic professionals should be equipped to provide treatment for OSA patients. Several treatment modalities exist to improve a patient's sleep pattern.[5-9] Successful treatment will improve a patient's subjective as well as objective assessment of their daytime alertness.[10-13]

DIAGNOSIS AND CLASSIFICATION

Adult orthodontics has become more common in recent years, and thus OSA patients are more likely to present at the orthodontic office for examination and consultation. The classic presenting symptom of OSA is excessive daytime sleepiness. The Epworth Sleepiness Scale is a simple, inexpensive screening tool.[14] Patients are asked a series of questions to assess their relative "sleep health." However, this test does not distinguish between OSA and the many other types of sleep-disordered breathing (e.g., restless legs syndrome).

Accurate diagnosis of OSA requires an overnight polysomnographic examination.[15] Independent sleep clinics and full-service hospitals with sleep clinics can perform the test. *Polysomnography* combines multiple tests, including electroencephalography (EEG), electrocardiography (ECG), electro-oculography (EOG), electromyography (EMG), respiratory rate, tidal volume, inspiratory/expiratory volume, as well as the number and severity of apneas and hypopneas. An *apnea* is defined as any cessation in breathing for 10 seconds or more with an arterial oxygen desaturation of 2% to 4%.[16] A *hypopnea* is defined as a 50% decrease in airflow for 10 seconds or more with a concomitant drop in arterial oxygen saturation.[16] The exact magnitude of desaturation for a hypopnea varies in the literature. Central apnea must also be differentiated from obstructive apnea.[17] Patients with *obstructive* apnea typically display respiratory effort without being able to ventilate adequately. Patients with *central apnea* exhibit decreased respiratory effort. The distinction between central and obstructive apnea is essential in determining the most appropriate treatment for the individual patient; certain treatments are effective only for obstructive apnea.

Polysomnography typically provides a patient score reflecting the number of apneas and hypopneas, called the *apnea/hypopnea index* (AHI). This may also be reported as the *respiratory disturbance index* (RDI). The AHI and RDI are slightly different but essentially interchangeable. Patients in normal sleep have an RDI of 5 or less. Patients with *mild* sleep apnea have an RDI of 5 to 15, with *moderate* sleep apnea typically 15 to 30 events and *severe* apnea 30 or more events per hour.[16] To illustrate the clinical significance of this scale, a patient with an RDI of 60 stops breathing or has a significant oxygen desaturation for at least 10 seconds every minute. Depending on the length of the apnea/hypopnea, significant reduction in oxygen perfusion to the brain can occur, causing increased risk of stroke, myocardial infarction, and other cardiac conditions.

The criteria used to determine successful treatment of OSA varies widely. For most successful outcomes, clinicians strive to achieve at least a 50% reduction in the RDI, or an

RDI of less than 20. More stringent criteria for success involve achieving a posttreatment RDI of less than 10. A recent report states that successfully treated patients have no increased morbidity or mortality.[18] Untreated individuals have 37% greater 5-year morbidity and mortality.[13] These statistics result from the higher incidence of motor vehicle accidents, heart attack, stroke, arrhythmia, and hypertension. One study concluded that the incidence of motor vehicle crashes in OSA patients can be compared with driving while intoxicated, which presents a major public health risk.[19,20]

NONDENTAL OR NONORTHODONTIC TREATMENT

Once a patient is diagnosed with obstructive sleep apnea, the most appropriate treatment is determined. Because many OSA patients are overweight, one treatment option includes weight loss. Reports vary, but some investigations have shown that significant weight loss can reduce a person's RDI as much as 50%.[5] In patients who are obese (>120% of ideal body weight, or body mass index [BMI] >30) or morbidly obese (>200% of ideal weight, or BMI >40), the weight loss can also help improve overall health status. Overweight patients who lose significant amounts of weight can greatly reduce or eliminate such problems as hypertension, type 2 diabetes, orthopedic conditions, and cardiac/stroke risks.

Other habits that can reduce the symptoms and severity of the sleep apnea include stopping alcohol consumption 3 hours before sleep.[6] Alcohol acts as a respiratory depressant. Studies show that mild or borderline OSA can become frank obstructive sleep apnea after the patient is challenged with 3 ounces of 80 proof alcohol. Both the duration and the depth of sleep are greatly reduced, as is the amount of time in rapid eye movement (REM) sleep.

Sleep position also can dramatically affect the amount and quality of sleep.[21] Patients sleeping in the supine position will notice that the laxity in the soft tissues combined with gravity often increases the number and severity of apneas and hypopneas. Positional aids to assist the patient in maintaining a lateral decubitus position for sleep can significantly improve the RDI.

Continuous Positive Air Pressure

A common treatment modality for OSA is continuous positive air pressure (CPAP)[7] (Fig. 20-1).

Whether the patient is diagnosed with obstructive or central apnea, CPAP can successfully reduce the symptoms. In addition, CPAP can effectively treat the mildest cases to the most severe cases of sleep apnea. CPAP works by forcing air into the nasopharynx and oropharynx to maintain airway patency.

After diagnosis, the clinician provides a prescription for a CPAP machine. To test the efficacy and to titrate to the proper settings, a second polysomnography is performed, or the second half of the diagnostic polysomnography is conducted with CPAP in place. The mask is fitted to the patient, and the patient is allowed to return to sleep. Once the apneas and hypopneas begin, the airflow and air pressure can be adjusted to bring the RDI into the normal range. The goal is to have the patient at the lowest possible flow rate and pressure that will ensure a patent airway. This allows an increase in the settings should the patient's airway accommodate over time and begin to collapse again.

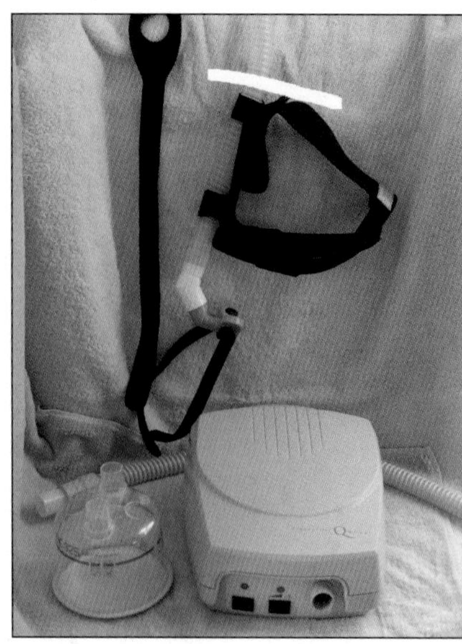

Fig. 20-1 Continuous positive air pressure (CPAP) machine can be worn at night to maintain airway patency. Air is pushed from the machine into one of many different styles of mask. Models vary; some warm and humidify the air to minimize patient discomfort and increase patient compliance.

ORTHODONTIC AND DENTAL TREATMENT

Oral appliances have repeatedly been shown to be an effective form of treatment for mild to moderate OSA.[22,23] If a patient with severe sleep apnea (RDI >30) cannot tolerate CPAP and is not a surgical candidate or refuses surgical correction, a dental appliance can be the most acceptable form of treatment. In fact, recent studies from the Cochrane Collaboration have shown higher efficacy with oral appliances than with uvulopalatopharyngoplasty or other forms of soft tissue surgery.[24]

Oral Appliances

Multiple appliance designs exist, both custom and stock. Before selecting a particular dental appliance, the patient must undergo the same polysomnography to determine the type, severity, and location of the obstruction. If the site is the upper airway (nasal cavity or retropalatal area), efficacy of mandibular protrusion appliances and tongue-retaining devices may be limited. In patients with hypertrophic tonsils and adenoids as well as a tongue obstruction, the efficacy of the dental appliance may be improved by tonsillectomy and adenoidectomy.

Tongue-positioning appliances

In the supine position, all gravity-dependent tissues, including the tongue, will tend to fall posteriorly unless otherwise supported. The tongue base is held anteriorly by the genial tubercles. If this support is insufficient, a tongue-retaining device can be used. To fit a tongue appliance, a piece of dental floss is gently wrapped around the tongue, removed, and measured (Fig. 20-2, *A*).

The appliance comes in three sizes: small, medium, and large. If the tongue is between two sizes, the manufacturer recommends using the larger of the two sizes. This appliance also comes in two styles: an intraoral appliance for patients with a full dentition and an extraoral design for patients with multiple missing teeth. The bulb of the appliance is moistened and compressed, and the tongue is inserted into the bulb. Both suction and the adhesion from the thin film of saliva on the plastic maintain the tongue in a more forward position, opening the oropharyngeal airway. This class of appliance is used infrequently because most patients find it uncomfortable and choose not to use it long term.

In rare cases the tongue can be surgically tethered to the genial tubercles, creating ankyloglossia ("tongue-tie"). Because of the associated speech defects, this is not usually performed.

Mandibular positioning appliances

A second class of appliances is available to protrude the mandible and assist in maintaining this forward position during sleep (Fig. 20-2, *B*). The appliances are removable, allowing the patient to use the appliance each night. Because it is smaller than a CPAP machine, the appliance is more mobile and can be taken on trips. The specific protrusion appliance can be individually selected for the patient using multiple factors, including cost, convenience, durability, adjustability, and patient comfort. Because anterior repositioning appliances function similarly, the patient and clinician can choose the most appropriate and comfortable appliance. Compliance is essential; for just as with CPAP, if the appliance is not worn, no improvement is observed.

Almeida, Lowe, et al.[25,26] studied potential side effects or changes to the bite resulting from long-term use of a dental sleep appliance. They observed tremendous variation, from minimal dental movement to both dental and apparent skeletal movement of the mandible. Many patients with more marked dental and skeletal changes had positive occlusal change with improvement of a Class II malocclusion. In some patients a Class I relationship was obtained. Some Class I patients became mildly Class III. Because the appliance's primary function was to cure the sleep apnea, occlusal changes usually were not treated. It is unclear whether occlusal changes would persist if appliance use were discontinued.

To fabricate these appliances, typically, upper and lower dental impressions are obtained. Range of motion is measured, including maximum opening, left and right lateral excursion, and maximum protrusion. The appliance is constructed using a position approximately one half to two thirds the patient's maximum protrusion and several millimeters open. Custom bite registrations in centric occlusion and the construction position are obtained. A George gauge can be helpful in stabilizing the patient in the construction bite position. The impressions and bite registrations can then be sent to a commercial laboratory for appliance fabrication, or an appliance may be made on site. In-house appliances may be fabricated and delivered more quickly and are more cost-effective for the patient. After delivery, the patient returns for assessment of appliance fit, comfort, and potential changes in the bite.

A positive-pressure thermoforming machine (e.g., BioStar, Great Lakes Orthodontics, Tonawanda, N.Y.) can be used to make a relatively inexpensive but effective mandibular positioning appliance (Fig. 20-2, *C*). A 2-mm-thick piece of thermoforming splint material can be formed over the maxillary model. Cold-cure acrylic can then be added to

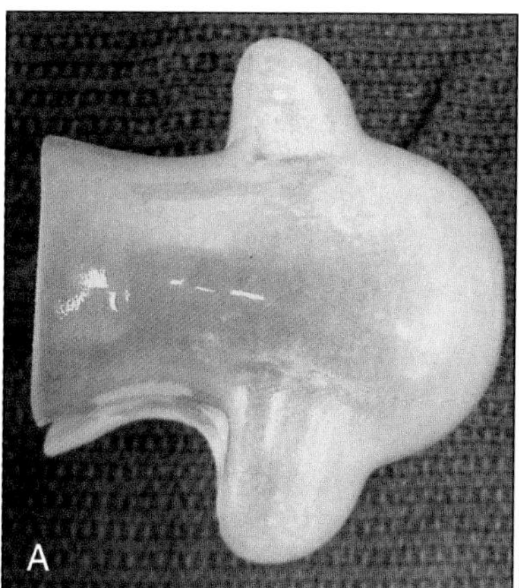

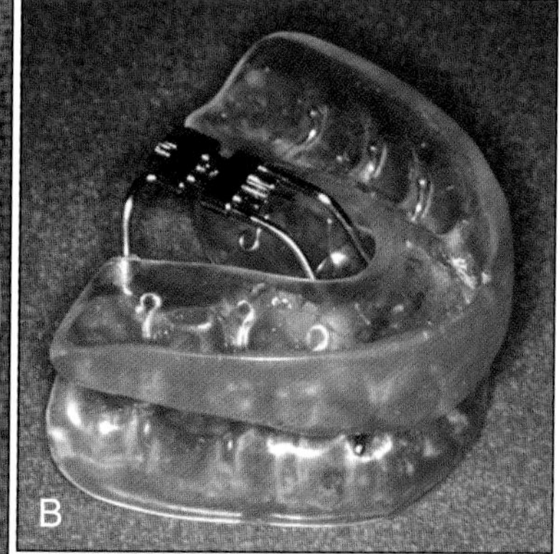

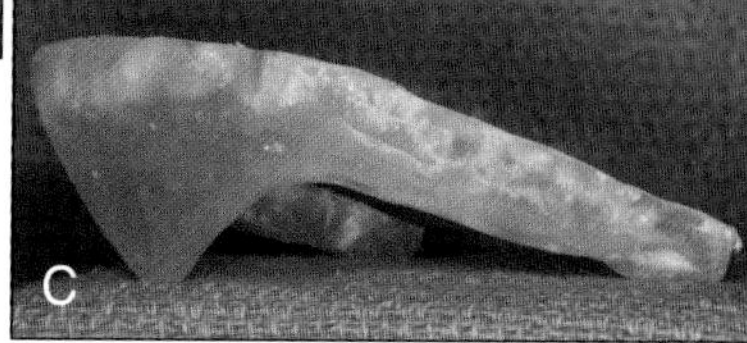

Fig. 20-2 **A,** Tongue-positioning bulbs can be used to hold the tongue in a more anterior position (Great Lakes Orthodontics, Tonawanda, N.Y.). Two styles are available: dentate and edentulous. **B,** Kleerway appliance acts to protrude the mandible during sleep (Great Lakes Orthodontics). **C,** Custom mandibular positioning appliance can be fabricated easily in-house to reduce patient costs. Each appliance should be evaluated with a follow-up sleep study and checked after the patient adequately acclimates, to assess the level of improvement. If incomplete correction is detected, alternate treatment therapies may be indicated.

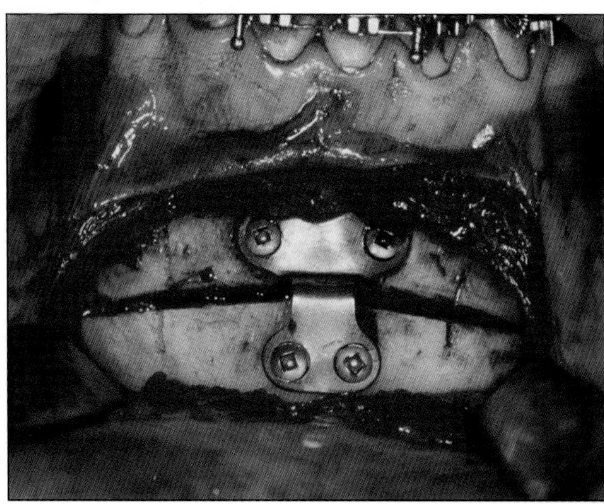

Fig. 20-3 Same advancement genioplasty done for esthetic reasons can also be done for the sleep apnea patient. The genial tubercles must be included in the "genial segment" so that both the genioglossus and the geniohyoid muscle are stretched. This increased stretch increases tissue tone and reduces the tendency for airway obstruction caused by the tongue falling against the back of the throat.

make a flange that extends inferiorly and palatally to rest gently against the lingual mucosa of the mandible in the protruded position. The flange can be altered by adding or removing the acrylic to advance or retract the mandible for patient comfort and additional symptom relief. A dental appliance also has the advantage of being relatively inexpensive and entirely reversible. If the patient does not obtain the desired and necessary improvement, no permanent changes have occurred, and alternative treatment options can be explored.

To measure the effect of the appliance, a lateral cephalometric radiograph taken in centric occlusion provides a baseline position for assessing later bite changes and determining the amount of airway opening. After appliance delivery and confirming patient comfort, a second radiograph can be taken to assess the two-dimensional change in the airway. Recent advances in three-dimensional imaging with cone-beam computed tomography may prove useful in the future to examine these airway changes with greater detail and accuracy.

Finally, it is important to obtain a follow-up sleep study with the appliance in place to objectively document the level of improvement. Some patients will report significant subjective change with the appliance, which may or may not be substantiated by the sleep test. If objective improvement is not observed, the patient should be provided alternate treatment options to improve the sleep apnea in measurable terms.

Surgical Orthodontic Options

Although dental appliances often work well in the patient with mild to moderate OSA, these devices are not universally effective and may not be appropriate in more severe cases. For patients with severe sleep apnea who do not want long-term CPAP, surgery is a viable treatment alternative. Surgery may be confined to the site of obstruction, such as with a uvulopalatopharyngoplasty (UPPP), or used as an aid in weight loss, such as bariatric surgery. Recent studies report only 40% long-term success with UPPP, however, and thus alternate forms of surgical intervention are being explored.

Genioplasty

An alternate first-tier surgical therapy for OSA is an advancement genioplasty.[27] The best candidates have a functional occlusion with good maxillomandibular skeletal positioning, but have deficient chin projection called *retrogenia* or microgenia. Retrogenia must be differentiated from retrognathia. With *retrognathia* the mandible is small and in a poor sagittal position, but the bony chin button may be adequate.

In some patients a standard genioplasty is performed, taking care to have the genial tubercles in the segment that is advanced (Fig. 20-3). Other osteotomy designs include advancing a full-thickness area of the mandibular symphysis containing the genial tubercles. Once the lingual cortex of the core of bone is buccal to the buccal cortex of the mandibular body, the core is rotated 90 degrees to maintain the advanced position.

Multiple minor variations in osteotomy design exist, based on anatomical restrictions and surgeon preference. If only partial resolution of the symptoms results from genioplasty alone, a second surgical phase of treatment that advances both the maxilla and the mandible can be performed.

Maxillomandibular advancement

Some OSA patients will elect to pursue maxillomandibular advancement (MMA) quickly because they want their symptoms resolved as soon as possible (Fig. 20-4). Because this does not allow presurgical orthodontic treatment, the published risks associated with MMA include postoperative malocclusion. The preferred approach should address the pretreatment malocclusion using presurgical orthodontic therapy to prepare the dental arches. CPAP or alternative forms of OSA treatment can be used to address the excessive daytime somnolence and the negative effects of OSA during this presurgical orthodontic phase. Once the dental arches complement each other, both an improved airway and an improved occlusion can be obtained concurrently.

Once MMA is complete and symptoms have resolved, CPAP can be discontinued.[28-30] Interestingly, patients undergoing orthognathic surgery often lose 10 or more pounds, which can be an additional source of health improvement and symptom resolution if maintained.

As with all surgical orthodontic patients, presurgical orthodontic therapy for MMA should focus on all three planes of space. The transverse, sagittal, and vertical relationship of the teeth and jaws should be assessed. The treatment plan must include where the teeth will be positioned in each jaw and where each jaw will be positioned relative to the cranial base. Special consideration is given to arch width, arch form, leveling, and arch length deficiency. Each aspect

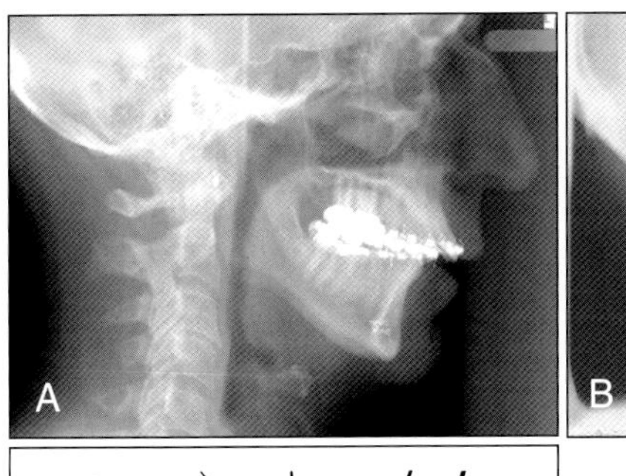

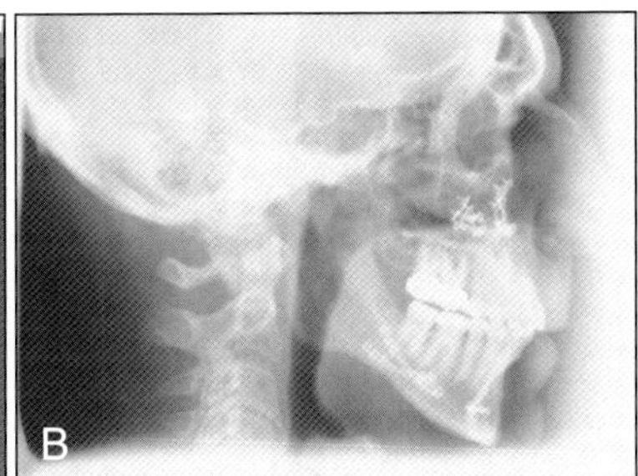

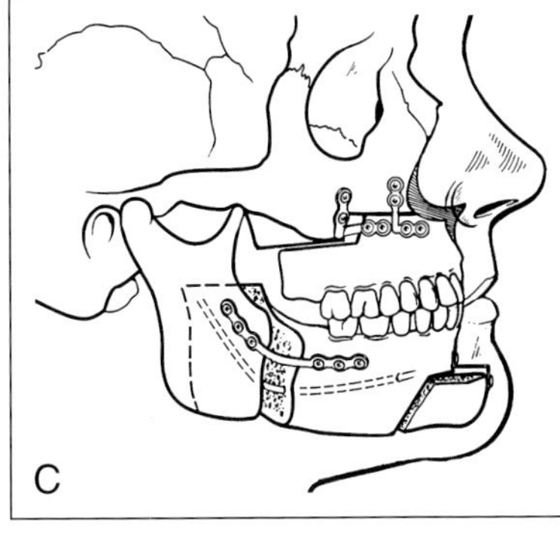

Fig. 20-4 Maxillomandibular advancement (MMA), one of the more successful treatments available for OSA patients. **A,** Pretreatment, and **B,** posttreatment, cephalograms demonstrating the magnitude of airway opening resulting from MMA. **C,** Diagrammatic representation of surgery and amount of advancement. (**C** courtesy Vanderbilt University Medical Arts Group, with consultation from Scott B. Boyd, DDS, PhD.)

is addressed separately here for ease of discussion but must be considered in a combined and coordinated manner.

Transverse dimension and arch form. The interarch transverse relationship is especially important in MMA. Without adequate attention to this dimension, the final position of the mandible relative to the maxilla may be adversely affected. To maximize improvement, when diagnostic models are taken, the orthodontist and oral surgeon should assess the transverse dimension in two positions: the current bite position and the anticipated final bite position. This is particularly important in significant Class II or Class III malocclusions. For example, a Class II patient may not have a frank crossbite in the presenting bite; however, as the mandible is advanced to Class I, either an edge-to-edge transverse relationship or a true crossbite may be observed. If undiagnosed, either the patient will have a crossbite postsurgically, or the mandible will not be advanced to Class I. Both leave the patient with a malocclusion. Conversely, Class III patients may demonstrate a crossbite during the initial examination, but when the maxilla is advanced relative to the mandible to Class I as part of the MMA, the patient may now have too much buccal overjet.

Although maxillary transverse excess can be easily managed by a .036-inch heat-treated stainless steel lingual arch to constrict the arch, the situation must be carefully evaluated before decreasing arch dimension in the OSA patient. Smaller arches leave less room for the tongue, which may exacerbate the sleep apnea. The planned orthodontic constriction might decrease the effectiveness of the MMA. This relationship is unclear at present, but a general rule with OSA should be to make *more* space, not less. Instead of constricting the maxilla, the clinician should consider increasing the dimension of the mandibular basal bone through transverse mandibular symphyseal distraction osteogenesis, as discussed later.

A useful tool to assist in the diagnosis of transverse problems is the occlusogram allows the practitioner to perform a treatment simulation on an acetate film[31-33] (Fig. 20-5). To construct this, all the teeth are traced on acetate. Orientation marks are made to establish the current anteroposterior (AP) position of the mandible to the maxilla. The ideal mandibular arch template is established first. AP changes in the mandible (relative to the maxilla) are performed by sliding the acetate forward to simulate a mandibular advancement or by sliding the mandibular acetate posteriorly to simulate a maxillary advancement. Now the ideal mandibular arch dimensions are transferred to the maxillary arch to establish the ideal maxillary arch size and arch form. Recent advances in modeling systems can allow this simulation to now be performed electronically.

Minor or mild maxillary or mandibular transverse deficiencies can be addressed with orthodontic therapy and mild (1-2 mm) arch and auxiliary wire expansion. In orthognathic surgery patients with smaller planned maxillary AP movement, moderate transverse deficiencies (e.g., 5-7 mm) can be addressed by segmenting the maxilla (Fig. 20-6, *A* and *B*). This enables both the AP and the transverse dimension to be corrected concurrently in a single stage segmental Le Fort I osteotomy.[34]

With the larger (10-12 mm) maxillary advancements routinely performed as a part of OSA treatment, many surgeons are hesitant to segment the maxillary arch at the same time as the advancement. If the maxillary transverse deficiency is severe (>7 mm), *transverse maxillary distraction osteogenesis* (previously "surgically assisted rapid maxillary expansion") is required as a first phase of surgery (Fig. 20-6, *C-E*). Following the expansion, a bite registration is recommended to accurately assess the magnitude of expansion that was achieved. It is important to ensure that adequate maxillary expansion was achieved at this stage while

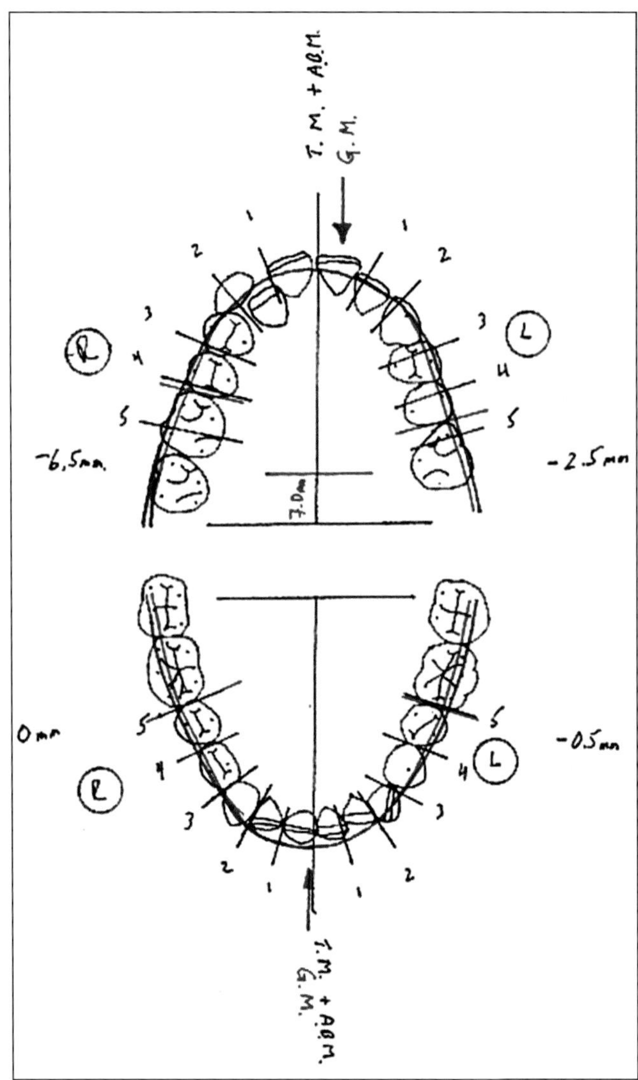

Fig. 20-5 Occlusogram, to assist in treatment planning. All the anticipated moves can be performed on the acetate film before placing bands and brackets. This can be regarded as a diagnostic wax-up performed on acetate.

additional expansion can still be obtained. It is recommended to mildly overexpand to allow for postsurgical relapse (taking care to keep teeth within alveolus).

Vertical dimension and leveling. Multiple orthodontic and surgical methods are available to achieve arch leveling. Some may produce the desired effect, whereas others may not. After determining the desired vertical position of the teeth within the face, the most appropriate orthodontic mechanics and type of surgical movement can be planned to achieve the stated goal. An important consideration to coordinate is the amount of vertical correction that will be performed by the orthodontist and how much will be performed by the oral surgeon. Both the method of leveling and the timing of leveling will be determined by the amount of leveling required. Various facial and occlusal patterns will somewhat dictate the most appropriate and most efficient time to level the dental arches.

Some orthodontic treatment plans state "place full fixed orthodontic appliances to level and align the dental arches." Although level arches will be present at surgery, this orthodontic plan is not specific enough; when, how, and where the leveling will be accomplished are important. If possible, a long face should not be lengthened unnecessarily with posterior extrusion. Similarly, the patient with a short face should not be forced to wait a year for surgery to obtain level arches if the teeth can be erupted more efficiently after surgery.

The short-face, deep-bite OSA patient can be viewed similarly to the classic surgical treatment of a short-face Class II mandibular advancement patient. Because of the tight orofacial musculature, if the bite can be opened during surgery, leveling within the mandible can be more efficiently performed postsurgically. Because the mandibular arch is not level at surgery, the interocclusal splint will be thicker, particularly in midarch. During the intermaxillary fixation period, the splint will remain in place. Once the intermaxillary fixation is removed, a heavy maxillary archwire and a relatively light mandibular archwire can be used. The patient is then given intermaxillary elastics to erupt the mandibular teeth into the interocclusal space (Fig. 20-7). This is extremely efficient because the impediment of the heavy occlusion has been removed. In addition, during this immediate postsurgical period, a *regional accelerative phenomenon* is observed.[35] It is especially important to ensure all the bands or brackets are firmly in place at this time. If a bracket or band is lost (or a hook becomes unusable), the tooth or group of teeth can remain gingival as the adjacent teeth are erupted. This vertical discrepancy can occur quickly and dramatically. It is advisable to see the patient more frequently during the immediate postoperative phase of treatment.

An alternative is *presurgical* leveling. Again, without special consideration and special techniques, presurgical leveling can be inefficient because of the heavy musculature and bite forces that are present. To increase efficiency, maxillary appliances with continuous archwires can be placed to align the arch. After a template arch is constructed, a maxillary impression can be taken. From this, a bite splint can be fabricated so that the mandibular incisors occlude on the acrylic of the bite splint and interocclusal space is created in the posterior. With a rigid maxillary arch and the bite splint, the mandibular dentition can be erupted in the same manner as described earlier for postsurgical leveling. The disadvantages of this second technique are the time required to enable insertion of a rigid maxillary archwire and patient compliance with the splint. In the presurgical patient without the bite splint (i.e., noncompliant patient), the heavy bite forces are still present, and only limited eruption will be observed. In addition, the advantage of the regional accelerative phenomenon is lost. The 6 to 9 months required to obtain the rigid maxillary archwire and no mandibular appliances in place delay the orthognathic surgery further. Sleep apnea patients need to proceed to surgery as quickly as reasonable, which this method does not accomplish.

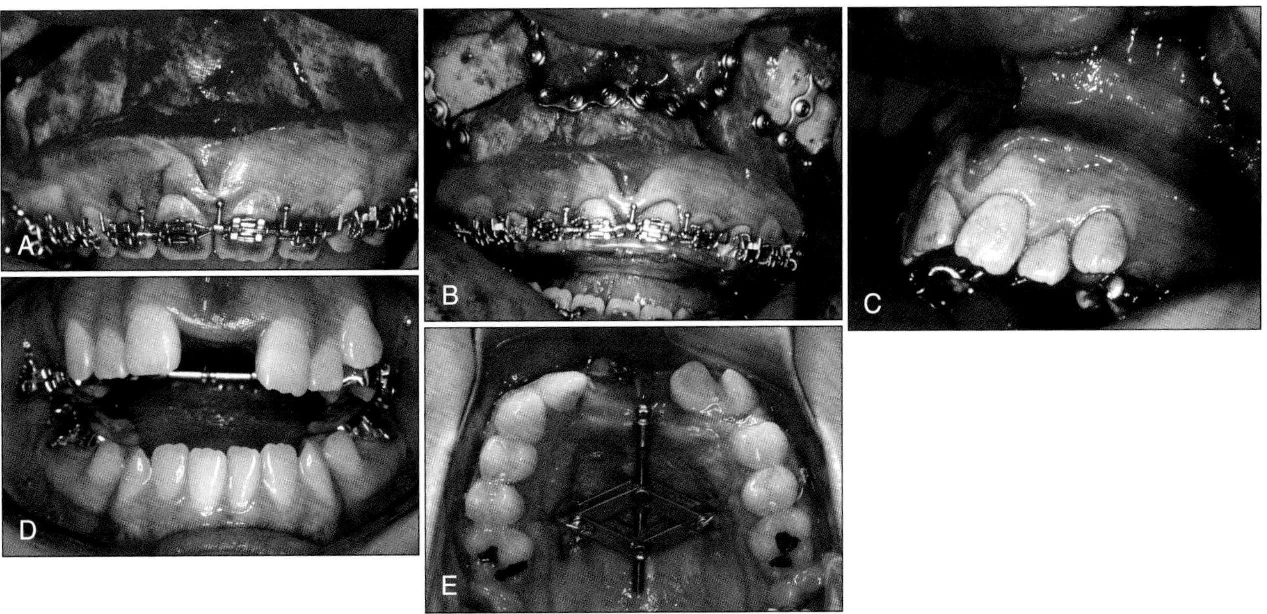

Fig. 20-6 Transverse dimension is often ignored, but several methods exist for evaluating and expanding the maxilla. **A** and **B,** Segmental maxillary osteotomy for expansion. **C** and **D,** Surgical-assist rapid palatal expander. **E,** Maxillary transverse distractor (KLS Martin Group, Tuttlingen, Germany).

An alternative to an acrylic bite splint is bonding composite buildups on the lingual surface of the upper incisors. Unfortunately, these can debond or break and are difficult to clean, and many adult patients complain and object to their placement. However, if the patient is not continually breaking them, the stops do give the practitioner the ability to place mandibular appliances at the same visit as the maxillary appliances resulting in less time lost in presurgical orthodontic treatment.

In some cases, it is not the mandibular curve of Spee that requires leveling, but a maxillary reverse curve of Spee that is most dramatically observed in Class II Division 2 patients. In this malocclusion, the maxillary incisors typically have erupted beyond the maxillary functional occlusal plane and are upright. This prohibits the mandibular advancement from occurring if the overbite is not corrected before surgery. A very effective way to improve the vertical position of the maxillary incisors is a segmental intrusive base arch.[40] In preparation for placing the intrusive base arch, brackets are placed in the upper arch. Wire segments are placed from the maxillary second molar to the canine or first premolar and from the lateral incisor to lateral incisor. A .017 × .025–inch stainless steel auxiliary wire can then be placed with two and a half helices. The intrusive base arch is then activated to deliver approximately 20 to 25 g of force per tooth (if incisor intrusion is desired) or higher forces (200+ g if posterior eruption is desired). These force levels can be measured with a Dontrix gauge. The helices bent into the intrusive base arch increase the length of the wire and improve the load deflection rate, which creates a longer acting and much more consistent force system.

The same type of leveling force system can be delivered with a beta titanium wire. Alternatively, there are commer-

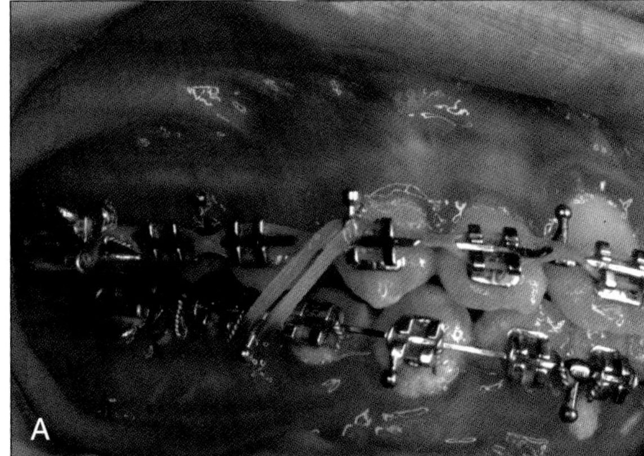

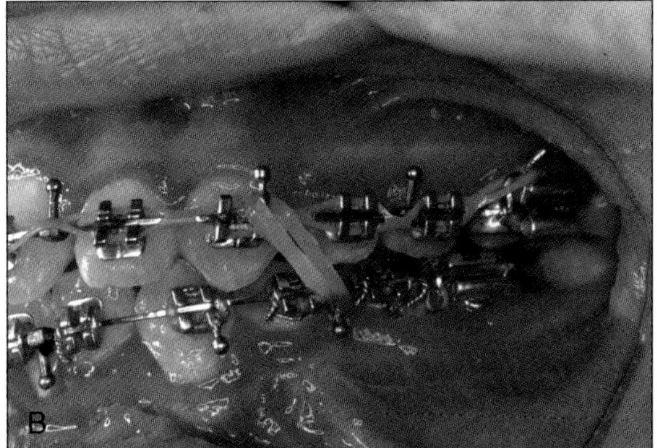

Fig. 20-7 Surgical leveling in the short-face patient can be more efficient in some cases when performed postsurgically. **A** and **B,** When rigid fixation is used, heavy elastics from the lower arch (which has lighter archwire) can be placed against the maxillary arch. The teeth are erupting into air rather than into the heavy forces of occlusion that were present before surgery.

cially available nickel-titanium (Ni-Ti) archwires that have been fabricated by the manufacturer with a V bend in the posterior aspect of the wire.

It is important to note that regardless of the wire material (stainless steel, beta titanium, or nickel titanium) the intrusive base archwire should not be placed into the bracket slots of the teeth to be intruded. Because the wire is rectangular, it can deliver torque in addition to the intrusive force. Depending on the wire bracket orientation, the torque can be additive (i.e., additional intrusion is present in the force system), or it can even negate the intrusive force system if a large amount of labial crown torque is present. It is impossible to know which situation is present. As a result, an indeterminate or unknown (and potentially undesirable) force system is present. To prevent this, the intrusive base arch should be ligated just gingival to the bracket.

Long-face patients may have deep overbite, moderate overbite, or an open bite. In addition, they may present with one occlusal plane or multiple occlusal planes. The long-face, open-bite patient with multiple occlusal planes and sleep apnea poses additional challenges. Typically, an open-bite patient's treatment plan consists of maxillary impaction, with or without a mandibular procedure depending on the amount of occlusal plane change. When the maxillary arch is at one consistent level, the patient is commonly planned for a single-piece Le Fort I osteotomy. When multiple occlusal planes are present, the non-OSA patient may be best treated with a three-segment Le Fort I osteotomy to assist with leveling the maxillary arch. In this plane of space, the segmentation site is primarily determined by the location of the different occlusal planes. If the occlusal plane "break" occurs in the canine area, the maxilla is segmented distal to the canine. If the "break" is instead in the incisor area only, the segments are made between the maxillary canine and lateral incisor. This must be planned in concert with the transverse considerations mentioned earlier in the chapter. Similarly, in the mandible the anterior portion of the dental arch can be repositioned surgically to aid leveling. The mandibular anterior subapical osteotomy can be performed to position the segment inferiorly in patients with extreme deep bite (Fig. 20-8).

With the significant 10- to 12-mm sagittal movements performed in sleep apnea surgery, many surgeons are uncomfortable with segmenting the maxilla as described previously and then advancing the segmented maxilla such a large distance. The primary surgical concern is that the pedicle providing the vascular support for the maxilla is being stretched significantly with the maxillary advancement alone. Additional stretching of the pedicle by segmenting the arch increases the risk of kinking the pedicle. Any kink in the pedicle decreases the vascular supply and increases the risk of necrosis of the affected maxillary segment(s). Instead, even though the stability of erupting the incisors may be less than the stability of surgically repositioning the anterior segment, the surgeon may want the incisors erupted to enable them to perform a single-piece Le Fort I osteotomy.

Because of the potential surgical segmentation restrictions with the OSA patient, an extrusive base arch may be used to erupt the maxillary incisors to obtain a uniform level for the maxillary arch. A similar segmental archwire setup can be placed, with the segment site determined by the location of the different occlusal planes. Once segmented, the same .017 × .025–inch stainless steel archwire with two and a half helices can be fabricated. The difference is that the wire will be positioned occlusal to the incisor brackets rather than gingival (Fig. 20-9). The extrusive base arch will then be ligated to the occlusal aspect of the maxillary incisor (and

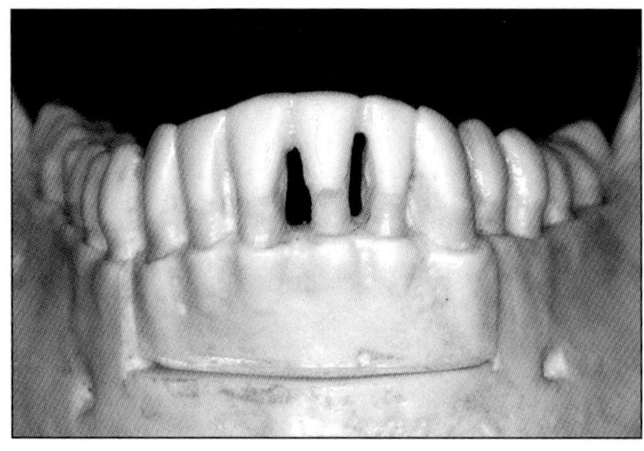

Fig. 20-8 Surgical leveling can also be obtained through segmental maxillary and mandibular subapical osteotomies. Care must be taken to avoid damage to the roots when making the interdental osteotomy, and occasionally roots must be diverged before surgery. The horizontal osteotomy is performed at least 5 mm apical to the root apices to minimize the risk of devitalizing the teeth. Although an excellent procedure, this is not routinely performed.

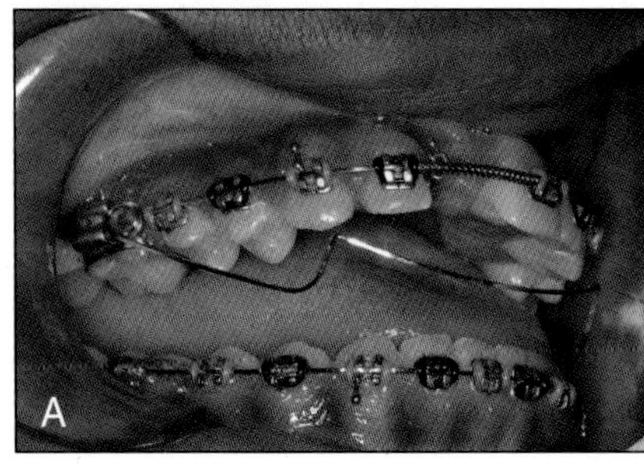

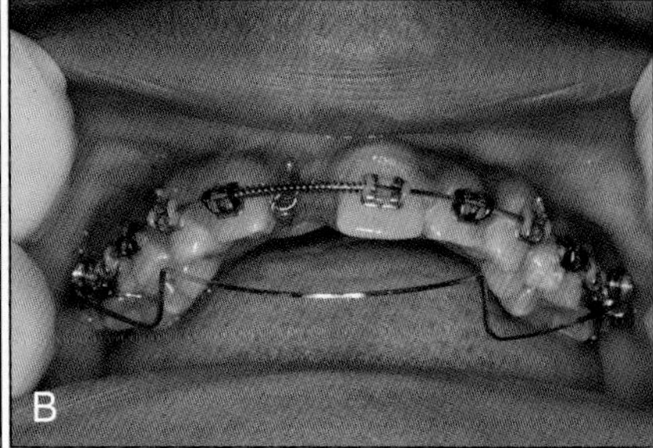

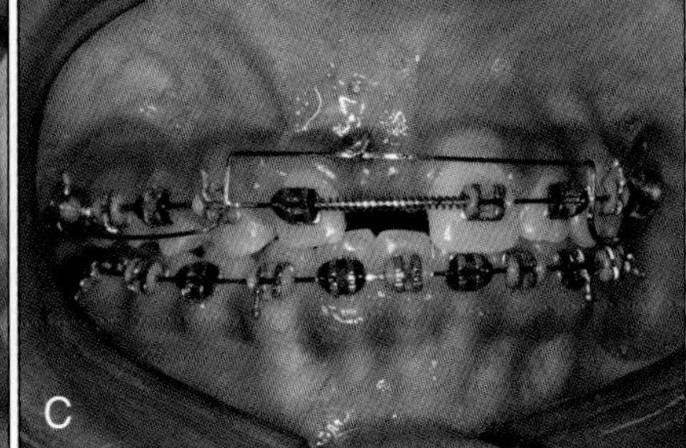

Fig. 20-9 Extrusive base arches are employed when eruption of one incisor is necessary.

perhaps canine) brackets. This can be augmented with interarch elastics if desired, but care should be taken not to deliver too much eruptive force, causing overeruption of the teeth. Once the teeth are all on the same level, a continuous stainless steel archwire can be placed to maintain the level occlusal plane. If not stabilized, the osteoid apical to the incisor tooth roots cannot mineralize. As a result, without the more rigid archwire, the newly erupted teeth can reintrude rather quickly.

Once the maxillary dentition is leveled orthodontically, the vertical position of the maxillary and mandibular dentition must be considered. If the incisor display is objectionable but the posterior maxillary position deemed appropriate, the anterior maxilla can be impacted as it is advanced (i.e., counterclockwise rotation of maxilla as viewed from right side of face). If the entire maxilla is inferiorly positioned, the whole maxilla may be impacted in parallel fashion. If the incisor display is not objectionable but a long face is present, the posterior maxilla can be impacted as the advancement occurs (i.e., clockwise rotation of maxilla). When performing differential or rotational impaction of the maxilla, the clinician must also examine the potential effect on chin projection. Even though the mandible is coming forward, the steepening of the occlusal plane (clockwise rotation of maxillary occlusal plane), tends to make the face more convex because the mandible must rotate clockwise as well. This may require either a vertical reduction genioplasty or an advancement genioplasty with vertical reduction to compensate.

Time and further study will determine whether presurgical leveling in the OSA patient with an open bite is more, less, or as stable as leveling through segmental osteotomies. Surgical technique to minimize compromise of the pedicle is always important. The amount of movement performed may or may not truly represent a reason to segment or not to segment the arch. Until further investigation is performed, it is unlikely that many surgeons will risk segmenting the maxilla in sleep apnea patients.

Sagittal dimension: molar classification and arch length. The pretreatment sagittal relationship will assist in determining the amount of differential jaw movement required for the MMA patient. Patients are typically planned for at least a 10-mm maxillary advancement.[28] If the patient presents with a Class I molar and canine relationship with minimal arch length deficiency or redundancy, the mandible should be advanced the same amount as the maxilla. The goals of the advancement should be resolution of the sleep apnea and maintenance of the pretreatment occlusion. This type of patient can potentially undergo jaw surgery with arch bars and not even require orthodontic treatment. Many patients, however, do not present with this type of occlusion.

More often, patients will present with some degree of Class II molar, canine, and skeletal relationship. In this situation, both the molar classification and any underlying arch length deficiency must be considered together to determine the surgical treatment plan. A general guideline for OSA patients is to *maintain or augment the dental arch, not diminish the dental arch dimension.* For debilitating and life-threatening obstructive sleep apnea, although important, postsurgical occlusion is a secondary goal. The most important factor is resolution of the sleep apnea. With smaller dental arches, there is less room for the tongue. Nonextraction orthodontic treatment (when possible) is preferred if a patient has sound periodontal health with mild to moderate arch length deficiency and the teeth can be maintained over basal bone. However, if the arch length deficiency is so significant that it is unreasonable to expect alignment of the teeth within basal bone, extractions must be considered.

If extractions are deemed appropriate, a second consideration is the anchorage requirement for extraction space management. The arch length deficiency, sagittal occlusal relationship, and skeletal relationship must guide the practitioner. Because a significant advancement of 10 to 12 mm is the goal of MMA, the anchorage requirements will often be different than with a nonsurgical case. A Class II patient with a Class II apical base relationship (AB-OP −6 or more), a Class II facial presentation, and 7 mm or more of arch length deficiency who does not have sleep apnea and *who will not undergo surgery* requires "maximum" anchorage in the maxilla and "minimum" anchorage in the mandible. The differential movement and space closure allows for the Class II relationship to be corrected. In the same patient *who will have surgery* for sleep apnea, the anchorage requirements are almost exactly opposite. With surgery, the goal in the maxilla is to place the upper teeth within basal bone while at least maintaining the Class II relationship and in some cases even make the Class II dental relationship worse. This allows the greatest mandibular advancement possible to be performed. If the Class II relationship is corrected orthodontically, both jaws will come forward, but the mandible will come forward only the same amount as the maxilla, which will not address the underlying apical base discrepancy. This potential decrease in mandibular advancement may also minimize the improvement in RDI and lead to unsuccessful surgical treatment for the sleep apnea.

One way to achieve the desired tooth position when extractions are necessary includes a segmental retraction assembly. A .036-inch heat-treated stainless steel transpalatal arch and lower lingual arch are fabricated. Then, posterior segments are created including the second molar, first molar, and second premolar. The incisors are not bonded initially to avoid proclining the teeth. An auxiliary .017 × .025–inch beta titanium "T" loop can be placed from the auxiliary tube of the maxillary first molar into the auxiliary tube of the canine or directly into the canine bracket. Precise activations can be placed to enable the clinician to create to desired moment to force ration for maximum, minimum, or reciprocal space closure. Typically, the canines are retracted only enough to address the incisor crowding but no further. At this point, the retraction spring is removed, the incisors are bracketed, and continuous archwires are placed. Now, any remaining space can be closed with minimal "C" anchorage. This has the overall effect of maintaining the dentition as far forward as possible (within the alveolar trough) and then moving the alveolar and basal bone forward with the surgical movement. Although one could argue that the overall dental arch dimension (arch perimeter arch depth, and arch length) is the same as an extraction arch with maximum or "A" anchorage, the difference is that the dentition itself is more forward with the maxilla and mandible.

Postsurgical finishing. Accomplishing presurgical orthodontic objectives helps the surgeon achieve the surgical objectives and in turn the postsurgical finishing of the occlusion. When the surgeon is able to obtain a strong Class I molar and canine relationship at surgery, finishing is similar to any other surgical orthodontic case. The main goals are final arch form coordination, interdigitation of the posterior occlusion, and use of postsurgical elastics to support the surgical move.

Arch form coordination in situations of extreme transverse discrepancies can be difficult to correct fully before surgery because the sagittal relationship may cause occlusal interferences. If nearly ideal coordination can be obtained before surgery, the final sagittal jaw position will facilitate final arch coordination. With the typical Class II presurgical relationship in a sleep apnea patient, the maxilla is mildly narrow. This can be adjusted easily with a transpalatal arch (TPA) activated for mild expansion and buccal root torque. If necessary, cross-arch elastics can be worn in addition to the TPA. If there has been a first stage of transverse maxillary distraction osteogenesis, mildly overexpanding the maxilla is preferable to underexpanding. It is typically easier to constrict an expanded arch than to expand an arch with insufficient surgical expansion further dentally. It should be emphasized that any overexpansion should be mild, not excessive. In addition, final archwire coordination can be assessed and achieved more efficiently once the final occlusion is visualized.

After the splint is removed, if mild maxillary transverse excess is present, a continuous round stainless steel archwire can be placed, maintaining the rectangular mandibular archwire. Vertical elastics can be worn to help roll in and interdigitate the occlusion. This often occurs in the Class III patient or the mildly overexpanded Class II patient.

When differential sagittal surgical movement has been performed (i.e., the mandible was advanced further than the maxilla or vice versa), elastic traction a few months following surgery is recommended to aid in stabilizing the jaws in the postsurgical position while bony healing and remodeling occur. In addition, it allows for mild callus manipulation during the healing phase so minor skeletal changes can be affected if necessary. Callus molding is more easily accomplished with wire osteosynthesis although this is rarely performed today and is almost never performed with the larger jaw movements used in correcting obstructive sleep apnea. However, even with the rigid internal fixation, there is some mild mobility to the jaws that the surgeon and the orthodontist can use to their advantage. It should be emphasized that when the splint is removed and if the occlusion is not what is expected, careful assessment by both the orthodontist and the surgeon should be performed. There is a limit to postsurgical manipulation with intermaxillary elastics. If the occlusion is outside this envelope, it is better to return to the operating room than try to manage the unexpected malocclusion with elastics. What the surgeon can achieve in a few hours may take the orthodontist months or years if it is even possible to accomplish with creative elastic patterns. Compliance by the patient with the prescribed elastic pattern is essential during this phase; incorrect or lack of usage may lead to incomplete correction of the malocclusion and a less desirable result.

Finally, at the end of postsurgical orthodontics, the patient's occlusion should be inspected closely. Light finishing wires can be placed for 2 to 4 weeks with individualized intermaxillary finishing elastics to achieve the final minute intercuspation that each patient requires.

Debonding and retention can then be performed. Depending on the amount of intercuspation, the orthodontist may select a positioner, Hawley retainers, or Essix retainers. The positioner and the Hawley allow for some active and passive settling, respectively, whereas the Essix retainer often fits so intimately against the teeth that the minor desired settling cannot occur. The retention decision should be made on an individualized basis to maximize treatment goals and patient compliance.

Maxillary and mandibular transverse distraction

Reports conflict regarding the size, shape, and form of the dental arches and facies of the average OSA patient. Anecdotal evidence from case series suggests a component of transverse deficiency in both jaws. The magnitude of the transverse deficiency varies, with some patients exhibiting extreme narrowness in both jaws. Some pediatric or adolescent reports theorize that expansion of the dental arches with rapid maxillary expansion can alleviate OSA in children.

Before the early 1990s, *distraction osteogenesis* as developed by Ilizarov[36] was confined to the long bones. One of the earliest reports of craniofacial distraction used mandibular symphyseal transverse distraction osteogenesis to widen the mandible concurrent with rapid maxillary expansion.[37] Before the development of mandibular transverse distraction osteogenesis, maxillary expansion was limited by the size, shape, and position of the mandible. If a crossbite was not present, the maxilla could not be expanded because there was no stable way to expand the mandible. Because of the encouraging results from rapid maxillary expansion in OSA children, maxillary and mandibular transverse distraction osteogenesis is anticipated to provide similar results in the adult population.[38] A recent case report illustrates the successful incorporation of transverse distraction osteogenesis in combination with MMA in an adult man with severe OSA.[39] The pretreatment RDI of 60 was reduced to 4 after treatment. Unfortunately, no interim sleep study was performed. As a result, one can only speculate regarding how

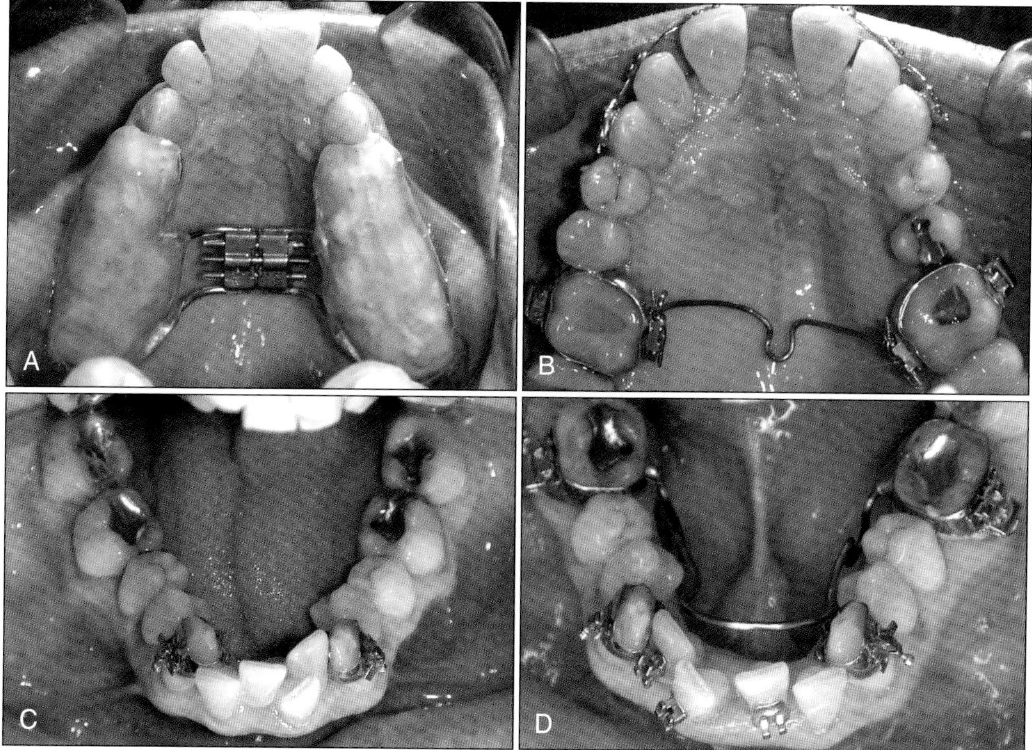

Fig. 20-10 Transverse dimension is often overlooked. For patients with severe arch constriction, maxillary and mandibular transverse distraction osteogenesis can be performed. Follow-up sleep studies are necessary to determine the effect on the overall correction of OSA. **A** and **B,** Arch expansion is possible using maxillary transverse distraction. **C** and **D,** Arch expansion is achieved using mandibular symphyseal distraction osteogenesis.

much of the correction was produced by the transverse distraction osteogenesis and how much correction was produced from the MMA.

When considering bimaxillary transverse distraction osteogenesis, the clinician first must determine how narrow the jaws are and how much they can be expanded (Fig. 20-10). A useful clinical guideline is that the mandible cannot be expanded more than about 10 mm. As a result, if the patient presents with a narrow maxilla and narrow mandible but no crossbite, no more than 10 mm of expansion in both arches should be planned. If the maxilla and mandible are narrow, however, and a crossbite exists, the mandible can be expanded 10 mm and the maxilla a greater amount. This can be assessed using diagnostic models, occlusogram, and posteroanterior (PA) cephalogram. Also, a set of normative values can be used to help determine the appropriate size of the maxilla and mandible. These should serve as clinical guidelines that are modified based on clinical experience and sound biomechanical and diagnostic principles.

Once transverse distraction osteogenesis is deemed appropriate for the patient and informed consent has been obtained, the maxillary and mandibular molars should be separated. Approximately 1 week later, bands should be fit to the maxillary and mandibular first molars and first premolars. Custom-made rapid maxillary and mandibular expansion appliances are constructed. In the mandible the expansion screw body should be placed lingual to the mandibular incisors and oriented approximately 45 degrees to the occlusal plane. This allows for easier activation of the appliance. If adequate interdental space is present between the maxillary and mandibular central incisors, limited predistraction movement will be required. Even if not needed to diverge the roots, it is helpful to have brackets on as many teeth as possible so that the central incisors can be held in place during the distraction and early consolidation periods. Movement too early into the distraction gap may lead to loss of periodontal attachment. Later in the consolidation period, the brackets can allow placement of an orthodontic archwire to serve as a track for the medial tooth movement. The increase in transverse dimension will provide additional arch perimeter, which can assist in initial alignment. The same space can also increase the ability to perform nonextraction orthodontic treatment where appropriate.

Transverse distraction osteogenesis should not be considered a panacea for arch length deficiencies.

Progress made with transverse distraction osteogenesis will provide additional results. A new testing protocol should be initiated with a sleep study before treatment, after transverse distraction osteogenesis, and after MMA. Such a protocol will lead to an improved understanding of the relative amount of OSA correction from the transverse distraction osteogenesis and from the MMA.

DIAGNOSIS AND TREATMENT IN ADOLESCENTS

Nonorthodontic Treatment Options

Typically, the most common cause of OSA in pediatric and adolescent patients is hypertrophic tonsils and adenoids.[40] Otolaryngologists have developed severity scales to assess the relative size of the lymphoid tissue.

The *tonsillar scale* ranges from types I to IV.[41] With type I the tonsils are barely visible in the pharyngeal pillars. Type II tonsils are visible, but the tissue remains confined to the crypts. With type III the tonsillar tissue is greatly increased and extends beyond the margins of the palatoglossus and palatopharyngeus muscles that make up the tonsillar pillars. With type IV the right and left tonsillar tissues almost approximate each other in the midline. Tonsillar hypertrophy can be seen on the lateral cephalometric radiograph and standard orthodontic clinical examination. Tonsillar tissue may shrink after age 6 years, and if the apnea/hypopnea is not severe, OSA can improve over time without treatment.

The lymphoid tissue of the adenoids can also be hypertrophic, but unlike the tonsils, this tissue cannot be visualized intraorally. It can be viewed on the lateral cephalogram as a moderately radiopaque mass above the soft palate. Depending on the severity of the apnea, parents may have difficulty finding an otolaryngologist (ear-nose-throat [ENT]) specialist who will remove the tonsils and the adenoids. As with the extraction/nonextraction debate, removal of the tonsils and adenoids has been controversial. In the 1950s and 1960s, tonsils and adenoids were routinely removed, even when asymptomatic or only mildly symptomatic. From the 1970s through the 1990s, however, even symptomatic tonsils were often managed medically with antibiotics, not surgically. Currently, mildly symptomatic and enlarged tonsils are being managed with antibiotics, with more severely affected and enlarged tonsils surgically excised.

One concern with tonsillectomy and adenoidectomy is the significant vascular supply of the tonsillar crypts. Surgery may traumatize a major vessel, leading to acute hemorrhage and death during the procedure. Also, slower extravasation of blood in the immediate postoperative period may lead to delayed pharyngeal swelling with potential airway obstruction. This is a particularly serious concern if the child is discharged from the hospital before the delayed inflammation is observed. Finally, the recovery period can be difficult for both the child and the parents because of the significant postoperative discomfort.

When properly performed and managed, however, the risks of surgery are reported to be small (often in the single digits), but not zero.

Historically, children are more active than adults and less prone to weight problems and obesity. However, over the past few generations, children have become increasingly sedentary, with overweight and obesity estimates ranging from one in four to one in three children.[42] With this earlier weight problem, children are experiencing OSA much earlier, leading to a lifetime of treatment with a much higher risk of being overweight or obese as adults. Therefore, even if they do not have OSA now, they are more likely to show signs and symptoms of OSA as adults. In addition, their weight can be a cofactor in other disease processes, such as hypertension, diabetes, and myocardial infarction.

Role of the Orthodontist

Because orthodontists see young patients frequently, they are able to build relationships and rapport with their patients. This rapport enables the orthodontists to motivate their young patients and encourage their compliance with headgear, tooth brushing, and other treatment-related concerns. As the patient relationship builds, the orthodontist and staff can also help guide the overweight child with nutritional counseling and diet modification. This is necessary not only to minimize decalcification and caries development during treatment, but also to assist the child maintain a healthy diet for life—an even greater benefit than the improved self-esteem or esthetic and functional improvement from orthodontic treatment. The orthodontist can also visibly demonstrate a healthy lifestyle by participating in community events in his or her town.

Certain craniofacial anomalies are another risk factor for pediatric sleep apnea. For severely affected children, CPAP has been advocated. Within the adult population, craniofacial side effects of CPAP have either not been observed or not been reported. Within the pediatric and adolescent population, there are concerns that growth disturbances may be caused by long-term CPAP use. Some clinicians have instituted daytime use of protraction headgear to mitigate the pressure placed on the maxilla from the mask with nightly CPAP.

These concerns have some biomechanical validity. The elastic strap that maintains the position of the CPAP mask does apply an inhibitory force on forward maxillomandibular development. This is similar to the effect a high-pull, cervical-pull, or Interlandi headgear has on maxillary growth in Class II children. However, when orthodontic headgear is used, force and direction of pull are measured, allowing precise resolution of the force system in all three planes of space. With CPAP, the elastic strap is adjusted to maintain the position of the mask, but the tension on the strap is assessed as either adequate or inadequate. "Adequate" means the mask is not displaced during the night, and a seal is obtained. "Inadequate" means some degree of displacement or loss of air seal is observed, decreasing the machine's efficiency.

At this point, it is unclear whether the midface deficiency observed in pediatric CPAP patients is caused by the CPAP or by the underlying craniofacial anomaly. To answer this question, a prospective randomized clinical evaluation is needed to determine the effect of CPAP on the developing face. If a negative effect is measured, the clinician must assess whether the potential growth disturbance from CPAP is more harmful than effect of untreated OSA. This requires an individualized plan for each affected child.

Besides diet modification and healthy lifestyle, is it possible during treatment in the adolescent period for the orthodontist to prevent or minimize the risk of developing OSA in later years? A recent report on the benefits of rapid maxillary expansion (RME) in OSA children has some limitations (e.g., small sample size, low RDI) but also some potentially important clinical implications.[38] If basal bone can be expanded in the maxilla, space in the oropharyngeal airway may increase. With an increased oropharyngeal airway, airflow should improve. If airflow improves, fewer hypopneas and apneas should occur. With fewer obstructive episodes, the condition should be minimized or potentially resolved, leading to increased daytime alertness and decreased morbidity from OSA.

The precise mechanisms for decreasing obstructive events are not fully understood at this time. The improvement may result from treating multiple causes and multiple sites. One site is the maxilla itself. As the maxilla expands, the palate and floor of the nasal cavity also expand, increasing the volume of the nasal cavity. In addition, the maxillary dentition is expanding at the same rate, assuming good skeletal expansion with the RME appliance. The maxilla provides additional room for the tongue, which may allow greater space and more forward positioning of the tongue. Finally, widening the maxillary basal bone has important effects on the velum of the palate, superior pharyngeal constrictors, and surrounding orofacial musculature. The combined contribution of these components appears to be clinically significant and extremely beneficial to the patient in samples studied to date.

In patients without a crossbite, rapid palatal expansion may not be indicated. A comprehensive, individualized analysis of tooth mass and arch length must be performed. Extraction therapy and nonextraction orthodontic therapy are excellent forms of treatment when indicated, but equally poor forms of treatment when performed inappropriately. Obstructive sleep apnea should not automatically place a patient into a nonextraction mode of treatment, and extraction therapy should not automatically be construed as having a negative effect on sleep architecture. The treatment goal in every patient should include a stable functional occlusion with the teeth positioned within the alveolus.

For a heavyset, borderline extraction/nonextraction adolescent patient, stably achieved nonextraction treatment may give the patient the largest reasonable arch dimension. Teeth should be extracted if this is not possible because of extreme crowding, or if negative esthetic concerns would result from a bimaxillary dentoalveolar protrusion.

Again, orthodontists should not consider OSA or the purported risk of developing it as an indication for nonextraction treatment in all patients. Sound clinical judgment based on biomechanics and the patient's desires, esthetics, and sleep health must inform the individualized extraction/nonextraction decision.

Another consideration is the evolution of diagnosis and treatment for Class III patients, particularly late-adolescent Class III surgical patients. The Class III malocclusion was once considered primarily a result of mandibular overgrowth, and the only surgical orthodontic treatment available was mandibular surgery to set the mandible back. As surgical techniques improved and maxillary surgery was made possible, the etiology of Class III malocclusion changed. Many currently believe that a Class III malocclusion results more from deficient maxillary growth, which may also have some component of mandibular overgrowth.[43] Each case must be diagnosed individually, but as a general rule, if airway concerns are present, surgically advancing the maxilla is recommended rather than setting the mandible back. Multiple studies in Class III patients examining the short-term airway changes after mandibular setback surgery demonstrated a decrease in airway size.[44,45] Most patients accommodated these changes well over the long term, but often these were not high-risk OSA patients. One study reported a sample size of only 10 patients, all young women of normal weight.

Finally, during diagnosis in patients who may have borderline OSA, a diagnostic sleep study should be performed in the process of planning treatment. Although this might add cost to the patient's treatment, if it aids in preventing iatrogenic OSA, the additional diagnostic cost would far outweigh the financial and other costs of doing mandibular setback surgery and transforming a borderline OSA patient to one with frank OSA.

If a patient is older than 21 years, an additional test is a "sleep challenge."[6] Studies have shown that consumption of 3 ounces of alcohol within 3 hours of going to bed can convert a patient from normal sleep architecture to OSA. Alternative medications may be used in patients under age 21 or those who do not consume alcoholic beverages. A borderline test result may indicate the need for a revised surgical treatment plan.

CONCLUSION

More and more people are being diagnosed with chronic obstructive sleep apnea. The dental community in general and the orthodontic community in particular need to be aware of the risk factors and ramifications of an OSA diagnosis. A focused health history helps the clinician begin to understand the potential for a patient to have OSA. An accurate and complete diagnosis can only be done with a polysomnography performed in an accredited sleep center by trained medical personnel. Following diagnosis, potential treatment options range from diet/behavior modification and CPAP to soft tissue surgery, dental/orthodontic appliance construction, and MMA surgery, provided by dentists, orthodontists, and oral surgeons. An orthodontic specialist should be able to perform dental sleep appliance construction, orthodontic therapy, and combined surgical-orthodontic treatment, as appropriate for each patient. Also, when treating adolescents, the clinician should not only focus on ideal occlusion and esthetics, but also consider the long-term health of the airway and prevention of OSA. Prevention is often the best and most cost-effective form of treatment.

References

1. Young T, Palta M, Dempsey J, et al: The occurrence of sleep-disordered breathing among middle-aged adults, *N Engl J Med* 328:1230-1235, 1993.
2. Strollo PJ, Rogers RM: Obstructive sleep apnea, *N Engl J Med* 334:99-104, 1996.
3. Marcus CL: Sleep-disordered breathing in children, *Am J Respir Crit Care Med* 164:1598-1603, 2001.
4. Smith R, Ronald J, Delaive K, et al: What are obstructive sleep apnea patients being treated for prior to this diagnosis? *Chest* 121:164-172, 2002.
5. Smith PL, Gold AR, Meyers DA, et al: Weight loss in mildly to moderately obese patients with obstructive sleep apnea, *Ann Intern Med* 103:850-855, 1985.
6. Scrima L, Broody M, Nay KN, Cohn MA: Increased severity of obstructive sleep apnea after bedtime alcohol ingestion: diagnosis and potential and proposed mechanisms of action, *Sleep* 5:318-328, 1982.
7. Sanders MH, Moore SE, Eveslace J: CPAP via nasal mask: a treatment for obstructive sleep apnea, *Chest* 83:144-145, 1983.
8. Coleman JA Jr: Laser-assisted uvulopalatoplasty: long-term results with a treatment for snoring, *Ear Nose Throat J* 77:22-34, 1998.
9. Prinsell JR: Maxillomandibular advancement surgery for obstructive sleep apnea syndrome, *J Am Dent Assoc* 133:1489-1497, 2002.
10. Campos-Rodriguez F, Pena-Grinan N, Reyes-Nunez N, et al: Mortality in obstructive sleep apnea/hypopnea patients treated with positive airway pressure, *Chest* 128:624-633, 2005.
11. Lavie P, Lavie L, Herer P: All-cause mortality in males with sleep apnea syndrome: declining mortality rates with age, *Eur Respir J* 25:514-520, 2005.
12. Milleron O, Pillière R, Foucher A, et al: Benefits of obstructive sleep apnea treatment in coronary artery disease: a long-term follow-up study, *Eur Heart J* 25:728-734, 2004.
13. Marti S, Sampol G, Muñoz X, et al: Mortality in severe sleep apnoea/hypopnoea syndrome patients: impact of treatment, *Eur Respir J* 20:1511-1518, 2002.
14. Johns MW: A new method for measuring daytime sleepiness: the Epworth Sleepiness Scale, *Sleep* 14(6):540-545, 1991.
15. Practice parameters for the indications for polysomnography and related procedures. Polysomnography Task Force, American Sleep Disorders Association Standards of Practice Committee, *Sleep* 206:406-422, 1997.
16. Flemmons WW, Buysse D, Redline S, et al: Sleep-related breathing disorders in adults: recommendations for syndrome definition and measurement techniques in clinical research—the report of an American Academy of Sleep Medicine task force, *Sleep* 22:667-689, 1999.
17. Abad VC, Guilleminault C: Neurological perspective on obstructive and nonobstructive sleep apnea, *Semin Neurol* 24:261-269, 2004.
18. Veale D, Chailleux E, Hoorelbeke-Ramon A, et al: Mortality of sleep apnoea patients treated by nasal continuous positive airway pressure registered in the ANTADIR observatory. Association Nationale pour le Traitement a Domicile de Insuffisance Respiratoire Chronique, *Eur Respir J* 15:326-331, 2000.
19. Horne JA, Reyner LA: Sleep related vehicle accidents, *BMJ* 310:565-567, 1995.
20. George CFP: Reduction in motor vehicle collisions following treatment of sleep apnoea with nasal CPAP, *Thorax* 56:508-512, 2001.
21. Phillips BA, Okeson J, Paesani D, Gilmore R: Effect of sleep position on sleep apnea and parafunctional activity, *Chest* 90:424-429, 1986.
22. Ferguson K, Ono T, Lowe A: A randomized cross-over study of an oral appliance vs. nasal CPAP in the treatment of mild-moderate OSA, *Chest* 190:1269-1275, 1996.
23. Cohen R: Obstructive sleep apnea: oral appliance therapy and severity of condition, *Oral Surg Oral Med Oral Pathol Oral Radiol Endod* 85:388-392, 1998.
24. Lim J, Lasserson TJ, Fleetham J, Wright J: Oral appliances for obstructive sleep apnoea, *Cochrane Database Syst Rev* Jan 25(1): CD004435, 2006. 10.1002/14651858.CD004435.pub3.
25. Almeida FR, Lowe AA, Sung JO, et al: Long-term sequelae of oral appliance therapy in obstructive sleep apnea patients. Part 1. Cephalometric analysis, *Am J Orthod Dentofacial Orthop* 129:195-204, 2006.
26. Almeida FR, Lowe AA, Otsuka R, et al: Long-term sequelae of oral appliance therapy in obstructive sleep apnea patients. Part 2. Study-model analysis, *Am J Orthod Dentofacial Orthop* 129:205-213, 2006.
27. Riley RW, Powell NB, Guilleminault C: Obstructive sleep apnea syndrome: a review of 306 consecutively treated surgical patients, *Otolaryngol Head Neck Surg* 108:117-125, 1993.
28. Hochban W, Brandenburg U, Peter JH: Surgical treatment of obstructive sleep apnea by maxillomandibular advancement, *Sleep* 17:624-629, 1994.
29. Waite PD, Shettar SM: Maxillomandibular advancement: a cure for obstructive sleep apnea, *Oral Maxillofac Surg Clin North Am* 7:327, 1995.
30. Prinsell JR: Maxillomandibular advancement surgery for obstructive sleep apnea syndrome, *J Am Dent Assoc* 133:1489-1497, 2002.
31. Marcotte MR: The use of the occlusogram in planning orthodontic treatment, *Am J Orthod* 69:655-667, 1976.
32. White LW: The clinical use of occlusograms, *J Clin Orthod* 16:92-103, 1982.
33. Faber RD: Occlusograms in orthodontic treatment planning, *J Clin Orthod* 26:389-401, 1992.
34. Jacobs JD, Bell WH, Williams CE, Kennedy JW: Control of the transverse dimension with surgery and orthodontics, *Am J Orthod* 77:284-306, 1980.
35. Frost HM: The biology of fracture healing: an overview for clinicians. Part I, *Clin Orthop Relat Res* (248):283-293, 1989.
36. Ilizarov GA: Basic principles of transosseous compression and distraction osteosynthesis, *Ortop Travmatol Protex* 32:7-15, 1971.
37. Guerrero C: Rapid mandibular expansion, *Rev Venez Ortod* 1:48, 1990.
38. Villa MP, Malagola C, Pagani J, et al: Rapid maxillary expansion in children with obstructive sleep apnea syndrome: 12-month follow-up, *Sleep* 8:128-134, 2007.

39. Conley RS, Legan HL: Correction of severe obstructive sleep apnea with bimaxillary transverse distraction osteogenesis and maxillomandibular advancement, *Am J Orthod Dentofacial Orthop* 129:283-292, 2006.
40. Potsic WP, Wetmore RF: Sleep disorders and airway obstruction in children, *Otolaryngol Clin North Am* 23:651-663, 1990.
41. Friedman M, Tanyeri H, La Rosa M, et al: Clinical predictors of obstructive sleep apnea, *Laryngoscope* 109:1901-1907, 1999.
42. Ogden CL et al: Prevalence of overweight and obesity in the United States, 1999–2004, *JAMA* 295:1549-1555, 2006.
43. Proffit WR, White RP Jr, Sarver DM: *Contemporary treatment of dentofacial deformity*, St Louis, 2003, Mosby.
44. Saitoh K: Long-term changes in pharyngeal airway morphology after mandibular setback surgery, *Am J Orthod Dentofacial Orthop* 125:556-561, 2004.
45. Kawamata A, Fujishita M, Ariji Y, Ariji EL: Three-dimensional computed tomographic evaluation of morphologic airway changes after mandibular setback osteotomy for prognathism, *Oral Surg Oral Med Oral Pathol Oral Radiol Endod* 89:278-287, 2000.

CHAPTER 21

Optimizing Esthetics for the Interdisciplinary Patient

Vincent G. Kokich

The focus in dentistry has gradually changed over the past 25 years. Dentists previously were in the "repair business." Routine dental treatment involved excavating dental caries and filling the enamel and dentinal defects with amalgam. Larger holes may have required more durable restorations, but the focus was the same: repair the effects of dental decay.

With the advent of fluorides and sealants, however, in addition to a better understanding of the role of bacteria in causing both caries and periodontal disease, patient needs have changed. Many young adults, who are products of the sealant generation, have little or no decay and few existing restorations. At the same time, the image of the value of teeth in Western society has also changed. The public still regards teeth as an important part of chewing, but the focus of many adults has shifted toward esthetics. They ask, "How can my teeth be made to look better?" Therefore the formerly independent disciplines of orthodontics, periodontics, restorative dentistry, and maxillofacial surgery must often join together to satisfy this desire to "look better."

This heightened awareness of esthetics has challenged dentistry to examine dental esthetics in a more systematic manner, to ensure that the health of patients and their teeth is still the most important underlying objective. Some existing dentitions simply cannot be restored to a more esthetic appearance without the assistance of several different dental disciplines. Every dental practitioner must now have a thorough understanding of the roles of these various disciplines in producing an "esthetic makeover," using the most conservative and biologically sound interdisciplinary treatment plan possible.

As an orthodontist, the author has worked with an interdisciplinary study group of nine dental specialists and one general dentist since 1984. The group has met monthly to educate the members about the advances in their respective areas of dentistry and to plan interdisciplinary treatment for the most challenging and complex dental situations.[1] One of these interdisciplinary areas is esthetics. The purpose of this chapter is to provide a systematic method of evaluating dentofacial esthetics in a logical, interdisciplinary manner.

SEQUENCING THE PLANNING PROCESS

Historically, the treatment-planning process in dentistry usually has begun with an assessment of the biology or biological aspects of a patient's dental problem. This might include the patient's caries susceptibility, periodontal health, endodontic needs, and general oral health. Once the biological health was reestablished through caries removal, modification of bone and gingiva, endodontic therapy, or tooth removal, the restoration of the resulting defects would be based on structural considerations. If teeth were to be restored or repositioned, the function of the teeth and condyles would be paramount in dictating occlusal form and occlusal relationships, respectively. Finally, esthetics would be addressed to provide a pleasing appearance of the teeth.

However, if the treatment-planning sequence proceeds from biology to structure to function and finally to esthetics, the eventual esthetic outcome could be compromised. The author proceeds in the opposite direction, starting with esthetics and proceeding to function, structure, and finally biology. None of the important parameters is left out; the planning process is merely sequenced from a different perspective. This sequence is chosen because the decisions made in each category, especially esthetics, will directly affect the subsequent categories.

BEGINNING WITH ESTHETICS

Maxillary Central Incisors Relative to Upper Lip

When beginning with esthetics, the first step is an appraisal of the position of the maxillary central incisors relative to the upper lip (Fig. 21-1). This assessment is made with the patient's upper lip at rest. Using a millimeter ruler or periodontal probe, the clinician determines the position of the incisal edge of the maxillary central incisor relative to the upper lip. The position of the maxillary central incisor can either be acceptable or unacceptable. An acceptable amount of incisal edge display at rest depends on the patient's age. Previous studies have shown that with advancing age, the amount of incisal display decreases proportionately.[2,3] For example, in a 30-year-old patient, 3 mm of incisal display at rest is appropriate, whereas in a 60-year-old patient, the incisal display could be 1 mm or less. The change in incisal display with time probably relates to the resiliency and tone of the upper lip, which tends to decrease with advancing age.

If the incisal edge display is *inadequate* (Fig. 21-2), a primary objective of interdisciplinary treatment may be to lengthen the maxillary incisal edges. This objective can be accomplished with restorative dentistry,[4] orthodontic extrusion,[5] or orthognathic surgery[6-8] (Fig. 21-2). Choosing the correct procedure will depend on the patient's facial proportions, existing crown length, and opposing occlusion. If the incisal edge display is *excessive,* an objective of treatment may be to move the maxillary incisors apically by equilibration,[9] restoration,[10] orthodontics,[11,12] or orthognathic surgery.[13] The treatment decision will depend on the patient's existing anterior occlusion and the facial proportions.

Maxillary Dental Midline

The second aspect of esthetic tooth positioning to be evaluated is the maxillary dental midline. Recent studies have shown that laypeople do not notice midline deviations of up to 3 or 4 mm if the long axes of the teeth are parallel with the long axis of the face.[14,15] Therefore the most important relationship to evaluate may be the mediolateral inclination

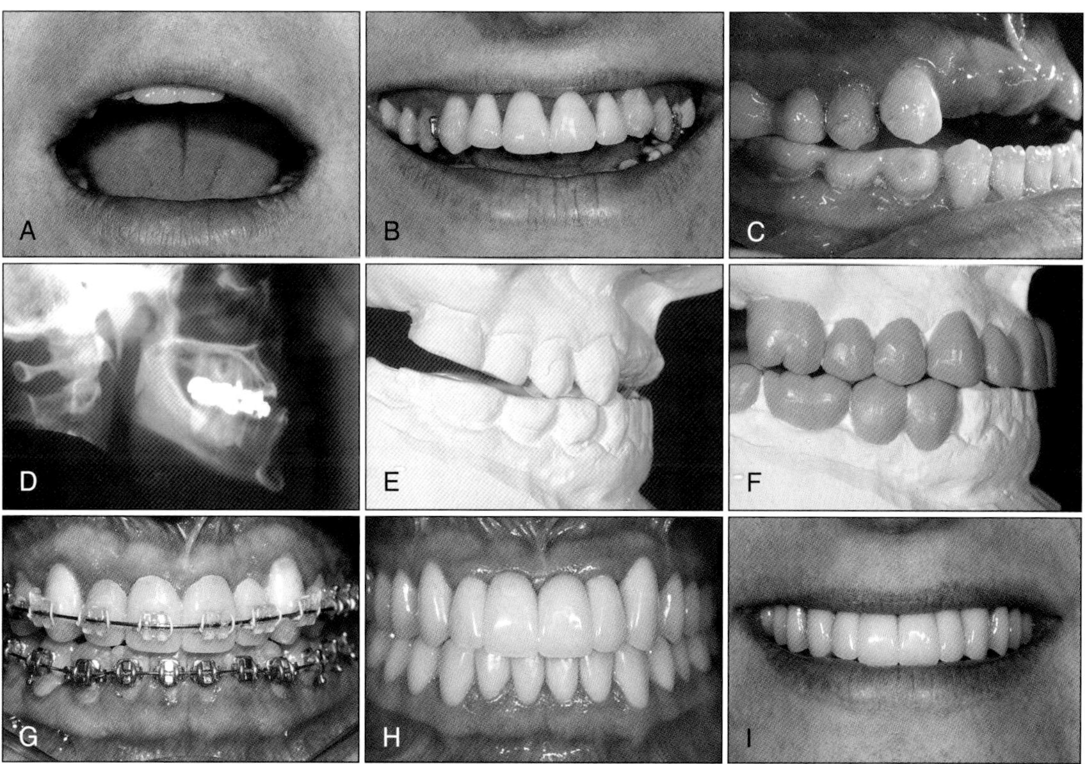

Fig. 21-1 This 35-year-old woman was missing her maxillary incisors. The incisal edge of her maxillary prosthesis was 2 mm from her upper lip at rest (**A**), and the gingival margins of the prosthetic teeth were at the level of the upper lip when smiling (**B**). She had an Angle Class III molar relationship (**C**) and maxillary retrognathism (**D**). She had severe wear of the posterior teeth, and the level of the maxillary posterior teeth was positioned too far coronally (**B** and **C**). Before Le Fort surgery, her entire dentition was provisionalized. The maxillary posterior interocclusal space was opened (**E**) to provide space for restorations (**F**). Orthodontic bracketing facilitated the finishing of the occlusion (**G**). Using the maxillary incisor position and the posterior occlusal plane as guides not only improved the occlusion (**H**), but also resulted in ideal smile esthetics after restoration (**I**).

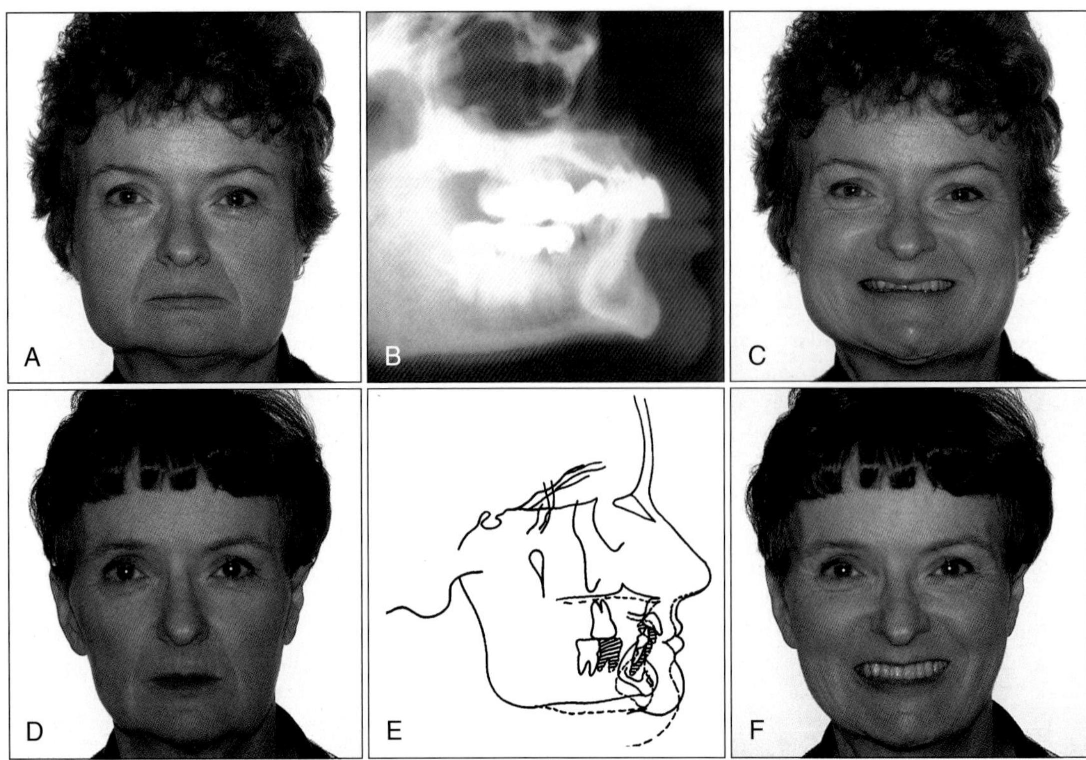

Fig. 21-2 This 61-year-old woman's chief esthetic complaint was that she did not show her teeth when speaking and smiling. She had a short lower facial height (**A**), and the maxillary incisal edges of her anterior bridge were 2 mm above the level of the upper lip at rest (**B**). As a result, she showed very little of her maxillary incisors on smiling (**C**). Both maxillary and mandibular osteotomies were used to rotate her maxilla and mandible downward in the anterior aspect to lengthen her lower facial height (**D** and **E**) and produce a much more esthetic smile (**F**). Her posterior facial height was not lengthened in order to maintain her vertical dimension of occlusion.

of the maxillary central incisors. If the incisors are inclined by 2 mm to the right or left (Fig. 21-3), laypeople regard this discrepancy as "unesthetic."[15,16] A canted midline can be corrected with orthodontics[17] or restorative dentistry.[18] Usually the decision depends on whether the maxillary incisors will require restoration.

Maxillary Incisor Inclination and Posterior Occlusal Plane

Once the correct incisal edge position and midline relationship of the maxillary incisors has been established, the next step is to evaluate the labiolingual inclination of the maxillary anterior teeth. Are they acceptable, proclined, or retroclined? When orthodontists evaluate labiolingual inclination, they rely on cephalometric radiographs to determine tooth inclination.[19] However, general dentists do not use cephalograms. Another method of assessing the inclination of the maxillary anterior teeth is to evaluate the labial surface of the existing maxillary central incisors relative to the patient's maxillary posterior occlusal plane. Generally, the labial surface of the maxillary central incisors should be perpendicular to the occlusal plane (Fig. 21-4). This relationship permits maximum direct light reflection from the labial surface of the maxillary central incisors, which enhances their esthetic appearance.[20] If teeth are retroclined (Fig. 21-5) or proclined (Fig. 21-6), correction may require either orthodontics or extensive restorative dentistry and possibly endodontics to establish a more ideal labiolingual inclination.[18]

The next step is to evaluate the maxillary posterior occlusal plane relative to the ideal location of the maxillary incisal edge. The maxillary incisal edge will be level with the posterior occlusal plane (see Fig. 21-4), coronal to the posterior occlusal plane (see Fig. 21-1), or apical to the posterior occlusal plane (see Fig. 21-2). Correcting the posterior occlusal plane position will require orthognathic surgery[21,22] (see Figs. 21-1 and 21-2) and/or restorative dentistry.[18] The amount of tooth abrasion, the patient's vertical facial proportions, and the position of the alveolar bone will help to determine the correct solution of posterior occlusal plane discrepancies.

After the position of the maxillary central incisal edges have been determined, the incisal edges of the maxillary lateral incisors and canines, as well as the buccal cusps of the maxillary premolars and molars, can be established

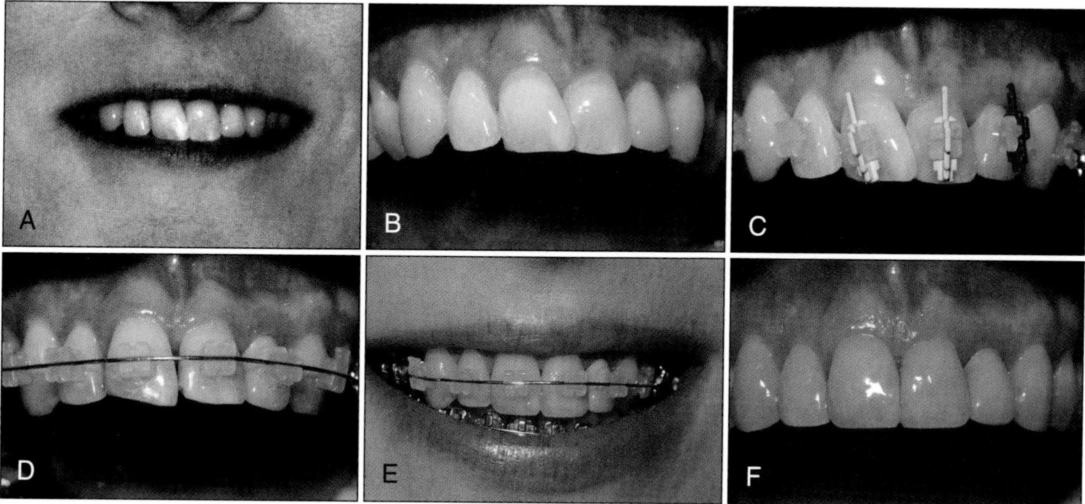

Fig. 21-3 This adult woman was dissatisfied with her smile. Her maxillary central incisors were inclined to her left (A), and the incisal edges had been abraded, producing a flat incisal edge relationship (B). To change the tooth inclination, the maxillary brackets were placed at an angle to the worn incisal edges, but perpendicular to the long axis of the roots (C). As the roots uprighted, the worn incisal edges became more apparent (D). Her general dentist added composite to the incisal edges during orthodontics (E) to restore the teeth to their normal size and proportion (F).

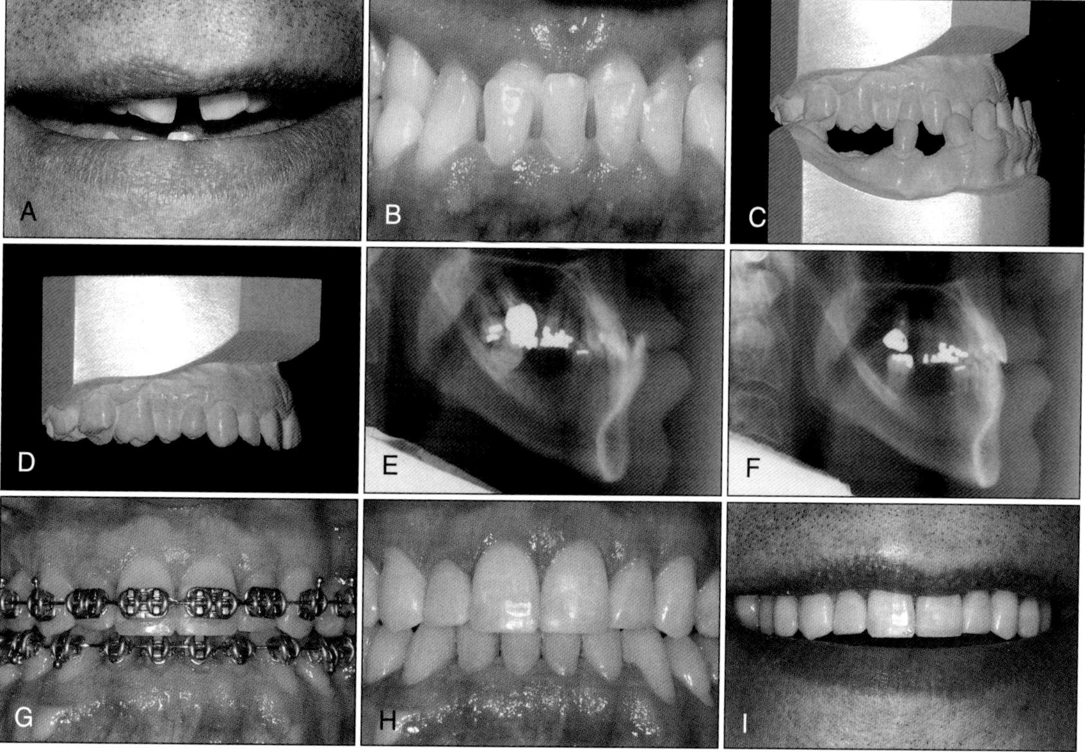

Fig. 21-4 The esthetic position of the maxillary incisal edges in this 52-year-old man was ideal relative to the upper lip (A). He had a significant malocclusion with anterior crossbite (B) and an Angle Class III posterior relationship in centric occlusion (C). With his condyles centered in the glenoid fossae, his maxillary and mandibular incisors were in an end-to-end anteroposterior relationship. His maxillary arch and the position of the maxillary posterior occlusal plane were ideal (D). His primary problem was the proclination of the mandibular incisors relative to the normally positioned maxillary incisors (E). His treatment involved nonsurgical orthodontics to retract the mandibular incisors and correct the crossbite (F). By maintaining the ideal relationship of the maxillary incisors during orthodontics (G), not only does he have good occlusion (H), but his incisal edge position and smile esthetics are ideal (I).

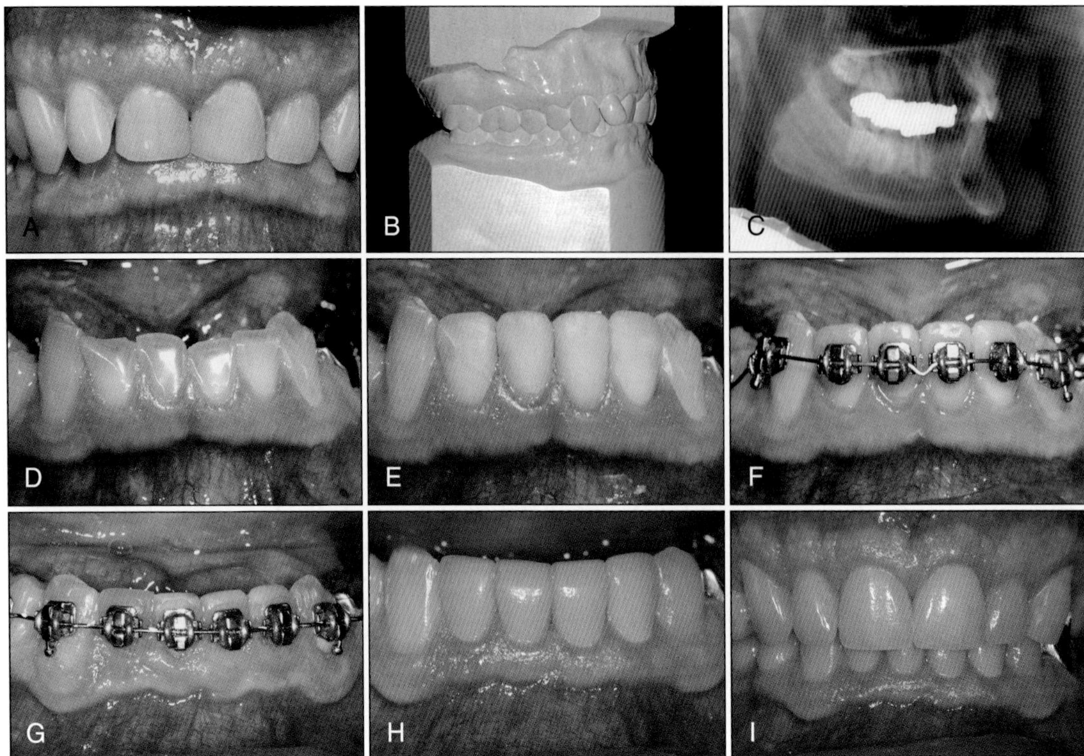

Fig. 21-5 This 54-year-old man had a deep anterior overbite **(A)** and retroclined maxillary incisors **(B)**. His occlusion was Angle Class I, but skeletally he had bimaxillary retrusion of both dental arches **(C)**. The position of the maxillary incisors was at the level of the upper lip **(C)**, which is normal for his age. The overbite problem was caused by overeruption of the mandibular incisors, which had also been abraded significantly **(D)**. Initially these teeth were built up with composite **(E)** so that brackets could be placed on these teeth **(F)** to intrude them into the alveolus **(G)**. This permitted the general dentist to restore these teeth **(H)** after the deep overbite had been corrected **(I)**.

(Fig. 21-7; see Fig. 21-4). The levels of these teeth generally are determined by their esthetic relationship to the lower lip when the patient smiles.[23,24] If the patient has an asymmetric lower lip, it may be more prudent to use the interpupillary line as a guide in establishing the posterior occlusal plane.[25]

Gingival Levels

The next step in the process of determining the esthetic relationship of the maxillary anterior teeth is to establish the gingival levels. The current gingival levels should be assessed relative to the projected incisal edge position. The key to determining the correct gingival levels is to determine the desired tooth size relative to the projected incisal edge position (Fig. 21-8). Remember, the incisal edge is not positioned to create the correct tooth size relative to the gingival margin levels. Using the gingiva as a reference to position the incisal edges is risky, because gingiva can move with eruption or recession. Thus the ideal gingival levels are determined by establishing the correct width/length ratio of the maxillary anterior teeth,[26-28] the desired amount of gingival display,[15] and symmetry between right and left sides of the maxillary dental arch.[18]

If the existing gingival levels will produce a tooth that is too short relative to the projected incisal edge position, the gingival margins must be moved apically (Fig. 21-9). This adjustment can be accomplished with gingival or osseous surgery (Fig. 21-9),[29,30] orthodontic intrusion,[11] or orthodontic intrusion and restoration[31-33] (see Figs. 21-6 and 21-9). The key factors that determine the most appropriate method of correction are the sulcus depth, location of the cementoenamel junction relative to the bone level, amount of existing tooth structure, root/crown ratio, and shape of the root.[34] In some situations, surgical crown lengthening of the maxillary incisors (see Fig. 21-9) is more appropriate to establish the correct gingival levels.[10] In other situations, orthodontic intrusion (see Fig. 21-6) and restoration of the incisal edge are more appropriate.[34]

The next step in the process of establishing the correct esthetic position of the maxillary anterior teeth is to assess the papillary levels relative to the overall crown length of the maxillary central incisors. Research has shown that the average ratio is about 50% contact and 50% papilla.[35] If the contact is significantly shorter than the papilla, it usually indicates moderate to significant incisor abrasion, which tends to shorten the crowns and therefore shortens the contact between the central incisors.[30] If the contact is

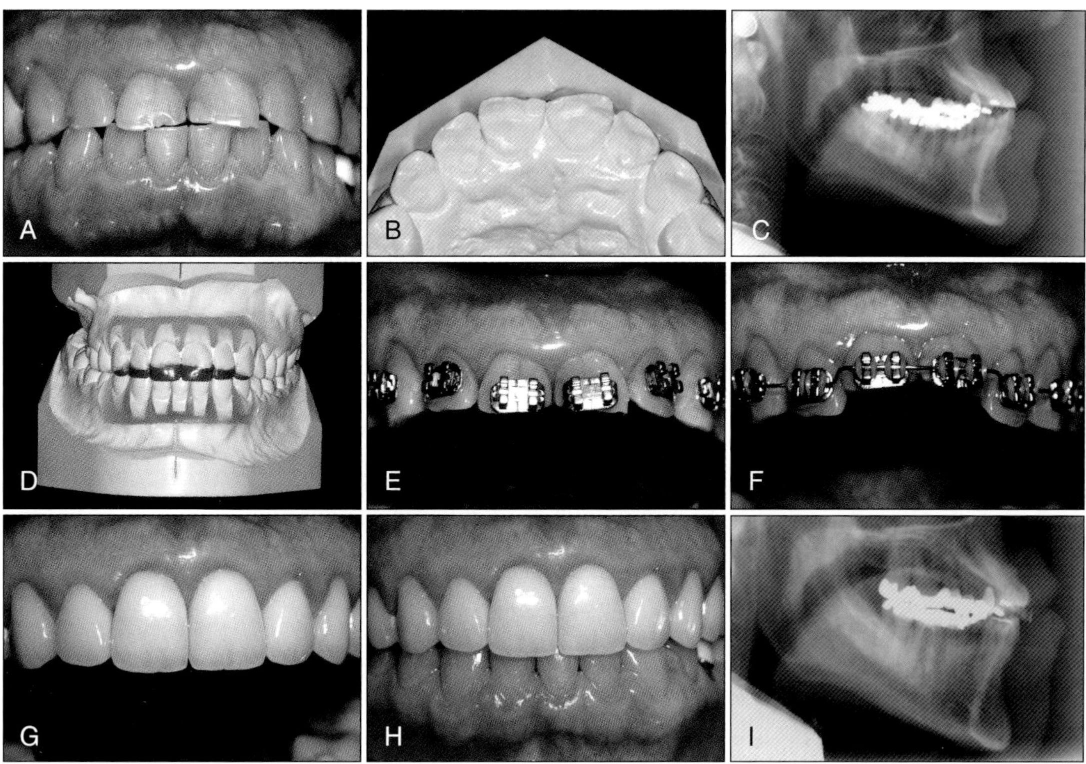

Fig. 21-6 This 52-year-old woman had short maxillary incisors that were positioned in an end-to-end relationship with the mandibular incisors (**A**). As a result, these teeth had worn significantly (**B**). Her general dentist could not restore these teeth because of her lack of overjet and because her maxillary incisal edge was at the level of the upper lip (**C**). Normal overjet for her age is 1 to 2 mm below the level of the upper lip. A diagnostic wax-up (**D**) showed that one lower incisor could be extracted to create the necessary overjet. To provide restorative space and the correct tooth proportions, the maxillary incisors were intruded (**E** and **F**) during orthodontics. This space allowed the dentist to restore length and proper proportion to the maxillary anterior teeth (**G**), but still create the proper overbite relationship (**H**) and improve her upper lip–to–incisal edge relationship after restorative treatment (**I**).

significantly longer than the papilla, the gingival contour or scallop over the central incisors might be flat, which could be caused by altered passive or altered active eruption of the teeth.[35] Gingival or osseous surgery[10] or orthodontic intrusion[13] or extrusion[34] (Fig. 21-10) may be necessary to correct the level of the papillae between the maxillary anterior teeth.[36]

MAXILLARY ARRANGEMENT, CONTOUR, AND SHADE

When the incisal edge position, the midline, the axial inclination, the gingival margins, and the papillary levels of the maxillary anterior teeth have been established, the next step is to determine if the arrangement of the maxillary anterior teeth can be accomplished restoratively. If not, the patient may require orthodontics to facilitate restoration. If in doubt, the clinician should perform a diagnostic wax-up (see Figs. 21-1, 21-6, and 21-8) to determine if the arrangement is possible restoratively.[18,34,37]

In addition, the contour and shade of the anterior teeth must be addressed. Does the patient have any specific requests concerning tooth shape or tooth shade? Remember, the more alterations made in these parameters, the more teeth will need to be treated, and the more involved the treatment plan will become. A good guide to esthetic treatment planning is to determine the ideal end point of treatment and then compare it to the patient's current condition. Treatment is indicated when the desired end point and the current condition do not match. The actual method of treatment can then be chosen based on the magnitude of the difference.

ESTHETIC PLAN FOR MANDIBULAR TEETH

After the esthetic relationship of the maxillary incisors has been established, the mandibular incisors must relate to the maxillary tooth position. First, evaluate the level of the mandibular incisal edges relative to the face. Do they have

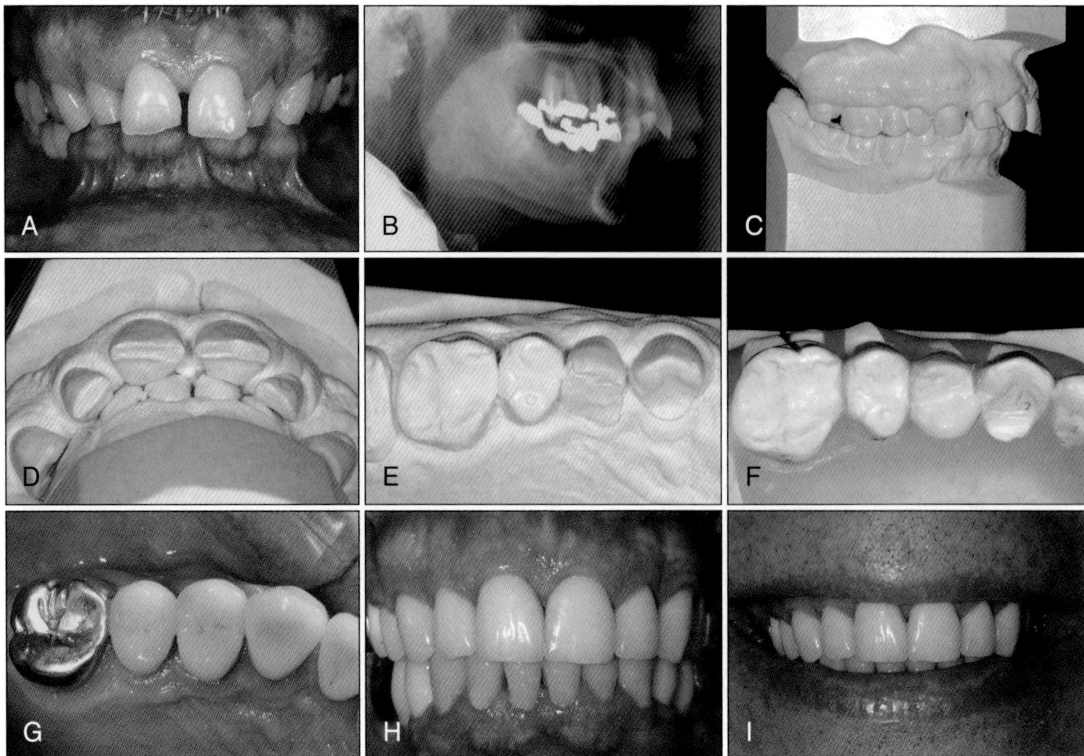

Fig. 21-7 This 61-year-old man was dissatisfied with the esthetic appearance of his teeth. He had an Angle Class II malocclusion with a deep anterior overbite **(A)** and mandibular retrusion **(B)**. His maxillary incisal edges were ideally positioned to the upper lip at rest for his age **(B)**, and the posterior occlusal plane was at the appropriate level relative to the anterior teeth **(C)**. The deep anterior overbite was caused by the mandibular incisor position **(D)**. He had significant wear of the posterior teeth **(E)**, which required restoration before orthodontics to place appliances on the teeth. A diagnostic wax-up **(F)** provided the guide for the restorative dentist before treatment and permitted ideal restoration of these teeth **(G)** after orthodontics and mandibular advancement to reposition the mandibular incisors relative to the maxillary arch. This change produced an ideal overbite and overjet **(H)** with excellent smile esthetics **(I)**.

acceptable display or excessive display, or are they not visible? If they have excessive display, equilibration, restoration, or orthodontic intrusion may correct the problem.[34] If they are not visible, either restoration or orthodontic extrusion may be necessary.[38,39]

Next, determine the relationship of the mandibular incisors relative to the posterior occlusal plane. Are the incisors level with the posterior occlusal plane? If not, they are either coronal or apical to the posterior occlusal plane. Correcting either of these relationships may require restoration, equilibration, orthodontics, or orthognathic surgery[4] (see Fig. 21-7).

Finally, the labiolingual inclination of the mandibular incisors must be evaluated. This relationship is partially determined by the projected position of the maxillary incisors. If the inclination is proclined (see Fig. 21-4) or retroclined (see Fig. 21-5), orthodontics could be a useful adjunct in adjusting the labiolingual position of the mandibular incisors.[34] The final mandibular incisal edge position is usually determined during the functional and structural phases of the treatment planning (see Figs. 21-6 and 21-8).

The gingival levels of the mandibular dentition may need to change when the different options for leveling the mandibular occlusal plane are considered. If orthodontics is selected to intrude (see Fig. 21-5) or extrude teeth, the gingival margins will move with the teeth.[40] However, if equilibration and restoration are necessary to level the mandibular occlusal plane, the gingival levels may need to be relocated with osseous surgery.[10]

At this point, based on the esthetic determination of the projected positions of the maxillary and mandibular teeth, the clinician should be able to determine which teeth will need restoration[41]: maxillary anterior, maxillary posterior, mandibular anterior, and/or mandibular posterior teeth. Once the maxillary and mandibular occlusal planes have been established through esthetic parameters, the clinician must then determine how to create an acceptable occlusal relationship between the arches.

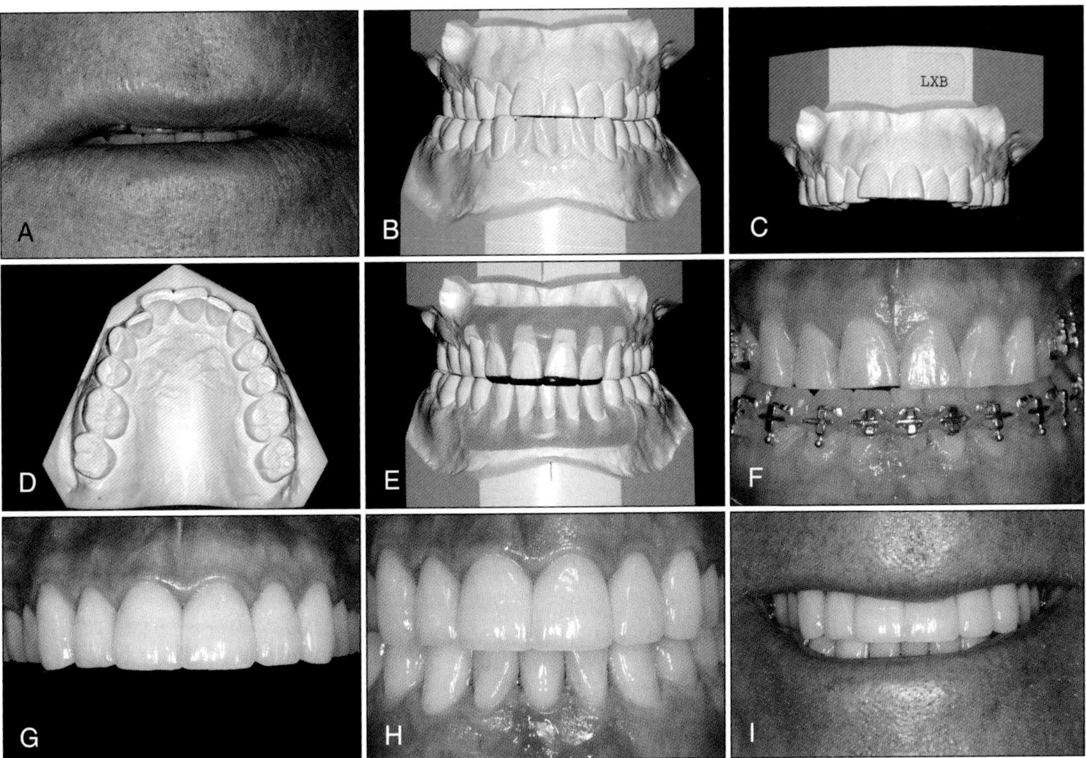

Fig. 21-8 This 62-year-old physician was dissatisfied with his smile esthetics and showed no maxillary incisal edge at rest (**A**) because of significant wear of the maxillary incisors (**B**). The tooth wear resulted from the end-to-end relationship of the maxillary and mandibular incisors (**B**). These teeth needed to be restored (**C** and **D**), but the mandibular incisors were in the way. A diagnostic wax-up (**E**) showed that extraction of one mandibular incisor would produce sufficient overjet (**F**), so that the maxillary incisors could be lengthened (**G**) and not only produce good anterior occlusion (**H**), but also improve this patient's smile esthetics (**I**).

INTEGRATING FUNCTION AND ESTHETICS

The first step to integrating the esthetic plan with the functioning occlusion is to evaluate the temporomandibular joints and muscles.[42] Does the patient have any joint or muscle symptoms? A key step in the process is to make centric relation records and mount the models. The author's definition of *centric relation* is the position of the condyles when the lateral pterygoid muscles are relaxed and the elevator muscles' contact with the disk is properly aligned.[42] The clinician must determine whether the desired esthetic changes can be made without altering the occlusion. If not, orthodontics and orthognathic surgery may be required to correct tooth position to facilitate the esthetic positioning of the teeth. To determine the impact of the esthetic plan on the function or occlusion, the esthetic changes in maxillary tooth position must be transferred to the maxillary dental cast.[42] This is accomplished with a combination of wax and adjustment of the plaster casts (see Fig. 21-1).

As the proposed esthetic treatment plan is transferred to the mounted casts, the clinician will be able to determine if only restoration will accomplish the desired occlusion, or if alteration of the occlusal scheme through orthodontics and orthognathic surgery will be necessary. This is especially true when the clinician is planning to level the occlusal planes. Will leveling of the occlusal planes create an acceptable anterior dental relationship? If the answer is "yes," and the leveling involves only the mandibular incisors, the patient's existing vertical dimension can be maintained. If the answer is "no," or the leveling involves mandibular posterior teeth, the existing vertical dimension may need to be altered. The clinician must determine whether altering the vertical dimension will result in acceptable tooth form and anterior relationships. There is no replacement for mounted dental casts and a diagnostic wax-up when these critical questions are being addressed.

DETERMINE IF ADEQUATE STRUCTURE EXISTS TO RESTORE TEETH

Once the esthetic treatment plan has been established, the projected tooth position verified on the diagnostic wax-up, and the functional relationships of the mounted dental casts assessed, the clinician must determine if adequate tooth structure exists to restore the teeth. If not, how will the clinician obtain adequate structure? What types of restorations

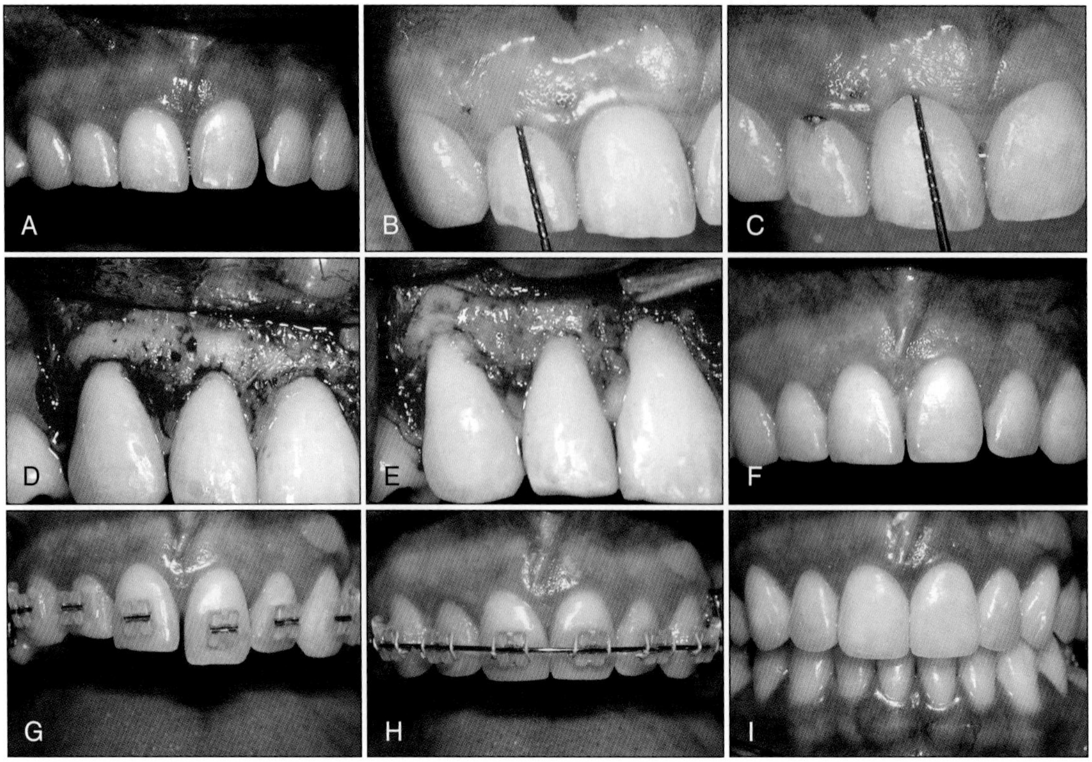

Fig. 21-9 This 35-year-old woman was uncomfortable with the uneven lengths of her maxillary anterior teeth (**A**). To determine the solution, a periodontal probe was used to push through the soft tissue attachment down to bone (sounding) over the right lateral (**B**) and central (**C**) incisors. This showed that the cementoenamel junctions were at the level of the bone (altered active eruption). This relationship was confirmed when a gingival flap was elevated (**D**). The bone was moved 2 mm from the cementoenamel junction (**E**). After healing there was still a discrepancy between the right and left incisor crown lengths (**F**). This difference was caused by uneven wear of the incisal edges and was corrected with intrusion of the right maxillary anterior teeth (**G**) to permit restoration of the incisal edges (**H**), which completed the correction of her uneven maxillary anterior tooth length (**I**).

will be placed? How will they be retained? How will any missing teeth be replaced?

Based on the clinician's assessment of the remaining tooth structure,[41] the choices for restoring anterior teeth may include composite bonding, porcelain veneers, bonded all-ceramic crowns, luted all-ceramic crowns, or metal-ceramic crowns (see Figs. 21-1 and 21-3 to 21-10). The posterior restorations may include direct restorations, inlays, onlays, or crowns. Missing teeth will be replaced with implants, fixed partial dentures, or removable partial dentures.

The criteria used to determine which restorations are appropriate include (1) the current clinical crown length; (2) the crown length after any gingival changes are performed for esthetics; (3) current amount of ferrule;[40] (4) whether sufficient space exists for a buildup; and (5) how crown lengthening for structural purposes will alter esthetics. The methods for increasing the retention of restorations are buildup, surgical crown lengthening,[10] orthodontic forced eruption,[33,40] and bonding the restoration. Each clinical situation must be carefully evaluated to determine the appropriate structural solution.

BIOLOGICAL CONSIDERATIONS

The esthetic plan has been established. The diagnostic wax-up confirms that the teeth will function properly. The restorative plan has taken into consideration the existing tooth structure. Now is the time to add the biological aspects of the treatment plan. These include endodontics, periodontics, and orthognathic surgery.

The primary objective of biological treatment planning is to establish a healthy oral environment with the tissue in the desired location. To accomplish this, endodontics may be necessary for teeth that are structurally and periodontally salvageable. In these patients the endodontic therapy must be completed first, before beginning the restorative phase of dentistry. The definitive periodontal therapy must be established to create a healthy periodontium based on the esthetic, functional, and structural needs of the restorations. Any elective periodontics must be completed next, in conjunction with the restorative plan. Finally, if any skeletal abnormalities require orthognathic surgical correction, this must be accomplished before the definitive restorative phase of treatment.

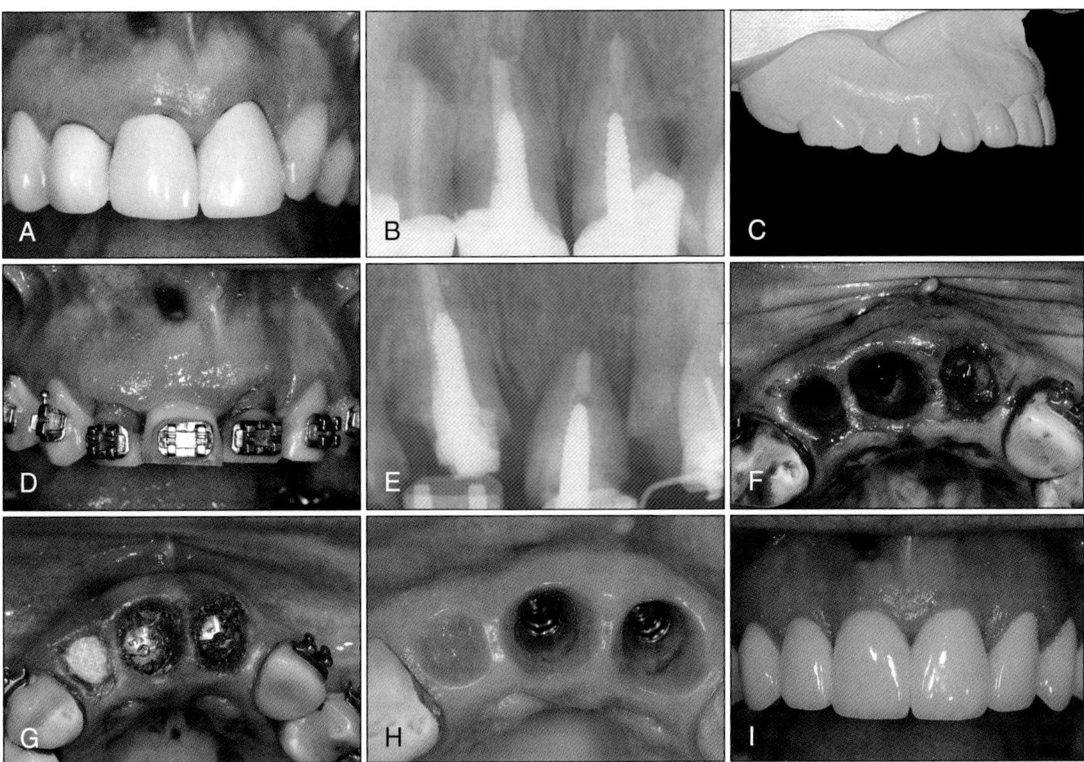

Fig. 21-10 This 42-year-old woman was dissatisfied with the esthetic appearance of her maxillary anterior teeth. She was missing her maxillary left lateral incisor (**A**), and the three remaining incisors had been restored with crowns. These teeth had short roots and had been treated endodontically (**B**). The maxillary incisors were positioned perpendicular to the occlusal plane (**C**), so they were in an ideal position to perform controlled extraction of the roots (**D**) to move the bone (**E**) and tissue incisally. After extraction of all three incisors (**F**), two immediate implants were placed in the central incisor sockets (**G**). After the implants had integrated, the soft tissue was molded with provisional crowns (**H**), so that the final restoration (**I**) produced ideal gingival margin relationships and tooth proportions.

SEQUENCING THE THERAPY

The plan is complete. It began with esthetics, was correlated to function, took into consideration the remaining tooth structure, and was facilitated by recognition of the patient's biological needs. Only two questions remain: How should this esthetically based treatment plan be sequenced? and, Can the patient afford the treatment?

The sequence of any treatment plan should always begin with the management or alleviation of acute problems. The remaining treatment plan can then be sequenced in a manner that seems the most logical and that facilitates the next phase of treatment, provided the result can be clearly identified, communicated, and achieved for the pertinent phase. When the author's group establishes the sequence of treatment for an interdisciplinary patient, they list the steps in the treatment plan based on their collective opinion before beginning treatment.[34,37] Every team member receives a copy of the treatment sequence. This step ensures that each member will be able to follow the steps in the esthetic, functional, structural, and biological rehabilitation of their mutual dental patient.

The economics of the interdisciplinary esthetic treatment plan is of primary importance. Patients in modern dental practice have been divided into four types.[43] Type I and II patients generally do not require significant esthetic restoration. Types III and IV typically will require the type of esthetic evaluation outlined in this chapter.

The type III patient is a healthy adult with no occlusal disease, no periodontal problems, but a desire for an esthetic change (see Figs. 21-2, 21-3, 21-6, 21-8, and 21-9). The type III patient could be described as the "cosmetic patient" who is dentally healthy, but wants to make a change in appearance. The hallmark of treating the true cosmetic patient is the requirement of time on the part of the dentist. The dentist must realize this commitment and charge a commensurate fee.

The most challenging situation is the type IV patient (see Figs. 21-1, 21-4, 21-5, 21-7, and 21-10), as outlined in this chapter. This is an adult whose dentition is failing and who may have occlusal disease, periodontal disease, multiple restorative needs, and missing teeth. The type IV patient is the complex reconstruction patient in any dental practice. The hallmark of this patient is multiple appointments over months or even years, depending on the patient's orthodontic, periodontal, endodontic, surgical, and restorative needs. Because of the increased number of appointments and laboratory fees, the clinician must adjust the fees to reflect the time commitment.[43]

CONCLUSION

"Esthetics" has become a respectable term in dentistry. In the past the importance of esthetics was discounted in favor of function, structure, and biology. If a treatment plan does not begin with a clear view of its esthetic impact on the patient, however, the outcome could be disastrous. In today's interdisciplinary dental world, treatment planning must begin with well-defined esthetic objectives. By beginning with esthetics and considering the impact on function, structure, and biology, the clinician can utilize the various disciplines in dentistry to deliver the highest level of dental care to each patient. This process of interdisciplinary esthetic dentistry serves the patient well.

REFERENCES

1. Spear F: My growing involvement in dental study groups, *J Am Coll Dent* 69:22-24, 2002.
2. Vig RG, Brundo GC: The kinetics of anterior tooth display, *J Prosthet Dent* 39:502-504, 1978.
3. Ackerman MB, Brensinger C, Landis JR: An evaluation of dynamic lip-tooth characteristics during speech and smile in adolescents, *Angle Orthod* 74:43-50, 2004.
4. Spear F, Kokich VG, Mathews D: An interdisciplinary case report, *Esthet Interdisc Dent* 1:12-18, 2005.
5. Lopez-Gavito G, Wallen TR, Little RM, Joondeph DR: Openbite malocclusion: a longitudinal 10-year post-retention evaluation of orthodontically treated patients, *Am J Orthod* 87:175-186, 1985.
6. De Mol van Otterloo JJ, Tuinzing DB, Kostense P: Inferior positioning of the maxilla by a Le Fort I osteotomy: a review of 25 patients with vertical maxillary deficiency, *J Craniomaxillofac Surg* 24:69-77, 1996.
7. Major PW, Phillippson GE, Glover KE, Grace MG: Stability of maxilla downgrafting after rigid or wire fixation, *J Oral Maxillofac Surg* 54:1287-1291, 1996.
8. Costa F, Robiony M, Zerman N, et al: Bone biological plate for stabilization of maxillary inferior repositioning, *Minerva Stomatol* 54:227-236, 2005.
9. Kokich VG: Maxillary lateral incisor implants: planning with the aid of orthodontics, *J Oral Maxillofac Surg* 62:48-56, 2004.
10. Spear F: Construction and use of a surgical guide for anterior periodontal surgery, *Contemp Esthet Restor Pract,* April 1999, pp 12-20.
11. Kokich VG: Anterior dental esthetics: an orthodontic perspective. II. Vertical relationships, *J Esthet. Dent* 5:174-178, 1993.
12. Nanda R: Correction of deep overbite in adults, *Dent Clin North Am* 41:67-87, 1997.
13. Kokich VG, Spear FM, Kokich VO: Maximizing anterior esthetics: an interdisciplinary approach. In McNamara JA Jr, editor: *Frontiers in dental and facial esthetics,* Craniofacial Growth Series, Center for Human Growth and Development, University of Michigan, Ann Arbor, 2001, Needham Press.
14. Beyer JW, Lindauer SJ: Evaluation of dental midline position, *Semin Orthod* 4:146-152, 1998.
15. Kokich VO, Kiyak HA, Shapiro PA: Comparing the perception of dentists and laypeople to altered dental esthetics, *J Esthet Dent* 11:311-324, 1999.
16. Thomas JL, Hayes C, Zawaideh S: The effect of axial midline angulation on dental esthetics, *Angle Orthod* 73:359-364, 2003.
17. Kokich VG: Anterior dental esthetics: an orthodontic perspective. III. Mediolateral relationships, *J Esthet Dent* 5:200-207, 1993.
18. Spear FM: The esthetic correction of anterior dental malalignment: conventional vs. instant (restorative) orthodontics, *J Calif Dent Assoc* 32:133-141, 2004.
19. Littlefield K: *A review of the literature of selected cephalometric analyses*, St Louis, 1992, St Louis University Press.
20. Rufenacht C: *Fundamentals of esthetics*, Carol Stream, Ill, 1990, Quintessence.
21. Denison TF, Kokich VG, Shapiro PA: Stability of maxillary surgery in openbite versus nonopenbite malocclusions, *Angle Orthod* 59:5-10, 1989.
22. Proffit WR, Bailey LJ, Phillips C, Turvey TA: Long-term stability of surgical open-bite correction by Le Fort I osteotomy, *Angle Orthod* 70:112-117, 2000.
23. Naylor CK: Esthetic treatment planning: the grid analysis system, *J Esthet Restor Dent* 14:76-84, 2002.
24. Van der Geld PA, van Waas MA: The smile line: a literature search, *Ned Tijdschr Tandheelkd* 110:350-354, 2003.
25. Chiche G, Kokich V, Caudill R: Diagnosis and treatment planning of esthetic problems. In Pinault A, Chiche G, editors: *Esthetics in fixed prosthodontics,* Carol Stream, Ill, 1994, Quintessence, pp 33-52.
26. Gillen RJ, Schwartz RS, Hilton TJ, Evans DB: An analysis of selected normative tooth proportions, *Int J Prosthod* 7:410-417, 1994.
27. Sterrett JD, Oliver T, Robinson F, et al: Width/length ratios of normal clinical crowns of the maxillary anterior dentition in man, *J Clin Periodontol* 26:153-157, 1999.
28. Wolfart S, Thormann H, Freitag S, Kern M: Assessment of dental appearance following changes in incisor proportions, *Eur J Oral Sci* 113:159-165, 2005.
29. Kokich VG: Esthetics: the ortho-perio-restorative connection, *Semin Orthod Dentofacial Orthop* 2:21-30, 1996.
30. Kokich VG, Kokich VO: Orthodontic therapy for the periodontal-restorative patient. In Rose L, Mealey B, Genco R, Cohen D, editors: *Periodontics: medicine, surgery, and implants,* St Louis, 2004, Mosby-Elsevier, pp 718-744.
31. Kokich VG: Anterior dental esthetics: an orthodontic perspective. I. Crown length, *J Esthet Dent* 5:19-23, 1993.
32. Kokich VG: Esthetics and vertical tooth position: the orthodontic possibilities, *Compend Contin Educ Dent* 18:1225-1231, 1997.
33. Kokich VG: Managing orthodontic-restorative treatment for the adolescent patient. In McNamara JA Jr, editor: *Orthodontics and dentofacial orthopedics,* Ann Arbor, Mich, 2001, Needham Press, pp 395-422.
34. Kokich VG, Kokich VO: Interrelationship of orthodontics with periodontics and restorative dentistry. In Nanda R, editor: *Bio-*

mechanics and esthetic strategies in clinical orthodontics, St Louis, 2005, Mosby-Elsevier, pp 348-373.

35. Kurth J, Kokich VG: Open gingival embrasures after orthodontic treatment in adults: prevalence and etiology, *Am J Orthod Dentofacial Orthop* 120:116-123, 2001.
36. Spear F: Maintenance of the interdental papilla following anterior tooth removal, *Pract Periodont Aesthet Dent* 11:21-28, 1999.
37. Kokich VG, Spear F: Guidelines for treating the orthodontic-restorative patient, *Semin Orthod Dentofacial Orthop* 3:3-20, 1999.
38. Emerich-Poplatek K, Sawicki L, Bodal M, Adamowicz-Klepalska B: Forced eruption after crown/root fracture with a simple and aesthetic method using the fractured crown, *Dent Traumatol* 21:165-169, 2005.
39. Koyuturk AE, Malkoc S: Orthodontic extrusion of subgingivally fractured incisor before restoration—a case report: 3-year follow-up, *Dent Traumatol* 21:174-178, 2005.
40. Spear F: When to restore and when to remove the tooth, *Insight and Innovation*: http://www.seattleinstitute.com/content/articles/B%26WWhentoRestoreWhentoRemove.pdf.
41. Spear F: A conversation with Dr. Frank Spear, *Dent Pract Rep* March:42-48, 2002.
42. Spear F: Occlusion in the new millennium: the controversy continues, *Signature* 7:18-21, 2002.
43. Spear F. Implementing the plan: the economics of restorative dentistry, *Insight and Innovation:* www.seattleinstitute.com/content/articles/ImplementingthePlanTheEconomicsofRestorativeDentistry.pdf.

CHAPTER 22

Temporary Anchorage Devices: Biomechanical Opportunities and Challenges

■ *Bhavna Shroff and Steven J. Lindauer*

Temporary anchorage devices (TADs) used to improve anchorage during routine orthodontic therapy have become popular in the past 5 years. Reasons for the increased interest in using such devices for anchorage include their commercial availability, the ease of placement, the lack of necessary patient cooperation, and the possibility of achieving better anchorage control during mechanotherapy.[1-5] This chapter discusses the use of TADs in specific orthodontic situations, presents appliance designs in use, and analyzes the biomechanics of the force systems involved. Recommendations are also included to optimize TAD placement to better control the force system generated by these appliances, thus improving quality of treatment outcome.

ANCHORAGE IN ORTHODONTICS

During orthodontic therapy, the movement of teeth is achieved through the application of a force system on the teeth and the transduction of that mechanical signal into a biological response. As orthodontic forces are applied to move teeth, anchorage is required from teeth in the same or opposing arch to achieve differential tooth movement. Anchorage can be obtained from adjacent teeth or groups of teeth consolidated as a unit. Anchorage to achieve a variety of tooth movements is also obtained extraorally through headgear (occipital, cervical, and combination) and requires significant patient compliance. Teeth that serve as anchorage units should ideally remain stationary; they should not express any of the forces or moments resulting from application of the desired force system to the teeth that need to be moved. In reality, however, anchorage teeth are subjected to the often-undesirable side effects of the mechanics used.

The introduction of implants in dentistry by Branemark[6] in 1969 led to the possibility of developing anchorage systems that could be used during orthodontics and remain stationary because of the implant's osseointegration.[6-8] Linkow[8] was the first author to report the use of implants in conjunction with orthodontic therapy. He advocated use of endosseous blade implants as space maintainers to avoid drifting of the teeth and as posterior anchorage in patients with posterior edentulous areas. He also reported the first clinical application of mandibular implants to support Class II mechanics through Class II elastics. Creekmore and Eklund[7] used bone screws as skeletal anchorage placed in the anterior nasal spine of patients who needed intrusion and torque control of the maxillary incisors.[7] Kanomi[9] described a mini-implant specifically designed to be used as direct anchorage for orthodontic purposes. Costa et al.[10] introduced the first miniscrew that could be used as direct or indirect anchorage because it incorporated a bracket configuration in the design of its head.[9,10]

Since these early reports on the use of skeletal anchorage to support orthodontic therapy, several authors have described the use of such anchorage devices in the hard palate, maxillary molar region, mandibular retromolar area, and maxillary tuberosity to achieve a variety of orthodontic tooth movements, including intrusion, distalization, uprighting, and space closure with torque control.[11-17] The use of endosseous dental implants, miniplates, and miniscrews has been described since the early 1980s, with miniscrews gaining popularity because they are easily placed by the orthodontist with minimal tissue invasion. The use of miniplates has been limited, however, because placement requires the intervention of an oral surgeon and a more invasive placement procedure.

Currently, several terms are used to refer to "skeletal anchorage devices," the most inclusive being *temporary anchorage devices.* Other names include implants, mini-implants, miniscrews, microscrews, screws, miniplates, and plates. *Implants* and *mini-implants* usually necessitate osseointegration for stability, whereas *screws, miniscrews,* and *microscrews* are generally loaded immediately after placement and receive their stability from mechanical retention in the bone. *Plates* are attached to the bone through a surgical procedure necessitating the elevation of a flap. A portion is left emerging in the oral cavity to serve as a point of application for the force system. According to Melsen,[2] these devices need to be classified into an osseointegrated or a nonosseointegrated group. Other authors consider that all these devices provide anchorage to bone and that all considered anchorage devices.

Definition of Anchorage

The concept of anchorage in orthodontics corresponds to the resistance (or lack of) that a tooth or group of teeth may provide when subjected to the application of a force. Clinically, anchorage control is central to achieving an ideal buccal occlusion with ideal overjet and overbite. The lack of posterior teeth can seriously jeopardize the type of tooth movement that can be achieved through orthodontics unless clinicians have options of additional anchorage techniques, such as incorporation of TADs, in treatment planning. Some orthodontic tooth movements (e.g., molar intrusion, mandibular molar distalization) are unpredictable when achieved through conventional orthodontics because of the side effects of the mechanics. Such movement can be achieved with simple force systems and essentially no undesirable side effects on adjacent teeth when TADs are incorporated in the treatment plan.[14,15,18-20]

Historically, the concept of anchorage was introduced by E.H. Angle,[21] and his classification recognized several different types of anchorage, including simple, stationary, reciprocal, intermaxillary, and occipital anchorage. Angle[21-23] distinguished among these different categories based on the treatment goals for tooth movement, as follows:

- *Simple anchorage* corresponded to a situation where an equivalent tooth or larger tooth was used as anchorage.
- *Stationary anchorage* was typically found where teeth were connected to each other in a rigid manner. In this clinical situation, teeth could not tip when subjected to orthodontic forces because of the rigidity of the attachment that connected them, but they translated slowly because of the resistance that the bone offered. The concept of stationary anchorage was primarily based on the rigidity of the anchorage unit.
- *Reciprocal anchorage* corresponded to an anchorage situation where two teeth were moved into their corrected position in the arch and acted as anchorage teeth to each other.
- *Intermaxillary anchorage,* first described by Angle in 1890, was defined as a situation where the anchorage necessary to move one tooth or a group of teeth was found in the opposite arch. A variation of the concept of intermaxillary anchorage included the "Baker anchorage" first introduced by H.A. Baker. In this specific situation, teeth of the entire arch were moved as a unit with respect to the teeth of the opposite arch in the sagittal plane to correct a Class II or III malocclusion, as described by Tweed (1966). The Baker anchorage corresponded to contemporary Class II or III mechanics.
- *Occipital anchorage* was the last type of anchorage described by Angle and corresponded to occipital extraoral anchorage. The anchorage required in these situations was attained by placing forces on the top and back of the patient's head using a headgear. When adequate patient compliance was achieved, this type of anchorage was particularly advantageous because the desired tooth movement was achieved without unfavorable movement of other teeth within the arch or on the opposing arch.

Optimum management of anchorage during orthodontic tooth movement was an important treatment step to ensure successful outcomes.[24]

Burstone[25,26] developed the segmented-arch technique in the early 1960s and introduced an anchorage classification based on the differential movement of the anterior and posterior segments of teeth when a force system was delivered to the dentition. The segmented-arch technique was developed to determine the optimal appliance design that delivered the desired force system to the teeth that needed to be moved. This technique introduced a systematic approach to analyze force systems applied to teeth to effectively control the undesirable side effects. This approach resulted in more predictable and reproducible tooth movement. The segmentation of the arch was a central feature in defining anterior and posterior segments of teeth between which a force system was delivered.

One of the advantages of such an approach to orthodontic mechanotherapy was the possibility of determining the force systems that act on the anterior and posterior segments of teeth, then identifying the desired forces and moments and the undesirable side effects generated by an appliance. This is more difficult to achieve with straight-wire mechanics because the force system generated by a continuous wire connecting multiple teeth is harder to determine than it is for two teeth. The force system delivered by a continuous arch is largely "indeterminate," and the advantage of a segmented approach is the delivery of a "determinate" and reproducible force system.[27] The segmented-arch technique also allows good control of the force and moment magnitudes on the different segments of teeth.[28,29] It uses wires of different cross sections, lengths, and configurations and different materials to combine high and low deflection rate appliances within one arch, allowing better control of the anchorage unit.[28] Finally, the segmented-arch technique introduced a novel way to manage anchorage by dividing the anchorage requirement in three groups: *group A* (or maximum) anchorage, *group B* (or reciprocal) anchorage, and *group C* anchorage (or en masse posterior protraction).

The utilization of the principles of the segmented-arch technique and a proper understanding of biomechanics have allowed for the delivery of the desired force systems, a better control of anchorage through the identification of the undesirable side effects, and an overall improved and more efficient appliance design.[30]

The TAD introduced a new way to incorporate the principles of the segmented-arch technique into a straight-wire system. Because TADs essentially provide an immediate absolute or stationary anchorage, it becomes possible for the clinician to deliver the desired force system using a TAD as anchorage without observing the undesirable side effects on the anchor teeth. In these situations, anchorage can be set up directly through the use of a TAD (direct anchorage) or indirectly through connecting teeth to a TAD and making this segment of teeth virtually stationary (indirect anchorage).

Also, TADs have become attractive alternatives to traditional anchorage that is subjected to undesired side effects and that highly relies highly on patient compliance. In clinical situations where maximum anchorage is required to retract anterior teeth (Burstone's group A anchorage), TADs can provide a simpler approach to anterior tooth retraction, applying the basic principles of biomechanics but simplifying the appliance design and activation. In this situation the clinician can use simple forces to retract the anterior segment of teeth, rather than elaborate retraction loops that need to incorporate appropriate moment of force ratios to control both anterior and posterior segments of teeth. The use of extraoral anchorage such as headgear provides good posterior anchorage but relies heavily on patient compliance and is thus unpopular. Nance appliances, which do not rely on patient cooperation, also provide posterior anchorage, but they can be uncomfortable and become embedded in the palatal mucosa. With headgear and Nance appliances, the anchorage unit of teeth is subjected to a force system and does not remain totally unaffected. TADs offer the possibility to manage anchorage differently because they replace the traditional use of teeth in their capacity as anchorage units. This allows the side effects from the mechanics to affect TADs, not teeth.

One of the keys to successful treatment is to understand and analyze the force system applied to the dentition, to predict and minimize the side effects. Planning to shift the expression of undesired side effects from teeth to TADs can increase the effectiveness of treatment and improve outcome. Again, a TAD in such clinical situations offers direct or indirect anchorage that does not affect tooth position (direct anchorage) or that can stabilize a group of teeth (indirect anchorage).

GENERAL CONSIDERATIONS FOR USE

The stability of TADs after implantation and during treatment and the location of their placement are critical in designing the proper appliance that delivers the appropriate force system. TADs are essentially used as stationary or *absolute* anchorage. TADs obtain their stability from mechanical retention and do not osseointegrate into bone. This stability is not absolute if the TADs fail, and this possibility necessitates attention. Studies in dogs have looked examined the pull-out strength of force necessary to dislodge the screw from its supporting bone and showed that screws placed in the anterior mandible required significantly less force to be pulled from bone than screws in the posterior mandibular regions. The correlation between the cortical bone thickness and the amount of force necessary was significant but weak.[31]

The stability of TADs also has been studied when implanted in the zygomatic buttresses for direct anchorage.[32] Miniscrews were stable but did not remain stationary when subjected to orthodontic forces. The screws showed about 0.4 mm of tipping forward at the level of the head of the screw and some signs of combined extrusion and tipping forward. The authors suggested that the movement of the screws was consistent with the loading pattern in some patients and recommended placement of screws in non–tooth-bearing areas or in tooth-bearing areas, allowing a minimum of 2 mm of safety clearance between the screws and the roots of the teeth.

Buchter et al.[33] evaluated the transverse loading of miniscrews and concluded the failure of implants was directly related to the magnitude of the moment applied. The value of the moment needed to be smaller than 900 centinewtons per millimeter (cN/mm) for immediate loading of the screws.

The stability of miniscrews is also related to the location of their insertion into the bone. Ishii et al.[34] measured the buccolingual and the mesiodistal lengths and areas of sectioned interalveolar septum from randomly selected maxillary bones using micro–computed tomography (micro-CT). They concluded that the safest position for implantation was the interalveolar septum between the maxillary first molar and the second premolar, 6 to 8 mm apical to the alveolar crest on the palatal side.

Poggio et al.[35] repeated the study using 25 maxillae and 25 mandibles retrieved from patients' records (data were collected with NewTom [DVT9000] Volume Scanner, QRsr1, Verona, Italy). They confirmed that the safest place in the maxilla to place a TAD was on the palatal side between the first permanent molars and the second premolars. The least amount of bone in the maxilla was found in the tuberosity area. The greatest thickness of bone measured buccopalatally was observed between the first and second molars. In the mandible, the least amount of bone was found between the first premolar and the canine, with the greatest bone thickness found between the first and second molars. The authors recommended a number of areas as safe for implant placement. They included the posterior aspect of the maxilla on the buccal and palatal aspects, and a generally more apical placement as the implantation site became more mesial. In the mandibular arch, the safest areas to place TADs were in the posterior areas, and implantation needed to be at least 11 mm from the alveolar crest as placement was performed in the premolar and canine areas.[35]

Wilmes et al.[36] reported on the potential factors affecting the primary stability of orthodontic mini-implants and concluded that the thickness of the compact bone, implant design, and implant site preparation were critical to the implant's stability.

Deciding on the appropriate placement of TADs is critical for safety and for the appropriate design and delivery of the desired force system. During the treatment planning of orthodontic therapy, the clinician needs to determine the desired force system and its equilibrium diagram to identify the force system acting on the *active* unit of teeth (the unit of teeth that needs movement) and the side effects affecting the anchorage unit of teeth. This will dictate ideal placement of the TAD to ensure safety and optimal appliance design.

Clinicians should be fully aware of the anatomical limitations to implantation of TADs. These limitations drive important decisions in appliance design and the resulting force system (e.g., point of force application, direction of force and moment generated). Also, the force system applied to the TAD needs to be carefully evaluated to control the moments generated that tend to unscrew the TAD, to prevent the miniscrew from loosening. If the application of such undesirable moments to the screw cannot be avoided, indirect anchorage is recommended to optimize the anchorage system and minimize the undesirable side effects resulting from the force system.[2]

INDICATIONS

The availability of TADs through various commercial companies has made their use in daily orthodontics very accessible. TAD use was initially limited to clinical situations where posterior teeth were missing and anchorage was necessary, as well as in posterior edentulous areas.[1,2,8] Use of TADs has since extended to facilitate a variety of tooth movements, including the following: intrusion of maxillary teeth,[11,15,37,38] distalization of teeth,[19] canine retraction and intrusion retraction mechanics,[13,39] anterior open-bite correction,* correction of deep overbite,[42] Class III correction combined with surgery,[12] and correction of canted occlusal planes.[43] Currently, TADs are available in a variety of shapes and include sophisticated head designs that offer multiple options in deciding on the point of force application.

In general, TADs have simplified orthodontic appliance design by allowing the direct application of the desired force system where needed, and they have tremendously improved the control of the anchorage. In some clinical situations, use of TADs has allowed orthodontic treatment and restoration of the dentition that would otherwise not be possible (e.g., intrusion of molars, distal movement of mandibular molars).[15,18-20] Some clinical reports have shown successful closure of anterior open bites using various mechanics incorporating TADs to intrude posterior teeth and redirect the cant of the occlusal plane.[14,15,17,18,41] Other clinical applications have been advocated and have been shown to be reasonably successful.[16,38,44]

The next section describes and analyzes the appliance design and the biomechanics of several clinical situations, including intrusion of molars, extrusion, and space closure. In each clinical case, a detailed analysis of the force system and its equilibrium helps the reader attain a better understanding of the strategic use of TADs and the resulting appliance design.

*References 14, 15, 17, 18, 40, and 41.

BIOMECHANICAL APPLICATION IN ORTHODONTICS

The use of temporary anchorage devices in orthodontics offers an exciting opportunity to achieve treatment results not previously possible with conventional mechanics. Because TADs do not move significantly, the unwanted side-effects of many biomechanical force systems used in orthodontic treatment can be eliminated, and tooth movements can be planned under the assumption of absolute anchorage conditions.

However, using TADs as anchors also presents new biomechanical challenges. Limitations arise because the locations available for TAD placement affect the direction of force application, which may or may not directly complement the tooth movement desired. Also, the design of most TADs currently available is not conducive for creating complex wire activations. Generally, direct force between the TAD and the target tooth is created by stretching an elastic chain or coil spring to move the tooth toward the TAD. Therefore, when using a TAD as a direct anchor, it is advantageous to place the TAD along the line of desired tooth movement. In this situation, force applied between the TAD and the tooth will cause the tooth to move as required. If a TAD cannot be placed in a favorable position for the desired force system, alternative configurations for force application must be devised, or untoward side effects may result.

Intrusion

An example of a favorable situation for TAD use is intrusion of overerupted posterior teeth.[3,45-47] Intrusion of posterior teeth is considered one of the most difficult types of tooth movement to achieve using conventional mechanics. Bite blocks, repelling magnets, and other interarch devices have been advocated and used with varying success in the past.[48-50] Figure 22-1 depicts how a TAD (miniplate or miniscrew) can be placed in the buccal vestibule apical to the posterior maxillary molars to be used as anchorage for molar intrusion. Analysis of the force system from the buccal view (Fig. 22-1, *A*) reveals a favorable force system for straight intrusion, with the effective intrusive force passing through the center of resistance of the molar segment. From the frontal view (Fig 22-1, *B*), however, it is apparent that the force passes buccal to the center of resistance and would result in buccal tipping of the molars (Fig 22-1, *C*). Three-dimensional analysis of the force systems created is often necessary for accurate prediction of the tooth movement that will occur.

Figure 22-2 illustrates successfully controlled intrusion of an overerupted molar. For this patient (Fig. 22-2, *A*), in

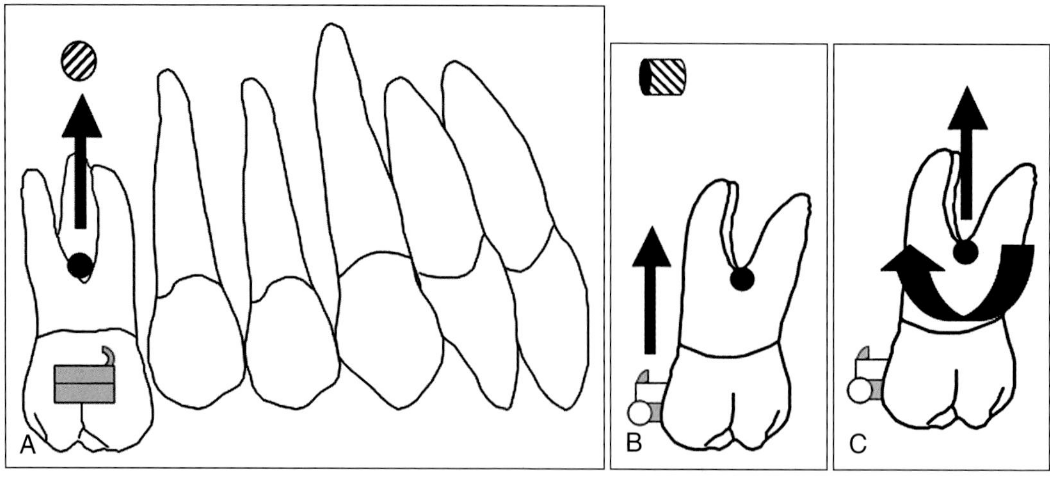

Fig. 22-1 Diagrammatic representation of maxillary molar intrusion using a temporary anchorage device (TAD) inserted on the buccal aspect. **A,** Buccal view. The intrusive force passes through the molar center of resistance *(black circle).* **B,** Frontal view. The force passes buccal to the center of resistance. **C,** The resultant force system would cause both intrusion of the molar and tipping of the crown to the buccal side.

addition to the buccal intrusive force *(B)*, a TAD was also placed on the palatal side to apply a palatal intrusive force *(C)*. The buccal attachment was a miniplate placed in the zygoma, and the palatal TAD was a miniscrew. By applying intrusive forces from both buccal and palatal aspects *(D)*, the resultant, effective intrusive force was redirected through the molar center of resistance *(E)* to achieve intrusion of the overerupted molar without tipping (*F* and *G*).

If posterior teeth are to be intruded bilaterally, then a transpalatal arch (TPA) can be used to avoid buccal tipping of the molars.[41,51] Figure 22-3 shows a patient with an anterior open bite *(A)*, and the plan is to intrude the molars to achieve a closing autorotation of the mandible. In this case, TADs (miniscrews) have been placed apical to the molars bilaterally (*B* and *C*). A TPA was inserted to negate the tendency of the molars to tip buccally as they intrude *(D)*. If some buccal tipping does occur during intrusion, it may be necessary to activate the TPA to produce equal and opposite couples in a crown palatal–root buccal direction[52] *(E)*. In addition, the TPA must be formed so that it is off of the palate when inserted to accommodate movement of the TPA apically as the molars intrude.

Intrusion of anterior teeth can often be accomplished successfully using conventional mechanics. Figure 22-4 shows an intrusion arch applying an apically directed force to the incisors along with an extrusive force and tip-back couple to the molars.[53-55] In a Class II patient (Fig. 22-4, *A*), these side effects can produce favorable tip-back of maxillary molars, allowing the crowns to become more Class I during the intrusion process *(B)*.[55] After the molar crowns are Class I *(C)*, the premolars may drift distally or can be retracted into a Class I relationship *(D)*.

If incisor intrusion is planned but the molar side effects from conventional mechanics are undesirable, TADs may be used to stabilize the molars during the incisor intrusion process. Alternatively, TADs can be placed anteriorly and used for direct application of the intrusive force to the incisors. Figure 22-5 shows mandibular anterior teeth being intruded using TADs placed distal to the canine roots in a patient missing several posterior teeth *(A)*. Although, the point of force application would have been more favorable if the TADs could have been placed closer to the midline for this patient, the location for TAD insertion was limited by bony architecture and a lack of space farther anteriorly *(B)*.

Extrusion

In much the same way that an intrusion arch can be used to intrude anterior teeth with conventional mechanics, an archwire with extrusive force can be used to extrude anterior teeth.[55,56] If a patient has an anterior open bite and the diagnosis is favorable for treating the condition dentally, extrusion can often be accomplished conventionally (Fig. 22-6). Activation of an extrusion arch results in a tip-forward couple and an intrusive force at the molar, along with extrusion anteriorly[55,56] (Fig. 22-6, *A*). Unless precautions are taken, a lateral open bite may occur over time as the molar tips forward, if a continuous wire or posterior segment is in place.[56] If the extrusive force is applied unilaterally, it can be used to correct an anterior cant of the occlusal plane (Fig. 22-6, *B*). In this patient the left anterior teeth are extruded to close the open bite and level the anterior occlusal plane by applying the extrusive force off-center (Fig. 22-6, *C*). In such situations, TADs can be used to stabilize against undesired tooth movements.

Applying extrusive force directly to teeth using a TAD can be challenging. Figure 22-7 shows a patient who had an ankylosed maxillary central incisor that was used as a TAD[57]

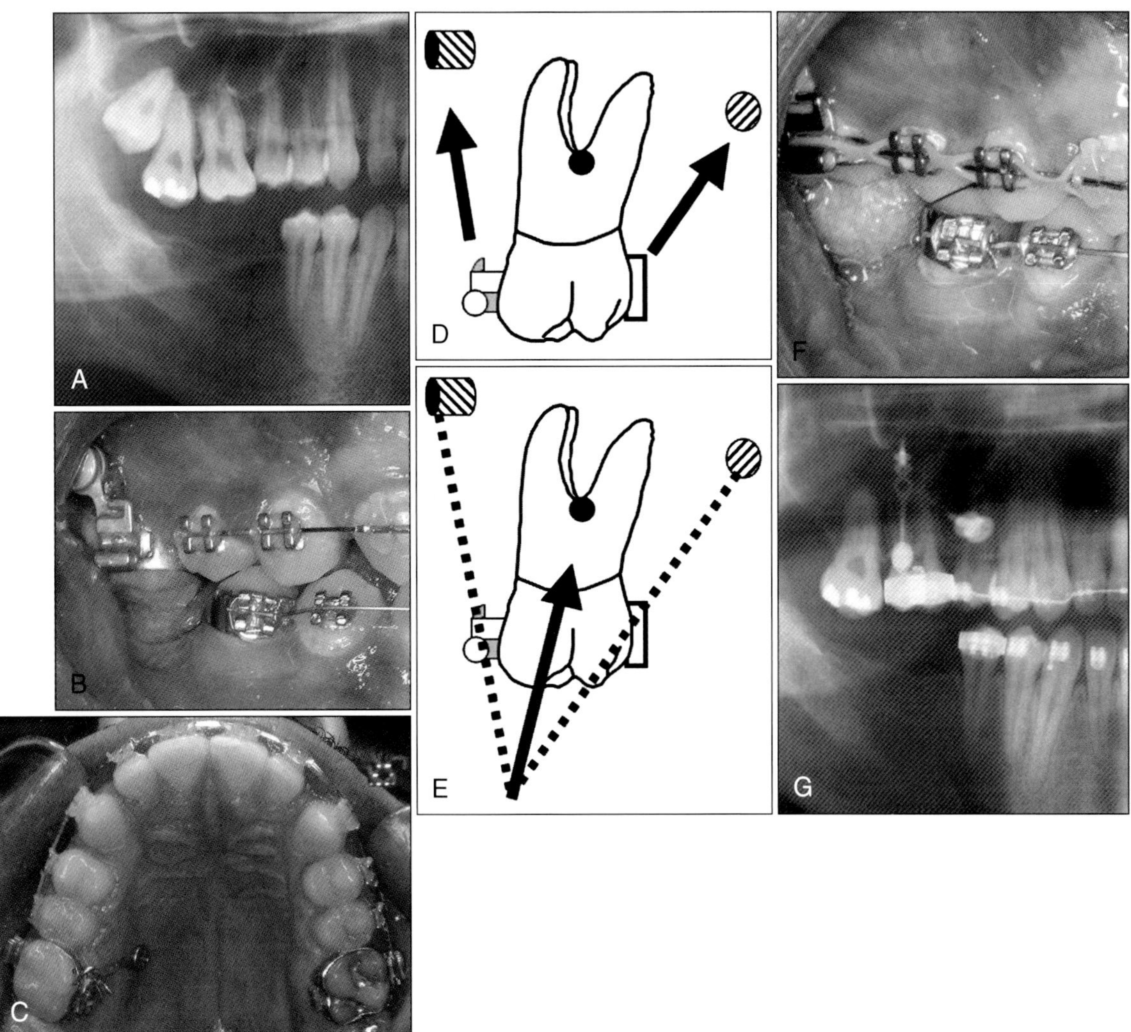

Fig. 22-2 Successful intrusion of overerupted molars. **A,** Panoramic radiograph showing overerupted maxillary right first and second molars. **B,** Buccal view showing elastic chain used to deliver an intrusive force to the molar from the buccal TAD. **C,** Occlusal view showing elastic chain used to deliver an intrusive force to the molar from the palatal TAD. **D,** The force system delivered to the buccal and lingual attachments on the molar. **E,** Resolution of the force system delivered shows that the net force is effective through the molar center of resistance, resulting in a pure translational intrusion of the molar (**F** and **G**).

to close an anterior open bite *(A)*. A spring was designed that would exert extrusive force on the adjacent lateral incisor when it was compressed *(B)*. Once the lateral incisor was at the desired vertical level, a rigid wire was used to hold the tooth in place relative to the ankylosed central incisor while the rest of the arch was aligned *(C)*. In this case the ankylosed incisor was used as stable anchorage, similar to how a TAD could have been used if an ankylosed tooth had not been available.

Space Closure

Using TADs to achieve absolute anchorage during space closure can be more difficult than it would first appear to be. To retract anterior teeth or to protract posterior teeth, it may be easier to use an indirect anchorage technique.[51] In this way the TAD is used to stop unwanted movements of segments of teeth while conventional mechanics are used to close the space. In Figure 22-8, for example, a miniscrew is used to prevent posterior movement of anterior teeth while elastic chain is being used to protract the first molar into the missing second premolar site *(A)*. To prevent movement of the anterior teeth, the extension from the TAD to the archwire has been activated slightly to exert an anteriorly directed force. This activation causes a clockwise couple at the TAD, thereby tightening the screw in a favorable direction for its stability *(B)*. A counterclockwise couple, on the other hand, would cause loosening of the screw. In this patient the TAD enabled maximum protraction of the posterior teeth with minimal patient compliance *(C)*.

Fig. 22-3 Molar intrusion to correct an anterior open bite. **A,** Frontal view showing a patient with an anterior open bite and TADs placed buccally bilaterally to deliver intrusive force to the molars. **B,** Right buccal view. **C,** Left buccal view. **D,** Occlusal view showing the transpalatal arch (TPA) used to prevent buccal tipping of the molar crowns as they intrude. **E,** Frontal view diagram showing the force systems delivered by the elastic chain from TADs and TPA activation.

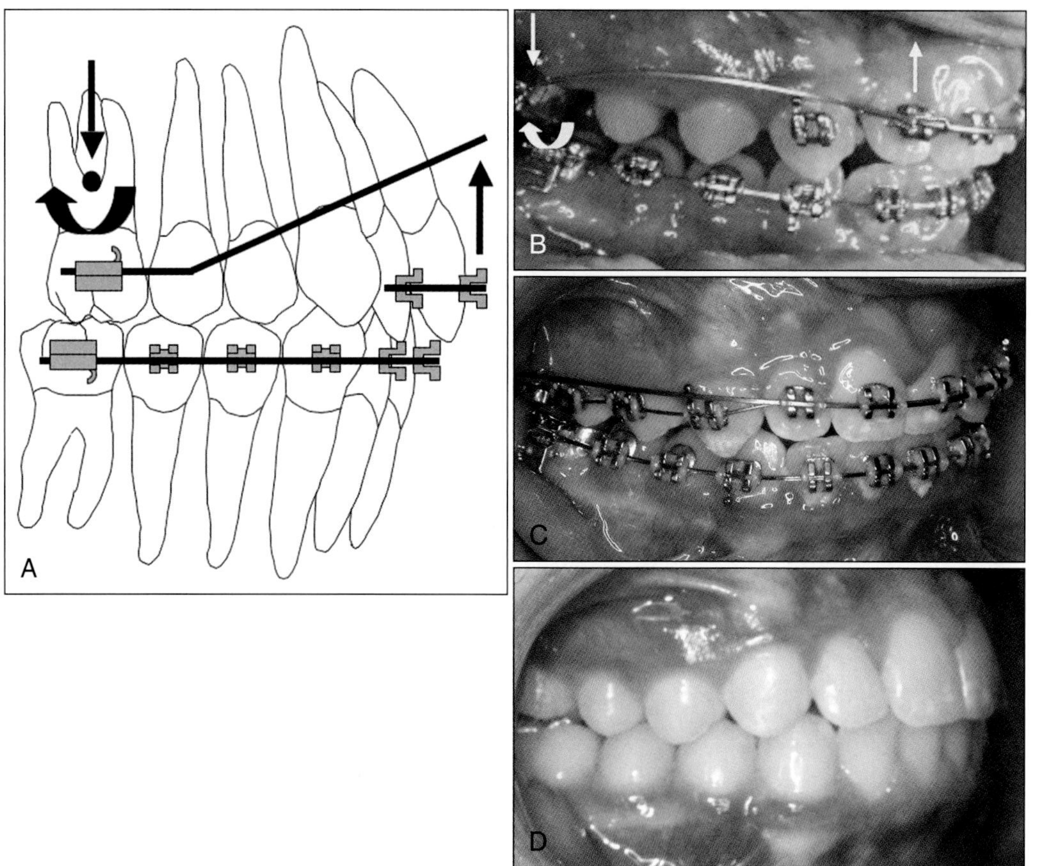

Fig. 22-4 Conventional intrusion arch mechanics to correct overbite and improve molar classification. **A,** The force system delivered by an intrusion arch. **B,** Right buccal view of a patient with an intrusion arch in place demonstrating incisor intrusion and molar tip-back to a Class I relationship. **C,** Right buccal view after the premolars are bonded and intrusion is complete. **D,** Right buccal view at the end of treatment.

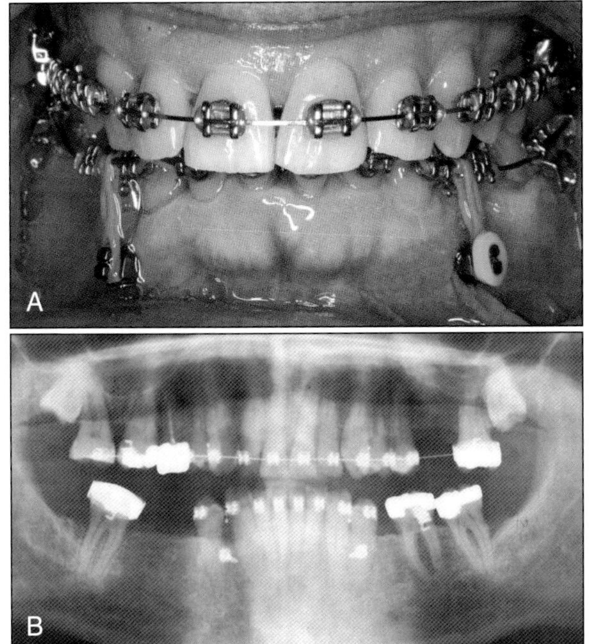

Fig. 22-5 Incisor intrusion using TADs as anchorage. **A,** Frontal view showing TADs used as anchorage to intrude lower anterior teeth in a patient with several missing posterior teeth. **B,** Panoramic radiograph showing TAD placement.

If direct anchorage is used to apply force to close space, the direction and point of force application become critical. Figure 22-9 shows a patient who required absolute posterior anchorage during space closure. TADs were placed mesial to the first molar roots, and chain elastic was used to apply force to the anterior brackets *(A)*. The force was directed in a distal and apical direction and passed well below the center of resistance of the anterior teeth *(B)*, resulting in significant and unfavorable uprighting of those teeth *(C)*. Alternatively, a segmented approach[25] could be used to redirect the force to a more favorable point of application. A distal extension to the anterior segment, bent apically so that the line of force is close to the center of resistance of the anterior teeth (Fig. 22-9, *D*),[58] allows for space closure to occur that approximates translation and minimizes tipping *(E)*.

To achieve certain sequences of tooth movement, a TAD may need to be removed and perhaps replaced if it physically impedes the progression of treatment. Figure 22-10 shows a patient in whom the plan was to protract the mandibular right second molar into the missing first molar position. However, the first step in treatment was to move the mandibular right canine and premolars anteriorly because they had tipped distally after the first molar was extracted. A TAD was placed between the first and second premolar roots and

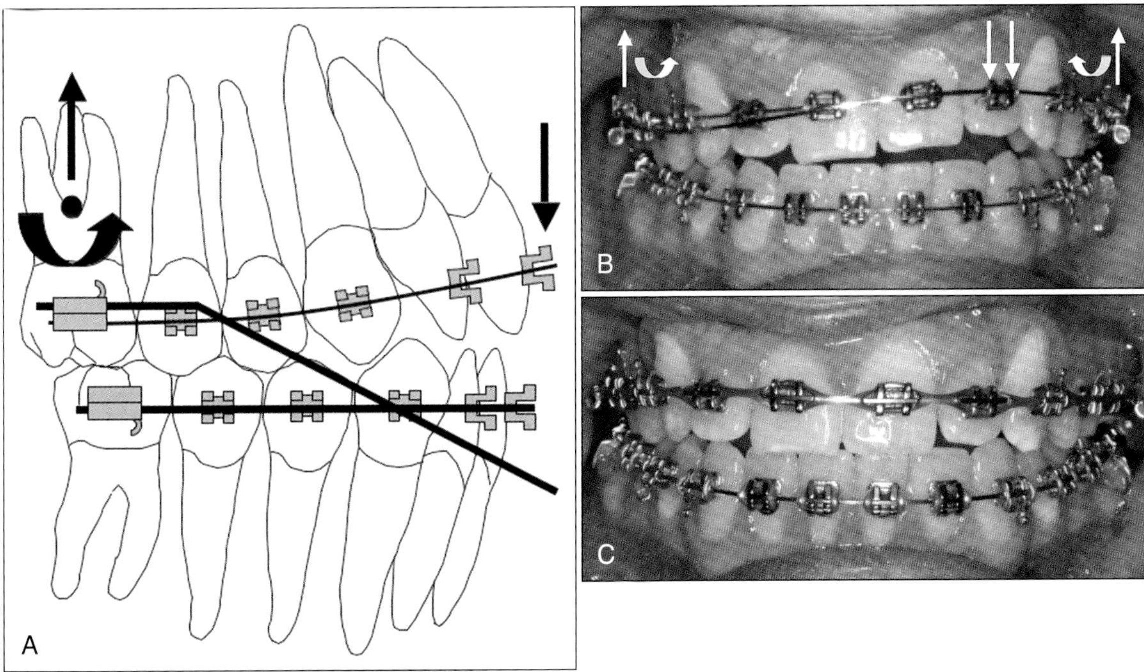

Fig. 22-6 Conventional extrusion arch mechanics to close an open bite and/or correct a cant of the anterior occlusal plane. **A,** The force system delivered by an extrusion arch. **B,** Frontal view showing a patient with a cant of the anterior occlusal plane and an extrusion arch tied only on the patient's left to deliver asymmetric force to correct the cant. **C,** Frontal view of the patient after the cant has been corrected.

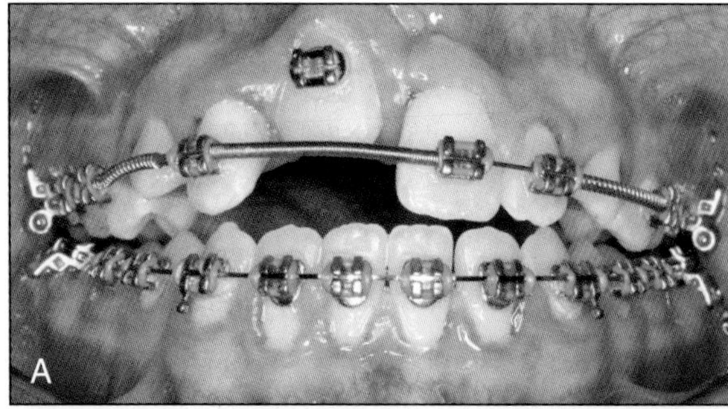

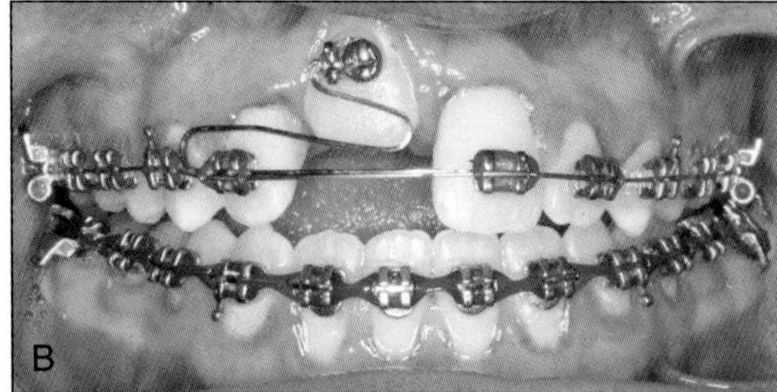

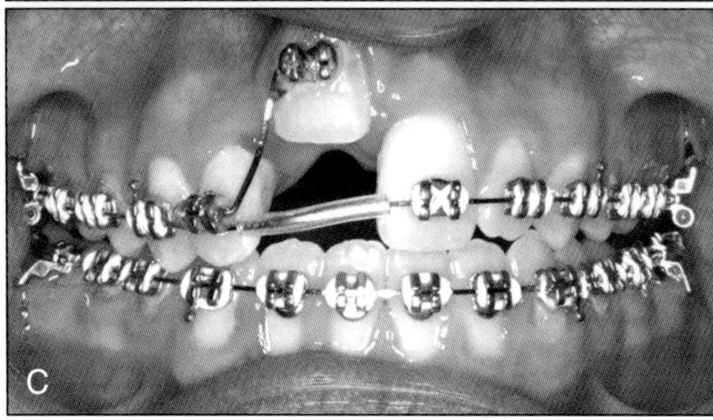

Fig. 22-7 Extrusion of teeth using a TAD as anchorage. **A,** Frontal view of a patient with an ankylosed maxillary right central incisor and an anterior open bite. **B,** Spring was designed to deliver extrusive force using the ankylosed tooth as anchorage. **C,** Rigid wire from the ankylosed tooth was used to maintain the vertical position of the extruded teeth as the arch was aligned.

tied to the second molar to prevent distal molar movement while the canine and first premolar were pushed anteriorly (Fig. 22-10, *A*). Later in treatment, however, when the TAD was being used as an anchor to protract the molar and second premolar, it was impeding movement of those teeth and had to be removed (Fig. 22-10, *B*). Another TAD was placed farther anteriorly, between the canine and first premolar, and used as an indirect anchor to support protraction of the second molar (Fig. 22-10, *C*).

In some patients, careful planning can help avoid situations where TADs will need to be moved during treatment. For other cases, it is always better to anticipate the need to remove and replace a TAD at some point so that the patient can be prepared before the situation arises.

CONCLUSION

The use of temporary anchorage devices has increased in popularity in recent years, and TADs have revolutionized the current approach to treatment planning and appliance design in orthodontics. Although TAD use was initially advocated as adjunctive and associated with every aspect of orthodontic mechanotherapy, it is now tailored to specific clinical applications that benefit from TAD implantation. The impressive number of clinical case studies published in the literature has also demonstrated that clinicians have become more experienced and more sophisticated in using TADs. Studies cited have also demonstrated that some applications are consistently successful with excellent treatment outcomes and some do not provide the reproducibility and predictability that are desired when treating patients. As orthodontics and dentistry in general has become more evidence based,[59] treatment techniques based on sound research have gained popularity in the past decade, and the use of TADs has not escaped this trend. Orthodontists have also become more educated on how to maximize the use of TADs to simplify their treatment mechanics based on a good understanding of biomechanical principles, as demonstrated by the clinical examples in this chapter.

The use of TADs is new and exciting, and most orthodontists currently in practice were not exposed to the use of such devices during their residency programs. Despite this lack of exposure, the use of TADs in clinical practice is experiencing an upward trend most likely because of the multidisciplinary approach to contemporary treatment planning, because of the expansion of the scope of treatment that orthodontists provide as specialists, and also because of the previously traditional surgical treatments that are now approached with orthodontic alternatives. Few residency programs have been proactive enough to systematically incorporate the use of TADs in their routine treatment, making them available to the population and to the future generations of orthodontists. As more research on the safety and efficacy of these devices becomes available, it is expected that more graduate programs will embrace this new area of orthodontic therapy. Just as the Human Genome Project had a significant impact on translating basic science research into clinically relevant applications,[60] TADs have had a profound impact on the way malocclusion is viewed and have provided alternative treatment modalities to those available through traditional orthodontics.

Further refinements in TAD design and a better understanding of how to maximize the use of TADs by analyzing the biomechanical force systems produced by various appliance designs will continue to make TADs a very attractive alternative to traditional anchorage techniques. Because the level of patient compliance is rapidly decreasing for clinicians, the option of using TADs will continue to grow, providing patients with desired treatment outcomes. TADs are not just a new appliance that is in fashion today; they are becoming part of an improved and sophisticated therapeutic strategy in orthodontics that will allow better treatment

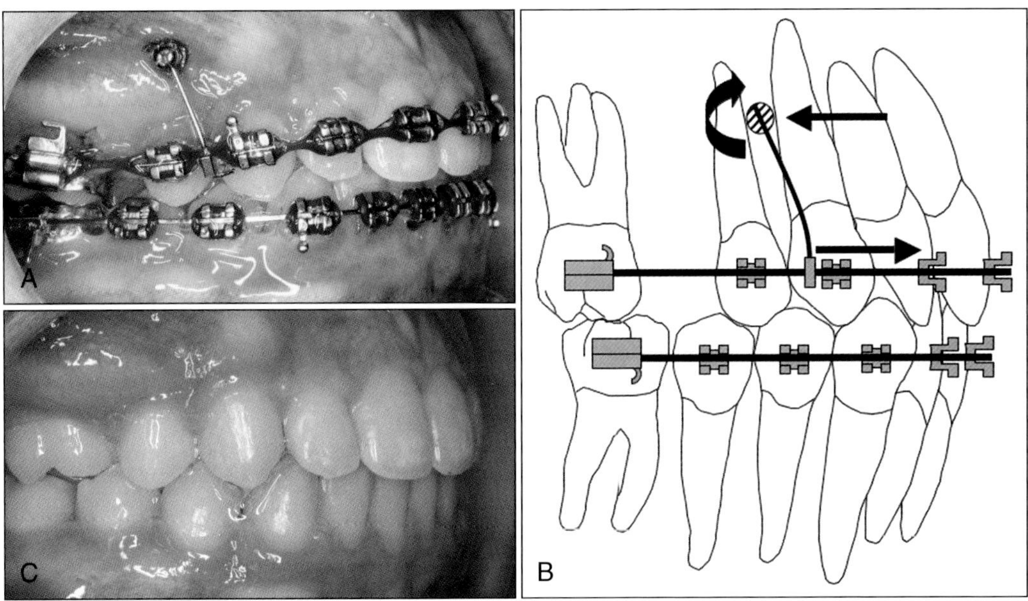

Fig. 22-8 Using a TAD for indirect anchorage during space closure. **A,** Wire extends from the TAD to a tube crimped to the archwire to prevent posterior movement of the anterior teeth during space closure to protract the maxillary first molar. **B,** Force-moment diagram illustrating that activating the wire to produce mesial force on the arch will cause the TAD to sustain a distal force and rotate clockwise, thereby tightening the screw slightly. **C,** Buccal view of the patient at the end of treatment demonstrating that the molar has been protracted into the missing second premolar space.

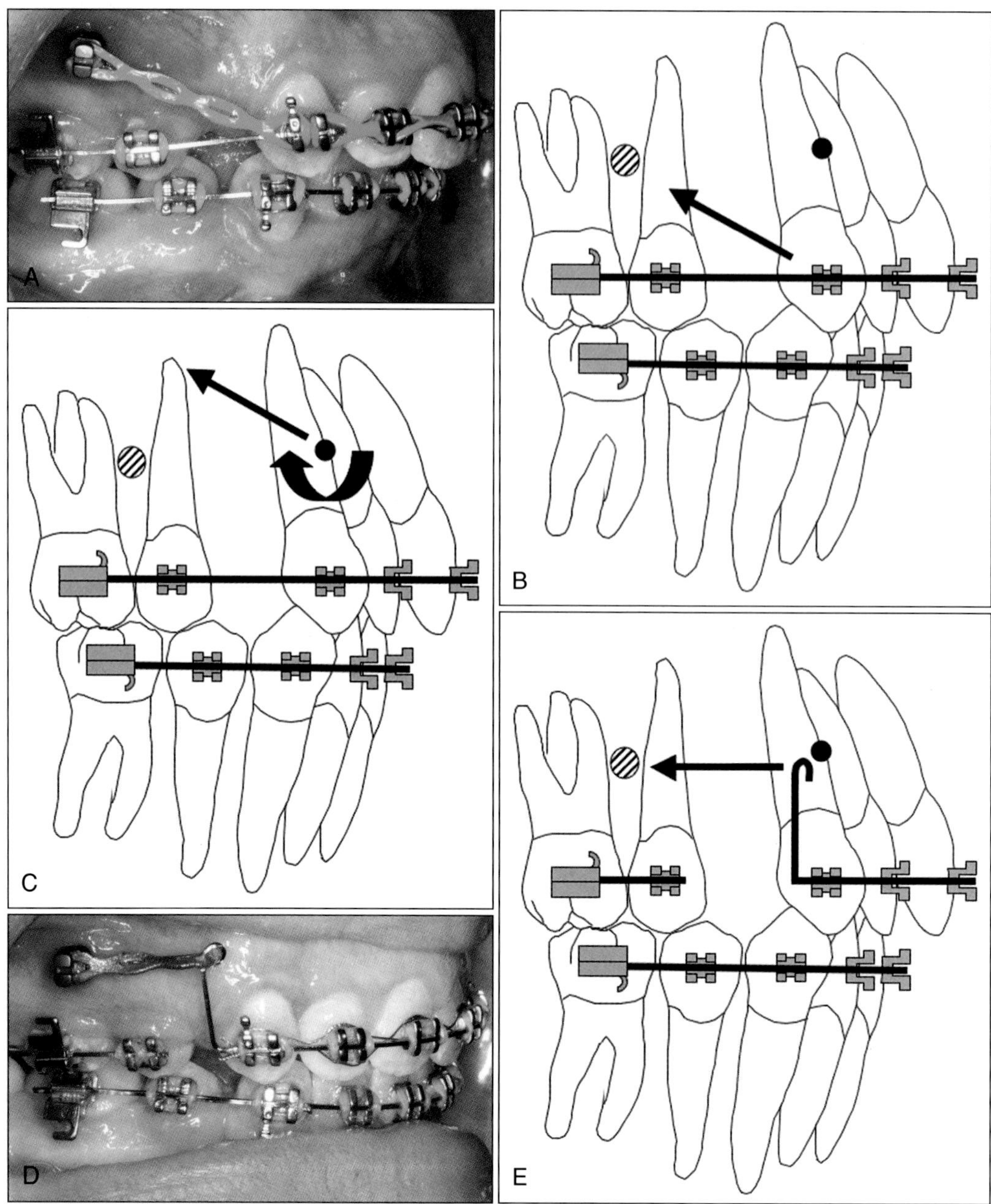

Fig. 22-9 Using a TAD for direct anchorage during space closure. **A,** Buccal view of a patient with elastic chain stretched from a TAD to the canine to retract anterior teeth. **B,** Force-moment diagram illustrating that the distal force from the elastic chain passes well below the center of resistance of the anterior teeth *(black circle).* **C,** Distal force causes the anterior teeth to move distally and intrusively as well as for their crowns to upright. **D,** Buccal view showing a TAD being used to deliver distal force to an anterior segment with a distal extension bent apically. **E,** Distal force passes close to the center of resistance of the anterior teeth.

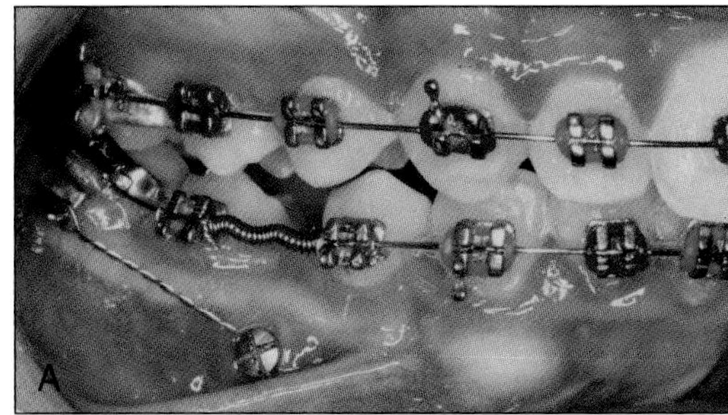

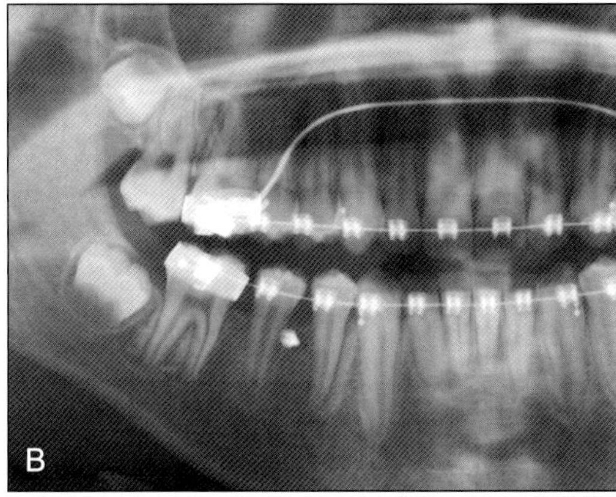

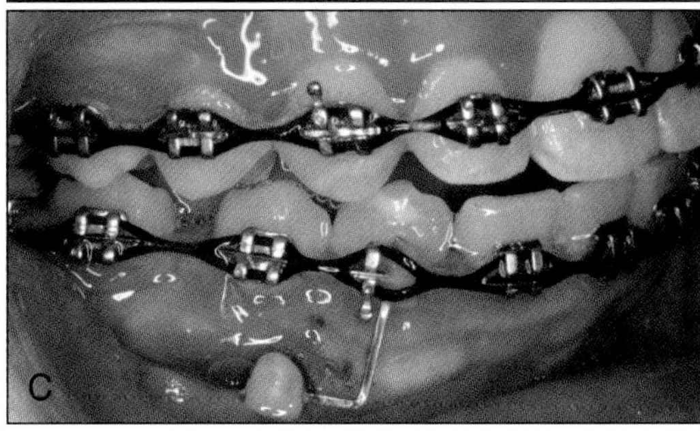

Fig. 22-10 Positioning a TAD can impede tooth movement. **A,** For this patient a TAD was first placed distal to the mandibular second premolar and used to prevent molar distal movement as the anterior teeth were being pushed forward. **B,** Panoramic radiograph showing that, later in treatment, the TAD impeded further anterior movement of the posterior teeth during space closure. **C,** Original TAD was removed. A new TAD was placed mesial to the first premolar and used as indirect anchorage to complete protraction of the posterior teeth mesially.

through simpler appliance designs. Temporary anchorage devices are here to stay.

ACKNOWLEDGMENTS

We wish to extend our thanks to Dr. Erica W. Reed and Dr. Robert E. Patterson for their assistance with this manuscript. We also thank Dr. Jason T. Gladwell, who inspired us to explore this new and exciting therapeutic alternative.

References

1. Huang LH, Shotwell JL, Wang HL: Dental implants for orthodontic anchorage, *Am J Orthod Dentofacial Orthop* 127:713-722, 2005.
2. Melsen B: Mini-implants: where are we? *J Clin Orthod* 39:539-547, 2005.
3. Mizrahi E, Mizrahi B: Mini-screw implants (temporary anchorage devices): orthodontic and pre-prosthetic applications, *J Orthod* 34:80-94, 2007.
4. Celenza F. Implant-enhanced tooth movement: indirect absolute anchorage, *Int J Periodont Restor Dent* 23:533-541, 2003.
5. Chen CH, Chang CS, Hsieh CH, et al: The use of microimplants in orthodontic anchorage, *J Oral Maxillofac Surg* 64:1209-1213, 2006.
6. Branemark PI, Adell R, Breine U, et al: Intra-osseous anchorage of dental prostheses. I. Experimental studies, *Scand J Plast Reconstr Surg* 3:81-100, 1969.
7. Creekmore TD, Eklund MK: The possibility of skeletal anchorage, *J Clin Orthod* 17:266-269, 1983.
8. Linkow LI: Implanto-orthodontics, *J Clin Orthod* 4:685-690, 1970.
9. Kanomi R: Mini-implant for orthodontic anchorage, *J Clin Orthod* 31:763-767, 1997.
10. Costa A, Raffainl M, Melsen B: Miniscrews as orthodontic anchorage: a preliminary report, *Int J Adult Orthod Orthog Surg* 13:201-209, 1998.
11. Kravitz ND, Kusnoto B, Tsay TP, Hohlt WF: The use of temporary anchorage devices for molar intrusion, *J Am Dent Assoc* 138:56-64, 2007.
12. Kuroda S, Sugawara Y, Yamashita K, et al: Skeletal Class III oligodontia patient treated with titanium screw anchorage and orthognathic surgery, *Am J Orthod Dentofacial Orthop* 127:730-738, 2005.
13. Park HS, Bae SM, Kyung HM, Sung JH: Simultaneous incisor retraction and distal molar movement with microimplant anchorage, *World J Orthod* 5:164-171, 2004.
14. Sugawara J, Daimaruya T, Umemori M, et al: Distal movement of mandibular molars in adult patients with the skeletal anchorage system, *Am J Orthod Dentofacial Orthop* 125:130-138, 2004.
15. Park YC, Lee SY, Kim DH, Jee SH: Intrusion of posterior teeth using mini-screw implants, *Am J Orthod Dentofacial Orthop* 123:690-694, 2003.
16. Hong RK, Heo JM, Ha YK: Lever-arm and mini-implant system for anterior torque control during retraction in lingual orthodontic treatment, *Angle Orthod* 75:129-141, 2005.
17. Umemori M, Sugawara J, Mitani H, et al: Skeletal anchorage system for open-bite correction, *Am J Orthod Dentofacial Orthop* 115:166-174, 1999.
18. Sugawara J, Baik UB, Umemori M, et al: Treatment and post-treatment dentoalveolar changes following intrusion of mandibular molars with application of a skeletal anchorage system (SAS) for open bite correction, *Int J Adult Orthod Orthog Surg* 17:243-253, 2002.
19. Park HS, Lee SK, Kwon OW: Group distal movement of teeth using microscrew implant anchorage, *Angle Orthod* 75:602-609, 2005.
20. Park HS, Jang BK, Kyung HM: Maxillary molar intrusion with micro-implant anchorage (MIA), *Aust Orthod J* 21:129-135, 2005.

21. Angle EH: *Treatment of malocclusion of teeth: Angle's system*, ed 7, Philadelphia, 1907, SS White Dental Manufacturing.
22. Angle EH: The latest and the best in orthodontic mechanism, *Dent Cosmos* 70:1143, 1928.
23. Angle EH: The latest and the best in orthodontic mechanism, *Dent Cosmos* 71:164, 260, 409, 1929.
24. Strang RH: Orthodontic anchorage, *Angle Orthod* 11:173, 1941.
25. Burstone CJ: Rationale of the segmented arch, *Am J Orthod* 48:805-822, 1962.
26. Burstone CJ: The mechanics of the segmented arch techniques, *Angle Orthod* 36:99-120, 1966.
27. Burstone CJ, Koenig HA: Force systems from an ideal arch, *Am J Orthod* 65:270-289, 1974.
28. Burstone CJ: Variable-modulus orthodontics, *Am J Orthod* 80:1-16, 1981.
29. Burstone CJ, Koenig HA: Optimizing anterior and canine retraction, *Am J Orthod* 70:1-19, 1976.
30. Burstone CJ: The segmented arch approach to space closure, *Am J Orthod* 82:361-378. 1982.
31. Huja SS, Litsky AS, Beck FM, et al: Pull-out strength of monocortical screws placed in the maxillae and mandibles of dogs, *Am J Orthod Dentofacial Orthop* 127:307-313, 2005.
32. Liou EJ, Pai BC, Lin JC: Do miniscrews remain stationary under orthodontic forces? *Am J Orthod Dentofacial Orthop* 126:42-47, 2004.
33. Buchter A, Wiechmann D, Koerdt S, et al: Load-related implant reaction of mini-implants used for orthodontic anchorage, *Clin Oral Implants Res* 16:473-479, 2005.
34. Ishii T, Nojima K, Nishii Y, et al: Evaluation of the implantation position of mini-screws for orthodontic treatment in the maxillary molar area by a micro CT, *Bull Tokyo Dent Coll* 45:165-172, 2004.
35. Poggio PM, Incorvati C, Velo S, Carano A: "Safe zones": a guide for miniscrew positioning in the maxillary and mandibular arch, *Angle Orthod* 76:191-197, 2006.
36. Wilmes B, Rademacher C, Olthoff G, Drescher D: Parameters affecting primary stability of orthodontic mini-implants, *J Orofac Orthop* 67:162-174, 2006.
37. Yao CC, Lee JJ, Chen HY, et al: Maxillary molar intrusion with fixed appliances and mini-implant anchorage studied in three dimensions, *Angle Orthod* 75:754-760, 2005.
38. Yao CC, Wu CB, Wu HY, et al: Intrusion of the overerupted upper left first and second molars by mini-implants with partial-fixed orthodontic appliances: a case report, *Angle Orthod* 74:550-557, 2004.
39. Park HS, Kwon OW, Sung JH: Microscrew implant anchorage sliding mechanics, *World J Orthod* 6:265-274, 2005.
40. Park HS, Kwon TG, Kwon OW: Treatment of open bite with microscrew implant anchorage, *Am J Orthod Dentofacial Orthop* 126:627-636, 2004.
41. Park HS, Kwon OW, Sung JH: Nonextraction treatment of an open bite with microscrew implant anchorage, *Am J Orthod Dentofacial Orthop* 130:391-402, 2006.
42. Ohnishi H, Yagi T, Yasuda Y, Takada K: A mini-implant for orthodontic anchorage in a deep overbite case, *Angle Orthod* 75:444-452, 2005.
43. Jeon YJ, Kim YH, Son WS, Hans MG: Correction of a canted occlusal plane with miniscrews in a patient with facial asymmetry, *Am J Orthod Dentofacial Orthop* 130:244-252, 2006.
44. Gibbons AJ, Cousley RR: Use of mini-implants in orthognathic surgery, *Br J Oral Maxillofac Surg* 45:406-407, 2007.
45. Herman R, Cope JB: Miniscrew implants: IMTEC mini ortho implants, *Semin Orthod* 11:32-39, 2005.
46. Kravitz ND, Kusnoto B: Posterior impaction with orthodontic miniscrews for openbite closure and improvement of facial profile, *World J Orthod* 8:157-166, 2007.
47. Sugawara J, Nishimura M: Minibone plates: the skeletal anchorage system, *Semin Orthod* 11:47-56, 2005.
48. Cinsar A, Alagha AR, Akyalcin S: Skeletal open bite correction with rapid molar intruder appliance in growing individuals, *Angle Orthod* 77:632-639, 2007.
49. Darendeliler MA, Darendeliler A, Mandurino M: Clinical application of magnets in orthodontics and biological implications: a review, *Eur J Orthod* 19:431-442, 1997.
50. Dellinger EL: A clinical assessment of the Active Vertical Corrector: a nonsurgical alternative for skeletal open bite treatment, *Am J Orthod* 89:428-436, 1986.
51. Maino GB, Mura P, Bednar J: Miniscrew implants: the Spider Screw Anchorage System, *Semin Orthod* 11:40-46, 2005.
52. Rebellato J: Two-couple orthodontic appliance systems: transpalatal arches, *Semin Orthod* 1:44-54, 1995.
53. Burstone CR: Deep overbite correction by intrusion, *Am J Orthod* 72:1-22, 1977.
54. Burtsone CJ: Biomechanics of deep overbite correction, *Semin Orthod* 7:26-33, 2001.
55. Lindauer SJ, Isaacson RJ: One-couple orthodontic appliance systems, *Semin Orthod* 1:12-24, 1995.
56. Isaacson RJ, Lindauer SJ: Closing anterior open bites: the extrusion arch, *Semin Orthod* 7:34-41, 2001.
57. Cope JB: Temporary anchorage devices in orthodontics: a paradigm shift, *Semin Orthod* 11:3-9, 2005.
58. Burstone CJ, Pryputniewicz RJ: Holographic determination of centers of rotation produced by orthodontic forces, *Am J Orthod* 77:396-409, 1980.
59. Richards D, Lawrence A: Evidence based dentistry, *Br Dent J* 179:270-273, 1995.
60. Slavkin HC: Toward molecular based diagnostics for the oral cavity, *J Am Dent Assoc* 129:1138-1143, 1998.

CHAPTER 23

THE USE OF MICROIMPLANTS IN ORTHODONTICS

Hyo-Sang Park

Numerous attempts have been made in the past to develop reliable sources of orthodontic anchorage. Recently, skeletal anchorage systems such as dental restorative implants,[1] miniscrew[2,3] or microscrew[4-6] implants, and miniplates[7] have been effectively used to obtain anchorage. However, because of their bulky size, the waiting period for osseointegration, and their high cost, dental implants have not been widely used. The extensive surgical procedure and high cost overshadow the use of plate-type anchorage, despite a high success rate. In the past decade, miniscrew or microscrew implants have gained wider acceptance because they are both easy and convenient to use. The application of skeletal anchorage has lead to a paradigm shift in orthodontic treatment from single-tooth movement to group-teeth movement.

This chapter addresses the development of microimplants, the surgical procedure involved in their placement, and the management of associated complications.

DEVELOPMENT OF MICROIMPLANTS

During the initial stages of development of microimplants, the author used a surgical microscrew for orthodontic anchorage, specifically the screws from Leibinger (now Stryker Osteosynthesis, a division of Stryker, Freiburg, Germany) and OsteoMed (Addison, Texas) (Fig. 23-1).[8] These screws were 1.2 mm in diameter and 5 to 10 mm in length. The success rate of these surgical screws varied from 80% to 90 %, depending on the site of placement.[9-10] One of the chief drawbacks of these surgical screws was a lack of any "superstructure" on the head for attaching elastics. To circumvent this problem, ligature wire was tied on the neck (under head of screw) and then bent up to make a hook. This hook caused persistent inflammation around microscrew implants.

Current microimplants have a hook, button, or bracket on the head for attaching elastic materials, which minimizes inflammation.[8,11] The tapered shape of trunk over head pushes the elastic material away from the soft tissue and prevents soft tissue impingement, especially around the canine eminence (Fig. 23-2). To simplify the placement of implants, self-drilling microimplants have also been developed.

Size of Microimplants

Microimplants ranging from 1.2 to 1.6 mm in diameter are small enough to be placed at most anatomical locations in the mouth, including the palate, chin, retromolar area, and interradicular spaces between teeth roots.[8,12] After placement, at least 6 mm of the total length of the microimplant should be embedded into the bone in the maxilla and 4 mm in the mandible. The author typically prefers to use microimplants 7 to 8 mm long in the maxillary buccal alveolar bone and 5 to 6 mm long in the mandibular buccal side. In the maxillary palatal alveolar bone, 10- to 12-mm-long microimplants need to be placed to compensate for the thick palatal soft tissue and to keep 6 mm of microimplants embedded in the bone. The most common diameter of the microimplants is 1.3 mm in the maxilla and 1.4 mm in the mandible and 1.5 or 1.6 mm in the midpalatal area where there are no teeth.

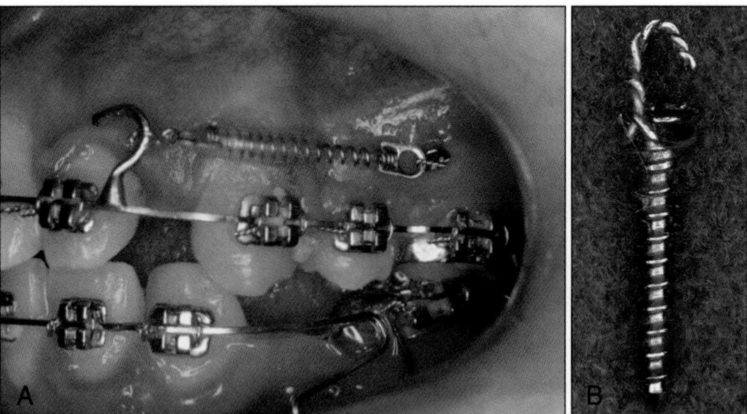

Fig. 23-1 **A,** Microscrew used as orthodontic anchorage. **B,** Ligature wire hook around neck of microscrew.

SURGICAL PROCEDURES FOR IMPLANT PLACEMENT

Anesthesia

Local anesthesia

Local anesthesia includes one-quarter ampoule for injection or application of anesthetic patch or topical anesthesia. Mild surface anesthesia of the oral mucosa maintains the sensitivity of nerve fiber in the periodontal ligament so that the patient is alert enough to know whether the pilot drill has impinged on the periodontal ligament. However, it is not always true that the pilot drill has impinged on the periodontal ligament, especially in the lower posterior teeth area. Occasionally there is pain despite no microimplant-root contact.

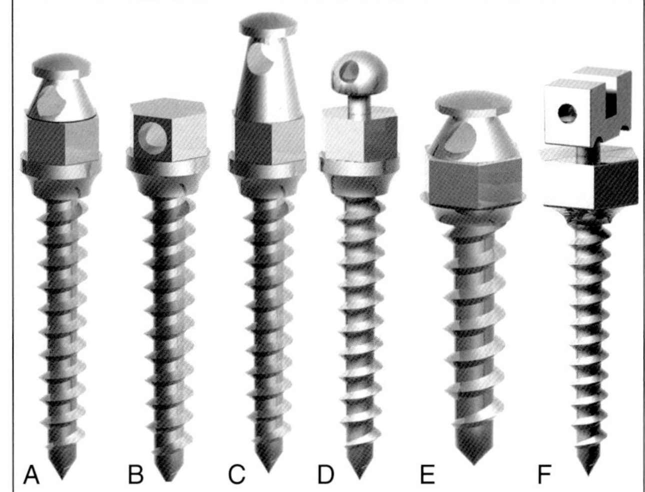

Fig. 23-2 Newly developed microimplants (Absoanchor): **A,** small head (SH); **B,** no head (NH); **C,** long head (LH); **D,** circular head (CH); **E,** fixation head (FH); **F,** bracket head (BH). (Courtesy Dentos Inc., Daegu, South Korea.)

Topical anesthesia

Topical anesthesia can also be used for this procedure. After drying the overlying soft tissue, topical anesthetic solution or patch can be applied (Fig. 23-3). Ten minutes of waiting time is required to obtain proper anesthesia.

Infiltration anesthesia

A one-third or one-quarter ampoule of anesthetic solution can be injected into mucosa (Fig. 23-4). Again, by depositing comparatively small amounts of anesthetic solution, clinicians can keep the nerve fibers in the periodontal ligament sensitive. If the microimplants touch the roots, the patient might show pain. At that moment the drill needs to be redirected in a different direction. Occasionally the patient might have pain even though the microimplant does not touch the root, especially in the lower jaw. Assessment of the position of microimplants relative to the roots is essential. The best was to assess this is by taking periapical radiographs.

Incision

Placing microimplants through the oral mucosa requires a 3-mm-long stab incision (Fig. 23-5). This incision can be omitted with placement in attached gingiva. The incision prevents the soft tissue from rolling up around the drill bit. Because of the small incision size, no sutures are required.

Drilling Method

There are two different methods to place microimplants: self-tapping and self-drilling. The self-tapping method requires a hole be predrilled before placing the microimplant. For placing microimplants in the mandibular posterior teeth area and maxillary palatal area (for all age groups) and in the maxillary buccal alveolar bone (for adult patients), the self-tapping method is a better option than the self drilling method. The self-drilling method can be used to place microimplants into the buccal alveolar bone in the maxillary jaw of young patients and the maxillary and mandibular anterior teeth area in all age groups.

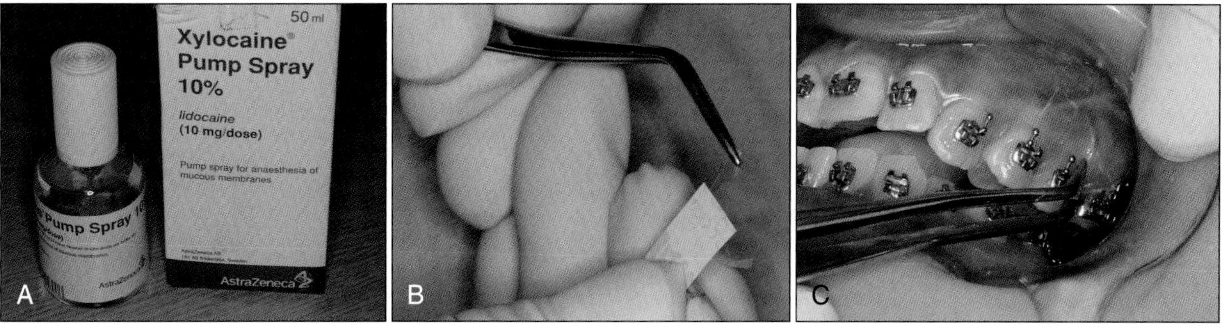

Fig. 23-3 Anesthesia with topical solution (A) or a patch (B) can be applied to soft tissue after drying (C).

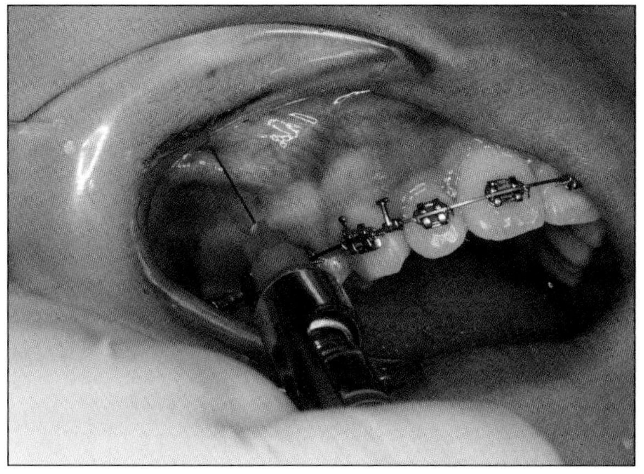

Fig. 23-4 Anesthesia by injection of anesthetic solution.

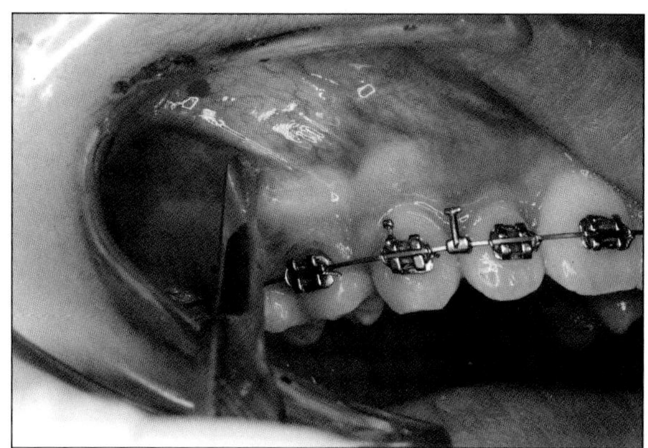

Fig. 23-5 Small vertical stab incision is made when placing a microimplant in oral mucosa.

Self-tapping method

After administering local anesthesia, a pilot drill is used to make a hole in the cortical bone, and the microimplant is introduced through this hole and screwed in with a hand driver (Fig. 23-6). When placing the microimplant into attached gingiva, the incision can be omitted, but when placing it in oral mucosa, a small, vertical incision is needed (see Fig. 23-4). Entrapping soft tissue in the hole when placing the microimplant without an incision is always a possibility and may compromise stability of the microimplant. An incision may also produce more postoperative pain and swelling.[13]

The diameter of the pilot drill should be slightly smaller than the inner (or core) diameter of the microimplant because it provides good purchase of bone.[14] During drilling, clinicians should abundantly irrigate with coolants to reduce heat generation.[15] The drill speed preferred is about 600 rpm. To minimize heat generation, clinicians need to move the drill in and out from the pilot hole when drilling into dense cortical bone. The heat generated is proportionate to the pressure applied;[16] therefore clinicians should not apply too much pressure while drilling. The drill hole should be made all the way through the cortical bone. Careful attention should be paid to keeping the axis of the drill stable so as not to enlarge the opening inadvertently.

Self-drilling method

Self-drilling is a simpler method for placing the microimplant than self-tapping. The microimplant is placed in the bone through the attached gingiva without drilling (Fig. 23-7). The microimplant is introduced at an angle of 90 degrees to the bone surface and screwed in with the hand driver. Placement at a certain angle requires a small indentation to be made to prevent slippage of the microimplant. The angular placement of microimplants with the self-drilling method can damage the cortical bone where it is dense and thick. If the microimplant is to be placed at an angle into dense cortical bone, the self-tapping method is always a better option.

After placement, it is important for the operator to check the three-dimensional relationship of the microimplant to the roots. Root contact can be noticeable or felt during the placement procedure because there is another strong resistance when the implant meets the root. The microimplants should be checked for firmness immediately after placement. If any mobility is detected, the implant needs to be removed

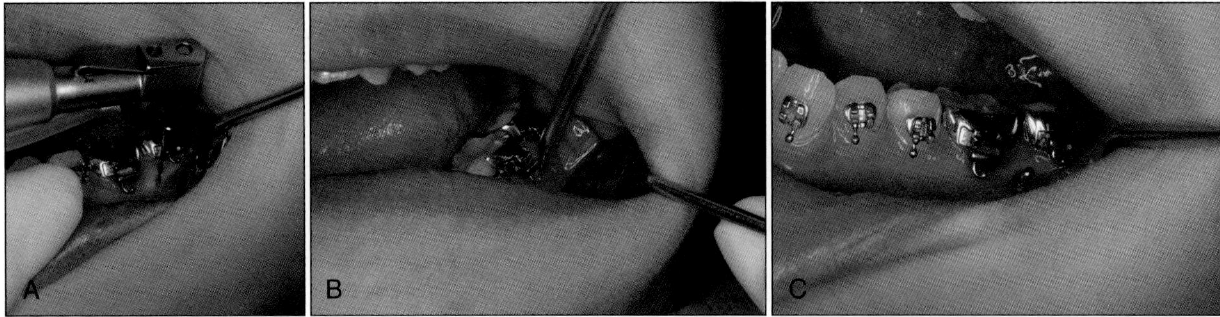

Fig. 23-6 Placement of microimplant with self-tapping method (drill method). **A,** Hole is made with a pilot drill. **B,** Microimplant is inserted and screwed in cortical bone. **C,** Microimplant after placement.

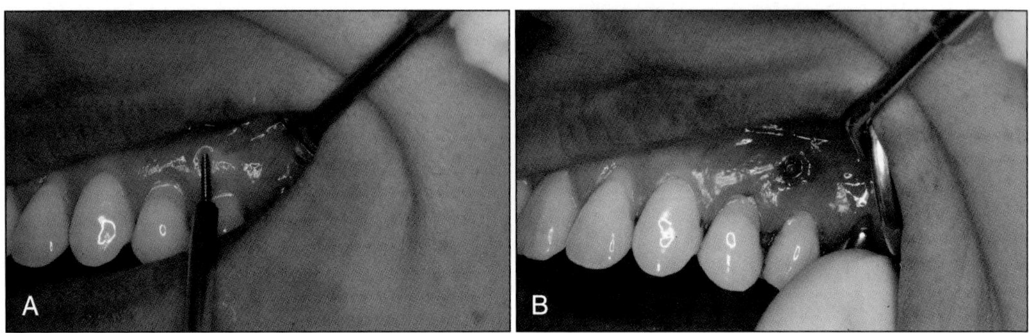

Fig. 23-7 Placement of microimplant with self-drilling method (drill-free method). **A,** Microimplant is screwed into alveolar bone without prior drilling. **B,** Microimplant after placement.

and replaced by a larger-diameter implant to obtain tighter purchase.

Placement Angle

Relative to the long axis of the teeth, microimplants can be placed at an angle of 30 to 40 degrees for the upper jaw (Fig. 23-8, *A*) and 20 to 60 degrees for the lower jaw (Fig. 23-8, *B*). This angular placement reduces the possibility of root contact by positioning the apex of the microimplants toward the apical portion of the roots, where there is relatively more space.[6,8,12,17] The advantages of angulating the microimplant during insertion are increased surface area of cortical bone contact with the microimplant and less chance of root contact or possible root damage (if any damage at all) if the implant hits root. Angulation also provides the operator with the option of placing longer microimplants, which may further enhance their stability. Perpendicular placement can also be done, but only after careful examination of the space between roots.

The angular placement into dense cortical bone with the self-drilling method may produce more bone fracture of the cortical bone than perpendicular placement (Fig. 23-9). Again, it is better to place microimplants with the self-tapping method in dense cortical bone.

Head Exposure

The heads of the microimplants can be exposed when placing them into attached gingiva, and the elastics or nickel-titanium (Ni-Ti) coil springs can be attached directly to the heads (Fig. 23-10). The head of the microimplants, when placed deep in the vestibule or retromolar area, may get embedded by the overgrowth of the surrounding soft tissue. The no-head (NH) type of microimplant is most suitable for this situation. To apply force, ligature wire extension tied around the neck of the microimplant can be used (Fig. 23-11). The Absoanchor microimplants (Dentos, Daegu, South Korea) have a small hole at the neck that can provide an attachment for engaging ligature wires.

Postoperative Management

Most patients experience no noticeable discomfort or infection after the placement and removal of microimplants. Antibiotics and antiinflammatory agents need to be prescribed to minimize postoperative discomfort. Patients need to be instructed to practice good oral hygiene by spraying water with a Water Pik (Fig. 23-12). Intentional or accidental application of heavy force on the microimplants during mastication should be avoided.

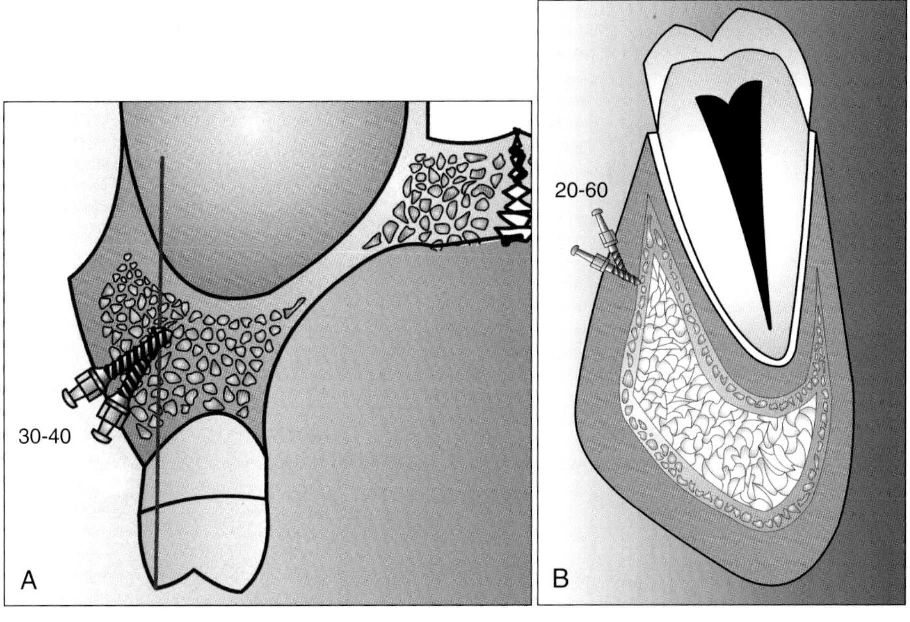

Fig. 23-8 **A,** Placement angle (30-40 degrees) in upper posterior teeth area to prevent root contact. **B,** Placement angle (20-60 degrees) in lower posterior teeth area.

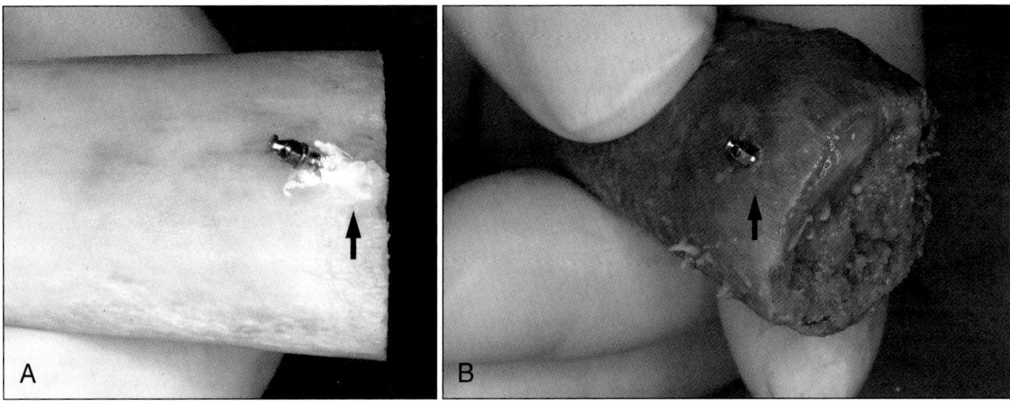

Fig. 23-9 Angular placement to the surface of the bone produces fractures in the thick cortical bone area (**A**), whereas no damage occurs in the thin cortical bone area (**B**).

Timing of Loading (Application of Force)

Miyawaki et al.[13] found no significant difference between loading at 1 to 2 months or at 3 months after placement. Melsen and Costa[18] found no significant difference between immediate loading and delayed loading in histological sections. The author prefers to load the microimplants immediately after placement and keep the force minimal (<70 g) until 2 months after placement. After 2 months the force can be increased up to 150 to 200 g. In young, growing patients the maximum force that can be used is 200 g for retraction of all the anterior teeth or the entire arch. In adults the force for retraction of anterior teeth need not exceed 200 g. For retraction of the entire arch, force can be increased to a maximum of 400 g.

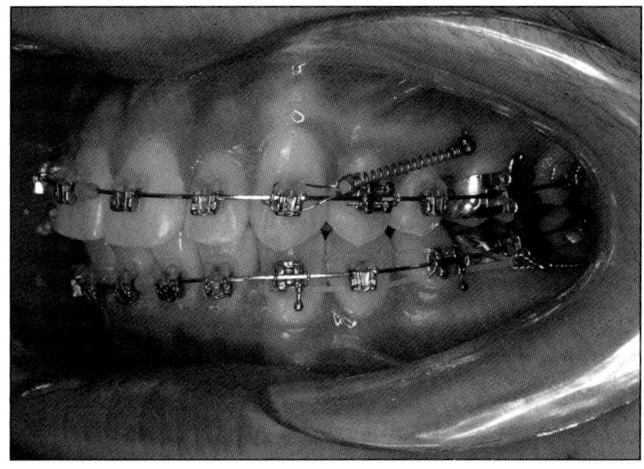

Fig. 23-10 Head of microimplants can be kept exposed when placed through attached gingiva so that Ni-Ti coil spring can be engaged directly.

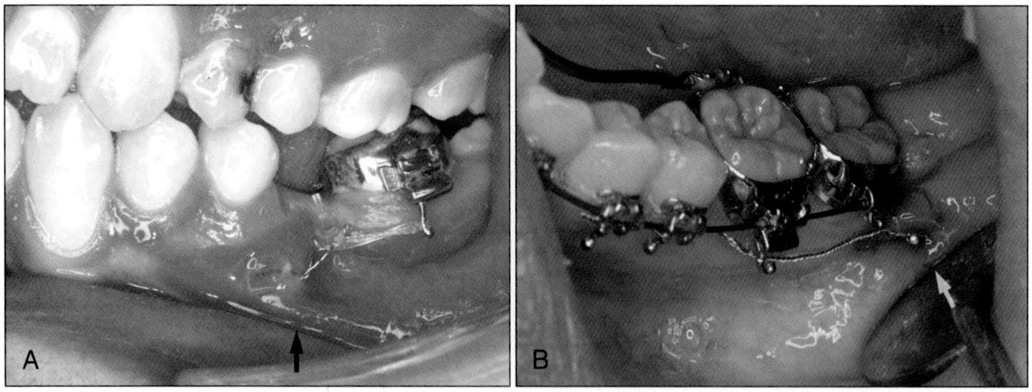

Fig. 23-11 Microimplants placed deep in the vestibule (**A**) and in the retromolar area (**B**) do not allow for the head to be exposed, and ligature wire extension is required to apply force.

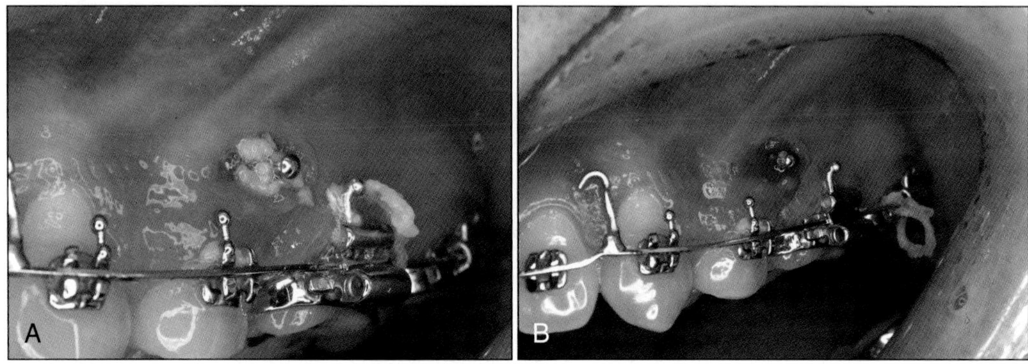

Fig. 23-12 Microimplant needs to be cleaned thoroughly with a Water Pik to minimize inflammation. **A,** Food impaction. **B,** Bleeding can result from inflammation.

Removal of Microimplants

The removal of microimplants is easily performed by turning them in the opposite direction of placement. If covered by overlying soft tissue, the head of the microimplant will need to be incised and reflected to expose the head of the implant. The shadow of the head can always be seen under the soft tissue covering. To eliminate any chance of fracture of the microimplant, the operator should apply light and gentle force until the interface between the microimplant and bone breaks. The operator needs to know the range of torque that might fracture the microimplant. If removal torque reaches fracture torque range, the clinician should wait 1 or 2 weeks, when the microimplant can be removed with lesser force.

COMPLICATIONS

The expected complications with microimplants include damage to adjacent anatomical structures while placing the implant, inflammation around microimplants, soft tissue impingement, irritation to tongue or cheek, and fracture of microimplants.

Inflammation

Periimplantitis is considered one of the major complications that can cause implant failure. This can be easily interpreted by observing that microimplants placed in thick and firm palatal mucosa have a higher success rate, almost 100%,[10,19] than those in other areas. Palatal masticatory mucosa is relatively more resistant to inflammation, and unattached, movable oral mucosa is considered a risk factor for implant failure.[20] The microimplants placed in the attached gingiva or in the palatal mucosa have less inflammation (Fig. 23-13). Microimplants placed in oral mucosa, deep in the vestibule, or near frenum can cause persistent inflammation[19,20] (Fig. 23-14).

From a biomechanical standpoint, some situations demand the placement of microimplants in the movable oral mucosa. In the author's experience, microimplants placed 1 mm below the mucogingival junction do not produce serious inflammation (see Fig. 23-13, *D*).

To prevent inflammation, microimplants need to be thoroughly cleaned. The author recommends compressed water spray with a Water Pik. The toothbrush is not a good option because the patient might inadvertently apply too

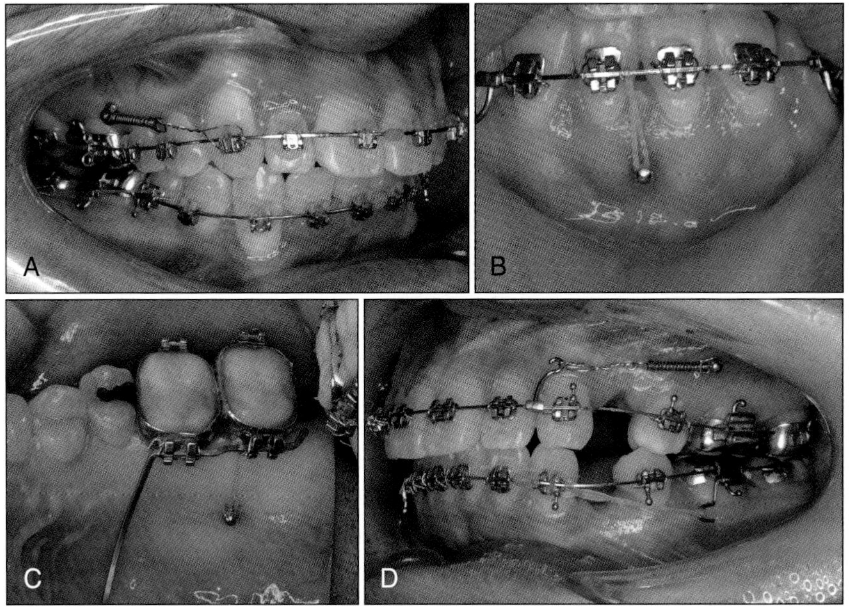

Fig. 23-13 Microimplants placed in attached gingiva on buccal side (**A** and **B**) and palate (**C**) do not produce inflammation. Also, microimplant near mucogingival junction, even in oral mucosa area, does not induce serious inflammation (**D**).

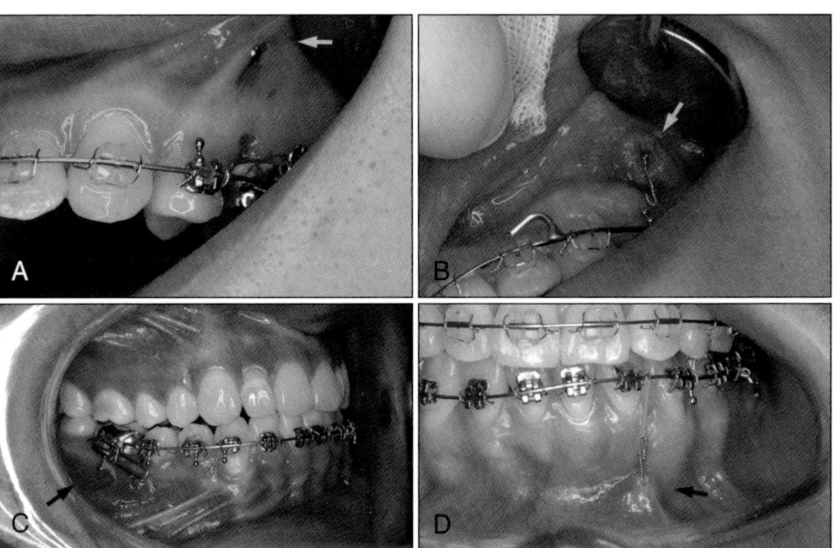

Fig. 23-14 Microimplant placed near the buccal frenum (**A**) produces inflammation (**B**). Microimplants placed deep in the vestibule (**C** and **D**) also result in inflammation.

much force on the microimplants during brushing or may accidentally dislodge the attached Ni-Ti coil spring or elastic material.

Soft Tissue Impingement

When retracting anterior teeth, the author often uses archwire with hooks crimped between the lateral incisors and canines and applies a distal force from the microimplants placed between the posterior teeth roots. Occasionally the Ni-Ti coil spring may impinge into the gingiva around the canine eminence and buccal mucosa of the first molars. The impingement around the canine eminence may in turn cause inflammation and gingival recession (Fig. 23-15). To prevent this, first the clinician should use the interradicular bone between the maxillary second premolars and first

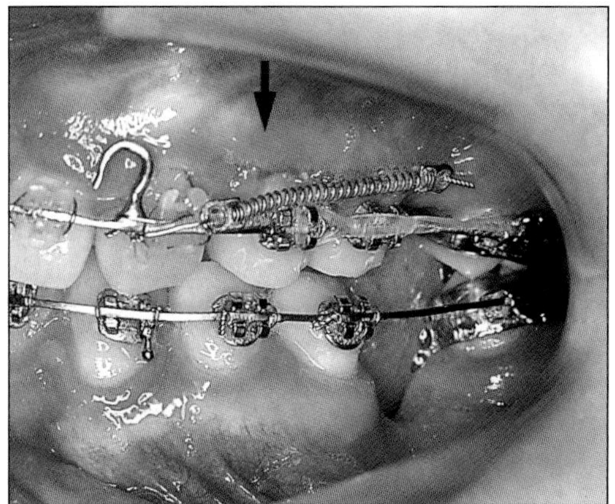

Fig. 23-15 Nickel-titanium coil spring impinging on soft tissue around canine eminence.

molars as the implant site rather than the location between the first and second molars. Second, the hooks attached to the archwire between the lateral incisors and canines must be bent out and bent in to move the point of force application outward. The new microimplants (e.g., Absoanchor) have tapered necks that push the Ni-Ti coil spring upward and outward away from the soft tissue.

Tongue and Cheek Irritation

Contrary to popular belief, microimplants placed in the buccal alveolar bone do not cause cheek irritation, although microimplants placed in the palatal area can cause tongue irritation. Bonding resin or a periodontal wound dressing can be applied on the head to minimize discomfort (Fig. 23-16).

Damage to Adjacent Structure

The inferior alveolar nerve runs lingual and inferior to the molar roots and moves buccally at the premolar area. When placed, microimplants remain confined within the alveolar bone space and do not cause damage to the inferior alveolar nerve. Even the microimplants placed deep into the vestibule are far above the inferior alveolar nerve.

Microimplants placed in the palatal alveolar bone may hit the greater palatine artery and nerve. The experienced operator, however, places the microimplant obliquely to the alveolar bone, near the apex of the roots of maxillary molars, staying clear of the greater palatine nerve and artery, which run higher. The risk of damage is at best minimal.

Root Damage

Root damage by a drill or microimplant is not common. In one study, among 232 miniscrews (2.0 mm in diameter) placed in 55 patients, 37 miniscrews (15.9%) produced minor root contact, of which 26 miniscrews (11.2%) had no serious complications, and only six screws producing pulp necrosis.[21] In another study, among 2300 surgical screws from 387 patients, only 13 (0.47%) had root contact but resulted in no serious complications.[22] The ratio of root contact between the mandible and the maxilla is 10:3.

The angular placement of the microimplants to the bone surface minimizes root contact. Typically, 6-mm-long microimplants are placed in the mandible at an angle of 20 to 30 degrees to the long axis of the teeth. By placing microimplants obliquely, the horizontal depth of insertion is less than 3 mm.[17] There is almost no root contact when considering that the cortical bone thickness in the mandibular posterior teeth reaches 3 mm (see Fig. 23-8, *B*).[23] Micromplants 7 to 8 mm long are placed in the maxillary interdental bone between the second premolar and first molar at an angle of 30 to 40 degrees to the long axis of the teeth (see Fig. 23-8, *A*). It is always a good idea to place the microimplants slightly mesial to the contact point of teeth because the distance from outer bone surface to buccal surface of the root of the second premolar is larger at the second premolars than that at the first molars.[17]

To minimize root contact during placement, clinicians need to evaluate the distance between roots from periapical radiographs. If the space is insufficient, alignment of the teeth should be undertaken to widen the interdental space before placement. Additionally, a surgical guide can be used to orient the pilot drill or microimplants into proper position and direction. Brass wire ligated between teeth can be used as a guide. Clinician can note root contact if they place the microimplants with a hand driver. The resistance of cortical bone is quite strong, but after penetrating the cortical bone, resistance is minimal until the end. If any strong resistance is felt, it may be a root surface, and at this point the clinician should remove the implant and change angulation to clear any root surface. Unabated pressure, even after encountering strong resistance, might result in microimplant fracture or root damage.

Despite all the precautions, what happens if the microimplant touches a root? Conclusions can be drawn by several studies. According to Andreasen,[24] less than 4 mm^2 of periodontal ligament damage was repaired at 8 weeks after transient ankylosis, whereas more than 4 mm^2 of damage produced ankylosis. The author typically uses a microimplant diameter of 1.2 to 1.5 mm, which cannot produce more than 4 mm^2 of damage. Bae[25] showed that periodontal damage by the microimplants did not produce serious consequences. Asscherickx et al.[26] reported that if damage does occur, the recovery time is relatively quick. Miniscrews that are 1.6 mm or more in diameter with a sharp cutting edge may produce root perforation.

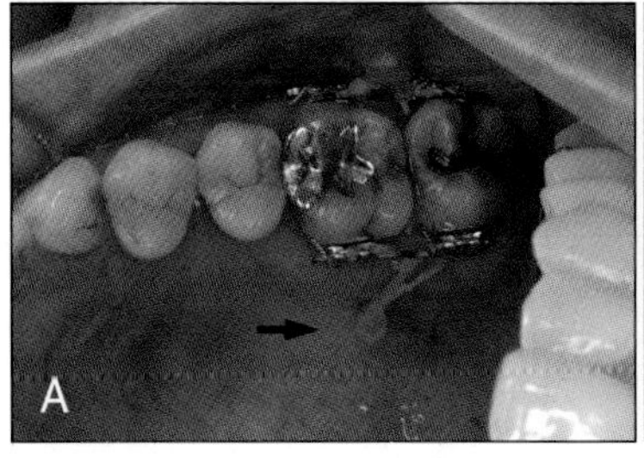

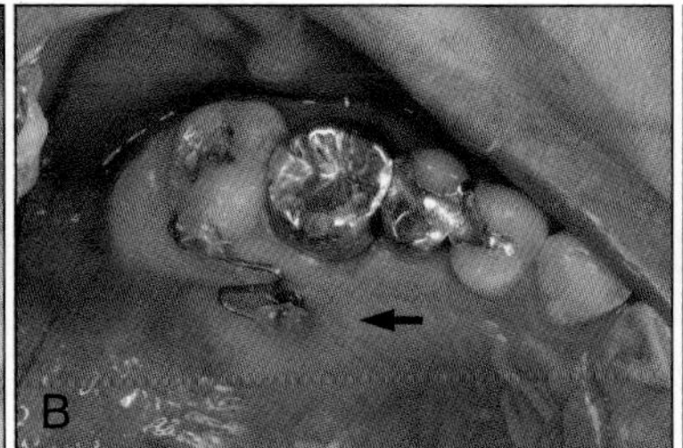

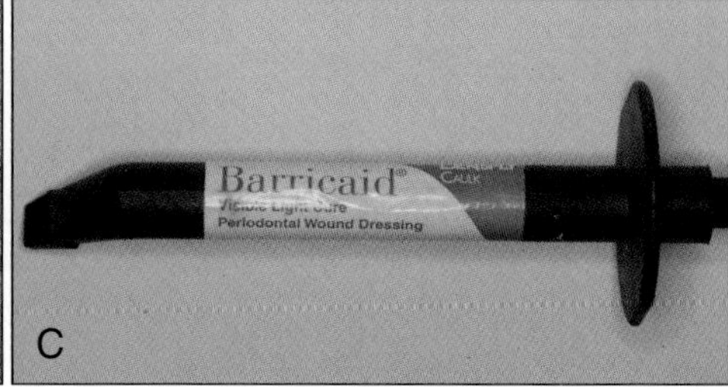

Fig. 23-16 Prevention of tongue irritation. **A,** Bonding resin covering the head. **B,** Periodontal wound dressing **(C)** applied on the head to reduce tongue irritation.

Fracture of Microimplants

The author has encountered less fracture with larger-diameter microimplants than with smaller diameters. In fact, the core (inner) diameter of the microimplants had a greater effect on fracture than the outer diameter. The material of the microimplants is also of importance. Although pure-titanium implants have better biocompatibility than titanium alloy, lower strength makes them more prone to fractures.

Fractures are most commonly seen during the last turn while inserting the microimplant and the first turn when removing. To minimize fracture of the microimplant, clinicians need to apply slow and gentle force. If the insertion resistance reaches the fracture strength of the implant, it is better to wait 1 to 2 minutes to relieve the internal stress accumulated in the microimplant and surrounding bone.

The level of fracture strength decreases when tightening the microimplant with a quick rotatory motion. Clinicians need to apply force with a slow rotatory motion of the hand driver and with finger pressure only, not with wrist pressure. By applying force with finger pressure, it is easier to keep the rotational axis of the hand driver stable and avoid any wobbling motion.

Microimplants placed in the mandible have higher removal torque than those placed in maxilla (unpublished data). Additionally, removal torque increases with increased duration of the micromplant in the bone and increased age of the patient. To remove such screws, the operator should apply gentle untightening pressure, or ultrasonic scaler on the head, partially break the bone-implant interface, and leave the screw for 1 to 2 weeks. Subsequently, the microimplant can be completely removed by applying minimal pressure.

FREQUENTLY ASKED QUESTIONS

How should mobile microimplants be managed after placement?

One or two months after placement, microimplants may show slight mobility. If this is evident, the clinician needs to tighten the microimplant and leave it for 1 to 2 months without loading, or if required, loading should be done with light force (Fig. 23-17). The microimplant should be firm after tightening. According to Ivanoff et al.,[27] noninfected dental implants can reintegrate after tightening. An accidentally avulsed bead implant can become firm after reimplantation and immediate loading.[28] In the author's experience, up to one third of all mobile microimplants can be salvaged by tightening.

How should incorrectly positioned microimplants with root contact be handled?

Clinicians may encounter the problem of microimplants hitting dental roots. In such a scenario the tooth will stop moving. Occasionally the microimplants may also become mobile. To continue planned tooth movement, microimplants must be removed and placed at a distant location (Fig. 23-18).

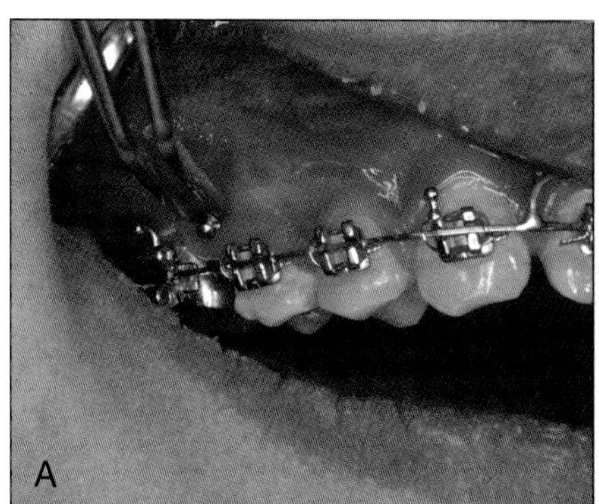

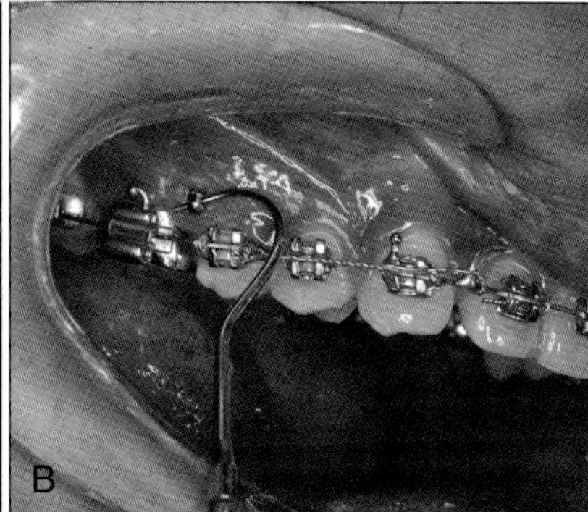

Fig. 23-17 After checking mobility (**A**), the microimplant can be tightened (**B**) when it is minimally mobile. It may become firm in 1 to 2 months.

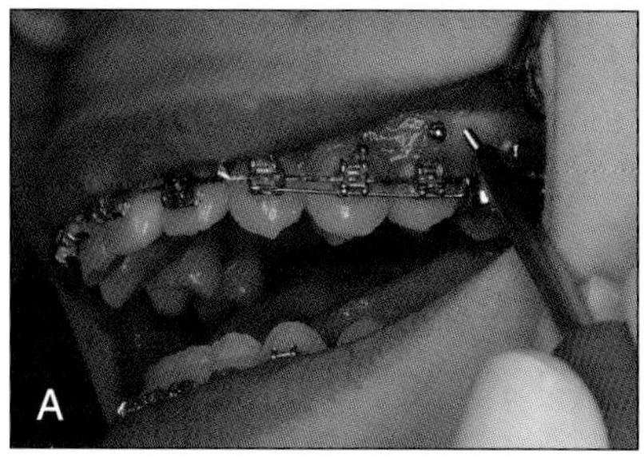

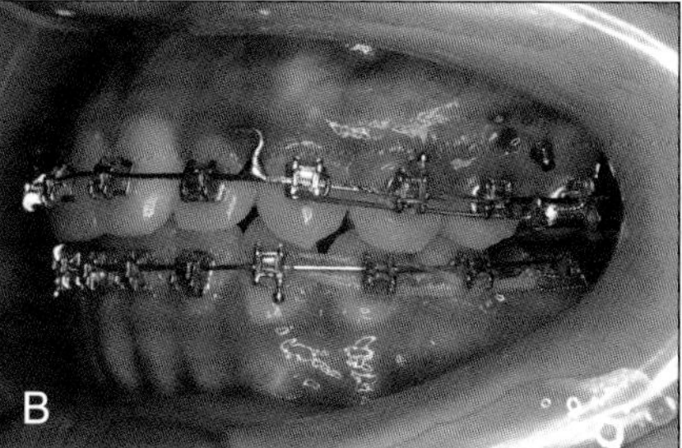

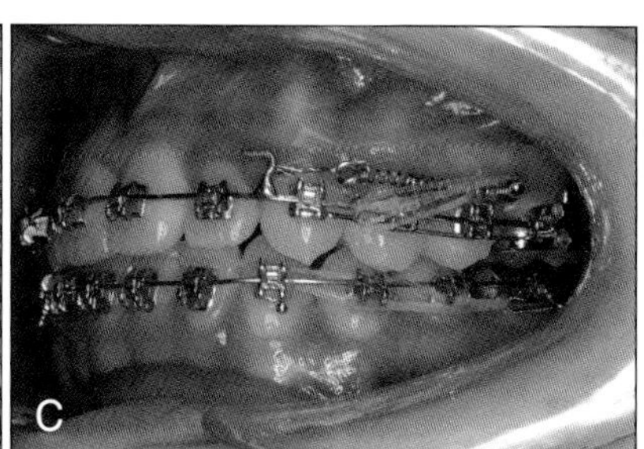

Fig. 23-18 When the microimplant interferes with teeth movement, another microimplant can be placed 2 mm distal to original site (**A** and **B**), and treatment can continue (**C**).

What success rate should be expected?

The success rate increases with time. Once clinicians become accustomed to using microimplants, they can achieve higher success; the success rate follows a "learning curve." The author had a success rate of 82% in 1999,[9] which increased to 93% in 2003.[10]

The author's 2003 study showed that the success rate of 180 microimplants was 93.3%, with a mean observation period of 15.76 months.[10] The microimplants placed in the upper buccal alveolar bone and the palatal alveolar bone had success rates of 94.6% and 100%, respectively. Implants placed in the lower buccal alveolar bone near second molars had 73.7% success. The low success rate in the lower jaw presumably was caused by inflammation resulting from a shallow vestibule and the movable oral mucosa surrounding the microimplants. This makes the microimplant more vulnerable to inflammation and minor trauma during chewing. Fifty-percent failure occurred within 2 months after placement and 75% failure within 6 months; all the other implants that failed did so within 10 months after insertion. Therefore proper surgical procedure is of greatest importance in success.

Cheng et al.[20] found that the posterior mandible and unattached gingiva were potential risk factors for failure. It is better to place microimplants through the attached gingiva than the oral mucosa, if acceptable from a biomechanical standpoint.

CONCLUSION

The use of microimplants has broadened the spectrum of orthodontic treatment. To have more consistent and successful use of microimplants, clinicians need to understand the underlying biological response of the bone surrounding the microimplants after placement, during active use, and on removal. Additionally, adequate steps should be taken to minimize surgical trauma and possible complications.

REFERENCES

1. Roberts WE, Nelsen CL, Goodacre CJ: Rigid implant anchorage to close a mandibular first molar extraction site, *J Clin Orthod* 28:693-704, 1994.
2. Creekmore TD, Eklund MK: The possibility of skeletal anchorage, *J Clin Orthod* 17:266-269, 1983.
3. Costa A, Raffainl M, Melsen B: Miniscrews as orthodontic anchorage; a preliminary report, *Int J Adult Orthod Orthog Surg* 13:201-209, 1998.
4. Kanomi R: Mini-implant for orthodontic anchorage, *J Clin Orthod* 31:763-767, 1997.
5. Park HS: The skeletal cortical anchorage using titanium microscrew implants, *Kor J Orthod* 29:699-706, 1999.
6. Park HS, Bae SM, Kyung HM, Sung JH: Micro-implant anchorage for treatment of skeletal Class I bialveolar protrusion, *J Clin Orthod* 35:417-422, 2001.
7. Umemori M, Sugawara J, Mitani H, et al: Skeletal anchorage system for open bite correction, *Am J Orthod Dentofacial Orthop* 115:166-174, 1999.
8. Park HS: *The use of micro-implant as orthodontic anchorage*, Seoul, South Korea, 2001, Narae.
9. Park HS, Kim JB: The use of titanium microscrew implant as orthodontic anchorage, *Keimyung Med J* 18:509-515, 1999.
10. Park HS: Clinical study on success rate of microscrew implants for orthodontic anchorage, *Kor J Orthod* 33:151-156, 2003.
11. Kyung HM, Park HS, Bae SM, et al: Development of orthodontic micro-implants for intraoral anchorage, *J Clin Orthod* 37:321-328, 2003.
12. Sung JH, Kyung HM, Bae SM, et al: *Microimplants in orthodontics*, Seoul, South Korea, 2006, Dentos.
13. Miyawaki S, Koyama I, Inoue M, et al: Factors associated with the stability of titanium screws placed in the posterior region for orthodontic anchorage, *Am J Orthod Dentofacial Orthop* 124:373-378, 2003.
14. Oktenoğlu BT, Ferrara LA, Andalkar N, et al: Effects of hole preparation on screw pullout resistance and insertional torque: a biomechanical study, *J Neurosurg* 94(Suppl 1):91-96, 2001.
15. Yacker MJ, Klein M: The effect of irrigation on osteotomy depth and bur diameter, *Int J Oral Maxillofac Implants* 11:634-638, 1996.
16. Matthews LS, Hirsch C: Temperatures measured in human cortical bone when drilling, *J Bone Joint Surg Am* 54:297-308, 1972.
17. Park HS. An anatomical study using CT images for the implantation of micro-implants, *Kor J Orthod* 32:435-441, 2002.
18. Melsen B, Costa A: Immediate loading of implants used for orthodontic anchorage, *Clin Orthod Res* 3:23-28, 2000.
19. Park HS, Jeong SH, Kwon OW: Factors affecting the clinical success of screw implants used as orthodontic anchorage, *Am J Orthod Dentofacial Orthop* 130:18-25, 2006.
20. Cheng SJ, Tseng IY, Lee JJ, Kok SH: A prospective study of the risk factors associated with failure of mini-implants used for orthodontic anchorage, *Int J Oral Maxillofac Implants* 19:100-106, 2004.
21. Fabbroni G, Aabed S, Mizen K, Starr DG: Transalveolar screws and the incidence of a dental damage: a prospective study, *Int J Oral Maxillofac Surg* 33:442-446, 2004.
22. Borah GL, Ashmead D: The fate of teeth transfixed by osteosynthesis screws, *Plast Reconstr Surg* 97:726-729, 1996.
23. Champy M, Pape H, Gerlach KL, Lodde JP: Mandibular fracture. In Kruger E, Schilli W, editors: *Oral and maxillofacial traumatology*, vol 2, Chicago, 1986, Quintessence, pp 19-43.
24. Andreasen JO: A time related study of periodontal healing and root resorption activity after replantation of mature permanent incisors in monkeys, *Swed Dent J* 4:101-110, 1980.
25. Bae SM: *Repair of pulp and periodontal tissue after intentional damage in adult dogs*, 2003, Kyungpook National University (thesis).
26. Asscherickx K, Vannet BV, Wehrbein H, Sabzevar MM: Root repair after injury from mini-screw, *Clin Oral Implants Res* 16:575-578, 2005.
27. Ivanoff CJ, Sennerby L, Lekholm U: Reintegration of mobilized titanium implants: an experimental study in rabbit tibia, *Int J Oral Maxillofac Surg* 26:310-315, 1997.
28. Ogunsalu C: Reimplantation and immediate loading of an accidentally avulsed beaded implant: case report, *Implant Dent* 13:54-57, 2004.

CHAPTER 24

Distalization of Molars in Nongrowing Patients with Skeletal Anchorage

■ *Junji Sugawara, Hiroshi Nagasaka, Hiroshi Kawamura, and Ravindra Nanda*

In adult orthodontics it is extremely difficult to correct malocclusions such as incisor crowding, maxillary protrusion, anterior crossbite, and bimaxillary protrusion without extracting bicuspids. The main reason for this difficulty is that in the adult patient the second molars have already fully erupted and any distalization approach will involve the distal movement of both the first and the second molars. Headgear has been a representative "distalizer" in traditional orthodontics and is frequently used to distalize the maxillary first molars in adolescent patients. This is seldom an option for adult patients, however, because of the possible impact on esthetics and compliance.[1-3]

To address these problems, various intraoral "noncompliance" appliances for maxillary molar distalization have been introduced and evaluated since the 1980s.[4-35] Although it is possible to distalize the maxillary molars with these appliances, two side effects have been reported: (1) anchorage loss of the maxillary premolars and flaring of the incisors in reaction to molar distalization and (2) considerable relapse, because the distalized molars must be used as part of anchorage during retraction of the premolars and the anterior teeth.[33] Moreover, most appliances used for molar distalization have been restricted to the maxilla; few effective noncompliance distalizers have been reported for the mandibular molars.[36-38] Simultaneous distalization of the maxillary and mandibular molars in adults has been almost impossible.

SKELETAL ANCHORAGE SYSTEM

To remedy the problems of previous noncompliance appliances, the authors developed the skeletal anchorage system (SAS) consisting of titanium miniplates and monocortical screws temporarily placed in either the maxilla or the mandible (or in both) as absolute anchorage units for adult orthodontics.[39-45] The SAS has been used as a multipurpose modality in combination with a multibracketed appliance, which makes it possible to move the maxillary and mandibular molars distally simultaneously. Although minor surgery for the implantation and removal of the miniplates are always necessary and infection can rarely occur (<10%), the SAS has a distinct advantage in that it enables distalization of the molars predictably in nongrowing patients. The SAS has been accepted as an effective modality for adult orthodontics and is expanding the envelope of nonextraction treatment modalities.

Recently, the authors conducted a study to verify the efficiency of the SAS. The purpose of this study was to investigate the following:

- Amount of distal movement of the maxillary and mandibular first molars
- Type of movement
- Difference between the predicted and actual amount of distalization
- Relationship between the amount of distalization and age of the patient

Three patients who underwent distalization of the maxillary and the mandibular posterior teeth at the same time utilizing SAS biomechanics are presented later in this chapter.

MATERIAL AND METHODS

Distalization of Maxillary Molars

Twenty-five nongrowing patients (22 females, 3 males) who had undergone SAS treatment for distalization of the maxillary molars were selected for the study. All the subjects met the following criteria for case selection:

1. Confirmation of cessation of active mandibular growth through analysis of serial cephalograms
2. Sufficient space behind the first molar for the second or third molars after distalization
3. Achievable individualized treatment goals based on the cephalometric and occlusogram predictions
4. Treatment executed through symmetrical distalization mechanics

The most common chief complaint of these patients was maxillary incisor crowding. Their average age at the beginning of treatment was 23 years, 11 months (range: 15 yr, 2 mo to 45 yr, 5 mo). The third molars were bilaterally extracted in 12 patients and bilaterally missing in five patients. The bilateral second molars were extracted in six patients because of anticipated difficulty in extracting the maxillary third molars. The average orthodontic treatment time using SAS was 19 months (range: 8-36 months).

Figure 24-1, *A*, shows the Y-type miniplates (Orthoanchor SMAP, Dentsply-Sankin, Tokyo, Japan) that were developed and used for distalization and intrusion for the maxillary posterior teeth.[42-45] The plates were made of pure titanium and were suitable for osseointegration and tissue integration. In addition, they were sufficiently strong to resist the usual orthodontic forces as well as the headgear force. The miniplates could be bent with ease for fitting the bone contour of the implantation site. Figure 24-1, *B*, shows the head portion intraorally exposed and positioned outside the dentition so that it never disturbed the distalization of the maxillary molars. Each head portion had three continuous hooks for easier application of the orthodontic force vectors. The arm portion was transmucosal and had three graduated lengths—short (6.5 mm), medium (9.5 mm), and long (12.5 mm)—to compensate for individual morphological differences (Fig. 24-1, *A*). The body portion was positioned subperiosteally.

The implantation sites of the miniplates required sufficiently thick cortical bone, at least 2 to 3 mm, to enable fixation of the miniplates with monocortical miniscrews. The screws were made of pure titanium. Each screw had a head with a tapered square inside and self-tapping thread. The diameter of the screw was 2 mm, and the available length was 5 mm. The miniplates were placed at the zygomatic buttress to distalize the maxillary posterior teeth (Fig. 24-1, *B*). Although the lateral wall of the maxilla was too thin to hold the screws of the miniplates, the bone of the zygomatic buttress was thick enough.

The operation was carried out under local anesthesia by oral surgeons. First, a mucoperiosteal incision was made at the buccal vestibule of the implantation site. A mucoperiosteal flap was elevated after subperiosteal ablation, and the surface of the cortical bone at the implantation site was exposed. The miniplate was selected according to the distance between the implantation site and the dentition, as shown on the panoramic x-ray film or the cone-beam computed tomography (CBCT) scan taken before surgery. The selected plate was contoured to fit the bone surface. A pilot hole was then drilled and a self-tapping monocortical screw inserted. After placement of the remaining screws, the miniplate was then firmly attached to the bone surface. The wound was closed and sutured with absorbable thread. The surgery took 10 to 15 minutes for each miniplate.

Orthodontic force was applied approximately 3 weeks after the implantation surgery, after soft tissue healing around the miniplates. It was unnecessary to wait for osseo-

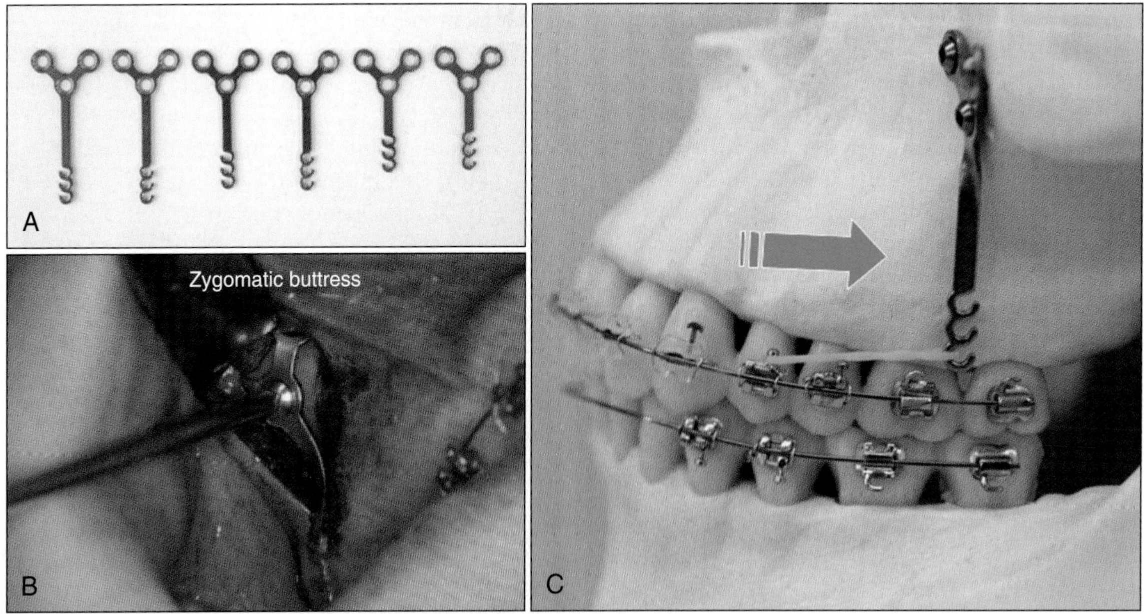

Fig. 24-1 **A,** Y-type miniplates. **B,** Miniplates implantation at the zygomatic buttress, and **C,** skeletal anchorage system (SAS) biomechanics for distal movement of maxillary posterior teeth.

integration of the titanium screws and miniplates. All miniplates were removed immediately after debonding.

Most patients who underwent the miniplates placement had mild to moderate facial swelling for several days after surgery. Infection occurred occasionally during orthodontic treatment (<10% of patients). Mild infections were controlled using antiseptic mouthwash and careful brushing techniques. In more severe cases, antibiotics were required.

Figure 24-1, *C*, shows the representative SAS mechanics for en masse distalization of the maxillary posterior teeth. All subjects were bonded with preadjusted multibracketed appliances with .022-inch slots. Heat-treated .018 × .025–inch Elgiloy (Rocky Mountain Orthodontics, Denver, Colo.) wires were used as the main archwires. The orthodontic forces were approximately 400 to 500 gf (grams force) for en masse distalization of posterior teeth. Orthodontic forces were mostly provided by nickel-titanium (Ni-Ti) open-coil springs (Tomy International, Tokyo, Japan) or elastic chain modules (Pro-Chain, Dentsply-Sankin, Tokyo, Japan).

Lateral cephalometric radiographs with wide-open mouths were used in this study to identify the crown shapes of the maxillary first molars without being obscured by the opposing teeth (Fig. 24-2). The radiographs were taken before treatment and immediately after debonding in all subjects. The cephalograms were traced, and the craniomaxillary tracings were carefully superimposed by using stable anatomical structures such as the cranium, anterior cranial base, and fine structures in the maxilla. The tracings of the left and right first molars were averaged.

Figure 24-2, *A*, shows the reference planes and landmarks for determining the distal movement of the maxillary first molars. The initial maxillary occlusal plane, defined by the first molar and the maxillary central incisor, served as the *x* axis, and the *y* axis was a perpendicular line drawn from the pterygomaxillary fissure. *C1* and *C2* were the most distal points of the maxillary first molar crown before treatment and at debonding, respectively. Similarly, *R1* and *R2* were the most distal points of the maxillary first molar root before treatment and at debonding, respectively. The *x* axis of each landmark was measured with calipers at a precision of 0.1 mm. The amount of posterior displacement at the crown (C1-C2) and root (R1-R2) was calculated, and the type of tooth movement was evaluated by the crown/root movement ratio. The difference from the predicted amount of the crown distalization (treatment goals) was then assessed. In addition, the relationship between the amount of posterior displacement of the crown and the patients' age (before treatment) was evaluated.

The Pearson correlation coefficient test was applied to evaluate the relationships between the amount of posterior displacement at the crown and root levels and the difference from the predicted crown movement.

Distalization of Mandibular Molars

Twenty-nine patients (24 females, 5 males) who had complained about lower anterior crowding or an anterior crossbite before orthodontic treatment were also selected for the study. The mandibular posterior teeth were symmetrically distalized with the SAS based on individualized treatment goals in all subjects. The criteria for case selection were the same as for the maxillary molars. The average age at the

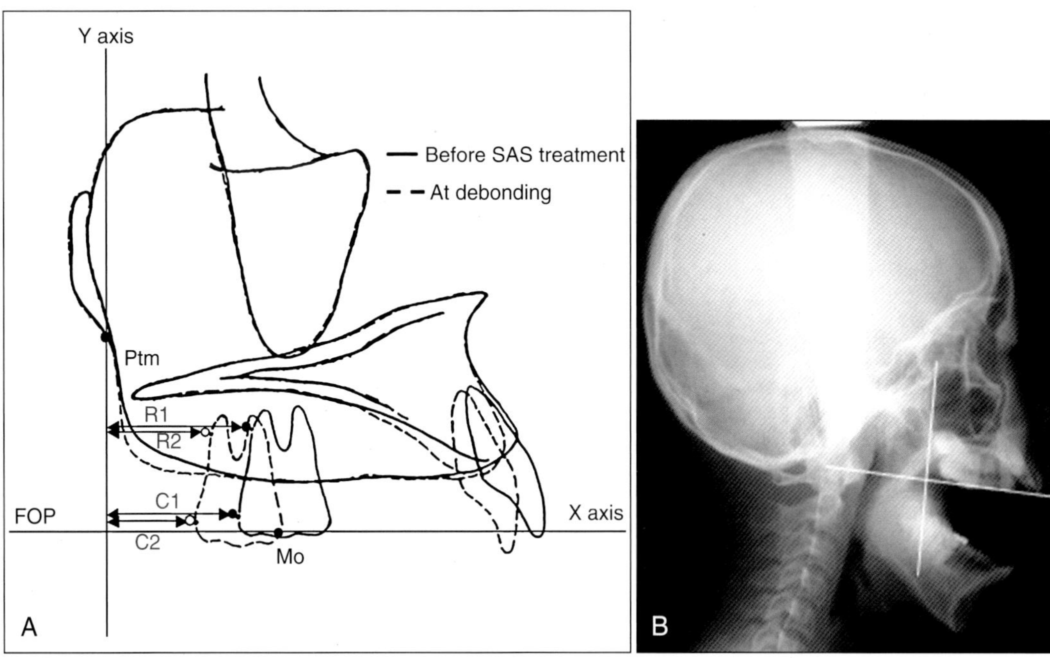

Fig. 24-2 **A,** Planes and landmarks used for determining distal movement of maxillary first molar (*Mo*). *C1-C2,* Crown distalization; *FOP,* functional occlusal plane; *Ptm,* pterygomaxillary fissure; *R1-R2,* root distalization. **B,** Lateral cephalometric film in wide-mouth opening.

beginning of treatment was 23 years, 10 months (range: 15 yr, 6 mo to 46 yr, 3 mo). The mandibular third molars were bilaterally extracted in 21 patients and were bilaterally missing in eight patients before orthodontic treatment.

Figure 24-3 shows T-type miniplates that are applied in the mandible and the biomechanics for en masse distalization of mandibular posterior teeth.[42-45] Generally, L-type miniplates are used by cutting off one of the circles of T-plates, which then are subperiosteally placed at the mandibular body between the first and second molars. Surgical procedures for implantation of miniplates in the mandible are almost the same as those for the maxilla.

Figure 24-4 shows the reference planes and landmarks for evaluation of distalization of the mandibular first molars. The mandibular cephalometric tracings were carefully superimposed by using fine anatomical structures of the mandible. The tracings of the left and right first molars were averaged. The initial functional occlusal plane in the mandible served as the *x* axis. The *y* axis was a perpendicular line drawn from the intersection point of the anterior border of the ramus

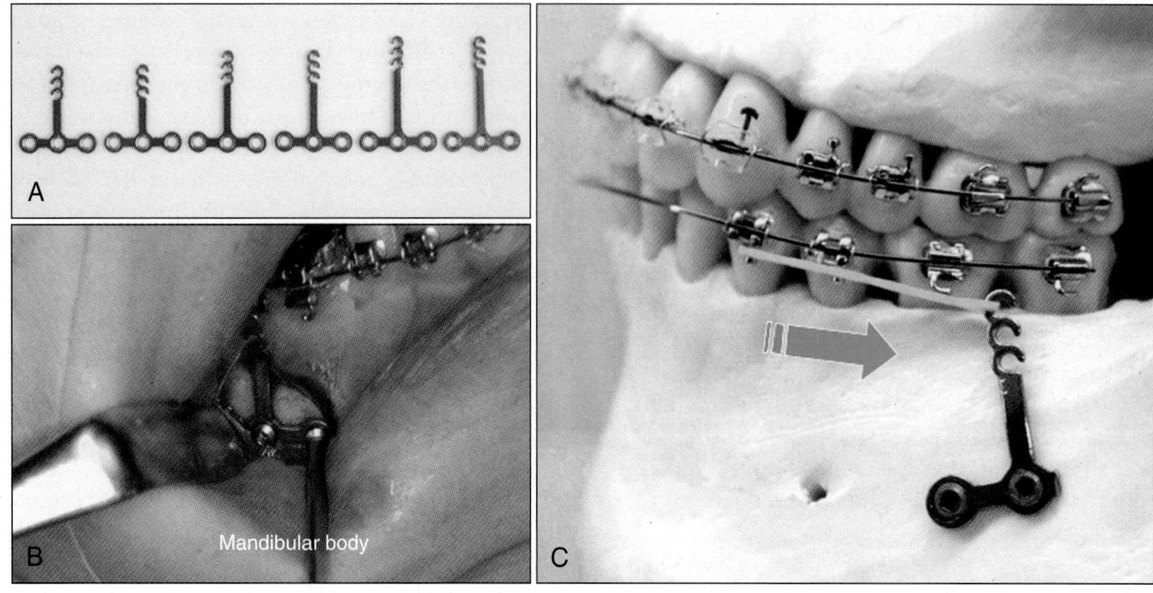

Fig. 24-3 **A,** T-type miniplates. **B,** Miniplates implantation at the mandibular body, and **C,** SAS biomechanics for distal movement of mandibular posterior teeth.

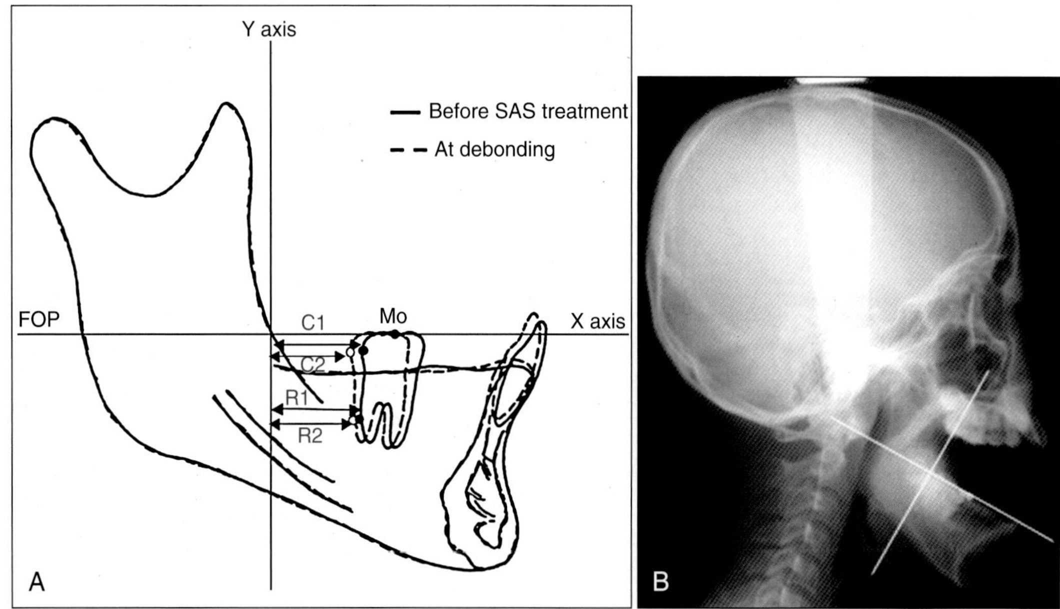

Fig. 24-4 **A,** Planes and landmarks for determining for distal movement of mandibular first molar. **B,** Lateral cephalometric film in wide-mouth opening.

with the occlusal plane. *C1* and *C2* were the most distal points of the mandibular first molar crown before treatment and at debonding, respectively. Similarly, *R1* and *R2* were the most distal points of the mandibular first molar root before treatment and at debonding, respectively. The *x* axis of each landmark and the amount of posterior displacement at the crown (C1-C2) and root (R1-R2) were measured. The types of distalization of the mandibular molars were evaluated following the same methods used for the maxillary molars.

Again, the Pearson correlation coefficient test was applied to evaluate the relationships between the amount of distal movement at the crown and root levels and the difference from the predicted amount of crown movement.

RESULTS

Amount and Type of Molar Distalization

Figure 24-5 is a scattergram of distal movement of the maxillary first molar crowns and roots of all study subjects. It shows the relationship between posterior displacement of the crowns and roots of the maxillary first molars individually. The average amount of distalization at the crown and root levels was 3.8 mm and 3.2 mm, respectively. The correlation coefficient between crown and root distalization was 0.78, indicating that the crown and root movements were significantly correlated. The maxillary molar tended to show almost bodily translation, with slight distal tipping.

Figure 24-6 shows a scattergram of distalization of the manibular first molar crowns and the roots. The average amount of distalization at the crown and root levels was 3.4 mm and 1.8 mm, respectively. The correlation coefficient between crown and root distalization was 0.64. The correlation between the crown and the root distalization was also significant.

Although the crown and the root movements were significantly correlated in the mandibular molar distalization, the mandibular molar tended to show more distal tipping than the maxillary molar.

Predictability of Molar Distalization

Distalization of the maxillary and the mandibular molars in all subjects was carried out in accordance with the individualized treatment goals established before the SAS treatment. In other words, the amount of the maxillary and mandibular molar distalization was predicted based on each patient's treatment goals.

Figure 24-7 shows the relationship between the predicted amount of crown distalization and the actual amount of distalization of the maxillary first molar crown. The average amount of predicted crown distalization and actual crown distalization was 3.6 mm and 3.8 mm, respectively. The correlation coefficient was 0.72 and statistically significant.

Figure 24-8 shows the difference between the predicted and the actual amounts of distalization of the mandibular first molar crown. The average amount of treatment goal and actual crown distalization was 3.2 mm and 3.4 mm, respectively. The correlation coefficient was 0.64, also significant.

Overall, distalization of the maxillary first molar was more predictable than that of the mandibular first molar.

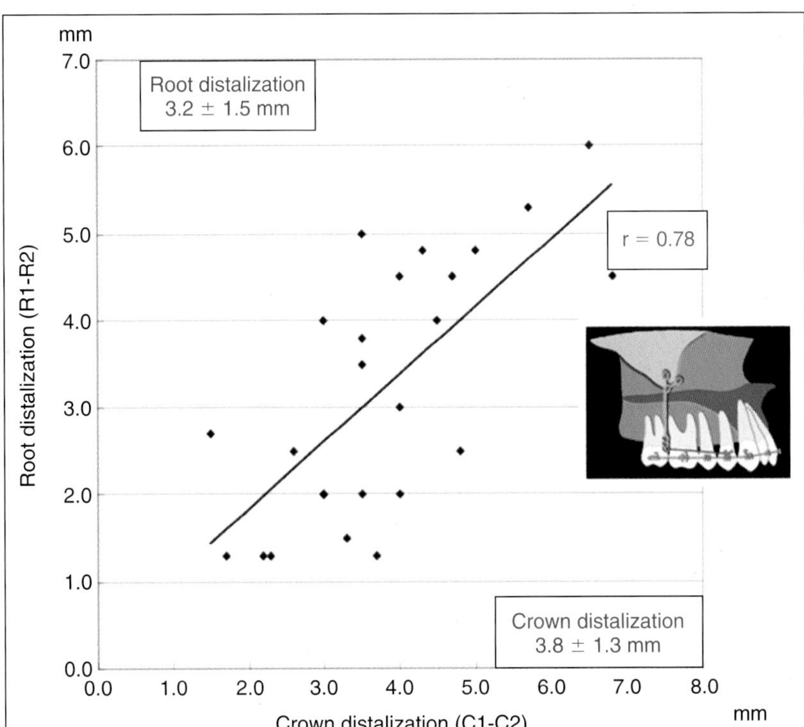

Fig. 24-5 Crown/root distalization ratio of maxillary first molar. *r*, Correlation coefficient.

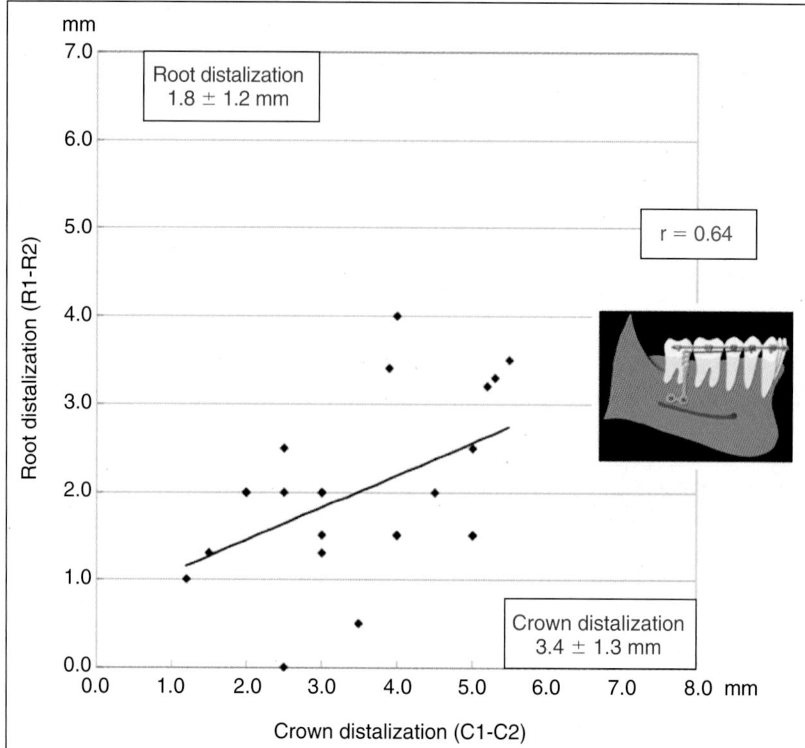

Fig. 24-6 Crown/root distalization ratio of mandibular first molar. *r*, Correlation coefficient.

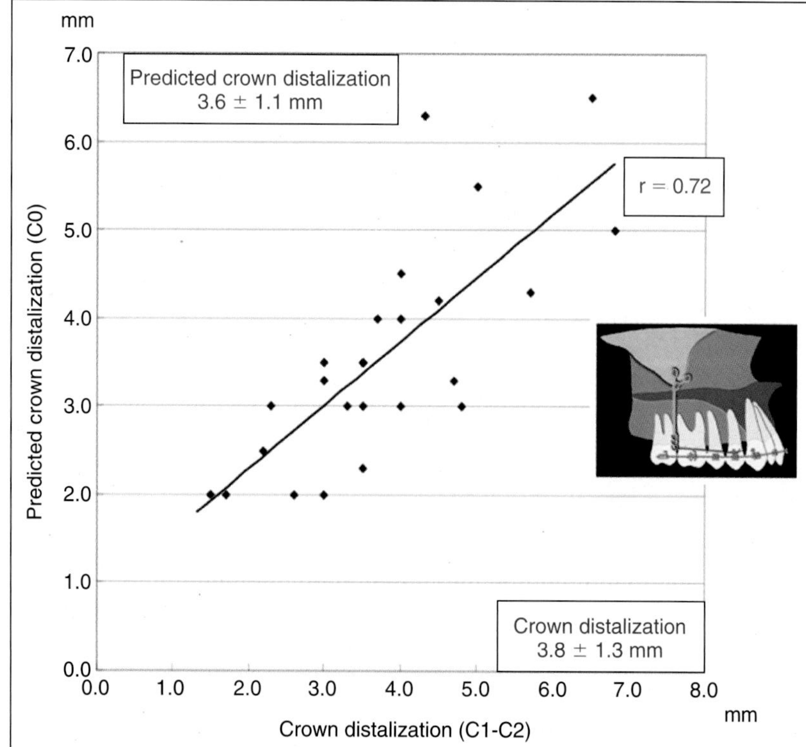

Fig. 24-7 Difference between actual and predicted crown distalization of maxillary first molar. *r*, Correlation coefficient.

Relationship Between Patients' Age and Distalization of Molars

The average age of patients at the start of treatment for the maxillary and mandibular molars was 23 years, 11 months and 23 years, 10 months, respectively. Therefore the subjects were simply divided into two age groups: those younger than 24 years ("younger group") and those older than 24 years ("elder group").

Figure 24-9 shows the relationship between the amount of distal movement of the maxillary first molar crowns and the age of the subjects. The average amount of distalization

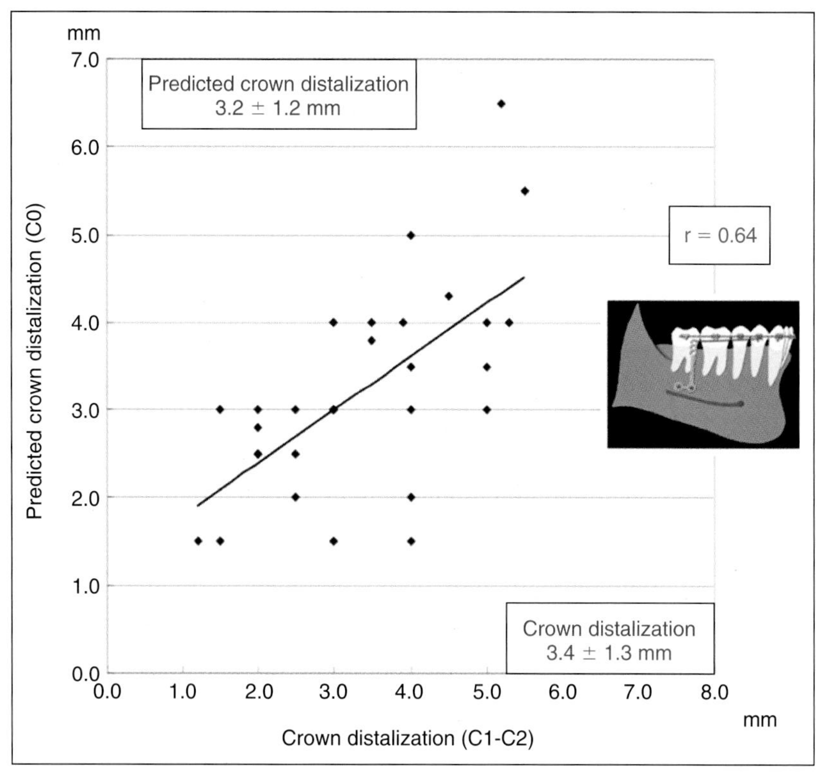

Fig. 24-8 Difference between actual and predicted crown distalization of mandibular first molar. *r*, Correlation coefficient.

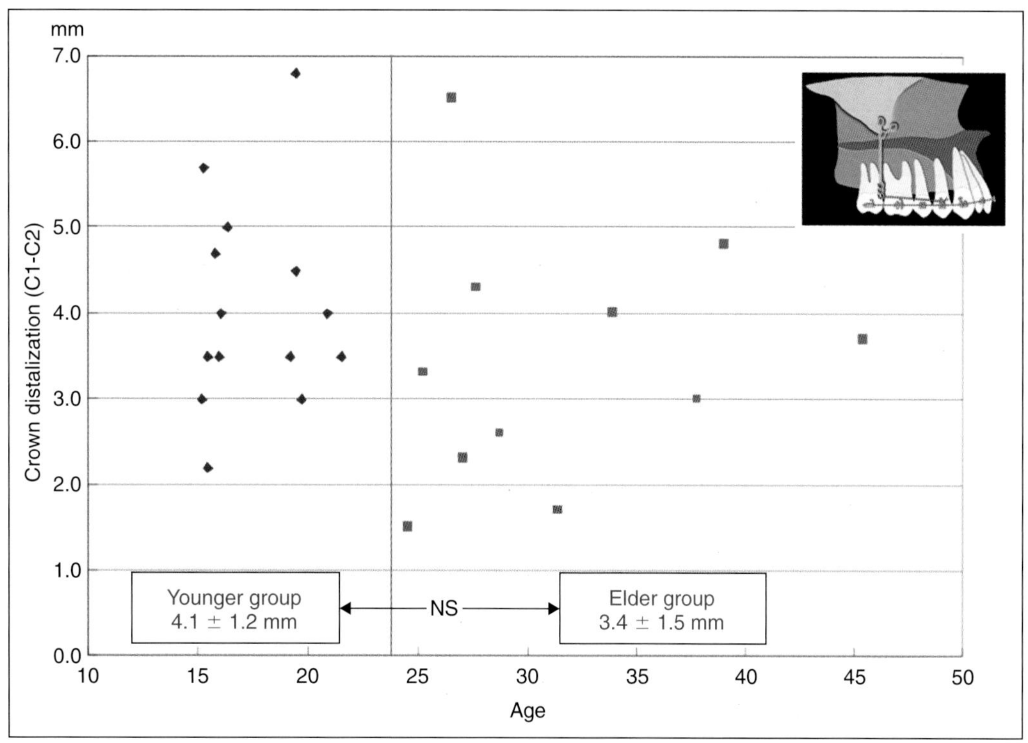

Fig. 24-9 Relationship between amount of crown distalization of maxillary first molar and patients' age. *NS*, Not significant.

in the maxillary first molar was 4.1 mm in the younger group and 3.4 mm in the elder group. There was no statistical difference between the younger and elder groups.

Figure 24-10 shows the relationship between the amount of distal movement of the mandibular first molar crowns and the age of the subjects. No statistical difference was found in the amount of distal movement of the mandibular first molars between the younger and elder groups.

Regardless of variations in age and extraction site, the maxillary and mandibular first molars could be distalized in accordance with individualized treatment goals with the SAS biomechanics.

Goal Achievement Ratio Between Younger and Elder Groups

Figure 24-11 shows the relationship between the goal achievement ratio of crown distalization of the maxillary first molar and the patients' age. The achievement ratio in the younger and elder groups was 77.7% and 80.3%, respectively. There was no statistical difference between the two groups.

Figure 24-12 shows the results for the amount of distalization of the mandibular first molars. The goal achievement ratio in the younger and elder groups was 71.6% and 77.9%, respectively. No significant difference was observed between the younger and elder groups.

CASE REPORTS: MAXILLARY AND MANDIBULAR DISTALIZATION WITH SKELETAL ANCHORAGE SYSTEM

It has been difficult to correct anterior crowding in non-growing patients without extracting bicuspids in traditional orthodontics, particularly in patients who have anterior crowding in both the maxillary and the mandibular dentition. However, after development of the skeletal anchorage system, it has become possible to move the maxillary and the mandibular molars distally at the same time. Three subjects who underwent simultaneous distalization of the maxillary and the mandibular posterior teeth with SAS application are described next.

Case 1

A 22-year-old woman presented with complaints of anterior crowding in the maxillary and mandibular dentitions at the initial consultation (Fig. 24-13, *A-F*). Although she had no skeletal problem, some denture problems were observed, including moderate anterior crowding, retroclination of bimaxillary incisors, lingoversion of tooth #12, and a deviation in the denture midline. According to the treatment goals, cephalometric prediction, and wax-up, it was necessary to distalize the maxillary and mandibular molars by 4.0 mm and 3.0 mm, respectively, to accomplish proper

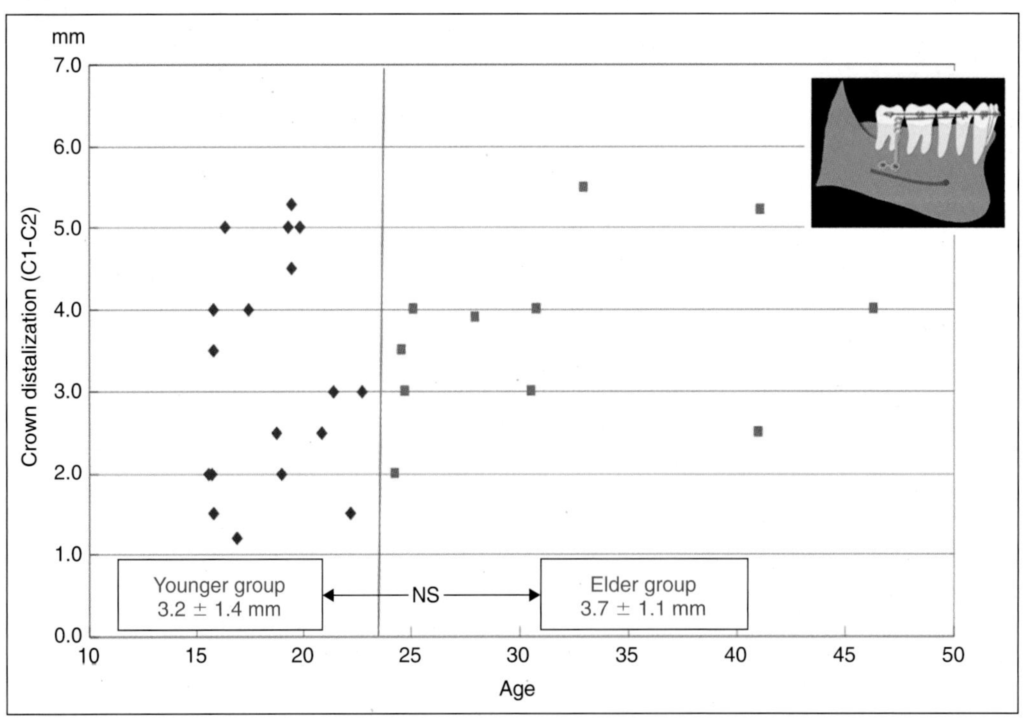

Fig. 24-10 Relationship between amount of crown distalization of mandibular first molar and patients' age. *NS,* Not significant.

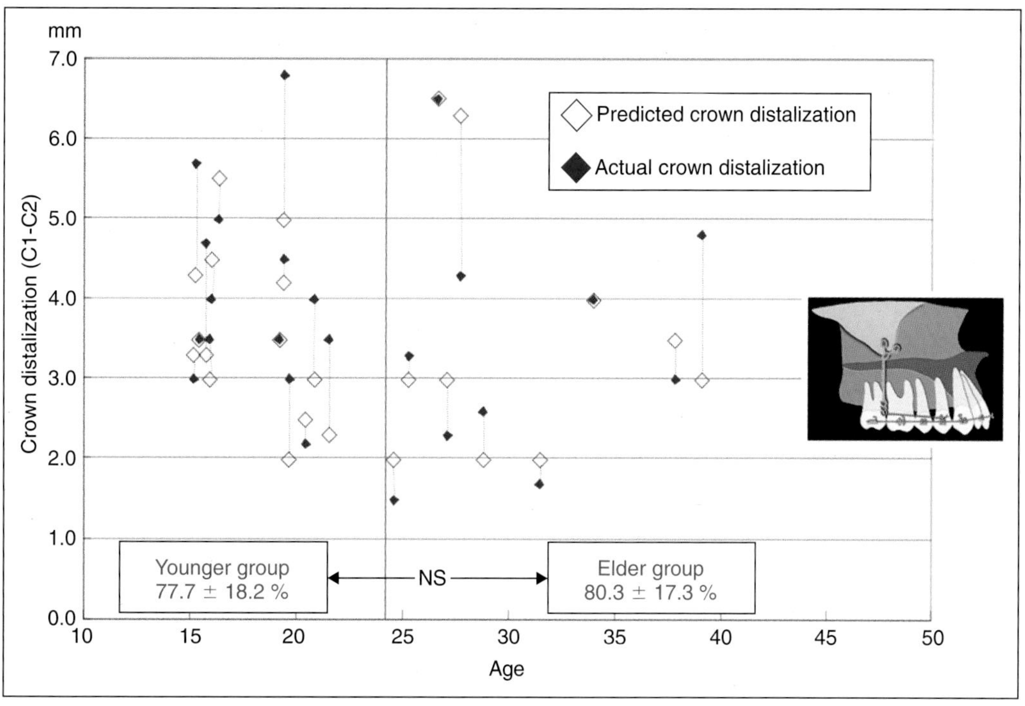

Fig. 24-11 Relationship between goal achievement ratio of crown distalization of maxillary first molar and patients' age. *NS,* Not significant.

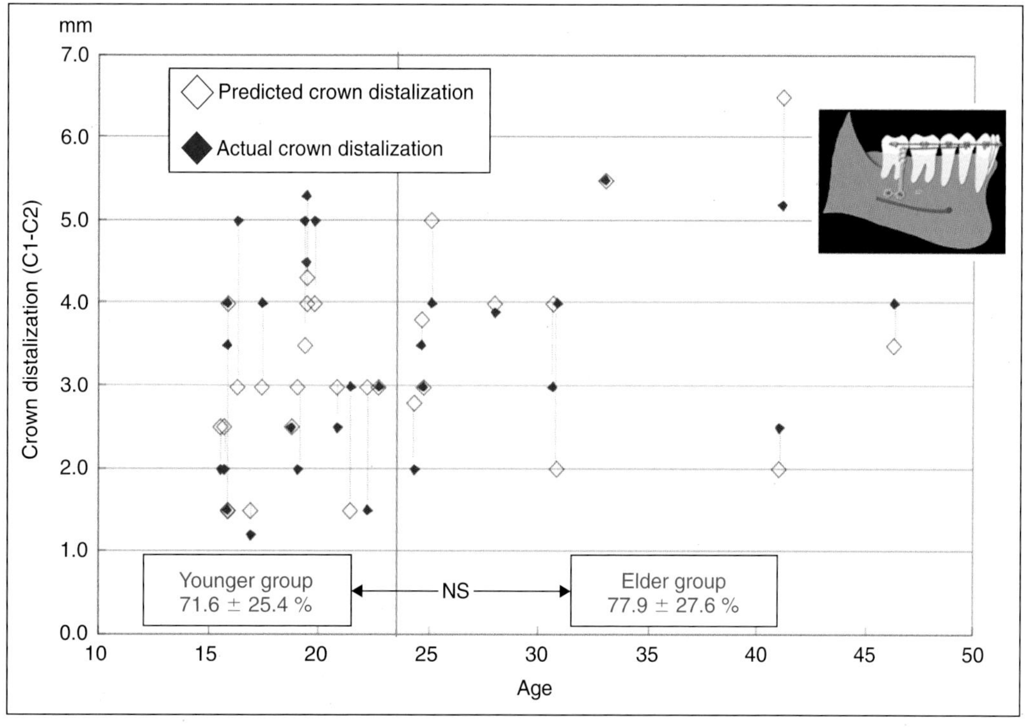

Fig. 24-12 Relationship between goal achievement ratio of crown distalization of mandibular first molar and patients' age. *NS,* Not significant.

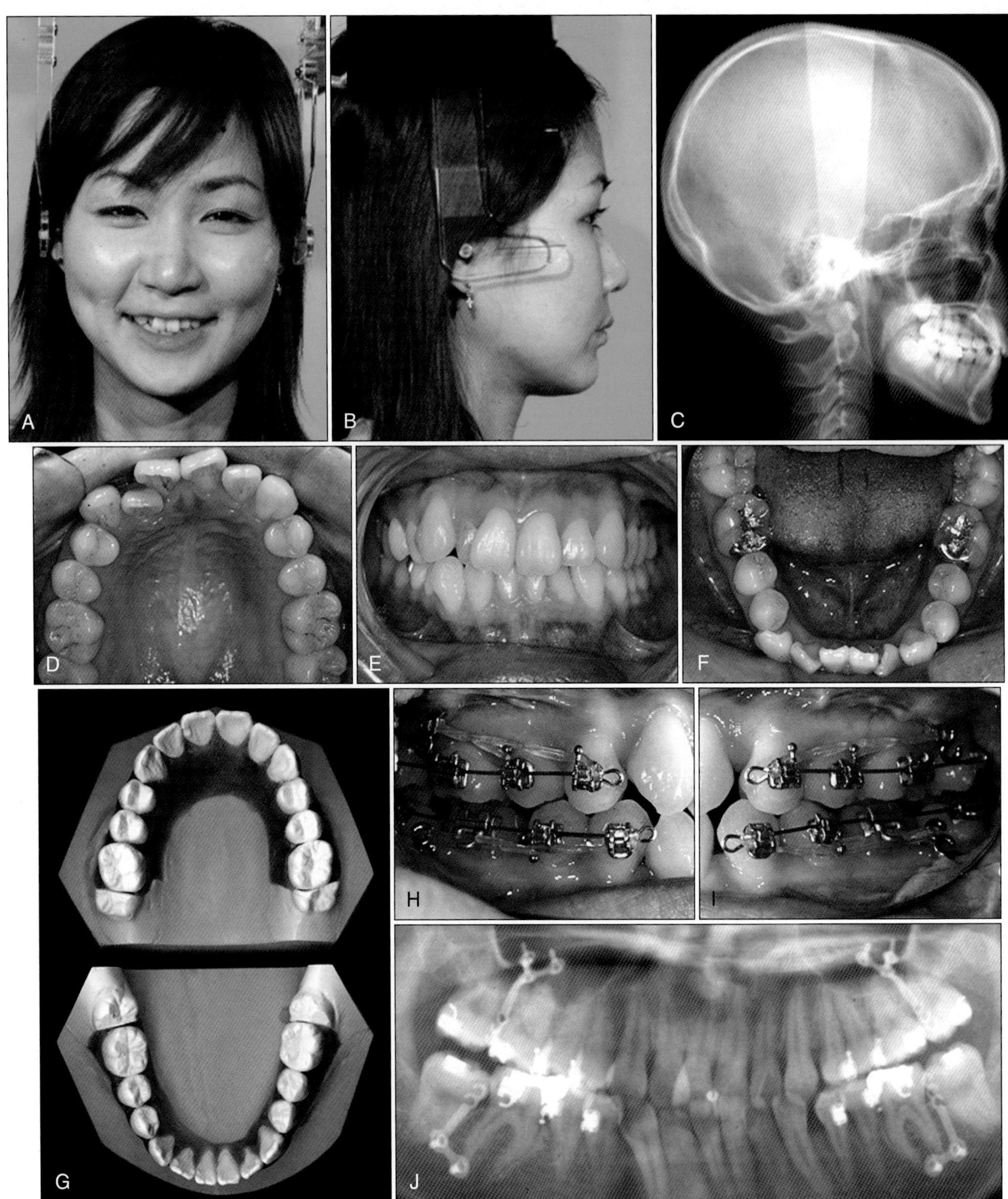

Fig. 24-13 Case #1. Nonextraction treatment of bimaxillary anterior crowding with SAS. **A** to **F**, Initial facial photographs (**A** and **B**), cephalometric radiograph (**C**), and intraoral photographs (**D-F**). **G** to **J**, Treatment goal (**G**) and SAS biomechanics in place (**H-J**).

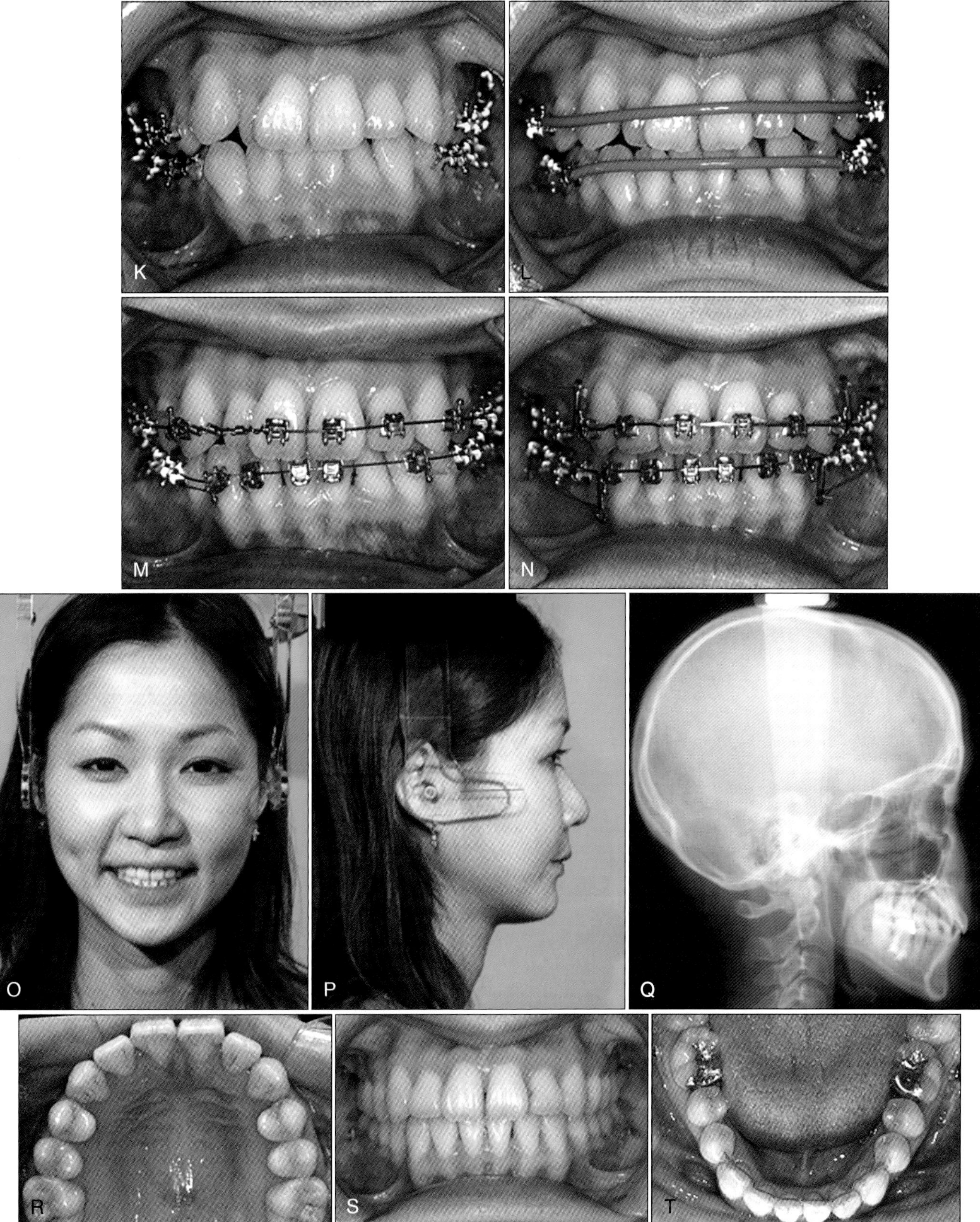

Fig. 24-13, cont'd **K** to **N**, Treatment progress: start of treatment (**K**), 5 months (**L**), 7 months (**M**), and 12 months (**N**). **O** to **T**, Debonding facial photographs (**O** and **P**), cephalometric radiograph (**Q**), and intraoral photographs (**R-T**).

Continued

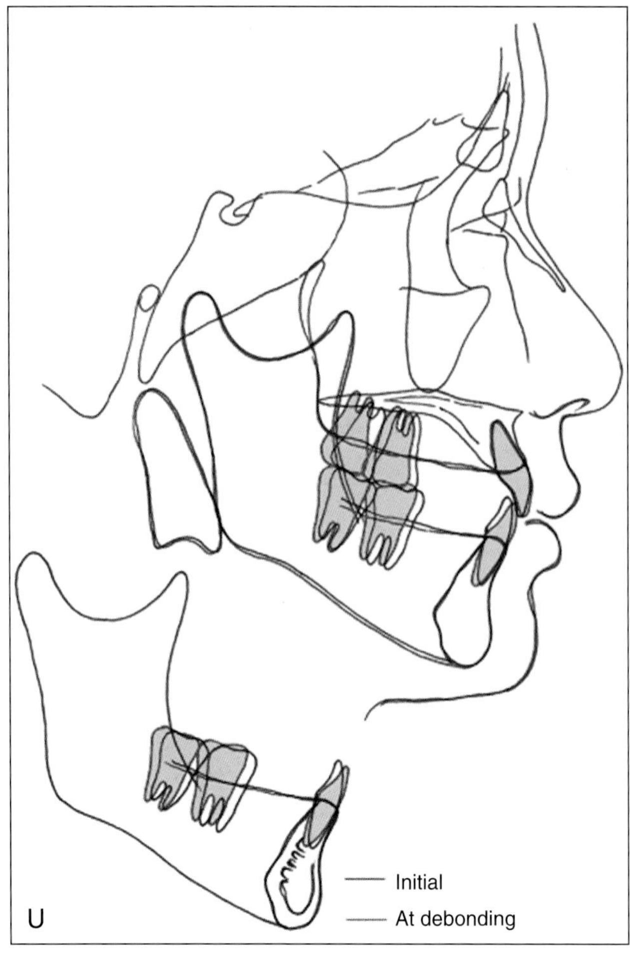

Fig. 24-13, cont'd U, Cephalometric superimpositions.

incisor relationship without extracting the bicuspids (Fig. 24-13, *G-J*).

After making spaces for distalization of the bimaxillary molars by means of third molar extraction, orthodontic treatment through a multibracketed system and the SAS was initiated. Two Y-type miniplates and two L-type miniplates were temporarily fixed at the zygomatic buttress and the mandibular body, respectively (Fig. 24-13, *J*). With the application of the SAS, the denture problems were successfully resolved in about 12 months (total treatment time) (Fig. 24-13, *K-N*). According to the cephalometric superimpositions, both the maxillary and the mandibular molar showed bodily movement, and the treatment goals were precisely accomplished (Fig. 24-13, *O-U*).

Case 2

A 21-year-old woman first presented with temporomandibular joint (TMJ) pain and anterior crowding in the maxillary and mandibular dentitions. Her orthodontic problems were mild skeletal Class II profile, TMJ disorders (internal derangement), a centric occlusion–centric relation (CO-CR) discrepancy, Class II denture bases, moderate anterior crowding, deviated dental midline, and open-bite tendency (Fig. 24-14, *A-F*). According to the individualized treatment goal, the predicted amount of molar distalization was 4.5 mm in the maxilla and 3.0 mm in the mandible bilaterally (Fig. 24-14, *G-J*).

As a result, all third molars were extracted before orthodontic treatment to obtain space for distalization of the molars. Subsequently, four miniplates were implanted at the zygomatic buttress and the mandibular body (Fig. 24-14, *J*). Using SAS distalizing mechanics, most of the orthodontic problems were significantly corrected in about 15 months without bicuspid extraction (Fig. 24-14, *K-N*). The treatment goals were predictably achieved and most of her complex orthodontic problems were successfully corrected with the application of SAS biomechanics (Fig. 24-14, *O-T*). According to cephalometric superimpositions, both the maxillary and the mandibular molar showed bodily translation (Fig. 24-14, *U*).

Case 3

A 24-year-old woman was initially seen to address the concern of anterior crowding. The following complex problems were observed at the initial examination: skeletal Class II jaw relationship, excessive lower facial height, TMJ disorders (osteoarthritis suspected), Class II denture bases, severe anterior crowding, and deviated maxillary dental midline (Fig. 24-15, *A-F*). Analysis of the dental arches revealed a space deficiency of 12.0 and 8.0 mm in the maxillary and the mandibular dentitions, respectively (Fig. 24-15, *G-J*).

In other words, distalization of 6 mm in the maxilla and 4 mm in the mandible bilaterally was required for a nonextraction treatment approach. From an anatomical viewpoint, it seemed possible to achieve the treatment goals by distalization of the maxillary and mandibular molars into the extraction spaces of the third molars. Nevertheless, the authors provided the patient with two treatment options: traditional four-bicuspid extraction or distalization of bimaxillary posterior teeth; she chose the latter. As shown in the previous cases, four miniplates were temporarily implanted and used as absolute anchorage for simultaneous distalization of the molars (Fig. 24-15, *G*).

Figure 24-15, *K* to *N*, show her treatment progress. Her complex orthodontic problems were significantly improved after about 23 months of treatment (Fig. 24-15, *O-T*). Figure 24-15, *U*, shows the cephalometric changes during the SAS treatment. With the application of distalization and intrusion biomechanics, her treatment goal was successfully achieved without flaring the incisors or increasing the lower facial height.

INDICATIONS FOR MOLAR DISTALIZATION

Numerous extraoral and intraoral mechanical modalities have been proposed for distalizing the maxillary molars. However, only a few appliances have been reported for the

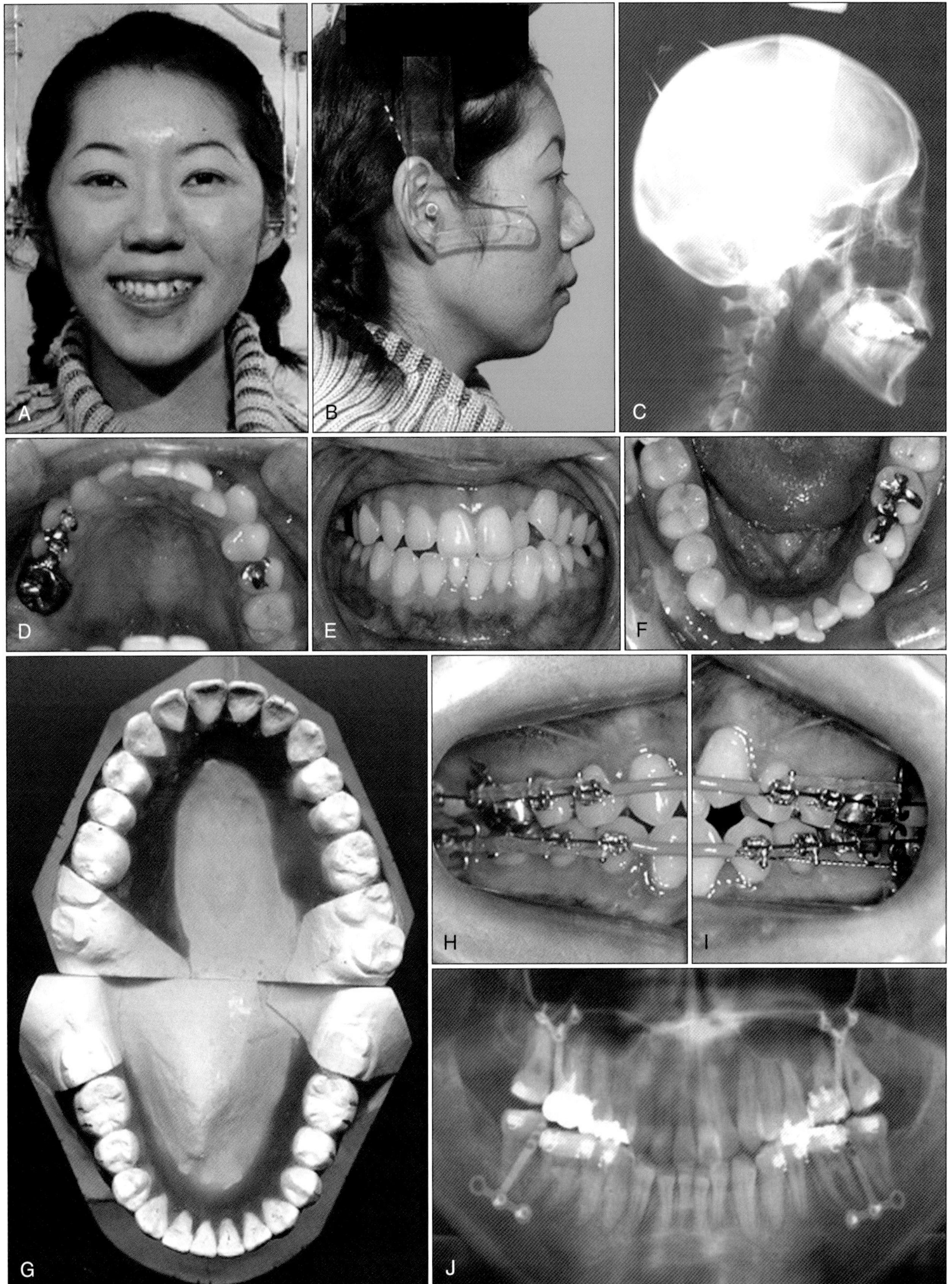

Fig. 24-14 Case #2. Nonextraction treatment of bimaxillary anterior crowding with SAS. **A** to **F**, Initial facial photographs (**A** and **B**), cephalometric radiograph (**C**), and intraoral photographs (**D-F**). **G** to **J**, Treatment goal (**G**) and SAS biomechanics in place (**H-J**).

Continued

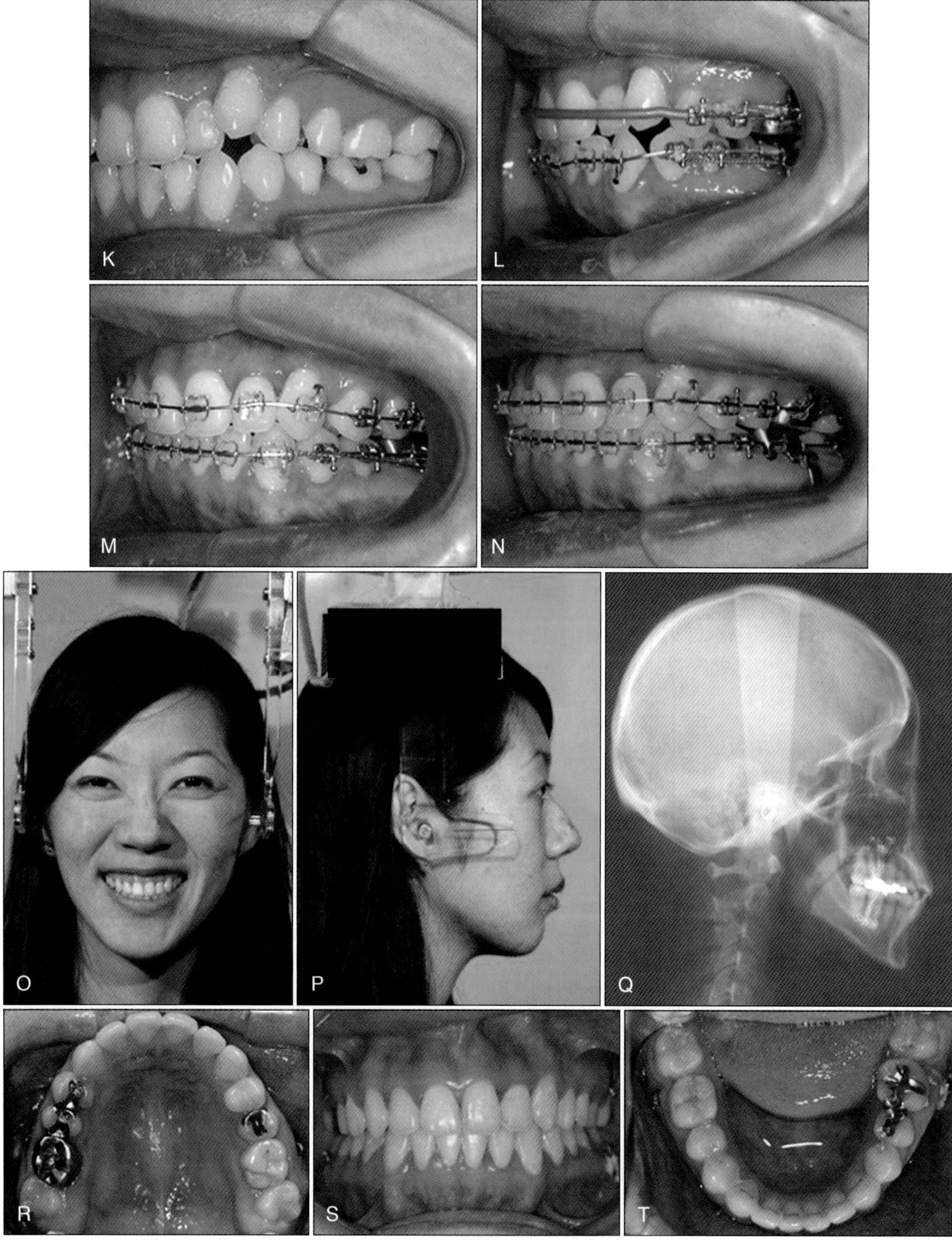

Fig. 24-14, cont'd K to N, Treatment progress: start of treatment (**K**), 3 months (**L**), 6 months (**M**), and 9 months (**N**). **O** to **T**, Debonding facial photographs (**O** and **P**), cephalometric radiograph (**Q**), and intraoral photographs (**R-T**).

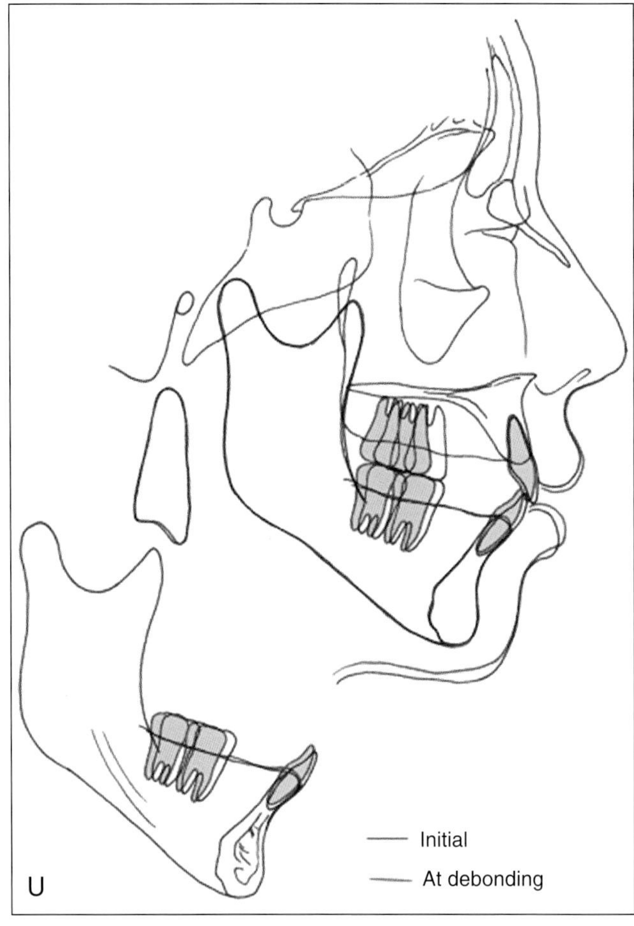

Fig. 24-14, cont'd U, Cephalometric superimpositions.

mandibular molars, which are more difficult to distalize than the maxillary molars. Nonetheless, as shown in the case reports, the SAS has enabled the authors to distalize the maxillary and the mandibular molars simultaneously. Accordingly, nonextraction therapy using the SAS distalizing biomechanics can resolve various types of malocclusion, including Class II and Class III malocclusions with or without asymmetric dentition and any malocclusion characterized by crowding of the dentition.

Open bite was a contraindication for previous intraoral distalizing appliances because of the tendency to increase the lower facial height and aggravation of open bite after distalization of the molars. In contrast, open bite might not be a contraindication for SAS treatment because it is now possible to intrude the molars simultaneously during molar distalization.[39-45] Indeed, 11 of the 54 subjects in the study were open-bite patients. Additionally, surgical patients who required decompensation of the maxillary or mandibular incisors in presurgical orthodontics are also candidates for distalization of the molars with the SAS biomechanics.

TIMING OF MOLAR DISTALIZATION

The prime candidates for the previously reported intraoral distalizing appliances were adolescent growing patients, because the distal movement of the first molars was thought to be easier to achieve before the eruption of the second molars. However, such an approach occasionally results in posterior crowding, eventually causing a disturbance in the establishment of posterior support at the second molars, ectopic eruption of the third molars, and root resorption of the second molars following the eruption of the third molars. Therefore the SAS has been used in nongrowing patients, taking into consideration the location and space for the third molars.

Usually it is recommended to extract the third molars immediately before distalization of the first molars with the SAS. However, for patients with other dental problems in the second molars, such as dental caries, endodontic/prosthetic problems, ectopic eruption (eruption at extremely unusual position), or extremely difficult third molar extraction, the second molars are extracted rather than the third molars. In addition, although the age of the subjects in this study varied from 15 to 46 years, individualized treatment goals were achieved in most patients regardless of age. Therefore the maxillary and the mandibular molar distalizing mechanics with the SAS can be used for a wide range of ages, including adults.

BIOMECHANICAL ADVANTAGES OF MOLAR DISTALIZATION WITH SKELETAL ANCHORAGE SYSTEM

A two-stage method was typically used to distalize the molars with intraoral distalizing appliances, as previously reported, particularly in the maxilla. The first molars were moved distally in the first stage. However, anchorage loss—mesial movement of the premolars and proclination of the incisors—generally occurred as a side effect during molar distalization, although sufficient anchorage support was provided by the second premolars. In the second stage, premolars, canines, and incisors were sequentially retracted after reinforcing the anchorage of the molars previously distalized in the first stage.

Although it is important to address the amount of distalization of the first molars and the anchorage loss at the first stage, a more important concern is the anchorage loss of the distalized molars during the second stage. Unfortunately, this problem has not been seriously discussed in previous reports. The progress of the molar distalization with the SAS is completely different from previous molar distalizing methods. The distalized molars are never required as a part of the anchorage during retraction of the premolars and the anterior teeth, because the orthodontic force can be directly applied from the miniplates. Accordingly, by using SAS biomechanics, it is possible to perform en masse movement of the posterior teeth and the anterior dentition together instead of a two-stage approach. This helps to save

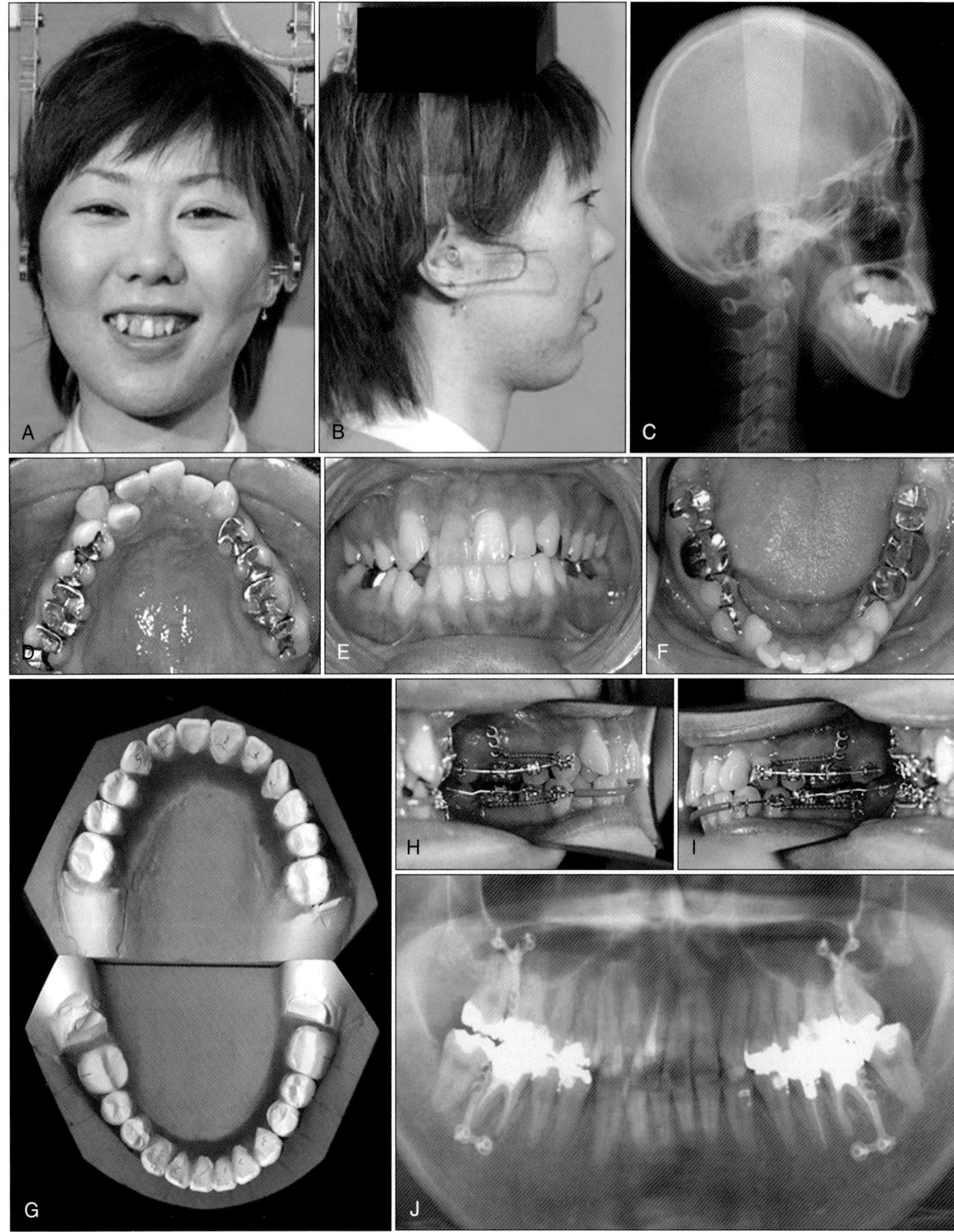

Fig. 24-15 Case #3. Nonextraction treatment of bimaxillary anterior crowding with SAS. **A** to **F**, Initial facial photographs (**A** and **B**), cephalometric radiograph (**C**), and intraoral photographs (**D-F**). **G** to **J**, Treatment goal (**G**) and SAS biomechanics in place (**H-J**).

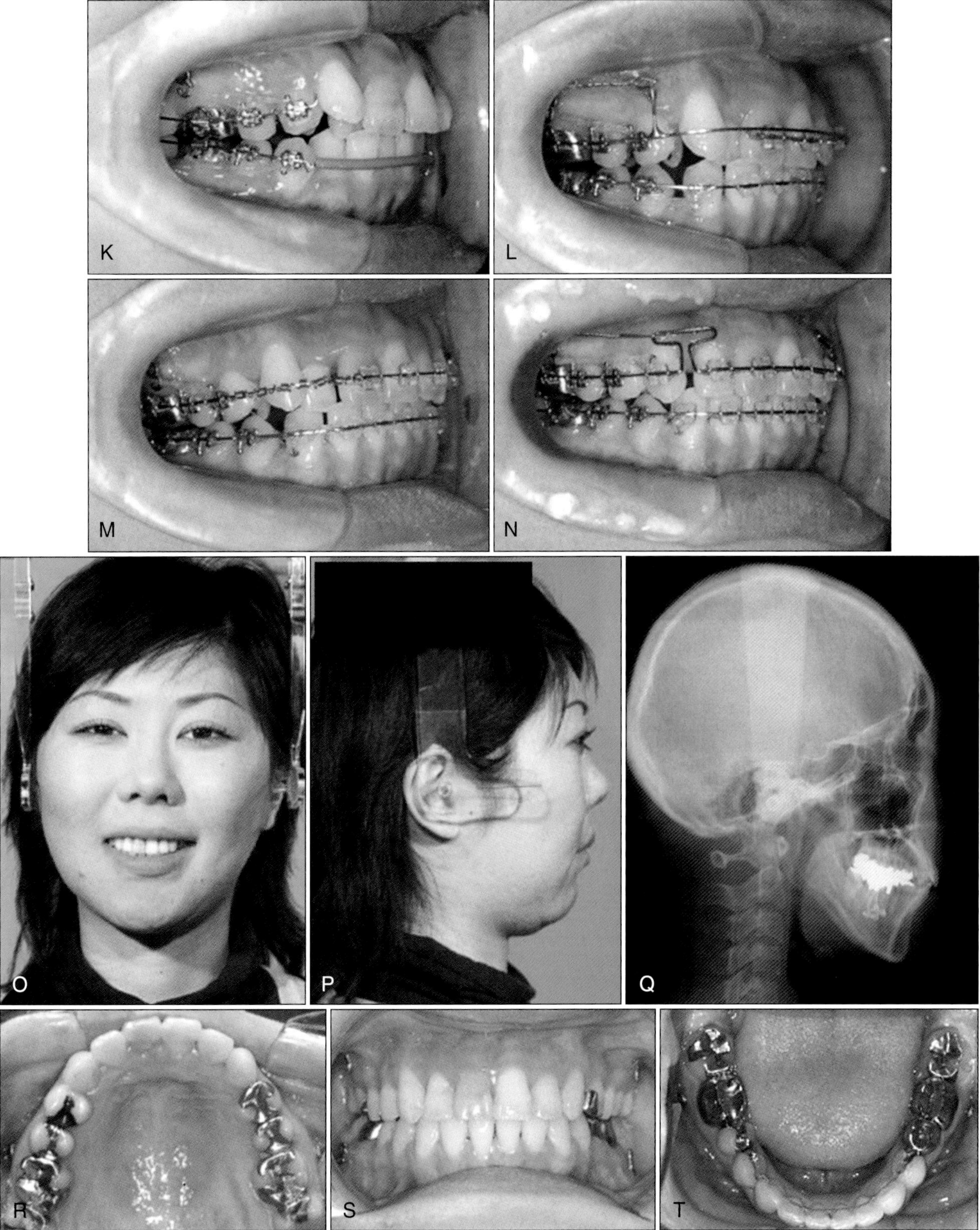

Fig. 24-15, cont'd **K** to **N**, Treatment progress: start of treatment (**K**), 6 months (**L**), 9 months (**M**), and 15 months (**N**). **O** to **T**, Debonding facial photographs (**O** and **P**), cephalometric radiograph (**Q**) and intraoral photographs (**R-T**). *Continued*

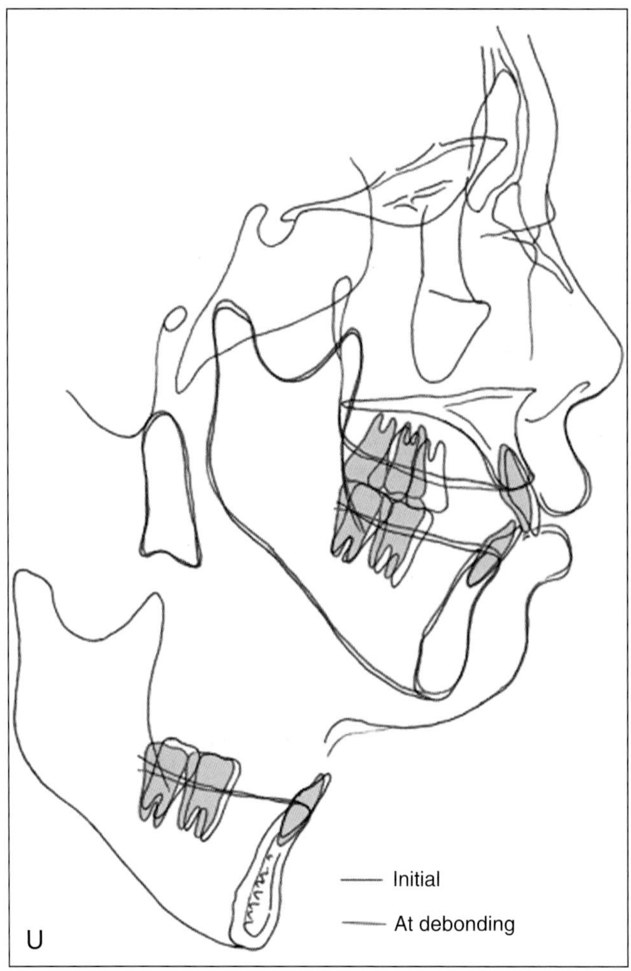

Fig. 24-15, cont'd U, Cephalometric superimpositions.

considerable treatment time and is therefore a distinct advantage of SAS biomechanics when compared with previous methods and techniques.

Amount of Molar Distalization

As the results of this study have shown, the average amount of the maxillary and mandibular molar distalization was 3.8 mm and 3.4 mm, respectively. This suggests that it might be possible to correct arch space deficiency of approximately 7 mm without the need for bicuspid extraction. In other words, the SAS biomechanics has significantly expanded the range of nonextraction treatment.

At the same time, it is important to realize that the "amount" of the molar distalization does not necessarily mean the *maximum* amount of molar distalization in each subject. Questions about the extent of maxillary and the mandibular molar distalization with SAS biomechanics have no "right" answer, partly because whenever SAS biomechanics is considered, individualized treatment goals must be established first.

It is essential to determine the posterior limits of the alveolar bone from an orthodontic, anatomical, or periodontal standpoint. For example, the location of the mandibular third molars should be a useful indicator for judging the posterior limit of the alveolar bone in the maxillary and mandibular dentitions. Currently, CBCT has become a useful diagnostic tool to determine the posterior limits of the alveolar bone.

Type of Molar Distalization

The type of molar distalization with SAS may be either a *translatory* or a *tipping* movement. The results of this study show differences between the type of distalization in the maxillary and mandibular molars. The maxillary molar represented almost a bodily distal translation, whereas the mandibular molar tended to represent tipping during distal movement. The authors believe that because the percentage of Class III malocclusion is relatively high in subjects requiring mandibular molar distalization, the mandibular occlusal plane must be rotated in a counterclockwise direction. Consequently, the mandibular molars might show a tipping distal movement.

It was not easy to prevent distal tipping completely with SAS treatment, but it was easier to obviate the distal tipping of the molars during the multibracketed treatment by considering the location of the center of resistance. Overall, in accordance with the individualized treatment goals, it is possible to control the type of molar distalization with the application of proper SAS biomechanics.

Predictability of Molar Distalization

Although goal-oriented strategies have been essential in contemporary orthodontics,[46,47] no previous report has mentioned treatment goals for distalization of the maxillary and mandibular molars. In this study, individualized treatment goals for distalization of the molars, incisor positions, and soft tissue profiles were established in all subjects before SAS treatment. Moreover, SAS treatment started after a careful evaluation of the three-dimensional treatment goals by using a wax-up. Consequently, the predicted amount of maxillary and mandibular first molar crown distalization was 3.6 mm and 3.2 mm, respectively, and was significantly correlated with the actual amount of distalization. Therefore the biomechanics of SAS treatment for distalization of the maxillary and mandibular molars seems quite predictable.

CONCLUSION

The skeletal anchorage system is a viable modality for distalizing the maxillary and the mandibular molars because it uses stable and reliable anchorage units. It enables not only single molar distalization but also en masse movement of the maxillary and the mandibular posterior teeth with only minor surgery to place the miniplates at the zygomatic buttress or the mandibular body. Therefore, this new noncompliance technique for adults is particularly useful for correcting Class II and Class III malocclusions with or without asymmetric dentition, decompensation for surgical patients, and other malocclusions characterized by anterior crowding. The SAS biomechanics should be evaluated as an indispensable modality in contemporary adult orthodontics.

References

1. Kloehn SJ: Evaluation of cervical traction of the maxilla and maxillary first permanent molar, *Angle Orthod* 31:91-104, 1961.
2. Wieslander L: The effect of force on craniofacial development, *Am J Orthod* 65:531-538, 1974.
3. Baumrind S, Korn EL, Isaacson RJ, et al: Quantitative analysis of the orthodontic and orthopedic effects of maxillary traction, *Am J Orthod* 84:384-393, 1983.
4. Cetlin NM, Ten Hoeve A: Nonextraction treatment, *J Clin Orthod* 17:396-403, 1983.
5. Gianelly AA, Vaitas AS, Thomas WM, Berger DG: The use of magnets to move molars distally, *Am J Orthod Dentofacial Orthop* 96:161-167, 1989.
6. Itoh T, Tokuda T, Kiyosue S, et al: Molar distalisation with repelling magnets, *J Clin Orthod* 25:611-617, 1991.
7. Jackel N, Rakosi T: Molar distalisation by intraoral force application, *Eur J Orthod* 13:43-45, 1991.
8. Gianelly AA, Bednar J, Dietz VS: Japanese NiTi coils used to move molars distally, *Am J Orthod Dentofacial Orthop* 99:564-566, 1991.
9. Jones RD, White JM: Rapid Class II molar correction using an open coil jig, *J Clin Orthod* 26:661-664, 1992.
10. Bondemark L, Kurol J: Distalization of maxillary first and second molars simultaneously with repelling magnets, *Eur J Orthod* 14:264-272, 1992.
11. Hilgers JJ: The Pendulum appliance for Class II non-compliance therapy, *J Clin Orthod* 26:706-714, 1992.
12. Locatelli R, Bednar J, Dietz VS, Gianelly AA: Molar distalization with superelastic NiTi wire, *J Clin Orthod* 26:277-279, 1992.
13. Muse DS, Fillman MJ, Emmerson WJ, Mitchell RD: Molar and incisor changes with Wilson rapid molar distalization, *Am J Orthod Dentofacial Orthop* 104:556-565, 1993.
14. Bondemark L, Kurol J, Bernhold M: Repelling magnets versus superelastic NiTi simultaneous distal movement of maxillary first and second molars, *Angle Orthod* 64:189-198, 1994.
15. Steger ER, Blechman AM: Case reports: molar distalization with static repelling magnets. Part I, *Am J Orthod Dentofacial Orthop* 108:547-555, 1995.
16. Carano A, Testa M: The distal jet for upper molar distalization, *J Clin Orthod* 30:374-380, 1996.
17. Ghosh J, Nanda RS: Evaluation of an intraoral maxillary molar distalization technique, *Am J Orthod Dentofacial Orthop* 110:639-646, 1996.
18. Basdra EK, Huber H, Komposch G: A clinical report for distalizing maxillary molars by using super-elastic wires, *J Orofac Orthop* 57:118-123, 1996.
19. Byloff FK, Darendeliler MA: Distal molar movement using the Pendulum appliance. Part 1. Clinical and radiological evaluation, *Angle Orthod* 67:249-260, 1997.
20. Byloff FK, Darendeliler MA, Clar E, Darendeliler A: Distal molar movement using the Pendulum appliance. Part 2. The effects of maxillary molar root uprighting bends, *Angle Orthod* 67:261-270, 1997.
21. Erverdi N, Koyuturk O, Kucukkeles N: Nickel-titanium coil springs and repelling magnets: a comparison of two different intra-molar distalization techniques, *Br J Orthod* 24:47-53, 1997.
22. Pieringer M, Droschl H, Permann R: Distalisation with a Nance appliance and coil spring, *J Clin Orthod* 31:321-326, 1997.
23. Gianelly AA: Distal movement of maxillary molars, *Am J Orthod Dentofacial Orthop* 114:66-72, 1998.
24. Gulati S, Kharbanda OP, Parkash H: Dental and skeletal changes after intraoral molar distalization with sectional jig assembly, *Am J Orthod Dentofacial Orthop* 114:319-327, 1998.
25. Bondemark L, Kurol J: Class II correction with magnets and superelastic coils followed by straight-wire mechanotherapy, *J Orofac Orthop* 59:127-138, 1998.
26. Runge ME, Martin JT, Bukai F: Analysis of rapid maxillary molar distal movement without patient cooperation, *Am J Orthod Dentofacial Orthop* 115:153-157, 1999.
27. Scuzzo G, Pisani F, Takemoto K: Maxillary molar distalization with a modified Pendulum appliance, *J Clin Orthod* 33:645-650, 1999.
28. Fortini A, Lupoli M, Parri M: The first class appliance for rapid molar distalization, *J Clin Orthod* 33:322-328, 1999.
29. Bussick T, McNamara JA Jr: Dentoalveolar and skeletal changes associated with the Pendulum appliance, *Am J Orthod Dentofacial Orthop* 117:333-343, 2000.
30. Brickman CD, Sinha PK, Nanda RS: Evaluation of the Jones Jig appliance for distal molar movement, *Am J Orthod Dentofacial Orthop* 118:526-534, 2000.
31. Keles A, Sayinsu K: A new approach in maxillary molar distalization: intraoral bodily molar distalizer, *Am J Orthod Dentofacial Orthop* 117:39-48, 2000.
32. Quick AN, Harris AMP: Molar distalization with a modified distal jet appliance, *J Clin Orthod* 34:419-423, 2000.
33. Ngantung V, Nanda RS, Bowman SJ: Posttreatment evaluation of the distal jet appliance, *Am J Orthod Dentofacial Orthop* 120:178-185, 2001.
34. Champagne M: The NiTi distalizer: a non-compliance maxillary molar distalizer, *Int J Orthod Milwaukee* 13:21-24, 2002.
35. Keles A, Pamukcu B, Tokmak EC: Bilateral maxillary molar distalization with sliding mechanics: Keles slider, *World J Orthod* 3:57-66, 2002.
36. Sakuda M, Taki S, Hayashi I, et al: An idea for distal movement of molar teeth: a distal extension lingual arch, *Nippon Kyosei Shika Gakkai Zasshi* 33:195-201, 1974.
37. Uner O, Haydar S: Mandibular molar distalization with the Jones Jig appliance, *Kieferorthop* 9:169-174, 1995.
38. Byloff F, Darendeliler MA, Stoff F: Mandibular molar distalization with the Franzulum appliance, *J Clin Orthod* 34:518-523, 2000.
39. Sugawara J: Dr. Junji Sugawara on the skeletal anchorage system, *J Clin Orthod* 33:689-696, 1999.
40. Umemori M, Sugawara J, Mitani H, et al: Skeletal anchorage system for open-bite correction, *Am J Orthod Dentofacial Orthop* 115:166-174, 1999.
41. Sugawara J, Daimaruya T, Umemori M, et al: Distal movement of mandibular molars in adult patients with the skeletal anchorage system, *Am J Orthod Dentofacial Orthop* 125:130-138, 2004.

42. Sugawara J, Nishimura M: Minibone plates: the Skeletal Anchorage System, *Semin Orthod* 11:47-56, 2005.
43. Sugawara J: A bioefficient skeletal anchorage system. In Nanda R, editor: *Biomechanics and strategies in clinical orthodontics,* St Louis, 2005, Saunders-Elsevier, pp 295-309.
44. Sugawara J, et al: The Skeletal Anchorage System. In Cope J, editor: *OrthoTADs: the clinical guide and atlas,* Dallas, 2007, Under Dog Media, pp 449-461.
45. Sugawara J, et al: Skeletal anchorage system using orthodontic miniplates. In Nanda R, Uribe F, editors: *Temporary anchorage devices in orthodontics,* St Louis, 2008, Mosby-Elsevier, pp 317-341.
46. Burstone CJ, Marcotte MR: *Problem solving in orthodontics,* Chicago, 2000, Quintessence.
47. Nanda R, editor: *Biomechanics and strategies in clinical orthodontics,* St Louis, 2005, Saunders-Elsevier.

CHAPTER 25

Biomechanics of Rapid Tooth Movement by Dentoalveolar Distraction Osteogenesis

■ *Haluk İşeri, Gökmen Kurt, and Reha Kişnişci*

Most orthodontic cases feature a shortage of space and some crowding. Although nonextraction treatment has become popular in the last decade, many patients still require treatment based on tooth extraction.

The first phase of treatment in premolar extraction cases is distalization of the canines. Using conventional orthodontic techniques, biological tooth movement can be achieved at a limited rate.[1,2] The canine retraction phase usually lasts about 6 to 8 months. In addition, extraoral or intraoral anchorage mechanics are required to keep the obtained space safe during canine distalization, particularly when maximum or moderate anchorage is required. Therefore, under normal circumstances, conventional treatment with fixed appliances is likely to last about 20 to 24 months. Unfortunately, duration of orthodontic treatment is the major complaint of patients, especially adults and young adults.

Many attempts have been made to shorten the time for orthodontic tooth movement and overall orthodontic treatment. In 1959, Köle[3] reported on a technique that combined orthodontics with "corticotomy" surgery to increase the rate of orthodontic tooth movement.[4-7] In 1980, Davidovitch et al.[8,9] studied how the rate of tooth movement and periodontal cyclic nucleotide levels could be increased by combined force and electrical currents. In 1998, Liou and Huang[10] introduced the technique of distraction of the periodontal ligament for rapid tooth movement.

In 1999, İşeri and Kişnişci introduced a technique called *dentoalveolar distraction* (DAD), which achieves rapid tooth movement by using the principles of distraction osteogenesis.[11-14] This chapter presents the associated biological principles, a detailed description of the DAD technique, the data regarding the effects of DAD on the dentofacial structures, and case reports.

BIOLOGICAL PRINCIPLES OF DISTRACTION OSTEOGENESIS

Distraction osteogenesis (DO) is a biological process involving new bone formation between the surfaces of bone segments that are gradually separated by incremental traction. The traction generates tension that stimulates bone formation parallel to the vector of distraction. Specifically, this process is initiated when distraction forces are applied to the callus tissues connecting the divided bone segments and continues as long as these tissues are stretched. DO begins with the development of a reparative callus. The callus is placed under tension by stretching, which generates new bone. DO consists of the following four sequential periods:

1. *Osteotomy* (or "corticotomy") means to fracture the bone into two segments. It should be vertical to the direction of distraction.
2. *Latency* is the period from bone division to the onset of traction (usually 5-7 days) and is the time required for callus formation.
3. *Distraction* is the period when gradual traction is applied and new bone, or *distraction regenerate,* is formed. DO has the benefit of simultaneously increasing bone length and the volume of surrounding soft tissues.
4. *Consolidation* is the period that allows healing and maturation and corticalization of the regenerate after traction forces are discontinued.

In 1988, Ilizarov[15] introduced two biological principles of distraction osteogenesis, known as the *Ilizarov effects:* (1) the tension stress effect on the genesis and growth of tissues and

(2) the influence of blood supply and loading on the shape of bones and joints.

The first Ilizarov principle postulates that gradual traction creates stress that can stimulate and maintain regeneration of living tissues. The newly formed bone rapidly remodels to conform to the bone's natural structure.

The second Ilizarov principle theorizes that the shape and mass of bones and joints depend on an interaction between mechanical loading and blood supply. Blood supply and mechanical loading have a significant influence on the shape and mass of the resulting bone. If the blood supply is inadequate to support normal and increased mechanical loading, the bone cannot respond favorably, leading to degenerative changes. In contrast, if blood supply is adequate to support increased mechanical loading, the bone will demonstrate compensatory hypertropic changes.

The principles of DO are as follows:

1. *Preservation of osteogenic tissues.* This is necessary during osteotomy, and periosteum, bone marrow, and the nutrient artery are equally important for new bone formation.
2. *Direction of distraction.* The regenerate within distraction gap was always formed along the axis of applied traction.
3. *Rate and rhythm.* Successful distraction depends on the rate and rhythm of the applied distraction force. Optimal rate of distraction is 1 mm per day. More frequent rhythms of distraction lead to more favorable regenerate formation and cause less soft tissue problems. If the rate of distraction is less than 0.5 mm per day, the bone may consolidate prematurely. If the rate of distraction is more than 1.5 mm per day, local ischemia in the interzone and delayed ossification or pseudoarthrosis may result.

Distraction osteogenesis was used as early as 1905 by Codivilla[16] and later popularized by the clinical and research studies of Ilizarov[15] in Russia. DO has been used mainly in the field of orthopedics. In fact, Ilizarov's concept of long-bone elongation by DO and its application to the craniofacial skeleton opened a new chapter in the treatment of craniofacial anomalies and various malocclusions.

The first report demonstrating the application of Ilizarov's principles to the dog mandible was published by Snyder et al.[17] in 1973. In this experimental study, the device was activated at a rate of 1 mm per day for 14 days after a 7-day latency period. Reestablishment of the mandibular cortex and medullar canal across the distraction gap was noted after 6 weeks of fixation. In 1977, Michieli and Miotti[18] demonstrated the feasibility of intraoral mandibular lengthening by using Ilizarov's principles and distraction protocol without damage to the mandible. Lengthening of the mandibular body in two dogs was achieved with a technique that involved osteotomies and the use of an experimental orthodontic appliance without any damage to the mandibular nerve and no conspicuous alterations of the nerve fibers.

Therefore the DO technique is proposed for use in *correction* of large discrepancies in length in patients with excessive mandibular retrusion. Guerrero[19] (1990) and McCarthy et al.[20] (1992) used DO in the human mandible. In 1999, dentoalveolar distraction (DAD) for rapid tooth movement was described and used by Iseri et al.[11-13] Since then, DO has been applied to various bones of the craniofacial skeleton.

RAPID TOOTH MOVEMENT BY DENTOALVEOLAR DISTRACTION OSTEOGENESIS

Appliance Design

A custom-made, rigid, tooth-borne, intraoral distraction device was designed and used in the DAD patients (Fig. 25-1). The device was made of stainless steel with one distraction screw, two guidance bars, and a special apparatus to activate the distractor by turning the screw clockwise.

The canines and the first molars were banded with .06 × 1.80–inch (.15 × 4.55–mm) band material, and an impression was made with the bands placed on the teeth (Fig. 25-2, *A* and *B*). The distractor was then soldered to the canine and first molar bands on the dental cast. The buccal location and angulation of the distractor is adjusted according to the position of the canine (Fig. 25-2, *C*). To minimize tipping, the distractor was positioned as high as possible buccally (Fig. 25-2, *D*).

Surgical Technique

Surgery was performed on an outpatient basis, with the patient under local anesthesia, sometimes supplemented with nitrous oxide sedation. A horizontal mucosal incision 2 to 2.5 cm in length was made parallel to the gingival margin of the canine and premolar beyond the depth of the vestibule (Fig. 25-3).

On the medial aspect of the canine tooth to be distracted posteriorly, multiple cortical holes were made on the alveolar bone between the canine and the lateral incisor with a

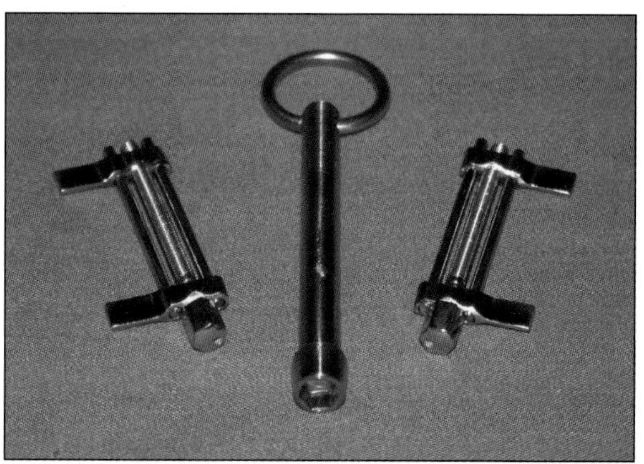

Fig. 25-1 Dentoalveolar distraction (DAD) device (distractor). This custom made, rigid, tooth-borne intraoral device is designed for DAD and rapid tooth movement. The stainless steel device has one distraction screw and two guidance bars. The patient or parent turns the screw clockwise with a special apparatus for rapid tooth movement.

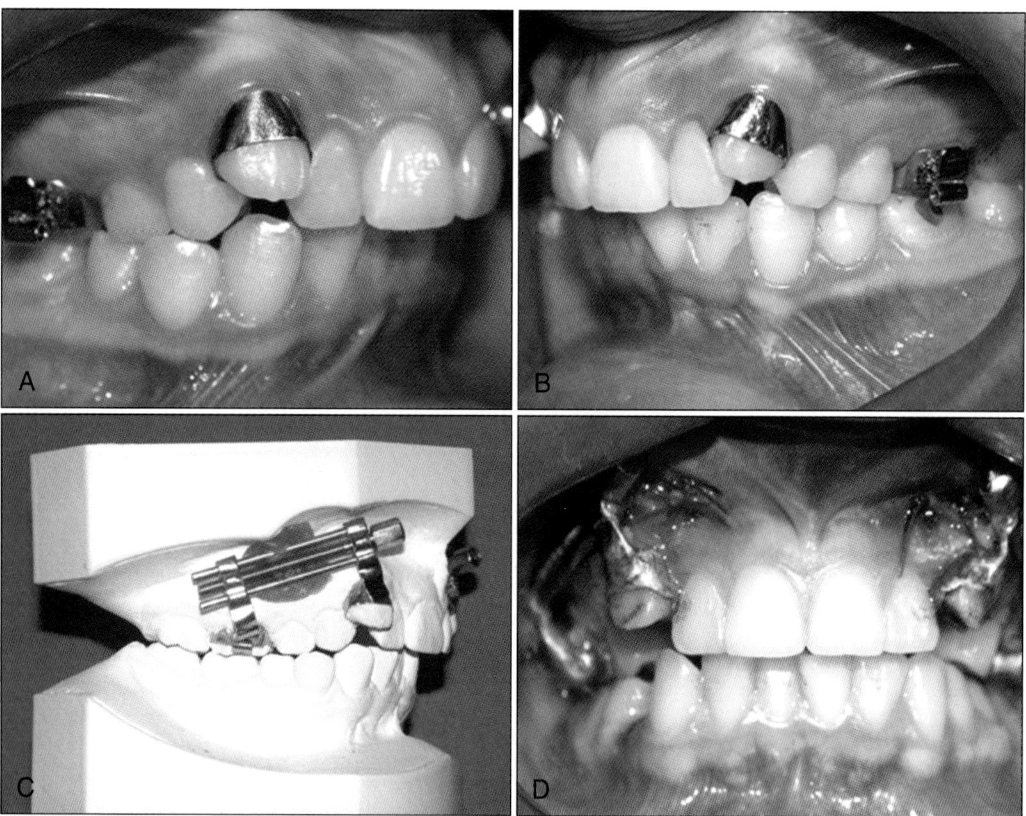

Fig. 25-2 Fabrication of DAD device. **A** and **B,** Intraoral views of fabricated molar and canine bands. **C,** Custom-made distractor is positioned using biomechanical principles of tooth movement, then soldered to the bands on the cast. **D,** Distractor is cemented on the canine and the first molar immediately after surgery.

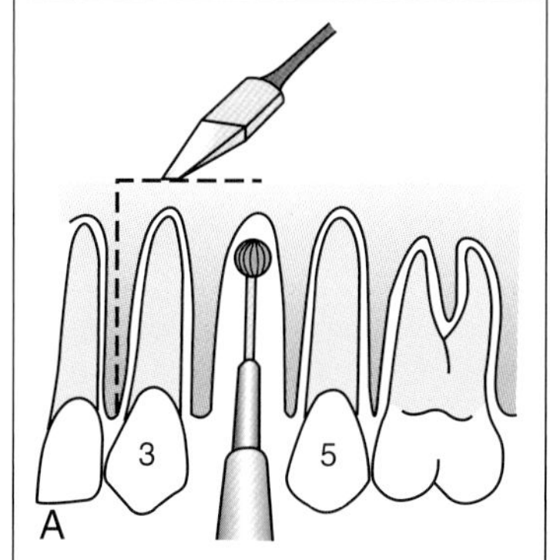

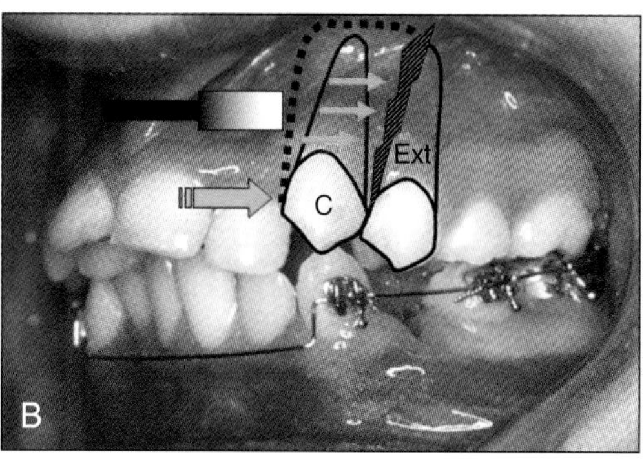

Fig. 25-3 **A** and **B,** Dentoalveolar distraction procedure. The first premolar was extracted. Bony interferences in the extraction socket were eliminated. Osteotomes were used to fully mobilize the alveolar segment, including the tooth (*C*, canine; *Ext*, extraction).

small, round carbide bur (Fig. 25-4, *A* and *B*). The same procedure was done on the distal aspect of the canine close to the extraction area. Subsequently, the holes around the canine root were connected by a thin, tapered fissure bur (Fig. 25-4, *C*).

The osteotomy curved apically at a distance of 3-5 mm from the apex. The fine osteotomes were then advanced in the coronal direction. The first premolar was extracted at this stage, and the buccal bone was removed between the outlined bone cut at the distal canine region anteriorly and the second premolar posteriorly by using a large, round bur. Larger osteotomes of appropriate sizes were then used to fully mobilize the alveolar segment, including the canine, by fracturing the spongy bone around its root of the lingual or palatal cortex (see Fig. 25-3). The buccal and apical bone through the extraction socket and bony interferences at the buccal aspect that might be encountered during the distraction process were eliminated or smoothed between the canine and the second premolar, preserving the palatal or lingual cortical shelves. Although the palatal shelf was

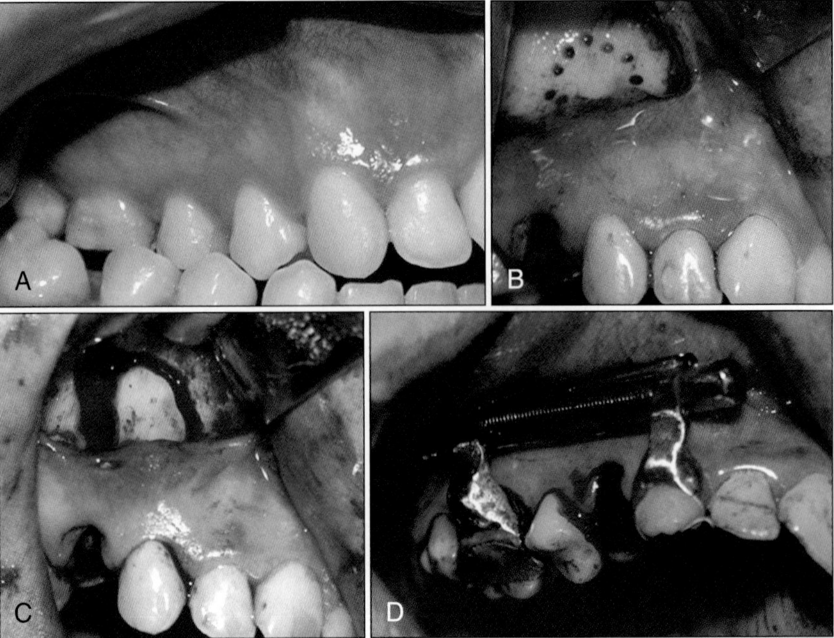

Fig. 25-4 **A,** Intraoral view of DAD surgical site. **B,** Multiple cortical holes were made on the alveolar bone with a small, round, carbide bur. **C,** View of osteotomy of cortical bone and extraction socket of first premolar. **D,** Distractor was cemented immediately after surgery, and the dentoalveolar segment, including the tooth, was used as a transport disk to carry the maxillary canine posteriorly.

preserved, apical bone near the sinus wall was removed, leaving the sinus membrane intact to avoid interferences during the active distraction process. (Fig. 25-4, *C*). Then, osteotomes along the anterior aspect of the canine were used to split the surrounding bone around its root from the palatal or lingual cortex and neighboring teeth. The transport dentoalveolar segment that included the canine also included the buccal and palatal cortex and the underlying spongy bone that envelopes the canine root, leaving an intact lingual or palatal cortical plate and the bone around the apex of the canine (see Fig. 25-4, *C*).

Finally, the DAD device was cemented on the canine and the first molar (Fig. 25-4, D). To ensure that the transport segment was fully mobilized, the alveolar segment carrying the canine had been fully mobilized intraoperatively, and the device was activated several millimeters and set back to its original position. The incision was closed with absorbable sutures, and an antibiotic and a nonsteroidal antiinflammatory drug (NSAID) were prescribed for 5 days.

The surgical procedure lasted approximately 30 minutes for each canine. The patients were instructed to discontinue tooth brushing to avoid trauma around the surgical site for 3 days. A 0.2% chlorhexidine gluconate (Klorhex, Drogsan, Ankara, Turkey) rinse was prescribed twice a day during the distraction period.[12,13]

Distraction Protocol

Distraction was initiated within 3 days after surgery. The distractor was activated twice daily, in the morning and in the evening, for a total of about 0.8 mm per day. DAD was based on movement of the alveolar bone as a "transport disk," which included the canine tooth (Fig. 25-5). This type of distraction is termed as a modification of *bifocal osteosynthesis* and consists of gradual movement of a vascularized bony segment (transport disk) previously separated from the residual bone segment (Fig. 25-6). New bone is formed during movement of the transport disk in the distraction site with simultaneous closing of the bony defect. In the authors' cases the alveolar bone was included with the canine.

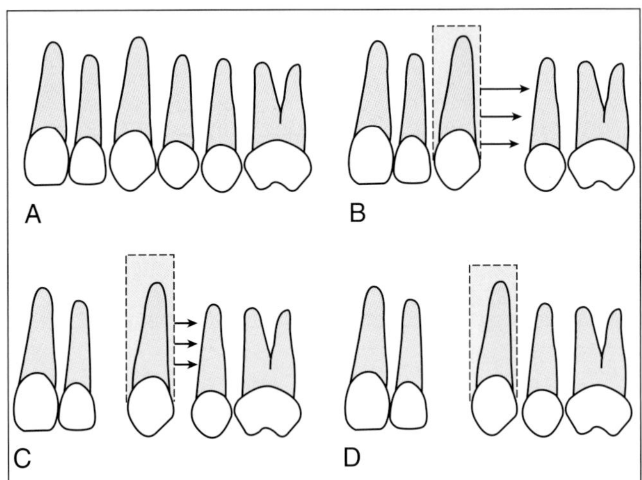

Fig. 25-5 **A** to **D,** Rapid canine movement using the principles of distraction osteogenesis (DO) by means of gradual movement of a vascularized bony segment (transport disk) previously separated from the residual bone segment (bifocal osteosynthesis). The transported dentoalveolar segment, including the canine, also includes the buccal cortex and the underlying spongy bone that envelopes the canine root, leaving intact the palatal or lingual cortical plate and the bone around the apex of the canine.

Dentoalveolar distraction was discontinued when the canine had moved posteriorly into the desired position or came into contact with the second premolar, if necessary. The DAD device (distractor) was then removed, and fixed-appliance orthodontic treatment was immediately initiated

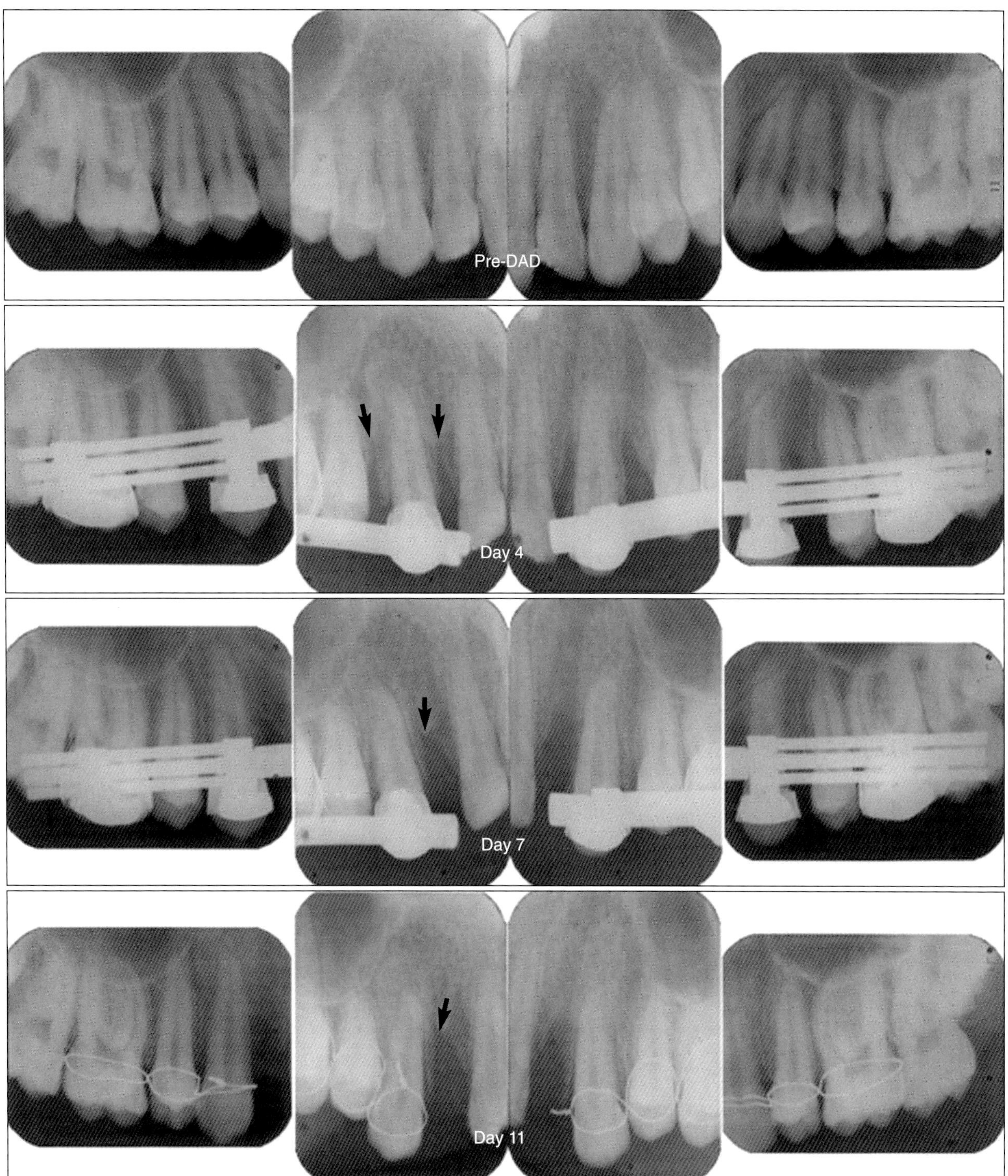

Fig. 25-6 Periapical views of rapid movement of the maxillary canines in 11 days using dentoalveolar distraction (DAD). The black arrows represent the movement of the canine in its surrounding alveolar bone as an alveolar bony transport disk, according to DO principles.

by the leveling of both dental arches particularly to benefit from the uncalcified distraction chamber to resolve anterior crowding and also to achieve incisor retraction if necessary. Ligatures were placed under the archwire between the distracted canine and the first molar and kept at least 3 months after the DAD procedure to avoid mesial movement of the canine.

All patients followed a program of meticulous oral hygiene, initiated before and after the DAD procedure and reinforced monthly during fixed-appliance orthodontic therapy, together with professional tooth cleaning.

Orthodontic Tooth Movement

Orthodontic tooth movement is a process in which the application of a force induces bone *resorption* on the pressure side and bone *apposition* on the tension side.[1,2] Thus, conventional tooth movement results from biological cascades of resorption and apposition caused by the mechanical forces. The term *physiological tooth movement* primarily refers to the slight tipping of the tooth in its socket and secondarily to the changes in tooth position that occur during and after tooth eruption.[21]

Basically, no significant difference exists between the tissue reactions observed in physiological tooth movement and those in orthodontic tooth movement. However, because the teeth are moved more rapidly during treatment, the tissue changes elicited by orthodontic forces are more marked and extensive. Classically, the typical rate of orthodontic tooth movement depends on magnitude and duration of force applied,[1] number and shape of roots, quality of bony trabeculae, individual response, and patient compliance. Presumably, application of force will result in hyalinization from both anatomical and mechanical factors.[22]

The hyalinization period usually lasts 2 to 3 weeks.[21] The rate of biological tooth movement with optimum mechanical force is about 1.0 to 1.5 mm in 4 to 5 weeks.[23] Therefore, in maximum anchorage premolar extraction cases, the canine distalization phase usually takes about 6 to 9 months, with an average overall treatment time of 2 years.

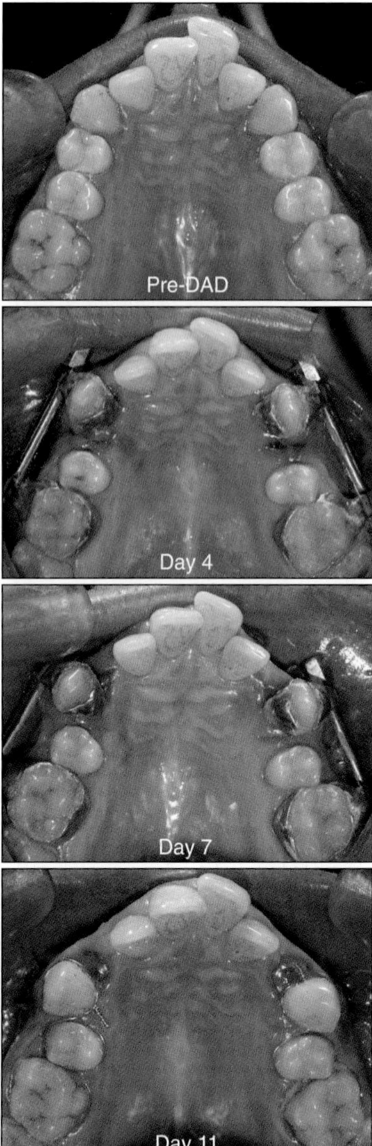

Fig. 25-7 Occlusal views of rapid movement of the maxillary canines by DAD. Full distraction of the canines was completed in 11 days.

Rapid Tooth Movement

Rapid tooth movement using DO principles is done to shorten the duration of orthodontic treatment. In 2005, İşeri et al.[13] published the duration of canine retraction and the effects of DAD on the dentofacial structures. The study sample consisted of 20 maxillary canines in 10 growing or adult subjects (mean age, 16.53 years; range, 13.08-25.67 years). The canines were moved rapidly into the sockets of the extracted first premolars in compliance with DO principles. The distraction procedure was completed in 8 to 14 days, with a screw-turning rate of 0.8 mm/day (Fig. 25-7). Full retractions of the canines were achieved in 10.05 (±2.01) days (Table 25-1). This was the most rapid orthodontic tooth movement demonstrated compared with previous studies.[10,23] The distal displacement of the canines was mainly a combination of tipping and translation, with a mean change in canine inclination of 13.15 (±4.65) degrees at the end of the distraction period.[13]

Posterior Anchorage Maintenance

No posterior anchorage loss was observed in any of the DAD cases. In 2005, İşeri et al.[13] reported the mean sagittal and vertical anchorage loss in molar teeth as 0.19 ± 0.31 mm and 0.51 ± 0.93 mm, respectively, during 10 days of rapid distraction of the canines, which was statistically insignificant (Table 25-2).

During orthodontic tooth movement, hyalinized tissue neighboring the tooth on the movement side must be undermined with indirect resorption. This period usually lasts 2 or 3 weeks;[21] again, rapid canine retraction with DAD was achieved in 8 to 14 days, a short period for molars to move mesially (see Figs. 25-6 and 25-7).

Root Resorption

Periapical radiographs of the canines and first molars and panoramic films were taken at the start and end of the distraction procedure to evaluate root structures. Root resorption scores were detected according to the scale modified from Sharpe et al.,[24] as follows:

- S0 = No apical root resorption
- S1 = Widening of periodontal ligament (PDL) space at the root apex
- S2 = Moderate blunting of the root apex up to one third of the root length
- S3 = Severe blunting of the root apex beyond one third of the root length

No clinical or radiographic evidence of complications (e.g., root fracture, root resorption, ankylosis, soft tissue dehiscence) was observed in the DAD patients (Fig. 25-8).[13]

Tooth Vitality

Pulp vitality was evaluated and recorded with an electronic digital pulp tester and a thermal pulp tester.[13] All teeth

TABLE 25-1

Survey of Age and Duration of Dentoalveolar Distraction*

	Mean	SD	Minimum	Maximum
Age, start of distraction (years)	16.53	3.76	13.08	25.67
Duration of distraction (days)	10.05	2.01	8.0	14
Rate of screw turning	0.8 mm/day			

From İşeri H, Kişnişci R, Bzeizi N, Tüz H: *Am J Orthod Dentofacial Orthop* 127:533-541, 2005.
*20 canines in 10 subjects.
SD, Standard deviation.

TABLE 25-2

Dentoskeletal Changes with Dentoalveolar Distraction of Canines

	Start of Distraction (mean ± SD)	End of Distraction (mean ± SD)	Difference (T Test) (mean ± SD)
MAXILLARY MEASUREMENTS (DEGREES)			
s n ss	77.58 ± 4.08	77.60 ± 4.11	0.05 ± 0.54
NSL/NL	8.90 ± 3.11	9.38 ± 2.45	0.49 ± 1.28
MANDIBULAR MEASUREMENTS (DEGREES)			
s n sm	73.57 ± 2.31	73.29 ± 2.41	−0.29 ± 0.63
NSL/ML	37.94 ± 5.84	38.61 ± 5.91	0.67 ± 0.80*
MAXILLOMANDIBULAR MEASUREMENTS			
ss n sm°	4.10 ± 2.43	4.65 ± 2.73	0.54 ± 0.97
n me (mm)	127.00 ± 8.12	128.00 ± 8.15	0.99 ± 0.57†
Overbite (mm)	3.19 ± 2.06	2.71 ± 1.64	−0.48 ± 1.20
Overjet (mm)	5.83 ± 4.16	5.50 ± 4.08	−0.34 ± 0.44*
DENTOALVEOLAR MEASUREMENTS			
NSL/can inc (degrees)	93.85 ± 9.82	84.20 ± 5.92	13.15 ± 4.65†
NSL-is (mm)	84.39 ± 3.86	84.68 ± 4.08	0.29 ± 0.62
NSL-ms (mm)	72.63 ± 3.62	73.14 ± 3.77	0.51 ± 0.93
NSLv-is (mm)	101.31 ± 5.40	101.31 ± 5.41	−0.01 ± 1.01
NSLv-ms (mm)	63.01 ± 7.93	62.82 ± 7.91	0.19 ± 0.31

From İşeri H, Kişnişci R, Bzeizi N, Tüz H: *Am J Orthod Dentofacial Orthop* 127:533-541, 2005.
*$p < 0.05$.
†$p < 0.01$.
Reference points and planes: *s,* sella; *n,* nasion; *ss,* A point; *is,* incisal edge of maxillary central incisor; *ms,* most anterior-inferior point of maxillary first molar; *sm,* B point; *me,* menton; *can inc,* canine inclination, line from most inferior point of maxillary canine tubercule and root apex of maxillary canine; *NSL,* s-n line represents anterior cranial base as horizontal reference plane; *NSLv,* vertical reference plane perpendicular to NSL at s; *NL,* nasal plane; *ML,* mandibular plane.

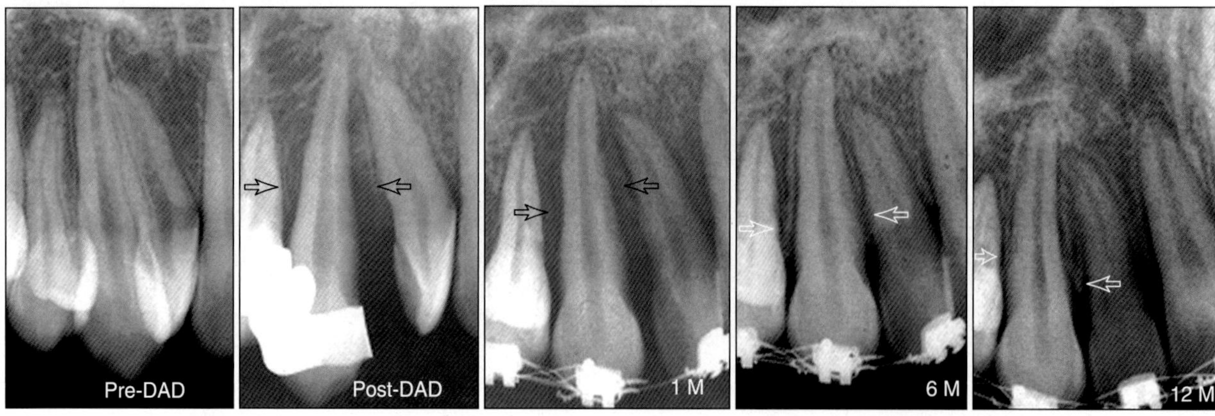

Fig. 25-8 Radiographic appearance of a maxillary canine on evaluation. Alterations in the alveolar bone at the proximal side were a loss *(black arrows)* and gain *(white arrows)* in mineralization. There is a clear view of the lamina dura at the proximal side of the canine on evaluation at 6 and 12 months *(M)*. There is no radiographic evidence of root fracture, root resorption, or ankylosis. (From Gürgan C, İşeri H, Kişnişci R: *Eur J Orthod* 27:324-332, 2005.)

subjected to pulp vitality tests (canines, incisors, second premolars, first molars) were cleaned and tested on the buccal surfaces.

Before the start of treatment, pulp vitality was tested with an electronic pulp tester. All teeth reacted positively, except for a right maxillary central incisor in a patient with previous root canal therapy. At the end of the DAD procedure and during the fixed-appliance orthodontic treatment, no reliable reactions to the pulp test were achieved in the study subjects. However, all teeth reacted positively at the 6-month evaluation after treatment.

Periodontal Status

In 2005, Gürgan et al.[14] evaluated the alterations that occurred in the gingival dimensions of canine teeth after DAD during a 12-month follow-up. Before surgery (pre-DAD), immediately after removal of the device (post-DAD), and at 1, 6, and 12 months post-DAD, the plaque index (PI), gingival index (GI), pocket depth (PD), and width of keratinized gingiva were recorded and the width of attached gingiva was calculated (Fig. 25-9).

There were significant differences between pre-DAD and post-DAD measurements for PD at all sites, with the highest at the distal site. The palatal sites likewise showed significant differences at the 1-, 6-, and 12-month follow-up compared with the post-DAD period. The buccal sites showed no significant changes at any time. The width of keratinized gingiva also showed no significant change during the follow-up period; the width of attached gingiva was significant only between the pre-DAD and post-DAD periods ($p < 0.01$). Periodontal status was normal in all cases at the end of the 1-year orthodontic treatment after DAD. The PI and GI values were increased after surgery and then gradually decreased through the 1-, 6-, and 12-month periods. The PD measurements on three sites other than the buccal site were increased by DAD, but decreased significantly during the follow-up period.

Therefore the DAD technique was found to be a viable innovative method to reduce the orthodontic treatment time without unfavorable long-term effects on the gingival tissues.

Fixed-Appliance Treatment in DAD Cases

Stages of fixed-appliance orthodontic treatment for the DAD patients were as follows:

1. End of DAD
2. Placement of .010-inch ligature between canine and first molar before removal of the distractor (see Figs. 25-6 and 25-7, day 11)
3. Initiation of fixed-appliance orthodontic treatment on the upper and lower dental arches
4. Removal of the .010-inch ligature and placement of a new, .008-inch ligature between the first molar tube and the canine bracket
5. Placement of .014-inch nickel-titanium (Ni-Ti) archwire for leveling (3-6 weeks)
6. Placement of .016-inch Ni-Ti archwire for leveling (if necessary, for 3 weeks)
7. Placement of .016 × .016–inch archwire with reverse closing loops for incisor retraction and torque control (3-4 months)
8. Placement of .017 × .025–inch or .018 × 025–inch finishing-phase archwires (3 months)
9. End of orthodontic treatment (9-12 months)

CASE 1

A Class II, Division 2 male patient age 14 years, 6 months presented with the chief complaint of anterior crowding in

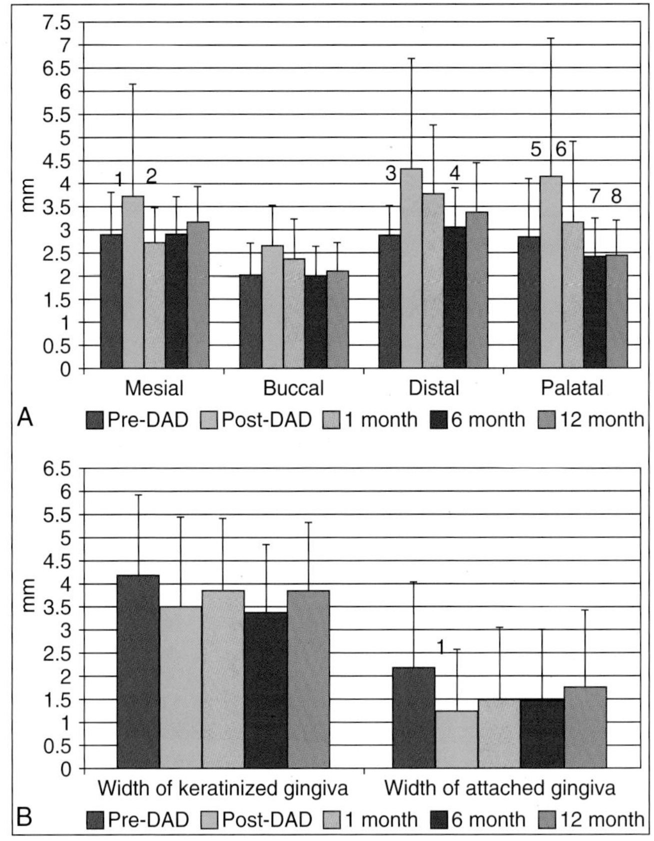

Fig. 25-9 Measurements of mesial, buccal, distal, and palatal pocket depth (**A**) and width of keratinized gingiva and attached gingiva (**B**) at each site during treatment and on evaluation. Means and standard deviations (SD) are presented in Table 25-2. *DAD,* Dentoalveolar distraction. **A,** *1, p* < 0.05, between pre- and post-DAD for mesial sites; *2, p* < 0.05, between post-DAD and 1 month for mesial sites; *3, p* < 0.001, between pre- and post-DAD for distal sites; *4, p* < 0.01, between post-DAD and 6 months for distal sites; *5, p* < 0.001, between pre- and post-DAD for palatal sites; *6, p* < 0.05, between post-DAD and 1 month for palatal sites; *7, p* < 0.001, between post-DAD and 6 months for palatal sites; *8, p* < 0.001, between post-DAD and 12 months for palatal sites; ⊤, SD. **B,** *p* < 0.01, between pre- and post-DAD; ⊤, SD. (Redrawn from Gürgan C, İşeri H, Kişnişci R: *Eur J Orthod* 27:324-332, 2005.)

upper maxillary dental arch and unesthetic tooth appearance on smiling (Fig. 25-10). He had Class II molar and canine relationship with 6 mm and 1 mm of overjet according to the right and the left maxillary central incisor, respectively. His profile was slightly convex. At the start of treatment, he had 4 mm of overbite and 8 mm and 2.5 mm of crowding in the maxilla and mandible, respectively. His maxillary right second lateral incisor was palatally located and blocked out, whereas the left maxillary lateral incisor was labially positioned. Intraoral evaluation showed that the maxillary midline shifted 1 mm to the right side and the mandibular midline shifted 1 mm to the left side. His left lower first molar was missing. Table 25-3 provides this patient's initial cephalometric values.

TABLE 25-3

Cephalometric Values for Case 1

	Pre-DAD	Post-DAD	End Treatment
Maxillary Measurements (degrees)			
s n ss	82.75	83.41	81.76
NSL/NL	11.24	10.53	12.57
Mandibular Measurements (degrees)			
s n sm	76.83	77.62	75.95
NSL/ML	34.95	36.35	35.83
Maxillomandibular Measurements			
ss n sm (degrees)	5.92	5.79	5.81
NL/ML (degrees)	23.71	21.61	23.27
Overbite (mm)	2.75	2.93	1.80
Overjet (mm)	6.07	5.88	2.45
Dentoalveolar Measurements			
NL/ILs (degrees)	113.93	114.83	108.69
NL/can inc (degrees)	119.50	103.81	102.77
NL/MLs (degrees)	100.78	100.70	101.11
NLv-is (mm)	1.82	1.86	5.60
NLv-uc (mm)	1.45	8.03	9.93
NLv-ms (mm)	25.17	25.37	25.66
NL-is (mm)	30.83	30.29	33.16
NL-uc (mm)	27.62	32.98	32.99
NL-ms (mm)	27.18	25.38	28.52

DAD, Dentoalveolar distraction; *End Treatment,* end of orthodontic treatment; *ILs,* maxillary central incisor inclination; *MLs,* maxillary molar inclination; *NLv,* vertical reference plane perpendicular to NL; *uc,* most inferior point of maxillary canine tubercule.

Treatment Plan

Bilateral maxillary premolar extraction was considered with the severe maxillary crowding and increased overjet. Conventional and rapid treatment options were explained to the patient and his parents, including cervical headgear for maximum anchorage to eliminate crowding and increased overjet, by means of maxillary canine and incisor retraction.

The patient preferred rapid orthodontic treatment of 1-year duration, without using extraoral anchorage appliances. The DAD surgery, DO protocol, and orthodontic procedures were described in detail, and an informed consent was signed by the patient and his father. The treatment plan was therefore bilateral maxillary first premolar extraction, followed by rapid canine retraction with DAD, then fixed-appliance orthodontic treatment, with no extraoral or intraoral anchorage appliances.

Treatment Progress

Dentoalveolar distraction surgery was performed and the distractor cemented on the canine and the first molar immediately after surgery. Distraction was initiated within 3 days

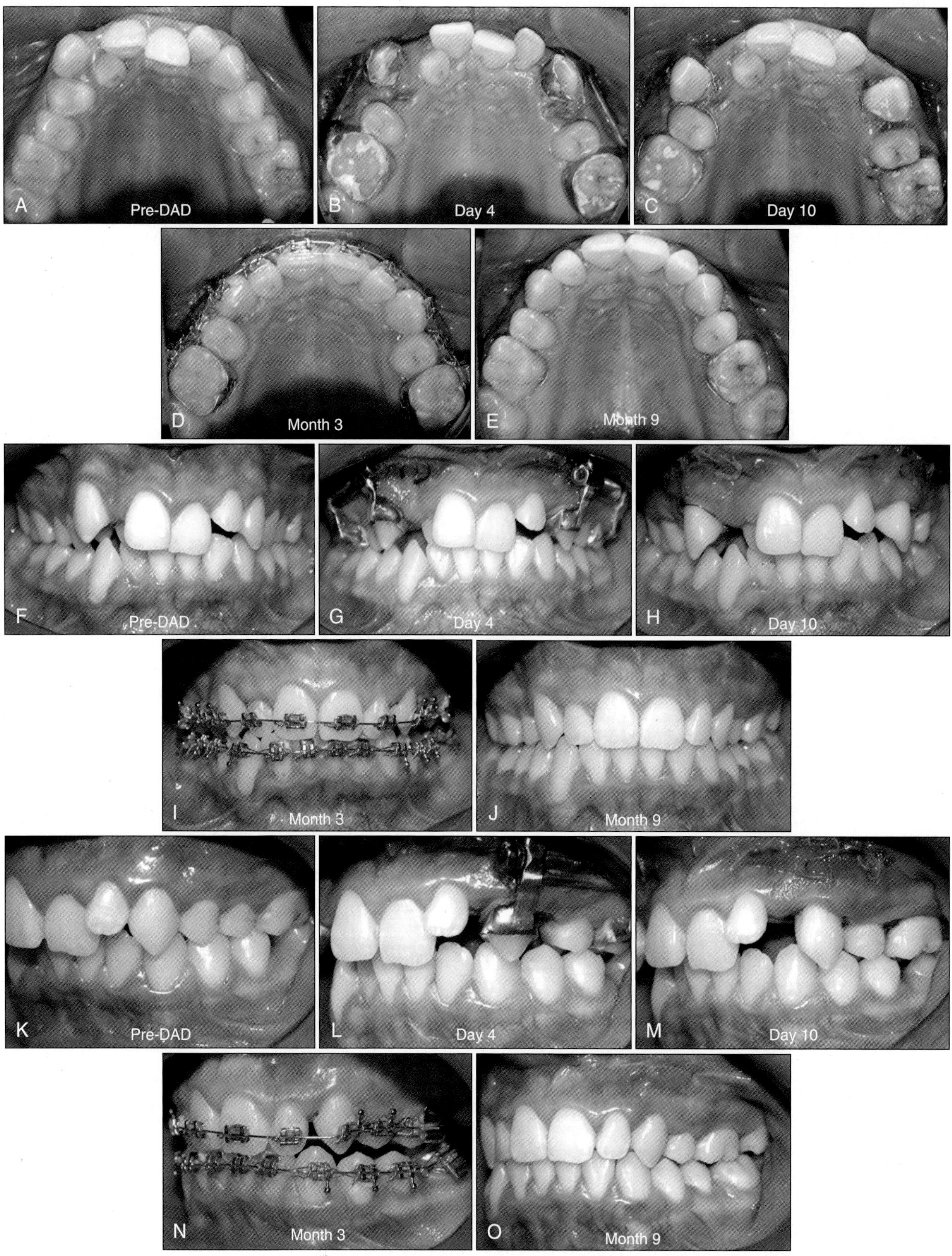

Fig. 25-10 Case #1. Dentoalveolar distraction of maxillary canines from start to end of distraction. Full distraction of the canines was completed in 10 days. **A** to **E,** Occlusal views. **F** to **J,** Frontal views from start of DAD to end of orthodontic treatment, which was completed in 9 months. DAD was completed in 10 days, and ligature was placed between canine and first molar before removal of distractor. Fixed appliances were initiated immediately after removal of distractor, and ligatures were then placed under the archwire between the distracted canine brackets and first molar tubes and kept in place for 3 months. **K** to **O,** Intraoral left views.

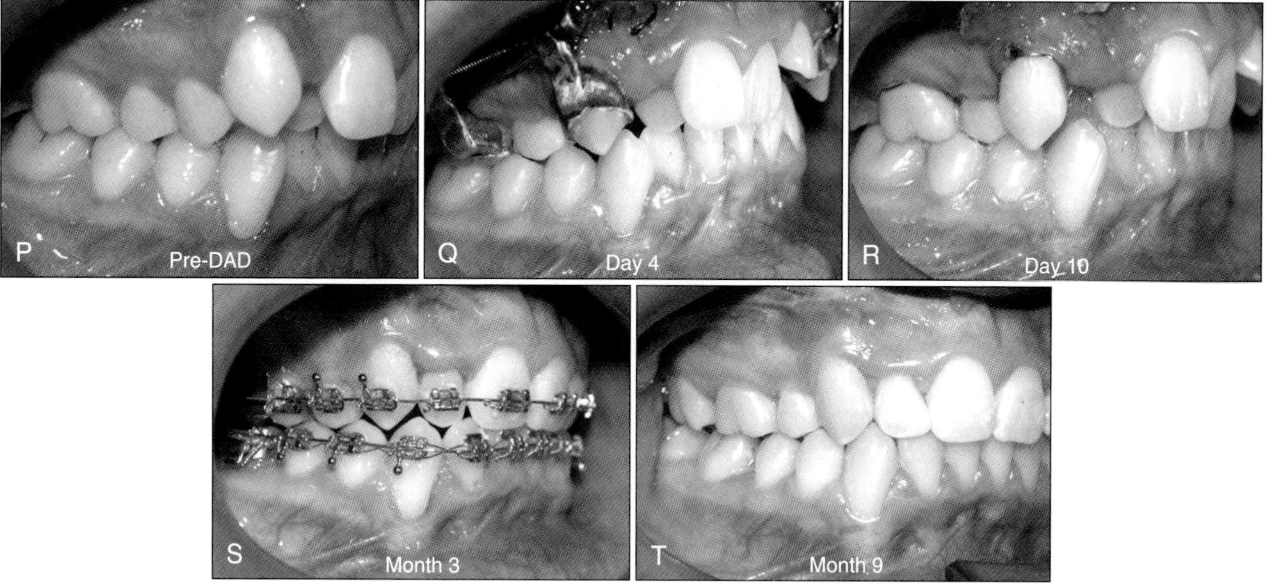

Fig. 25-10, cont'd **P** to **T**, Intraoral right views.

Continued

after surgery. The distractor was activated twice daily, in the morning and in the evening, for a total of 0.8 mm/day. Rapid canine movement using DO principles was completed in 10 days, and the distractors were removed when the canine teeth came into contact with the second premolars.

Mild edema was observed after the DAD surgery, but no significant soft tissue changes were seen at the end of 10 days.

After removal of the distractors, fixed-appliance orthodontic treatment was immediately initiated. First a .014-inch and then a .016-inch Ni-Ti archwire was placed in the upper and lower dental arches for leveling. In the next appointment, a .016 × .016–inch stainless steel archwire with reverse closing loop was used to close the mild extraction space in the maxillary left side. After closure of the extraction space, .017 × .025–inch stainless steel archwires were used for maintaining adequate torque in both dental arches. Class II elastic traction from the left lower second molar was used to close the space of the missing left lower first molar and to correct the shifted midline as well.

Treatment Outcome

Class I canine and Class II molar relationship was achieved at the end of orthodontic treatment. The patient's cephalometric values after DAD and at the end of orthodontic treatment are given in Table 25-3. Cephalometric measurement and superimposition showed no sagittal or vertical posterior anchorage loss at the upper first molar region during DAD and fixed treatment. Canine teeth moved 6.6 mm posteriorly, 5.4 mm vertically, and inclined 15.7 degrees (right maxillary canine) during DAD (10 days). Class I canine and Class II molar relationship and ideal overbite and overjet were achieved after orthodontic treatment in 9 months.

Cephalometric superimposition on the maxillary structures indicated full distalization of the canines as well as marked incisor retraction (Fig. 25-11). No posterior anchorage loss was seen, even though no extraoral or intraoral anchorage device was used during the DAD and fixed-appliance orthodontic treatment.

Radiographic analysis of maxillary canines before and after DAD and after orthodontic treatment (9 months) indicated no evidence of complications such as root resorption, root fracture, or ankylosis (Fig. 25-12).

CASE 2

A female patient age 16 years, 9 months presented with the main complaint of an increased overjet (Fig. 25-13). Her profile was convex, and she had an increased interlabial gap caused by the upper incisor proclination. The patient exhibited 10-mm overjet, Class II molar and canine relationship, and a narrow maxillary dental arch at the start of treatment. She had 4-mm overbite and 3-mm and 0.5-mm crowding in the maxilla and mandible, respectively. The mandibular midline was shifted 4 mm to the left side. There was an amalgam restoration on the lower-left first molar. Table 25-4 provides this patient's initial cephalometric measurements.

Treatment Plan

Detailed explanation regarding conventional and rapid treatment options was given to the patient and her parents. Because of 10-mm overjet, the patient was informed about the possible use of cervical headgear for maximum anchorage reasons related to maxillary canine distalization and incisor retraction. Extraction of the maxillary first premolars and use of extraoral anchorage appliances for retraction of

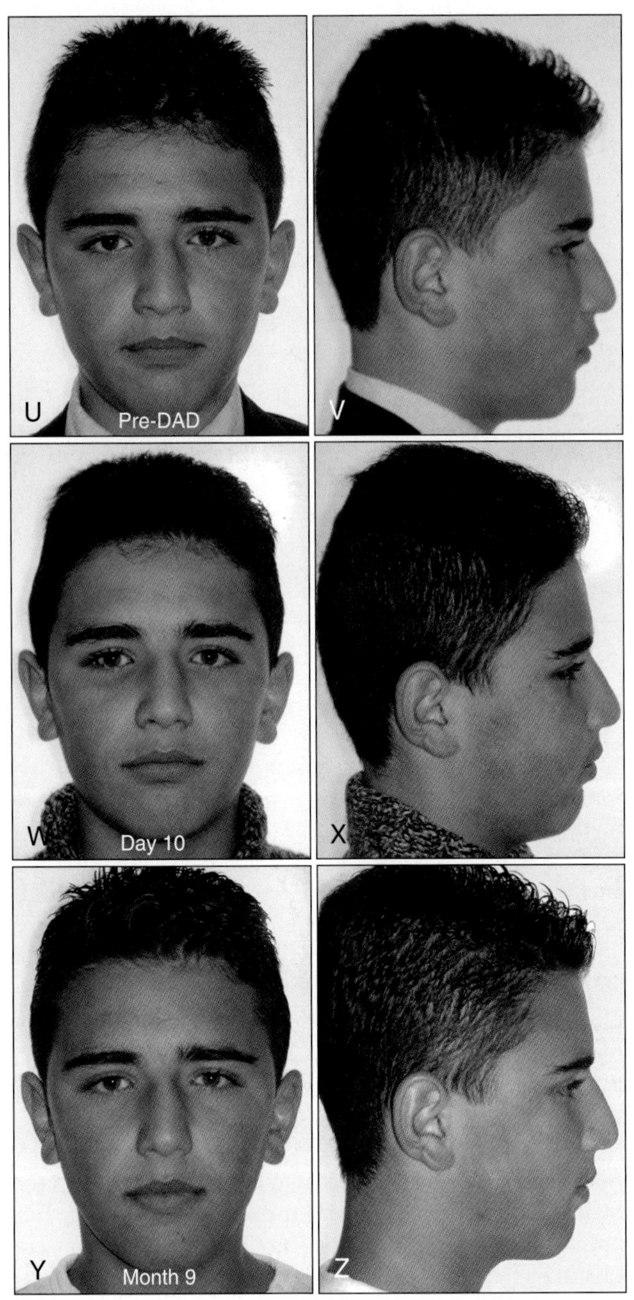

Fig. 25-10, cont'd **U** to **Z**, Facial photographs at start of DAD (**U** and **V**), end of DAD (**W** and **X**), and end of orthodontic treatment (**Y** and **Z**). No significant soft tissue change (edema) was observed after surgery.

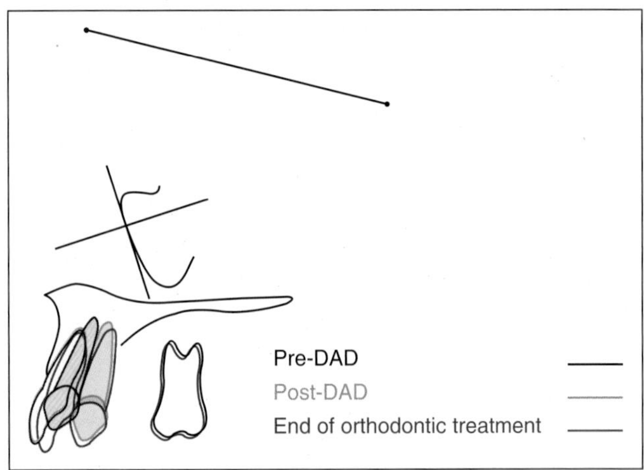

Fig. 25-11 Maxillary superimposition for Case #1 indicates full retraction of the canines and elimination of severe crowding without any posterior anchorage loss during DAD and fixed-appliance orthodontic treatment. *Black line,* Before DAD; *blue line,* after DAD (10 days); *red line,* end of orthodontic treatment (9 months).

TABLE **25-4**

Cephalometric Values for Case 2

	Pre-DAD	Post-DAD	End Treatment
Maxillary Measurements (degrees)			
s n ss	73.74	73.60	73.42
NSL/NL	12.13	11.50	10.96
Mandibular Measurements (degrees)			
s n sm	70.84	70.47	69.26
NSL/ML	40.23	40.26	42.41
Maxillomandibular Measurements			
ss n sm (degrees)	2.90	3.13	4.16
NL/ML (degrees)	28.10	28.76	31.45
Overbite (mm)	4.23	4.31	1.54
Overjet (mm)	9.73	9.61	3.20
Dentoalveolar Measurements			
NL/ILs (degrees)	118.07	118.02	100.73
NL/can inc (degrees)	105.63	93.40	94.81
NL/MLs (degrees)	88.48	90.05	90.88
NLv-is (mm)	1.65	1.46	7.68
NLv-uc (mm)	5.71	13.39	13.70
NLv-ms (mm)	30.74	30.58	29.22
NL-is (mm)	31.08	30.04	30.39
NL-uc (mm)	29.75	27.86	27.77
NL-ms (mm)	118.07	118.02	100.73

the maxillary canines and incisors to eliminate the increased overjet were presented as the conventional treatment modality. Different options were offered to maintain adequate posterior anchorage during the canine and incisor retraction, including extraoral (headgear) and intraoral (TPA and mini-implants or zygomatic implants) mechanics.

The patient preferred rapid orthodontic treatment of 1-year duration with no use of extraoral or intraoral anchorage appliances. Information about DAD surgery, DO protocol, and orthodontic procedures was then provided, and an informed consent was signed by the patient and her parent. The treatment plan was therefore bilateral maxillary first premolar extraction, followed by rapid canine retraction with DAD, then fixed-appliance orthodontic treatment, with no extra or intraoral anchorage appliances.

Treatment Progress

Dentoalveolar distraction was performed and the distractor cemented on the canine and the first molar immediately after surgery. Distraction was initiated within 3 days after surgery. The distractor was activated twice daily, in the morning and in the evening, for a total of 0.8 mm/day. When the canine teeth came into contact with the second premolars, the distractors were removed. Distraction phase continued 13 days.

Mild edema was observed after DAD surgery, but no significant soft tissue changes were seen at the end of 13 days.

The fixed-appliance orthodontic treatment was immediately started after removal of the distractors, and .016-inch Ni-Ti archwires were initiated on both dental arches. At the end of leveling stage (2 months after DAD), a .016 × .022–inch stainless steel archwire with reverse closing loop was used for retraction of the maxillary anterior teeth. At the end of maxillary incisor retraction, .017 × .025–inch stainless steel archwires were placed on both dental arches for the finishing phase. Overall orthodontic treatment time was 10 months. Table 25-4 provides the patient's cephalometric values after DAD and at the end of orthodontic treatment.

Treatment Outcome

Overjet was eliminated and a Class I canine and Class II molar relationship achieved at the end of orthodontic treatment. According to the cephalometric analysis, the canines moved 7.7 mm posteriorly, 1.9 mm vertically, and inclined 12.2 degrees by DAD in 13 days. The upper first molars did not exhibit significant mesial, vertical, or angular changes during or after DAD. Cephalometric superimposition indicated marked maxillary canine distalization and incisor retraction (see Table 25-4). There was no sagittal or vertical posterior anchorage loss during DAD and fixed-appliance orthodontic treatment (Fig. 25-14).

Radiographic analysis of maxillary canines before and after DAD and after orthodontic treatment (10 months) indicated no evidence of complications, such as root resorption, root fracture, or ankylosis (Fig. 25-15).

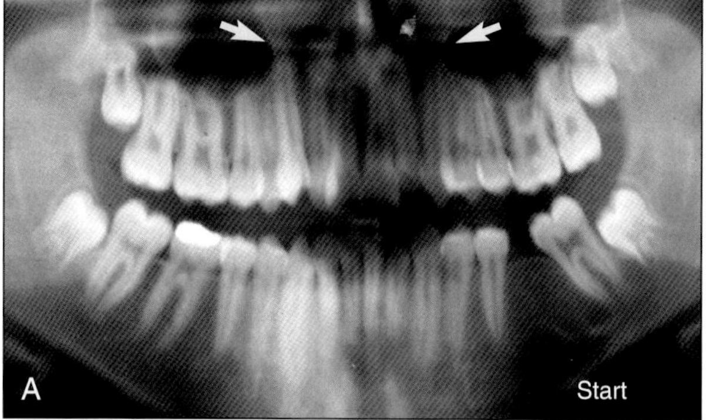

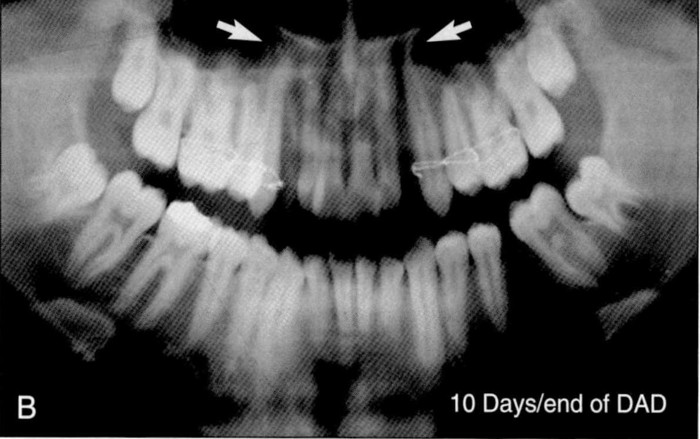

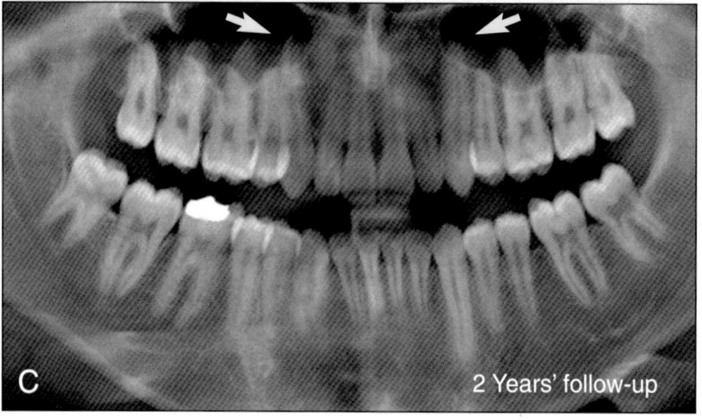

Fig. 25-12 Radiographic appearance of maxillary canines in Case #1 before and after DAD and after orthodontic treatment of 9 months. **A,** Start of treatment; **B,** 10 days into treatment (end of DAD); **C,** 2 years after treatment. There was no radiographic evidence of root resorption, root fracture, or ankylosis.

INDICATIONS OF DAD

The following patients would be good candidates for rapid tooth movement using DAD:

1. Patients with compliance problems (for social and professional reasons)
2. Older adolescent and adult patients with moderate or severe crowding
3. Adult Class II, Division 1 patients
4. Bimaxillary dental protrusion patients
5. Orthognathic surgery patients needing dental decompensation
6. Patients with root shape malformations, short roots, and periodontal problems
7. Patients with ankylosed teeth

CONCLUSION

Dentoalveolar distraction (DAD) for rapid orthodontic tooth movement is based on the principles of distraction osteogenesis (DO). DAD shortens overall orthodontic treatment time in extraction cases. Rapid canine retraction by DAD is based on four sequential DO periods: osteotomy, short-term latency, distraction, and consolidation including active orthodontic treatment particularly to benefit from the uncalcified distraction chamber to resolve anterior crowding and incisor protrusion if necessary. After DAD surgery, distraction is initiated within 3 days. The distractor is activated twice daily, in the morning and in the evening, for a total of about 0.8 mm/day. The tooth (canine) is moved in its

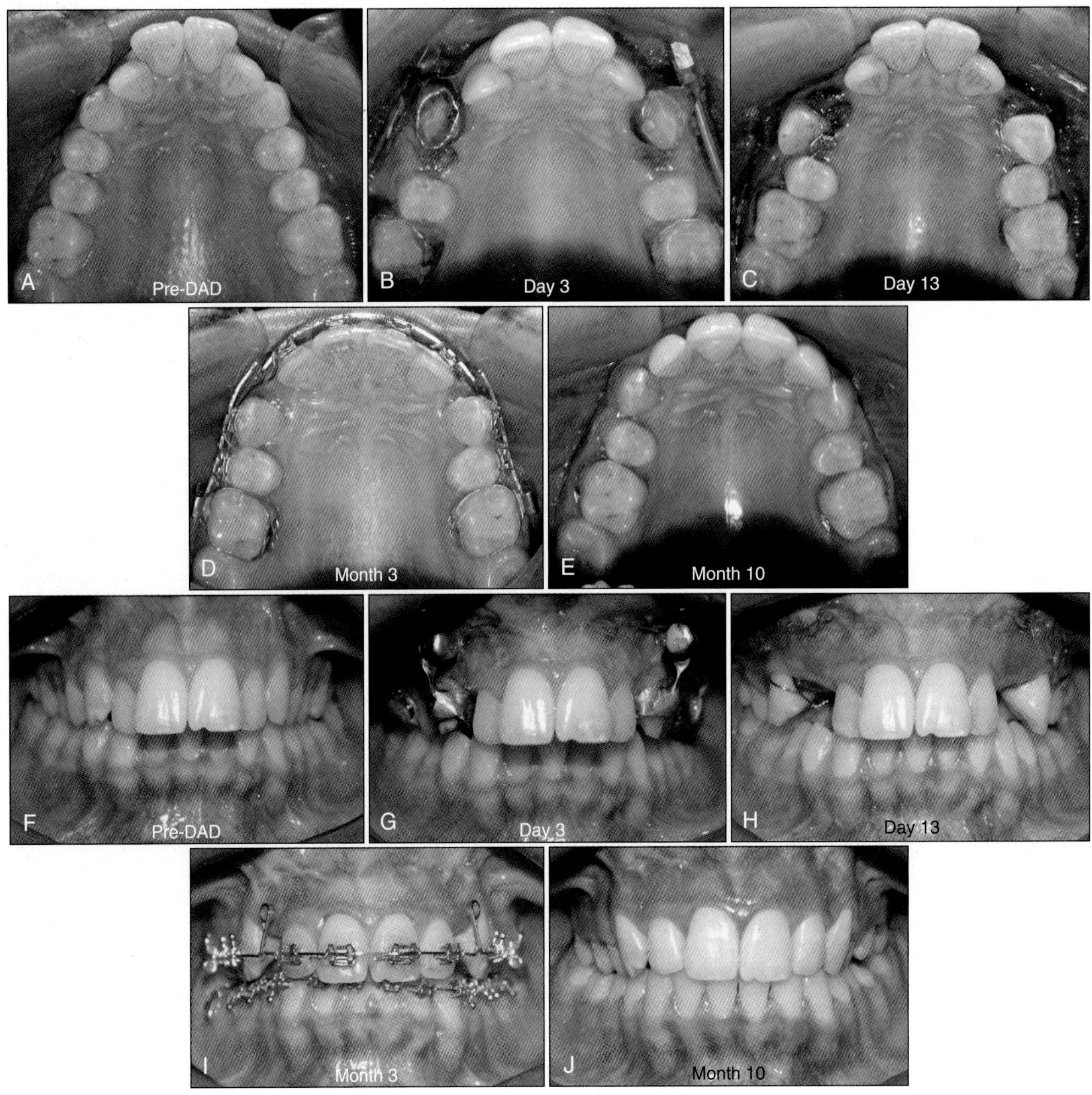

Fig. 25-13 Case #2. Dentoalveolar distraction of maxillary canines from start to end of distraction. Full distraction of the canines was completed in 13 days. **A** to **E,** Occlusal views. **F** to **J,** Frontal views from start of DAD to end of orthodontic treatment, which was completed in 9 months. DAD was completed in 13 days. Fixed appliances were initiated immediately after removal of distractor, and ligatures were kept between the distracted canine brackets and first molar tubes for 3 months.

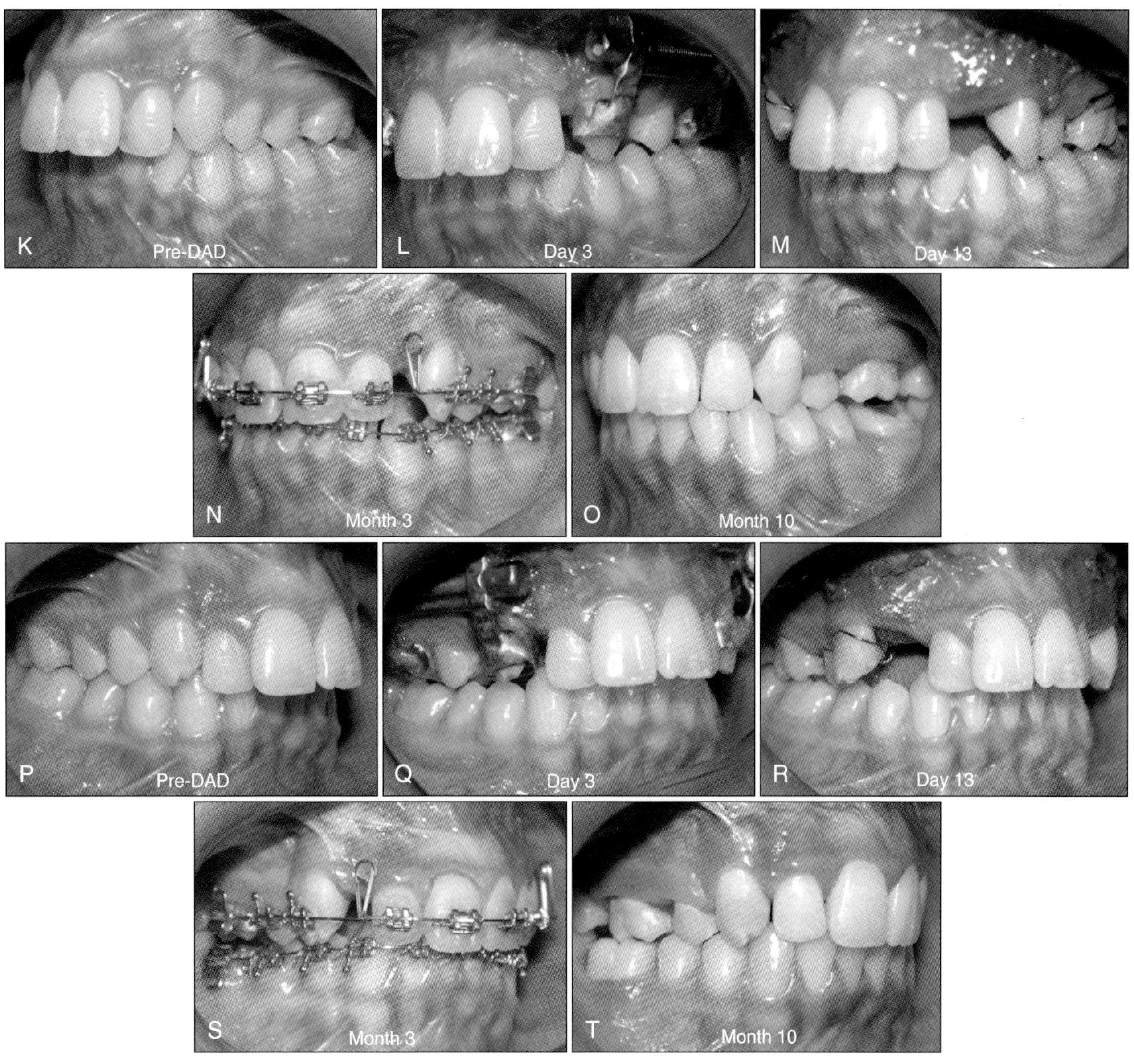

Fig. 25-13, cont'd **K** to **O**, Intraoral left views. **P** to **T**, Intraoral right views.

Continued

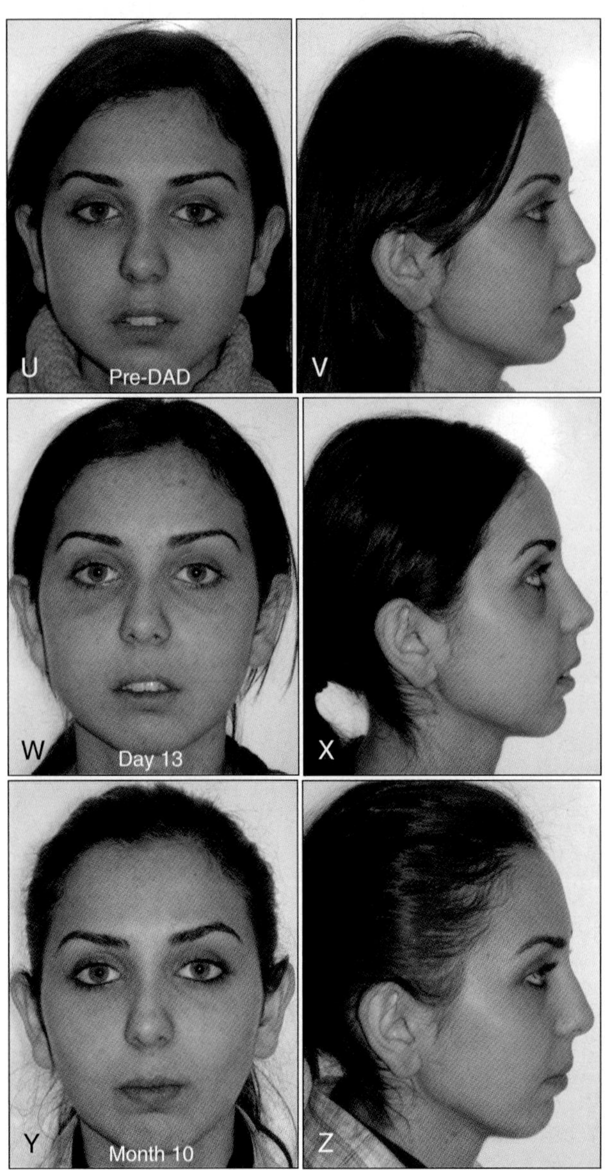

Fig. 25-13, cont'd **U** to **Z,** Facial photographs at start of DAD (**U** and **V**), end of DAD (**W** and **X**), and end of orthodontic treatment (**Y** and **Z**). Mild edema was observed after surgery.

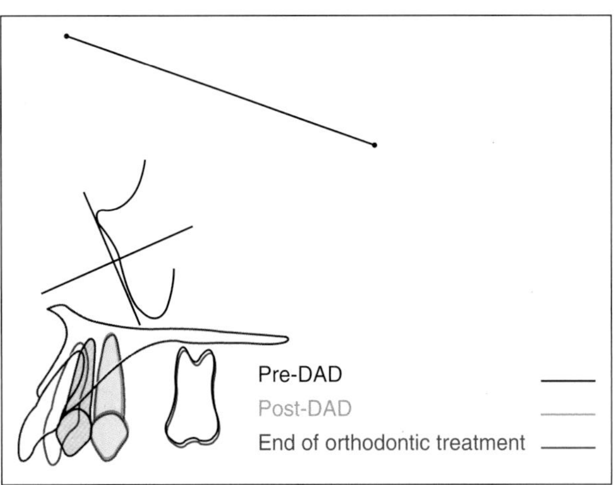

Fig. 25-14 Maxillary superimposition for Case #2 shows the full retraction of the canines with no posterior anchorage loss during DAD and fixed-appliance orthodontic treatment. Significant maxillary incisor retraction was also achieved without posterior anchorage loss during the orthodontic treatment. *Black line,* Before DAD; *blue line,* after DAD (13 days); *red line,* end of orthodontic treatment (10 months).

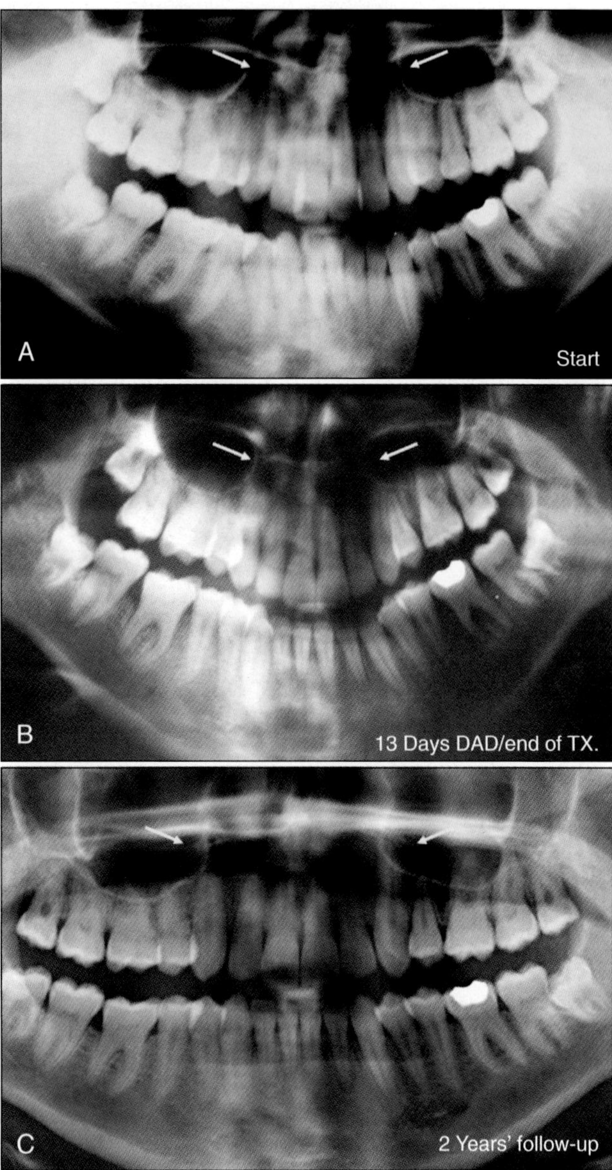

Fig. 25-15 Radiographic appearance of maxillary canines in Case #2 at different stages of orthodontic treatment. **A,** Start of treatment. **B,** 10 months into treatment (end of fixed appliance orthodontic treatment). **C,** 2 years after treatment. There was no radiographic evidence of root resorption, root fracture, or ankylosis.

surrounding alveolar bone as an alveolar bony "transport disk." Canines can be fully retracted into extraction spaces of the premolars in 8 to 14 days.

With the DAD technique, anchorage teeth can withstand the retraction forces with no anchorage loss, and teeth can be moved rapidly without complications (root resorption, root fracture, ankylosis, periodontal/soft tissue problems). DAD reduces overall orthodontic treatment time by about 50%; duration is 9 to 12 months in moderate to severe malocclusion cases, with no unfavorable long term effects on the surrounding hard and soft (gingival) tissues. Using DAD requires no extraoral or intraoral anchorage mechanics, even in maximum anchorage cases.

REFERENCES

1. Reitan K: Clinical and histological observations on tooth movement during and after orthodontic treatment, *Am J Orthod* 53:721-745, 1967.
2. Rygh P: Elimination of hyalinized periodontal tissues associated with orthodontic tooth movement, *Scand J Dent Res* 80:57-73, 1974.
3. Köle H: Surgical operations of the alveolar ridge to correct occlusal abnormalities, *Oral Surg Oral Med Oral Pathol* 12:515-529, 1959.
4. Anholm M, Crites D, Hoff R, Rathbun E: Corticotomy-facilitated orthodontics, *Calif Dent Assoc J* 7:8-11, 1986.
5. Gantes B, Rathburn E, Anholm M: Effects on the periodontium following corticotomy-facilitated orthodontics: case reports, *J Periodontol* 61:234-238, 1990.
6. Suya H: Corticotomy in orthodontics. In Hösl E, Baldauf A, editors: *Mechanical and biological basics in orthodontic therapy,* Heidelberg, Germany, 1991, Hütlig Buch, pp 207-226.
7. Wilcko WM, Wilcko T, Bouquot JE, Ferguson DJ: Rapid orthodontics with alveolar reshaping: two case reports of decrowding, *Int J Periodont Restor Dent* 21:9-19, 2001.
8. Davidovitch Z, Finkelson MD, Steigman S, et al: Electric currents, bone remodeling and orthodontic tooth movement. I. The effect of electric currents on periodontal cyclic nucleotides, *Am J Orthod* 77:14-32, 1980.
9. Davidovitch Z, Finkelson MD, Steigman S, et al: Electric currents, bone remodeling and orthodontic tooth movement. II. Increase in rate of tooth movement and periodontal cyclic nucleotide levels by combined force and electric currents, *Am J Orthod* 77:33-47, 1980.
10. Liou EJW, Huang CS. Rapid canine retraction through distraction of the periodontal ligament, *Am J Orthod Dentofac Orthop* 114:372-381, 1998.
11. İşeri H, Bzeizi N, Kişnişci R: Rapid canine retraction using dentoalveolar distraction osteogenesis, *Eur J Orthod* 23:453, 2001 (abstract).
12. Kişnişci R, İşeri H, Tüz H, Altuğ A: Dentoalveolar distraction osteogenesis for rapid orthodontic canine retraction, *J Oral Maxillofac Surg* 60:389-394, 2002.
13. İşeri H, Kişnişci R, Bzeizi N, Tüz H: Rapid canine retraction and orthodontic treatment with dentoalveolar distraction osteogenesis, *Am J Orthod Dentofacial Orthop* 127:533-541, 2005.
14. Gürgan C, İşeri H, Kişnişci R: Alterations of gingival dimensions following rapid canine retraction using dentoalveolar distraction osteogenesis, *Eur J Orthod* 27:324-332, 2005.
15. Ilizarov GA: The principles of Ilizarov method, *Bull Hosp Joint Dis Orthop Inst* 48:1-11, 1988.
16. Codivilla A: On THA means of lengthening in THA lower limbs, THA muscles and tissues which are shortened through deformity, *Am J Orthop Surg* 2:353-369, 1905.
17. Snyder CC, Levine GA, Swanson HM, Browne EZ Jr: Mandibular lengthening by gradual distraction, *Plast Reconstr Surg* 51:506-508, 1973.
18. Michieli S, Miotti B: Lengthening of mandibular body by gradual surgical-orthodontic distraction, *J Oral Surg* 35:187-192, 1977.
19. Guerrero C: Expansion mandibular quirurgica, *Rev Venez Ortod* 1-2:48-50, 1990.
20. McCarthy JG, Schreiber JS, Karp NS, et al: Lengthening the human mandible by gradual distraction, *Plast Reconstr Surg* 89:1-10, 1992.
21. Reitan K: Initial tissue behaviour during apical root resorption, *Angle Orthod* 44:68-82, 1974.
22. Reitan K: Biomechanical principles and reactions. In Graber TM, Swain BF, editors: *Current principles and techniques,* St Louis, 1985, Mosby, pp 108-123.
23. Pilon JJGM, Kuijpersa-Jagtman AM, Maltha JC: Magnitude of orthodontic forces and rate of bodily tooth movement, an experimental study in beagle dogs, *Am J Orthod Dentofac Orthop* 110:16-23, 1996.
24. Sharpe W, Reed B, Subtelny JD, Polson A: Orthodontic relapse, apical root resorption, and crestal alveolar bone level, *Am J Orthod Dentofac Orthop* 91:252-258, 1987.

PART IV

Applications of Biomedicine to Orthodontics

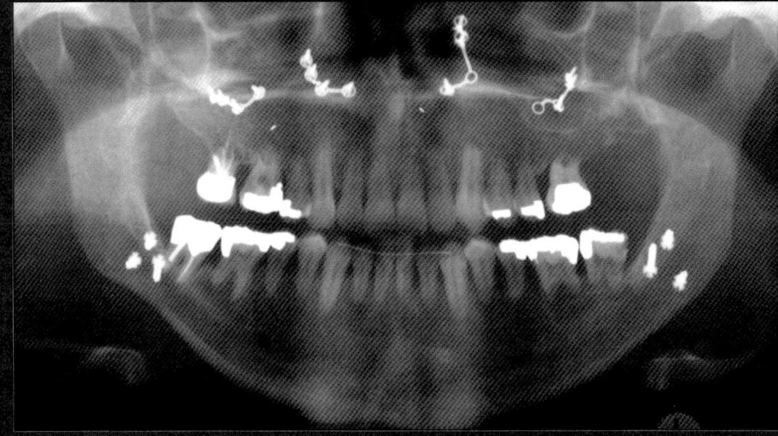

CHAPTER 26

Mechanotransduction of Orthodontic Forces

■ *Sunil Wadhwa, Ravindra Nanda, and Carol Pilbeam*

Mechanical loading of bone is essential for maintaining bone mass and integrity. Conceptually, bone adapts to natural (weight bearing, muscle pull) and therapeutic (orthodontic) mechanical strains to achieve a better balance between mechanical stress and the load-bearing capacity of the bone tissue.[1,2] For example, increased loading, as seen in the arms of tennis players, results in increased bone formation.[3] In contrast, loss of loading, as during immobilization[4] or spaceflight,[5] can decrease bone formation and increase bone resorption, resulting in bone loss.

When an external force is applied to a bone, it results in displacement of particles from their original positions. Displacement differs from one particle to the next and results in deformation of shape or volume of the bone. This deformation is called strain. In a simple one-dimensional linear system, such as the uniform stretching of a wire, *strain* is defined as the fractional change in the length, ε = (change in length)/(original length). Although strain is dimensionless, it is common to measure it in *microstrain* ($\mu\varepsilon$), or 10^{-6} mm/mm. For example, a strain of 0.01 mm/mm would be equivalent to 10,000 $\mu\varepsilon$, or 1%, which would be considered a large strain in bone. These displacements generate stresses equivalent to force per unit area (σ) at internal surfaces within the bone. For linear elastic solids, stress and strain are proportional, σ = (constant) $\times$ (ε).

For alveolar bone tissue subjected to mechanical loading, orthodontic forces must be converted into intracellular signals in mechanosensitive cells. This information must then be communicated to other nonmechanosensitive cells to produce a coordinated response. For this to occur, the following events must take place:

1. External orthodontic forces must be converted into a signal detectable by the cell (transduction mechanism).
2. The periodontal ligament (PDL) and alveolar bone must have cells that are able to detect mechanical loading–induced signals (mechanosensitive cells).
3. Mechanosensitive cells must have a mechanism to sense the signal (mechanoreceptor).
4. Mechanoreceptors must transduce loading information to intracellular signals.
5. Intracellular signals within mechanosensitive cells must lead to the production and release of cellular mediators to communicate mechanical loading information to other cells.

Major responses of mechanosensitive bone and PDL cells to mechanical loading include activation of signaling pathways and new gene transcription, leading to the production of cellular mediators, such as *nitric oxide* (NO) and *prostaglandin E_2* (PGE_2), which are thought to play a role in the local regulation of bone formation and resorption seen in orthodontic tooth movement.

MECHANOTRANSDUCTION

Transduction Mechanisms

When an orthodontic force is placed on teeth, it must be transduced into a signal detectable by mechanosensitive cells. Three possible transduction mechanisms have been proposed (Fig. 26-1). First, loading of the periodontal ligament and bone causes deformation of the matrix. The mechanosensitivity of PDL cells, osteoblasts, and osteocytes is related to the amount of deformation or strain they experience.

Second, it has been proposed that cells themselves do not undergo significant deformation but are responsive to fluid shear stress generated by the deformation of matrix. Bone

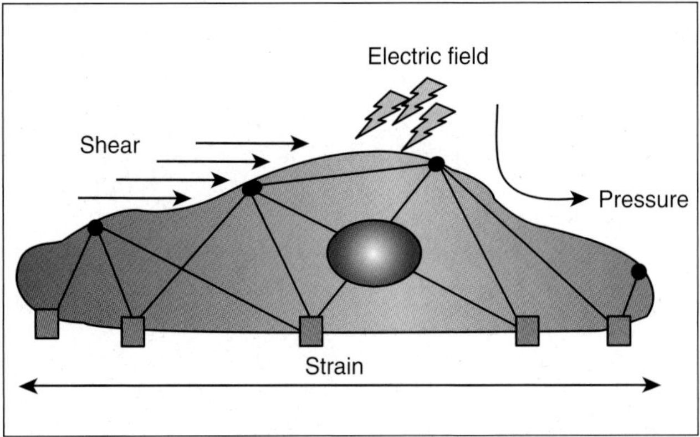

Fig. 26-1 Mechanical force in the cellular environment. Skeletal loading generates deformation of the hard tissue, causing strain across the cell's surface and fluid flow through the canalicular-lacunar network, which causes shear forces to drag over the cells and dynamic electric fields to form as the interstitial fluid flows past charged bone crystals. (Redrawn from Rubin J, Rubin C, Jacobs CR: Molecular pathways mediating mechanical signaling in bone, *Gene* 15:367:1-16, 2006.)

has been described as a "water-soaked sponge," such that a compressive force on one side drives interstitial fluid toward the other side. The velocity with which the fluid flows is related to the rate at which the force is applied. This fluid flow through the canalicular-lacunar network creates shear stress on the surface of the osteocytes and bone-lining cells.

Third, it has been proposed that stress-generated potentials are responsible for the effects of mechanical loading on bone. The fluid in bone contains various ions. Movement of the ions by mechanical loads creates a stress-generated potential, and it has been shown that bone cells are responsive to electric fields. Current research indicates, though, that the actual changes in potential difference produced by streaming potentials are small compared with the electric potential difference induced by muscle contractions.[6] The electric potential difference from the muscles completely overwhelms the local potential difference at the bone surface. Because the stimulus to bone remodeling from loading is usually associated with muscular activity, the effect of streaming potentials appears to be of minor importance in the mechanical loading–induced cell signaling in bone.[7,8]

Whether the transduction mechanism is primarily caused by fluid flow or the actual deformation of the cell by the orthodontic force is still unknown. In the PDL, mechanical loading by the application of compression or tension has been shown to cause the upregulation of a variety of genes.[9-11] In addition, pulsating-fluid shear stress of 0.6 MPa has been shown to cause upregulation of interleukin-8 (IL-8) gene expression,[12] NO,[13] and prostaglandin production,[13] but whether orthodontic tooth movement produces this level of fluid shear stress in the PDL is debatable.

Evidence that strain by itself is not the mechanotransducer in bone cells comes from in vitro experiments. In one study, osteoblastic cells were incubated on polystyrene film and subjected to unidirectional linear strains by stretching of the film in the range of 500 to 5000 $\mu\varepsilon$. There was no increase in the production of two factors thought to be important in mediating loading effects on bone, NO and PGE_2, after loading. In contrast, the investigators found that exposure of osteoblastic cells to increased fluid flow induced both PGE_2 and NO production.[14] Another study used a technique that produces uniform levels of strain and fluid shear stress and that permitted both shear stress and strain to be varied independently.[15] *Osteopontin* (OPN) messenger ribonucleic acid (mRNA) expression, a marker of osteoblastic differentiation, was used to assess the anabolic response of MC3T3-E1 osteoblastic cells. When fluid forces were low, neither strain magnitude nor strain rate was correlated with OPN expression. Higher magnitudes of fluid shear stress, however, significantly increased OPN message levels independently of the strain magnitude or rate. The study suggests that fluid shear stress may play a more important role than strain in the bone response to mechanical loading.

Further evidence that strain alone is not the mechanotransducer comes from comparing in vivo to in vitro data. Customary strains in whole bone in vivo are typically in the range of 0.04% to 0.3% (400-3000 $\mu\varepsilon$) for animal and human locomotion but seldom exceed 0.1% (1000 $\mu\varepsilon$).[16,17] Assuming that cell membrane stretch directly results from surrounding tissue deformation, strain on osteocyte/osteoblast membranes should be comparable to the bone tissue strain. However, in vitro studies show that to induce any cellular response by direct mechanical deformation of bone cells, deformations need to be one to two orders of magnitude larger than the bone tissue strains normally experienced by the whole bone in vivo.[18] The larger strains needed to stimulate osteocytes/osteoblasts cannot be derived directly from matrix deformations because they would cause bone fracture.[19]

A recent model by Weinbaum suggests that the amount of strain the osteoblastic cells experience in vivo may be amplified by the action of fluid flow on pericellular matrix and its coupling to the intracellular actin cytoskeleton.[19,20] This model predicts that physiological levels of fluid shear stress could produce cellular levels of strain in bone up to 100-fold greater than normal levels of strain in tissues (0.04%-0.3%, or 400-3000 $\mu\varepsilon$). Weinbaum concludes that the strain in the membrane of cell processes caused by the loading can be of the same order as the in vitro strains measured in cell culture studies where intracellular biochemical responses are observed for cells on stretched elastic substrates.[19]

Mechanosensitive Cells

The PDL and bone contain a variety of cell types, and there is debate about which cells are mechanosensitive. *Osteocytes,* terminally differentiated osteoblasts housed in mineralized lacunae and communicating with each other via processes extending through narrow canaliculi, are considered to form the major strain-sensing network in bone.[21] A theoretical model for flow-generated shear stresses in lacunar-canicular spaces developed by Weinbaum et al.[22] predicts physiological fluid-induced shear stresses of 8 to 30 dynes/cm^2 in the proteoglycan-filled fluid annuli around osteocyte processes.

It is generally assumed that the marrow sinusoids enclosing *osteoblasts* are much too wide to generate meaningful levels of shear stress during physiological loading. However, recent studies have indicated that very low levels of shear stress are able to induce gene expression of a major enzyme needed for PGE_2 production, *cyclooxygenase-2* (COX-2), in osteoblastic cells,[23] suggesting a role for osteoblastic cells in the detection of mechanical forces. When rats are reloaded after 2 weeks of tail suspension, there is a transient increase on c-Fos expression in periosteal cells and an increase in COX-2 expression in osteocytic cells within the femur, suggesting that both osteoblasts and osteocytes are mechanosensitive.[24]

Interestingly, bone marrow pre-osteoclasts and osteoclast cells may also be mechanosensitive,[25,26] although the physiological significance of these effects remains unclear. Current thinking is that all or most cells are mechanosensitive, and their in vivo context determines the physiological significance of their responses to mechanical loading.

Mechanoreceptors

Bone and PDL cells must be able to convert external signals, fluid shear stress, and strain into intracellular signals. For this to occur, the PDL and bone cells must have a mechanism that is sensitive to external forces. Proposed mechanosensitive mechanisms include the integrin-cytoskeleton–nuclear matrix structure, G-protein–dependent pathways, stretch-activated ion channels within the cell membrane, and plasma disruption. Recent evidence suggests that the entire cell is a mechanosensor and that many different pathways are available for the transduction of a mechanical signal.[27]

Integrins and tensegrity model

Integrins are the major family of cell surface receptors that mediate attachment to the extracellular matrix (ECM). They are composed of alpha (α)and beta (β)transmembrane subunits. There are currently 16 known α and eight known β subunits that heterodimerize to produce more than 20 different receptors. Most integrins bind ligands that are components of the extracellular matrices (e.g., collagen, fibronectin, vitronectin). These ligands cross-link or cluster integrins by binding to adjacent integrin molecules on the cell surface.[28] The localized attachment domains within which integrin receptors cluster are referred to as *focal adhesions.* Focal adhesions form complexes that contain actin-associated proteins, such as talin, vinculin, paxillin and α-actinin. Focal adhesion complex proteins interact with the cytoplasmic portions of integrins and physically interconnect the ECM with the actin cytoskeleton.[29] This structural interconnection not only serves as an anchor, but also is hypothesized to mediate mechanosensation[30] (Fig. 26-2). Also associated with these complexes are kinases, which can be either targets or initiators of various signaling pathways.

According to the *tensegrity model,* mechanical forces in the cell are balanced between tensile actin filaments, microtubular struts, and ECM anchoring supports.[31] Integrins are

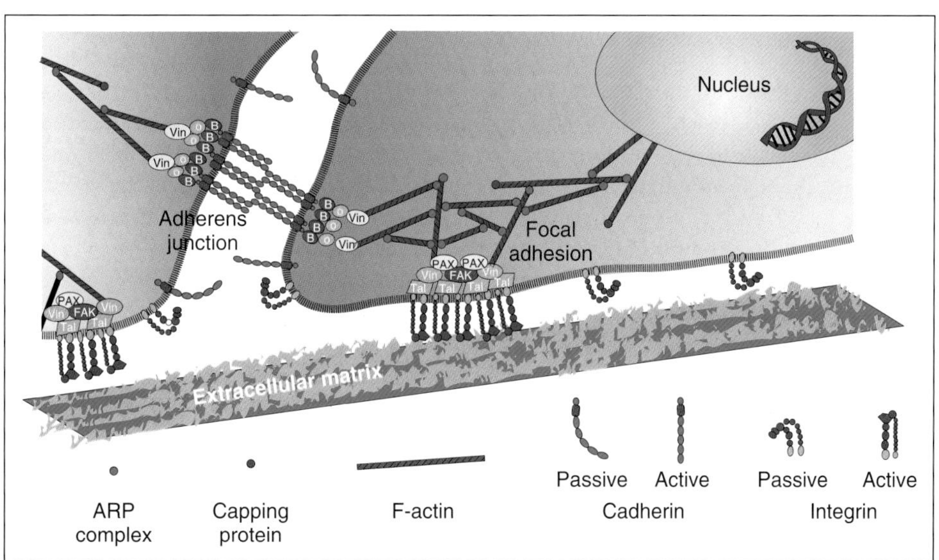

Fig. 26-2 Focal adhesion complex proteins physically interconnect the extracellular matrix with the actin cytoskeleton by activated integrin attachments. This structural interconnection not only serves as an anchor, but also may mediate mechanosensation. *ARP,* Actin-related protein. (Redrawn from Girard PP, Cavalcanti-Adam EA, Kemkemer R, et al: Cellular chemomechanics at interfaces: sensing, integration and response, *Soft Matter* 3:307-326, 2007. Reproduced by permission of The Royal Society of Chemistry.)

responsible for maintaining the stability of this equilibrium. When external forces are applied to cells, the internal cellular tension changes to equalize the external forces by coordinate changes in actin bundle assembly.[30] Prolonged exposure of cells to steady fluid flow results in their realignment in the direction of flow, a process driven by the rearrangement of the cytoskeleton. The actin cytoskeleton of cells exposed to flow changes from a disorganized banding pattern to almost-parallel fibers (stress fibers) aligned to the direction of flow.[32,33] It is believed that actin cytoskeletal changes initiate protein *phosphorylation* cascades within focal contacts. Shear stress applied to the luminal surface of endothelial cells results in directional remodeling of abluminal focal adhesion sites[34] and causes the activation of cellular signaling.[35] Initiation of cell signaling involves a nonreceptor tyrosine kinase called *focal adhesion kinase* (FAK). FAK is tyrosine phosphorylated and localizes to focal adhesions after exposure to fluid shear stress.[35] FAK activation by mechanical forces leads to activation of the *mitogen-activated protein* (MAP) kinase signaling pathway.[35,36] Also, integrins are involved in fluid shear stress induction of new gene expression in osteoblastic cells.[33,37]

Transmembrane G-protein receptor pathways

Another proposed mechanosensory pathway within the cell is through transmembrane G-protein receptors. G-protein receptors contain seven transmembrane hydrophobic domains associated with α, β, or gamma (γ) subunits, each encoded by separate gene families. The family that encodes the α subunit is especially diverse. In the resting state, guanine diphosphate (GDP) is bound to the α subunit. On binding of the ligand, the GDP is released and guanine triphosphate (GTP) is bound. This causes a conformational change and the disassociation of the α-GTP subunit from the β and γ subunits. The subunits then regulate metabolic pathways, resulting in the activation of various second messengers, enzymes, and ion channels. Inactivation is caused by hydrolysis of the GTP, which leads to reassociation of the α subunit with GDP and the β and γ subunits.

It has been proposed that transmembrane G-protein receptors are activated indirectly by fluid flow. In this model, shear stress is transduced via the cell membrane's lipid bilayer to activate G proteins on the cytosolic face of the plasma membrane in the absence of a ligand.[38,39] Recent studies have shown that fluid shear stress increases the fluidity of the cell membrane.[39] The increase in membrane fluidity is hypothesized to cause an increase in the intramolecular dynamics and diffusivity of membrane-bound enzymes, such as G proteins, leading to their activation. In a study designed to test this model, purified G proteins were reconstituted into phospholipid vesicles of defined composition.[40] The reconstituted vesicles were then loaded with labeled GTP and subjected to shear stress using the cone-and-plate viscometer. It was found that shear stress activated GTP hydrolysis by G proteins, which were located inside the vesicle. In addition, the activation of GTP hydrolysis by shear stress was modulated by membrane lipid composition. The more fluid the membrane bilayer, the greater was the GTP hydrolysis when exposed to shear stress. These results suggest that fluid shear stress can decrease the lipid bilayer's viscosity. This decrease in viscosity alters the physical properties of the membrane bilayer, which changes the functions of the membrane proteins, allowing activation of membrane-bound G proteins in the absence of a ligand.

Another study showed that G-protein activation and NO production by fluid shear stress did not require an intact cellular cytoskeleton in endothelial cells but was dependent on the membrane fluidity.[41]

These observations indicate that transmembrane G proteins can be activated by fluid shear stress independently of a ligand and an intact cytoskeleton, suggesting a role of transmembrane G proteins as possible mechanoreceptors. Furthermore, it has been shown that the fluid shear stress induction of prostaglandin production in osteoblastic cells depends on a pertussis toxin–sensitive G protein.[42] However, whether all transmembrane G proteins are mechanosensitive, or whether other non–G-protein transmembrane receptors are mechanosensitive, remains unknown. Interestingly, a non–G-protein receptor, a membrane-bound receptor tyrosine kinase, can be activated without a ligand by fluid shear stress in endothelial cells.[43]

Stretch-sensitive ion channels

Another proposed mechanosensitive pathway within bone cells is through stretch-sensitive ion channels. Ion channels exist in the cell membrane that are sensitive to mechanical stress.[44] The existence of these channels has been found using patch clamp procedures in a variety of organisms, from mammals to bacteria. Recently, a stretch-activated ion channel was identified in osteoblastic cells.[45] This study found that osteoblastic cells express the alpha subunit of the epithelial sodium channel (α-ENaC), which has been shown to be closely related to known stretch-activated ion channels in *Caenorhabditis elegans.* Furthermore, this study cloned and transfected the osteoblastic α-EnaC into a fibroblastic cell line that had no stretch-activated cation activity. The reconstituted osteoblastic α-EnaC caused stretch-activated cation activity in the null fibroblastic cell line. However, the physiological role of this channel in osteoblasts has not been reported.

Additional evidence for stretch-activated channels being involved in the response of osteoblasts to mechanical loading comes from experiments using *gadolinium,* a presumed specific stretch-activated ion channel inhibitor. Gadolinium inhibits strain-induced *c-fos* expression[46] and fluid shear stress–induced transforming growth factor beta-1 expression[47] in osteoblastic cells. Gadolinium has been reported to be nonspecific for stretch-activated ion channels and has been shown to cause blockage of voltage-gated calcium ion (Ca^{++}) channels, rendering its use as a specific stretch-activated channel inhibitor problematic.[48]

Thus the physiological role and the existence of stretch-activated channels in bone cells are debatable.

Plasma disruption

Another potential mechanoreceptor in the PDL during tooth movement is sublethal plasma disruption. When mechanical stress is imposed on various tissues in vivo, transient, survivable disruptions of the plasma membrane are created, called *sublethal plasma disruption.* To examine if this occurs during orthodontic tooth movement, investigators placed a 50-g orthodontic force for 5 minutes on rat molar teeth and found that it caused a significant increase in sublethal plasma disruption within the PDL of the tension side. The authors hypothesized that the disruption of plasma membrane enables the release of growth factors and cytokines that do not contain a signal peptide sequence, such as interleukin-1 beta (IL-1β) and basic fibroblast growth factor (FGF-2), from within the cell to the ECM.[49,50]

Intracellular Signaling Pathways

For cells to respond to mechanical forces, activation of mechanoreceptors must lead to the activation of intercellular second messengers and/or protein kinases. The signaling pathways can then lead to the activation of transcription factors and new gene transcription. Some parts of the signaling pathways leading to new gene transcription have been identified.

Mechanical loading of osteoblastic and PDL cells has been reported to cause the activation of a number of second messengers. In vitro mechanical loading causes an increase in intracellular Ca^{++} concentrations in PDL[51] and osteoblastic cells.[52] In addition, mechanical loading causes an increase in cyclic adenosine monophosphate (cAMP) levels and NO production in PDL[13,53] and osteoblastic cells.[54,55]

The activation by mechanical loading of various protein kinases has been demonstrated in PDL and osteoblastic cells. The protein kinase C (PKC) signaling pathway has been reported to be activated by mechanical loading in osteoblastic cells.[56] Involvement of the PKC pathway by mechanical loading in osteoblastic cells has also been reported.[57,58] In addition, studies using specific inhibitors have implicated the phospholipase C (PLC) signaling pathway in the response to mechanical loading in osteoblastic cells[52,58] and the rho kinase signaling pathway in the response to mechanical loading in PDL cells.[59]

Mitogen-activated protein kinases (MAPKs) are a family of serine/threonine protein kinases organized into hierarchical cascades. MAPKs are phosphorylated and activated by MAPK kinases (MAPKKs), which in turn are activated by MAPKK kinases (MAPKKKs). MAPKKKs are activated by a variety of interactions with small GTPases and other protein kinases, which can interconnect this pathway with other signaling pathways. The three major MAPKs are extracellular-regulated kinase (ERK), stress-activated protein kinase (JNK/SAPK), and p38 kinase. ERK is thought to be activated by growth factors and G proteins and to mediate proliferation and differentiation. On the other hand, JNK and p38 are thought to be activated by physiological stress and to mediate apoptosis.[60] Mechanical loading has been shown to activate the ERK[61,62] and JNK pathway[63] in PDL cells and the ERK,[64] JNK,[65] and p38[66,67] pathway in osteoblastic cells (Fig. 26-3).

Mechanical loading of bone and PDL has been shown to cause new gene transcription. Various transcription factors have been implicated in this process. One of the key transcription factors regulating osteoblast differentiation is Runx2/Cbfa1. Mechanical stretch of osteoblastic cells has been shown to upregulate the expression and binding activity of Cbfa1.[68]

In addition, orthodontic tooth movement in rats has been shown to cause an upregulation of Cbfa1 protein expression in PDL of the tension side.[61] In vitro experiments have shown that mechanical stretch causes the activation of the *activator protein-1* (AP-1) transcription factor in osteoblastic and PDL cells.[69] The AP-1 transcription factor is made up of dimers of c-Fos and c-Jun. Mechanical stretch has also been shown to cause the upregulation of c-Fos and c-Jun expression in osteoblastic and PDL cells.[70] The AP-1 binding site has been shown to be important in the fluid shear stress induction of COX-2 in osteoblastic cells.[23] Mechanical loading of bone has also been shown to stimulate other transcription factors, including Egr-1,[71,72] p57kip2 (a cyclin-dependent kinase inhibitor),[73] and nuclear factor kappa B (NF-κB).[71]

Coordinated Response

For bone to respond to external loading, cells that are able to sense mechanical loads, such as PDL cells, osteocytes and osteoblasts, must be able to communicate information about the external environment to nonmechanosensitive or nonstimulated cells, such as osteoclasts. This communication may occur through direct cell-cell interactions or soluble mediators.

One way in which bone and PDL cells respond to mechanical loading is by increasing channels that connect adjacent cells. *Gap junctions* are transmembrane protein channels that enable neighboring cells to link physically. *Connexins,* a type of gap junction, form by the docking of head-to-head partner connexin hemichannels positioned on neighboring cells.[74] The formation of connexin gap junctions allows the rapid diffusion of small molecules and ions, thereby facilitating the communication of neighboring cells.[75] In experimental tooth movement models, orthodontic forces have been shown to cause an increase in connexin-43 mRNA expression in osteoblasts and in connexin-43 protein expression in osteocytes,[76] as well as in PDL cells.[77] Interestingly, recent reports have shown that the induction of unopposed connexin-43 hemichannels in osteocytic cell lines may be responsible for adenosine triphosphate (ATP)[78] and prostaglandin (PG)[79] release in response to mechanical loading.

Mechanical loading of bone has been shown to cause an increase in NO[80-82] and PG,[83-85] both of which have been proposed as soluble mediators of the effects of loading (Fig. 26-4). Their induction is especially important for orthodontic tooth movement because specific inhibitors of NO[86-88]

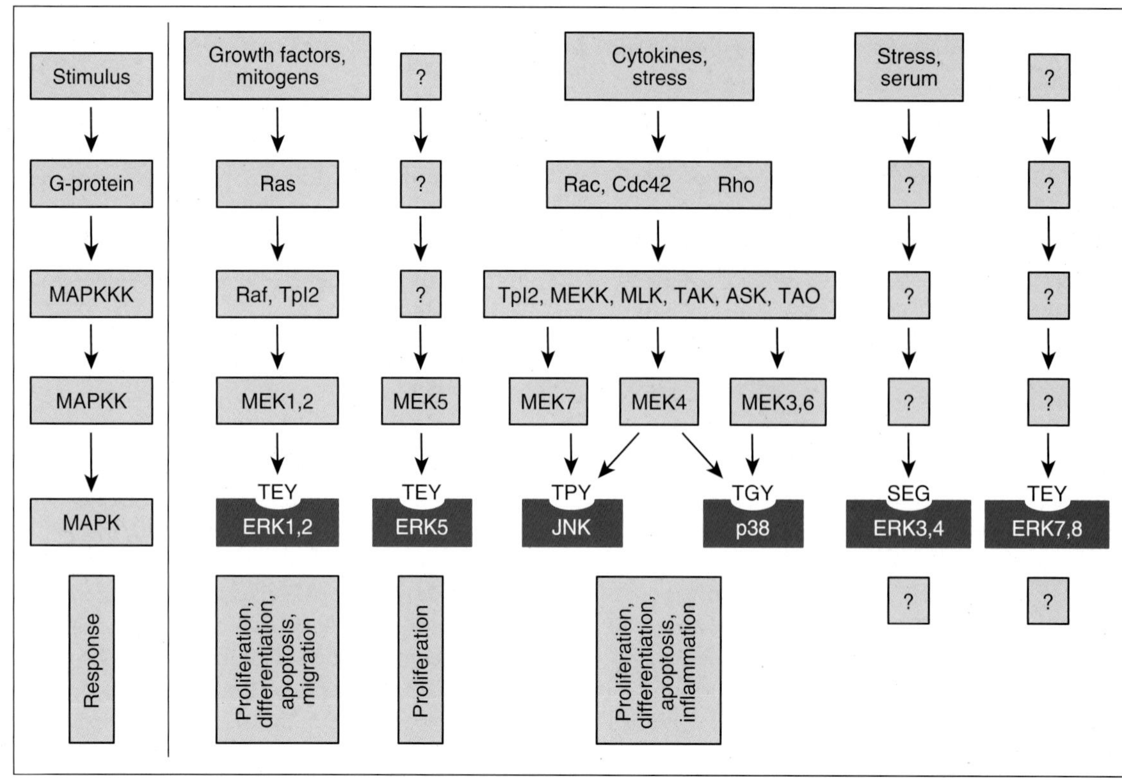

Fig. 26-3 Mitogen-activated protein (MAP) kinase signaling pathway. (Redrawn from Dhillon AS, Hagan S, Rath O, Kolch W: MAP kinase signalling pathways in cancer, *Oncogene* 26:3279-3290, 2007.)

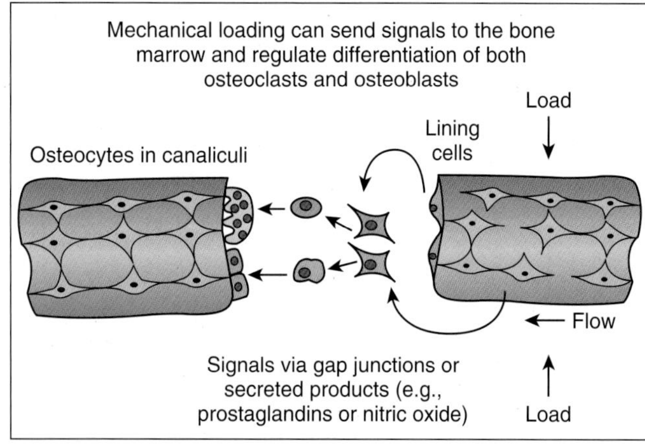

Fig. 26-4 Mechanical loading in bone causes signals that can regulate both osteoblast and osteoclast differentiation. Through the secretion of prostaglandins and nitric oxide, osteocytes are thought to mediate the mechanical loading response in bone.

cause a significant decrease in the rate of tooth movement. In addition, PG inhibitors have been shown to decrease both the total amount of orthodontic tooth movement and the number of osteoclasts on the compression surface.[89-93] Other studies have shown that administration of PGE_1 locally causes an increase in orthodontic bone resorption[94] and tooth movement.[95-97]

ALTERATIONS OF MECHANICAL LOADING

Response of Bone to External Mechanical Loading

The adaptation of bone to mechanical forces has been recognized for more than 100 years. In 1892, Wolff, the first to report on the association of bone biology and mechanical forces, stated in his law of bone remodeling, "Every change in the form and function of bones or of their function alone is followed by certain definite changes in their internal architecture, and equally definite alterations in their external conformation."[98] In the past few years, much experimental evidence has been gathered about the way bone adapts to mechanical forces, and some common threads have emerged. For example, Turner[99] believes that (1) bone adaptation is driven by dynamic, rather than static, loading; (2) only a short duration of mechanical loading is necessary to initiate an adaptive response; and (3) bone cells accommodate to a customary mechanical loading environment, making them less responsive to routine loading signals.

Frost[100] hypothesized that mechanically induced bone remodeling was dependent on the strain, not the stress, or more specifically, on a *minimum effective strain* (MES). Experimental evidence has suggested that the MES range is about 0.0008 to 0.002 units bone surface strain, and that strains below the MES do not cause bone remodeling.[100] In

1971, Liskova and Hert[101] showed that dynamic, but not static, strains caused increased bone formation in rabbits. Since then, a number of studies have shown that the anabolic effects of mechanical loading of bone are more likely to be the result of dynamic rather than static strains.[102-105] In fact, static loading may actually suppress both appositional and longitudinal bone formation.[106]

Increased duration of loading does not cause increased bone formation. Several studies have even shown that, as loading duration is increased, the bone formation response tends to saturate. In one study the effects of jump training on bone morphological and mechanical properties were investigated in immature rat bone.[107] The rats were divided into control or 5, 10, 20, 40, or 100 jumps per day. It was found that 5-jumps/day group generated the same amount of new bone formation as the groups with more jumps. Another study investigated the effects of the number of load cycles per day on new bone formation in an isolated avian bone preparation to which external loads could be applied in vivo.[108] Neither the extent nor the character of the mechanically induced bone changes was affected by additional increases in the number of load cycles, from 36 to 1800.

These observations have led to the hypothesis that bone cells are able to sense and respond to mechanical forces, but that the mechanosensitivity of bone declines soon after the application of the force. Therefore, under continued stimulation, bone is desensitized to mechanical stimuli. In support of this hypothesis, it has been shown that if bone is given a sufficient recovery period between loading regimens (8 hours), it is able to regain its mechanosensitivity.[109]

Activities that produce large strains in bone seem to cause a more anabolic response than activities that produce smaller strains. A current hypothesis is that the adaptive response of bone is predominantly a result not of the numerous cycles of "small" strains during routine activity, but rather of the far fewer cycles of relatively "large" strains produced during unusual loading situations.[110] One study found that in a variety of animals during daily activity, large strains (>1000 με) occurred relatively few times a day, whereas very small strains (<10 με) from activities such as standing occurred thousands of times a day.[16] Several studies have shown that large applied strains to bone at low loading frequencies cause more bone formation than smaller strains at higher loading frequencies.[104,111] Also, girls who have a greater number of large-strain occurrences by being active in impact-loading sports (gymnastics, volleyball) have a higher bone mineral density than girls who are active in nonimpact sports (swimming).[112-114]

This is not to say that small strains have no influence on bone. Muscle contractions from activities such as standing and talking create small strains on the relevant bones. These strains occur thousands of times a day. A role of these strains in the maintenance of the skeletal structure has been recently shown. One study found that very-low-magnitude strains at high-frequency vibrations applied only 20 minutes a day to sheep caused a 34% increase in trabecular femur bone density compared to control sheep.[115] It is important to note that the strain (5 με) the animals received through the high-frequency vibrations was 20-fold higher than that normally occurring in the sheep at the same frequency from activities such as standing. Therefore, even though the stimulus was for only 20 minutes, it still represents an order-of-magnitude increase in the total strain energy induced at that frequency from routine activities over a 12-hour period.[115]

Alterations in Orthodontic Forces

When a mesial force is placed on a tooth, it causes the tooth to move in that direction. For this to occur, bone must be resorbed on the mesial surface *(compression side)* and laid down on its distal surface *(tension side)*. Melsen[116] describes two types of orthodontic tooth movement: tooth movement *through* the bone and tooth movement *with* the bone. Orthodontic forces create *compression* of the PDL space on the side in which the tooth moves and *tension* of the PDL on the other side. If this orthodontic force is large enough, it creates ischemia within the PDL on the compression side and hyalinization of the PDL space. In this case the tooth is moving *through* the bone, and bone resorption begins outside the hyalinized PDL space. If the orthodontic force is not excessive, it does not create hyalinization of the PDL space of the compression side, and bone resorption begins within the PDL space. In this case the tooth is moving *with* the bone. In both types of tooth movement, new bone is being laid down of the tension side.

Recent research has indicated that factors that increase bone resorption increase the rate of tooth movement, and factors that inhibit resorption delay tooth movement.[117,118] The formation of mature bone-resorbing osteoclasts from hematopoietic precursors requires cell-cell interaction with cells from the osteoblastic lineage[119] (Fig. 26-5). Osteoblastic cells are therefore said to be necessary to "support" osteoclastogenesis. The molecule mediating this interaction is *receptor activator of NF-κB* (RANK) ligand, or RANKL.[120] Osteoblastic cells express RANKL as a membrane-associated factor, and expression of RANKL is induced by multiple stimulators of resorption, including PGE_2.[121] Osteoclast precursors express RANK, the receptor for RANKL. RANKL is also a ligand for *osteoprotegerin* (OPG).[122] OPG, which is produced by osteoblastic cells, acts as a decoy receptor for RANKL, thus preventing RANKL-RANK binding (Fig. 26-6). Increased OPG expression can therefore suppress osteoclast formation.[123] Not surprisingly, recent in vivo experiments have shown that exogenously added OPG decreases the rate of orthodontic tooth movement,[124,125] and that exogenously added RANKL increases the rate of orthodontic tooth movement.[126]

The expression of RANKL and OPG in the PDL seems to depend on the type of mechanical loading (i.e., compression vs. tension) but not on duration or magnitude of the force. Compressive forces on PDL cells cause the induction of RANKL expression,[127,128] with little changes in OPG expression.[129] In contrast, tensile forces on PDL cells cause the

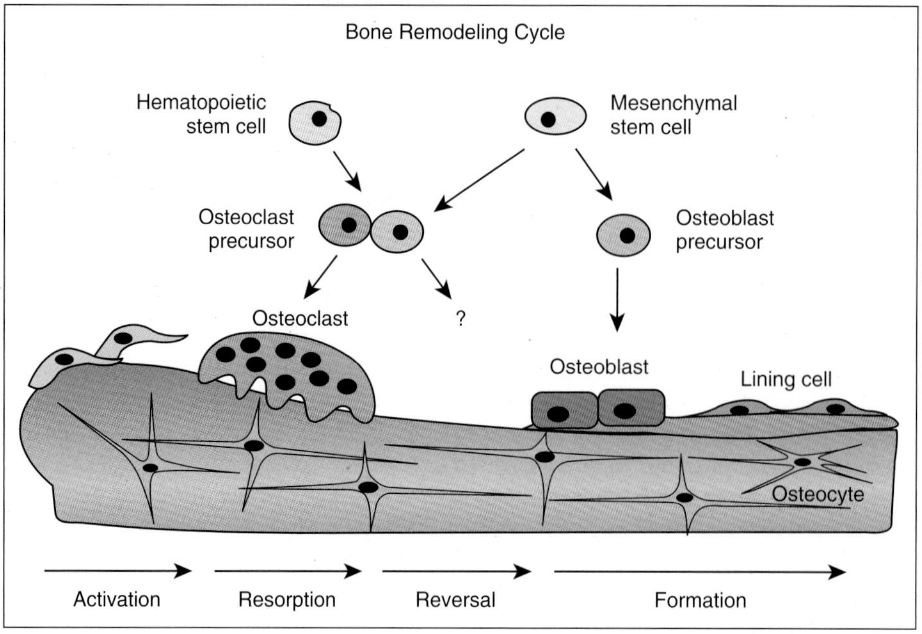

Fig. 26-5 Bone remodeling involves four steps—activation, resorption, reversal, and formation—that involve cells from both the hematopoietic (osteoclasts) and the mesenchymal (osteoblasts) cell lineage.

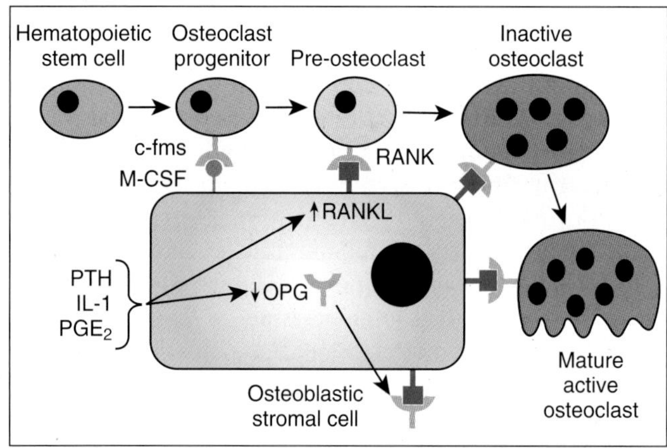

Fig. 26-6 Osteoclastogenesis. Osteoblast stromal cells express RANK ligand *(RANKL),* which binds either receptor activator of nuclear factor kappa B *(RANK)* on osteoclast precursors, promoting osteoclastogenesis, or osteoprotegerin *(OPG),* which prevents binding of RANKL to RANK. *M-CSF,* Macrophage colony-stimulating factor; *IL-1,* interleukin-1; *PGE$_2$,* prostaglandin E$_2$.

upregulation of both OPG[130] and RANKL[131] expression. These differences may explain why the compression side of orthodontic tooth movement is associated with an increase in bone resorption.

Unlike the anabolic actions of mechanical loading in bone, studies have shown that continuous orthodontic forces increase the rate of tooth movement compared to noncontinuous orthodontic forces.[132-136] Interestingly, continuous loading does not cause an increase in RANKL expression in the PDL[127] or in osteoblastic cells[137] compared to short loading or intermittent loading. Furthermore, despite a difference in the amount of tooth movement, the number of osteoclasts was no different in a rat model comparing continuous versus intermittent orthodontic forces.[133] These results suggest that intermittent versus continuous forces in orthodontic tooth movement may effect osteoclast activation rather than formation. Additionally, increased magnitudes of compressive forces do not lead to increased expression of RANKL in PDL cells.[127] Therefore it is not surprising that the magnitude of orthodontic forces plays little role in the rate of orthodontic tooth movement, with a wide range of orthodontic forces leading to maximum rates of tooth movement.[138,139]

CONCLUSION

Orthodontic tooth movement requires a remarkably complicated cascade of molecular and cellular events to occur, to convert orthodontic forces into alveolar bone formation and resorption. During the last 10 years, a lot of these pathways have been elucidated, and soon some of this new biological information may be applied into clinical settings.

REFERENCES

1. Turner CH, Woltman TA, Belongia DA: Structural changes in rat bone subjected to long-term, in vivo mechanical loading, *Bone* 13:417-422, 1992.

2. Rubin CT, Gross TS, McLeod KJ, et al: Morphologic stages in lamellar bone formation stimulated by a potent mechanical stimulus, *J Bone Miner Res* 10:488-495, 1995.
3. Jones HH, Priest JD, Hayes WC, et al: Humeral hypertrophy in response to exercise, *J Bone Joint Surg Am* 59:204-208, 1977.
4. Leblanc AD, Schneider VS, Evans HJ, et al: Bone mineral loss and recovery after 17 weeks of bed rest, *J Bone Miner Res* 5:843-850, 1990.
5. Collet P, Uebelhart D, Vico L, et al: Effects of 1- and 6-month spaceflight on bone mass and biochemistry in two humans, *Bone* 20:547-551, 1997.
6. McDonald F, Houston WJ: An in vivo assessment of muscular activity and the importance of electrical phenomena in bone remodeling, *J Anat* 172:165-175, 1990.
7. McDonald F: Electrical effects at the bone surface, *Eur J Orthod* 15:175-183, 1993.
8. Hung CT, Allen FD, Pollack SR, et al: What is the role of the convective current density in the real-time calcium response of cultured bone cells to fluid flow? *J Biomech* 29:1403-1409, 1996.
9. Yamashiro K, Myokai F, Hiratsuka K, et al: Oligonucleotide array analysis of cyclic tension-responsive genes in human periodontal ligament fibroblasts, *Int J Biochem Cell Biol* 39:910-921, 2007.
10. Lee YH, Nahm DS, Jung YK, et al: Differential gene expression of periodontal ligament cells after loading of static compressive force, *J Periodontol* 78:446-452, 2007.
11. De Araujo RM, Oba Y, Moriyama K: Identification of genes related to mechanical stress in human periodontal ligament cells using microarray analysis, *J Periodont Res* 42:15-22, 2007.
12. Maeda A, Soejima K, Bandow K, et al: Force-induced IL-8 from periodontal ligament cells requires IL-1β, *J Dent Res* 86:629-634, 2007.
13. Van der Pauw MT, Klein-Nulend J, Van den Bos T, et al: Response of periodontal ligament fibroblasts and gingival fibroblasts to pulsating fluid flow: nitric oxide and prostaglandin E_2 release and expression of tissue non-specific alkaline phosphatase activity, *J Periodont Res* 35:335-343, 2000.
14. Smalt R et al: Induction of NO and prostaglandin E_2 in osteoblasts by wall-shear stress but not mechanical strain, *Am J Physiol* 273(4 Pt 1):E751-E758, 1997.
15. Owan I, Burr DB, Turner CH, et al: Mechanotransduction in bone: osteoblasts are more responsive to fluid forces than mechanical strain, *Am J Physiol* 273(3 Pt 1):C810-C815, 1997.
16. Fritton SP, McLeod KJ, Rubin CT: Quantifying the strain history of bone: spatial uniformity and self-similarity of low-magnitude strains, *J Biomech* 33:317-325, 2000.
17. Burr DB, Milgrom C, Fyhrie D, et al: In vivo measurement of human tibial strains during vigorous activity, *Bone* 18:405-410, 1996.
18. You J, Yellowley CE, Donahue HJ, et al: Substrate deformation levels associated with routine physical activity are less stimulatory to bone cells relative to loading-induced oscillatory fluid flow, *J Biomech Eng* 122:387-393, 2000.
19. You L, Cowin SC, Schaffler MB, et al: A model for strain amplification in the actin cytoskeleton of osteocytes due to fluid drag on pericellular matrix, *J Biomech* 34:1375-1386, 2001.
20. Han Y, Cowin SC, Schaffler MB, et al: Mechanotransduction and strain amplification in osteocyte cell processes, *Proc Natl Acad Sci USA* 101:16689-16694, 2004.
21. Klein-Nulend J, Van der Plas A, Semeins CM, et al: Sensitivity of osteocytes to biomechanical stress in vitro, *Faseb J* 9:441-445, 1995.
22. Weinbaum S, Cowin SC, Zeng Y: A model for the excitation of osteocytes by mechanical loading-induced bone fluid shear stresses, *J Biomech* 27:339-360, 1994.
23. Ogasawara A, Arakawa T, Kaneda T, et al: Fluid shear stress-induced cyclooxygenase-2 expression is mediated by C/EBP beta, cAMP-response element-binding protein, and AP-1 in osteoblastic MC3T3-E1 cells, *J Biol Chem* 276:7048-7054, 2000.
24. Matsumoto T, Nakayama K, Kodama Y, et al: Effect of mechanical unloading and reloading on periosteal bone formation and gene expression in tail-suspended rapidly growing rats, *Bone* 22(Suppl 5):89S-93S, 1998.
25. Kim CH, You L, Yellowley CE, et al: Oscillatory fluid flow-induced shear stress decreases osteoclastogenesis through RANKL and OPG signaling, *Bone* 39:1043-1047, 2006.
26. McAllister TN, Du T, Frangos JA: Fluid shear stress stimulates prostaglandin and nitric oxide release in bone marrow-derived preosteoclast-like cells, *Biochem Biophys Res Commun* 270:643-648, 2000.
27. Duncan RL, Turner CH: Mechanotransduction and the functional response of bone to mechanical strain, *Calcif Tissue Int* 57:344-358, 1995.
28. Clark EA, Brugge JS: Integrins and signal transduction pathways: the road taken, *Science* 268:233-239, 1995.
29. Plopper G, Ingber DE: Rapid induction and isolation of focal adhesion complexes, *Biochem Biophys Res Commun* 193:571-578, 1993.
30. Ingber D: Integrins as mechanochemical transducers, *Curr Opin Cell Biol* 3:841-848, 1991.
31. Stamenović D, Fredberg JJ, Wang N, et al: A microstructural approach to cytoskeletal mechanics based on tensegrity, *J Theor Biol* 181:125-136, 1996.
32. Davies PF: Flow-mediated endothelial mechanotransduction, *Physiol Rev* 75:519-560, 1995.
33. Pavalko FM, Chen NX, Turner CH, et al: Fluid shear-induced mechanical signaling in MC3T3-E1 osteoblasts requires cytoskeleton-integrin interactions, *Am J Physiol* 275(6 Pt 1):C1591-C1601, 1998.
34. Davies PF Robotewskyj A, Griem ML: Quantitative studies of endothelial cell adhesion: directional remodeling of focal adhesion sites in response to flow forces, *J Clin Invest* 93:2031-2038, 1994.
35. Li S, Kim M, Hu YL, et al: Fluid shear stress activation of focal adhesion kinase: linking to mitogen-activated protein kinases, *J Biol Chem* 272:30455-30462, 1997.
36. Pommerenke H, Schmidt C, Durr F, et al: The mode of mechanical integrin stressing controls intracellular signaling in osteoblasts, *J Bone Miner Res* 17:603-611, 2002.
37. Carvalho RS, Schaffer JL, Gerstenfeld LC: Osteoblasts induce osteopontin expression in response to attachment on fibronectin: demonstration of a common role for integrin receptors in the signal transduction processes of cell attachment and mechanical stimulation, *J Cell Biochem* 70:376-390, 1998.
38. Butler PJ, Norwich G, Weinbaum S, Chien S: Shear stress induces a time- and position-dependent increase in endothe-

lial cell membrane fluidity, *Am J Physiol Cell Physiol* 280:C962-C969, 2001.
39. Haidekker MA, L'Heureux N, Frangos JA: Fluid shear stress increases membrane fluidity in endothelial cells: a study with DCVJ fluorescence, *Am J Physiol Heart Circ Physiol* 278: H1401-H1406, 2000.
40. Gudi S, Nolan JP, Frangos JA: Modulation of GTPase activity of G proteins by fluid shear stress and phospholipid composition, *Proc Natl Acad Sci USA* 95:2515-2519, 1998.
41. Knudsen HL, Frangos JA: Role of cytoskeleton in shear stress-induced endothelial nitric oxide production, *Am J Physiol* 273(1 Pt 2):H347-H355, 1997.
42. Reich KM, McAllister TN, Gudi SRP, Frangos JA: Activation of G proteins mediates flow-induced prostaglandin E_2 production in osteoblasts, *Endocrinology* 138:1014-1018, 1997.
43. Chen KD, Li YS, Kim M, et al: Mechanotransduction in response to shear stress: roles of receptor tyrosine kinases, integrins, and Shc, *J Biol Chem* 274:18393-18400, 1999.
44. Sackin H: Stretch-activated ion channels, *Kidney Int* 48:1134-1147, 1995.
45. Kizer N, Guo XL, Hruska K: Reconstitution of stretch-activated cation channels by expression of the alpha-subunit of the epithelial sodium channel cloned from osteoblasts, *Proc Natl Acad Sci USA* 94:1013-1018, 1997.
46. Peake MA, Cooling LM, Magnay JL, et al: Selected contribution: regulatory pathways involved in mechanical induction of *c-fos* gene expression in bone cells, *J Appl Physiol* 89:2498-2507, 2000.
47. Sakai K, Mohtai M, Iwamoto Y: Fluid shear stress increases transforming growth factor beta 1 expression in human osteoblast-like cells: modulation by cation channel blockades, *Calcif Tissue Int* 63:515-520, 1998.
48. Lacampagne A, Gannier F, Argibay J, et al: The stretch-activated ion channel blocker gadolinium also blocks L-type calcium channels in isolated ventricular myocytes of the guinea-pig, *Biochim Biophys Acta* 1191:205-208, 1994.
49. Orellana MF, Smith AK, Waller JL, et al: Plasma membrane disruption in orthodontic tooth movement in rats, *J Dent Res* 81:43-47, 2002.
50. Orellana-Lezcano MF, Major PW, McNeil PL, Borke JL: Temporary loss of plasma membrane integrity in orthodontic tooth movement, *Orthod Craniofac Res* 8:106-113, 2005.
51. Nakago-Matsuo C, Matsuo T, Nakago T: Intracellular calcium response to hydraulic pressure in human periodontal ligament fibroblasts, *Am J Orthod Dentofacial Orthop* 109:244-248, 1996.
52. Chen NX, Ryder KD, Pavalko FM, et al: Ca(2+) regulates fluid shear-induced cytoskeletal reorganization and gene expression in osteoblasts, *Am J Physiol Cell Physiol* 278:C989-C997, 2000.
53. Santos de Araujo RM, Oba Y, Moriyama K: Role of regulator of G-protein signaling 2 (RGS2) in periodontal ligament cells under mechanical stress, *Cell Biochem Funct* 25:753-758, 2007.
54. Reich KM, Gay CV, Frangos JA: Fluid shear stress as a mediator of osteoblast cyclic adenosine monophosphate production, *J Cell Physiol* 143:100-104, 1990.
55. McAllister TN, Frangos JA: Steady and transient fluid shear stress stimulate NO release in osteoblasts through distinct biochemical pathways, *J Bone Miner Res* 14:930-936, 1999.
56. Geng WD, Boskovic G, Fultz ME, et al: Regulation of expression and activity of four PKC isozymes in confluent and mechanically stimulated UMR-108 osteoblastic cells, *J Cell Physiol* 189:216-228, 2001.
57. Reich KM, Frangos JA: Protein kinase C mediates flow-induced prostaglandin E_2 production in osteoblasts, *Calcif Tissue Int* 52:62-66, 1993.
58. Ajubi NE, Klein-Nulend J, Alblas MJ, et al: Signal transduction pathways involved in fluid flow-induced PGE_2 production by cultured osteocytes, *Am J Physiol* 276(1 Pt 1):E171-E178, 1999.
59. Wongkhantee S, Yongchaitrakul T, Pavasant P: Mechanical stress induces osteopontin expression in human periodontal ligament cells through rho kinase, *J Periodontol* 78:1113-1119, 2007.
60. Hipskind RA, Bilbe G: MAP kinase signaling cascades and gene expression in osteoblasts, *Front Biosci* 3:D804-D816, 1998.
61. Kawarizadeh A, Bourauel C, Gotz W, Jager A: Early responses of periodontal ligament cells to mechanical stimulus in vivo, *J Dent Res* 84:902-906, 2005.
62. Danciu TE, Gagari E, Adam RM, et al: Mechanical strain delivers anti-apoptotic and proliferative signals to gingival fibroblasts, *J Dent Res* 83:596-601, 2004.
63. Matsuda N, Morita N, Matsuda K, Watanabe M: Proliferation and differentiation of human osteoblastic cells associated with differential activation of MAP kinases in response to epidermal growth factor, hypoxia, and mechanical stress in vitro, *Biochem Biophys Res Commun* 249:350-354, 1998.
64. Wadhwa S, Godwin SL, Peterson DR, et al: Fluid flow induction of cyclo-oxygenase 2 gene expression in osteoblasts is dependent on an extracellular signal-regulated kinase signaling pathway, *J Bone Miner Res* 17:266-274, 2002.
65. Wu CC, Li YS, Haga JH, et al: Roles of MAP kinases in the regulation of bone matrix gene expressions in human osteoblasts by oscillatory fluid flow, *J Cell Biochem* 98:632-641, 2006.
66. You J, Reilly GC, Zhen X, et al: Osteopontin gene regulation by oscillatory fluid flow via intracellular calcium mobilization and activation of mitogen-activated protein kinase in MC3T3-E1 osteoblasts, *J Biol Chem* 276:13365-13371, 2001.
67. Kusumi A, Sakaki H, Kusumi T, et al: Regulation of synthesis of osteoprotegerin and soluble receptor activator of nuclear factor-kappa B ligand in normal human osteoblasts via the p38 mitogen-activated protein kinase pathway by the application of cyclic tensile strain, *J Bone Miner Metab* 23:373-381, 2005.
68. Ziros PG, Gil APR, Georgakopoulos T, et al: The bone-specific transcriptional regulator Cbfa1 is a target of mechanical signals in osteoblastic cells, *J Biol Chem* 277:23934-23941, 2002.
69. Peverali FA, Basdra EK, Papavassiliou AG: Stretch-mediated activation of selective MAPK subtypes and potentiation of AP-1 binding in human osteoblastic cells, *Mol Med* 7:68-78, 2001.
70. Kletsas D, Basdra EK, Papavassiliou AG: Effect of protein kinase inhibitors on the stretch-elicited c-Fos and c-Jun up-regulation in human PDL osteoblast-like cells, *J Cell Physiol* 190:313-321, 2002.
71. Granet C, Vico AGL, Alexandre C, Lafage-Proust MH: MAPK and SRC-kinases control EGR-1 and NF-κB inductions by changes in mechanical environment in osteoblasts, *Biochem Biophys Res Commun* 284:622-631, 2001.

72. Ogata T: Fluid flow induces enhancement of the Egr-1 mRNA level in osteoblast-like cells: involvement of tyrosine kinase and serum, *J Cell Physiol* 170:27-34, 1997.
73. Billotte WG, Dumas K, Hofmann MC: Transcriptional pathways induced by fluid shear stress in mouse preosteoblast cells, *Biomed Sci Instrum* 37:1-6, 2001.
74. Evans WH, de Vuyst E, Leybaert L: The gap junction cellular internet: connexin hemichannels enter the signalling limelight, *Biochem J* 397:1-14, 2006.
75. Saunders MM, You J, Trosko JE, et al: Gap junctions and fluid flow response in MC3T3-E1 cells, *Am J Physiol Cell Physiol* 281:C1917-C1925, 2001.
76. Gluhak-Heinrich J, Gu S, Pavlin D, Jiang JX: Mechanical loading stimulates expression of connexin 43 in alveolar bone cells in the tooth movement model, *Cell Commun Adhes* 13:115-125, 2006.
77. Su M et al: Expression of connexin 43 in rat mandibular bone and periodontal ligament (PDL) cells during experimental tooth movement, *J Dent Res* 76:1357-1366, 1997.
78. Genetos DC, Kephart CJ, Zhang Y, et al: Oscillating fluid flow activation of gap junction hemichannels induces ATP release from MLO-Y4 osteocytes, *J Cell Physiol* 212:207-214, 2007.
79. Cherian PP, Siller-Jackson AJ, Gu S, et al: Mechanical strain opens connexin 43 hemichannels in osteocytes: a novel mechanism for the release of prostaglandin, *Mol Biol Cell* 16:3100-3106, 2005.
80. Pitsillides AA, Rawlinson SC, Suswillo RF, et al: Mechanical strain-induced NO production by bone cells: a possible role in adaptive bone (re)modeling? *FASEB J* 9:1614-1622, 1995.
81. Klein-Nulend J, Semeins CM, Ajubi NE, et al: Pulsating fluid flow increases nitric oxide (NO) synthesis by osteocytes but not periosteal fibroblasts: correlation with prostaglandin upregulation, *Biochem Biophys Res Commun* 217:640-648, 1995.
82. Johnson DL, McAllister TN, Frangos JA: Fluid flow stimulates rapid and continuous release of nitric oxide in osteoblasts, *Am J Physiol* 271(1 Pt 1):E205-E208, 1996.
83. Reich KM, Frangos JA: Effect of flow on prostaglandin E_2 and inositol trisphosphate levels in osteoblasts, *Am J Physiol* 261(3 Pt 1):C428-C432, 1991.
84. Smalt R, Mitchell FT, Howard RL, et al: Mechanotransduction in bone cells: induction of nitric oxide and prostaglandin synthesis by fluid shear stress, but not by mechanical strain, *Adv Exp Med Biol* 433:311-314, 1997.
85. Klein-Nulend J, Semeins CM, Ajubi NE, et al: Pulsating fluid flow stimulates prostaglandin release and inducible prostaglandin G/H synthase mRNA expression in primary mouse bone cells, *J Bone Miner Res* 12:45-51, 1997.
86. Akin E, Gurton AU, Olmez H: Effects of nitric oxide in orthodontic tooth movement in rats, *Am J Orthod Dentofacial Orthop* 126:608-614, 2004.
87. Hayashi K, Igarashi K, Miyoshi K, et al: Involvement of nitric oxide in orthodontic tooth movement in rats, *Am J Orthod Dentofacial Orthop* 122:306-309, 2002.
88. Shirazi M, Nilforoushan D, Alghasi H, et al: The role of nitric oxide in orthodontic tooth movement in rats, *Angle Orthod* 72:211-215, 2002.
89. Zhou D, Hughes B, King GJ: Histomorphometric and biochemical study of osteoclasts at orthodontic compression sites in the rat during indomethacin inhibition, *Arch Oral Biol* 42:717-726, 1997.
90. Sandy JR, Harris M: Prostaglandins and tooth movement, *Eur J Orthod* 6:175-182, 1984.
91. Kehoe MJ, Cohen SM, Zarrinnia K, et al: The effect of acetaminophen, ibuprofen, and misoprostol on prostaglandin E_2 synthesis and the degree and rate of orthodontic tooth movement, *Angle Orthod* 66:339-349, 1996.
92. Chumbley AB, Tuncay OC: The effect of indomethacin (an aspirin-like drug) on the rate of orthodontic tooth movement, *Am J Orthod* 89:312-314, 1986.
93. Giunta D, Keller J, Nielsen FF, Melsen B: Influence of indomethacin on bone turnover related to orthodontic tooth movement in miniature pigs, *Am J Orthod Dentofacial Orthop* 108:361-366, 1995.
94. Lee WC: Experimental study of the effect of prostaglandin administration on tooth movement: with particular emphasis on the relationship to the method of PGE_1 administration, *Am J Orthod Dentofacial Orthop* 98:231-241, 1990.
95. Leiker BJ, Nanda RS, Currier GF, et al: The effects of exogenous prostaglandins on orthodontic tooth movement in rats, *Am J Orthod Dentofacial Orthop* 108:380-388, 1995.
96. Yamasaki K, Shibata Y, Fukuhara T: The effect of prostaglandins on experimental tooth movement in monkeys *(Macaca fuscata)*, *J Dent Res* 61:1444-1446, 1982.
97. Yamasaki K, Shibata Y, Imai S, et al: Clinical application of prostaglandin E_1 (PGE_1) upon orthodontic tooth movement, *Am J Orthod* 85:508-518, 1984.
98. Wolff J: *The law of bone remodeling*, New York, 1986, Springer-Verlag.
99. Turner CH: Three rules for bone adaptation to mechanical stimuli, *Bone* 23:399-407, 1998.
100. Frost HM: A determinant of bone architecture: the minimum effective strain, *Clin Orthop* 175:286-292, 1983.
101. Liskova M, Hert J: Reaction of bone to mechanical stimuli. 2. Periosteal and endosteal reaction of tibial diaphysis in rabbit to intermittent loading, *Folia Morphol Praha* 19:301-317, 1971.
102. Forwood MR, Turner CH: Skeletal adaptations to mechanical usage: results from tibial loading studies in rats, *Bone* 17(Suppl 4):197S-205S, 1995.
103. Hsieh YF, Turner CH: Effects of loading frequency on mechanically induced bone formation, *J Bone Miner Res* 16:918-924, 2001.
104. Rubin CT, Lanyon LE: Regulation of bone formation by applied dynamic loads, *J Bone Joint Surg Am* 66:397-402, 1984.
105. Gross TS, Srinivasan S, Liu CC, et al: Noninvasive loading of the murine tibia: an in vivo model for the study of mechanotransduction, *J Bone Miner Res* 17:493-501, 2002.
106. Robling AG, Duijvelaar KM, Geevers JV, et al: Modulation of appositional and longitudinal bone growth in the rat ulna by applied static and dynamic force, *Bone* 29:105-113, 2001.
107. Umemura Y, Ishiko T, Yamauchi T, et al: Five jumps per day increase bone mass and breaking force in rats, *J Bone Miner Res* 12:1480-1485, 1997.
108. Lanyon LE: Functional strain as a determinant for bone remodeling, *Calcif Tissue Int* 36(Suppl 1):56-61, 1984.
109. Robling AG, Burr DB, Turner CH: Recovery periods restore mechanosensitivity to dynamically loaded bone, *J Exp Biol* 204(Pt 19):3389-3899, 2001.
110. Lanyon LE: The success and failure of the adaptive response to functional load-bearing in averting bone fracture, *Bone* 13(Suppl 2):17-21, 1992.

111. Cullen DM, Smith RT, Akhter MP: Bone-loading response varies with strain magnitude and cycle number, *J Appl Physiol* 91:1971-1976, 2001.
112. Grimston SK, Willows ND, Hanley DA: Mechanical loading regime and its relationship to bone mineral density in children, *Med Sci Sports Exerc* 25:1203-1210, 1993.
113. Fehling PC, Alekel L, Clasey J, et al: A comparison of bone mineral densities among female athletes in impact loading and active loading sports, *Bone* 17:205-210, 1995.
114. Courteix D, Lespessailles E, Peres SL, et al: Effect of physical training on bone mineral density in prepubertal girls: a comparative study between impact-loading and non-impact-loading sports, *Osteoporos Int* 8:152-158, 1998.
115. Rubin C, Turner S, Mallinckrodt C, et al: Mechanical strain, induced noninvasively in the high-frequency domain, is anabolic to cancellous bone, but not cortical bone, *Bone* 30:445-452, 2002.
116. Melsen B: Biological reaction of alveolar bone to orthodontic tooth movement, *Angle Orthod* 69:151-158, 1999.
117. Keles A, Grunes B, DiFuria C, et al: Inhibition of tooth movement by osteoprotegerin vs. pamidronate under conditions of constant orthodontic force, *Eur J Oral Sci* 115:131-136, 2007.
118. Liu L, Igarashi K, Haruyama N, et al: Effects of local administration of clodronate on orthodontic tooth movement and root resorption in rats, *Eur J Orthod* 26:469-473, 2004.
119. Suda T, Takahashi N, Udagawa N, et al: Modulation of osteoclast differentiation and function by the new members of the tumor necrosis factor receptor and ligand families, *Endocr Rev* 20:345-357, 1999.
120. Anderson DM, Maraskovsky E, Billingsley WL, et al: A homologue of the TNF receptor and its ligand enhance T-cell growth and dendritic-cell function, *Nature* 390:175-179, 1997.
121. Tsukii K, Shima N, Mochizuki S, et al: Osteoclast differentiation factor mediates an essential signal for bone resorption induced by 1-alpha,25-dihydroxyvitamin D_3, prostaglandin E_2, or parathyroid hormone in the microenvironment of bone, *Biochem Biophys Res Commun* 246:337-341, 1998.
122. Yasuda H, Shima N, Nakagawa N, et al: Osteoclast differentiation factor is a ligand for osteoprotegerin/osteoclastogenesis-inhibitory factor and is identical to TRANCE/RANKL, *Proc Natl Acad Sci USA* 95:3597-3602, 1998.
123. Suda T, Kobayashi K, Jimi E, et al: The molecular basis of osteoclast differentiation and activation, *Novartis Found Symp* 232:235-247 (discussion, 247-250), 2001.
124. Dunn MD, Park CH, Kostenuik PJ, et al: Local delivery of osteoprotegerin inhibits mechanically mediated bone modeling in orthodontic tooth movement, *Bone* 41:446-455, 2007.
125. Kanzaki H, Chiba M, Takahashi I, et al: Local OPG gene transfer to periodontal tissue inhibits orthodontic tooth movement, *J Dent Res* 83:920-925, 2004.
126. Kanzaki H, Chiba M, Arai K, et al: Local RANKL gene transfer to the periodontal tissue accelerates orthodontic tooth movement, *Gene Ther* 13:678-685, 2006.
127. Nakao K, Goto T, Gunjigake KK, et al: Intermittent force induces high RANKL expression in human periodontal ligament cells, *J Dent Res* 86:623-628, 2007.
128. Kim T, Handa A, Iida J, Yoshida S: RANKL expression in rat periodontal ligament subjected to a continuous orthodontic force, *Arch Oral Biol* 52:244-250, 2007.
129. Kanzaki H, Chiba M, Shimizu Y, et al: Periodontal ligament cells under mechanical stress induce osteoclastogenesis by receptor activator of nuclear factor kappa B ligand up-regulation via prostaglandin E_2 synthesis, *J Bone Miner Res* 17:210-220, 2002.
130. Tsuji K, Uno K, Zhang GX, Tamura M: Periodontal ligament cells under intermittent tensile stress regulate mRNA expression of osteoprotegerin and tissue inhibitor of matrix metalloprotease-1 and -2, *J Bone Miner Metab* 22:94-103, 2004.
131. Kanzaki H, Chiba M, Sato A, et al: Cyclical tensile force on periodontal ligament cells inhibits osteoclastogenesis through OPG induction, *J Dent Res* 85:457-462, 2006.
132. Hayashi H, Konoo T, Yamaguchi K: Intermittent 8-hour activation in orthodontic molar movement, *Am J Orthod Dentofacial Orthop* 125:302-309, 2004.
133. Konoo T, Kim YJ, Gu GM, King GJ: Intermittent force in orthodontic tooth movement, *J Dent Res* 80:457-460, 2001.
134. Owman-Moll P, Kurol J, Lundgren D: Continuous versus interrupted continuous orthodontic force related to early tooth movement and root resorption, *Angle Orthod* 65:395-401 (discussion, 401-402), 1995.
135. Van Leeuwen EJ, Maltha JC, Kuijpers-Jagtman AM: Tooth movement with light continuous and discontinuous forces in beagle dogs, *Eur J Oral Sci* 107:468-474, 1999.
136. Kameyama T, Matsumoto Y, Warita H, Soma K: Inactivated periods of constant orthodontic forces related to desirable tooth movement in rats, *J Orthod* 30:31-37 (discussion, 21-22), 2003.
137. Mehrotra M, Saegusa M, Wadhwa S, et al: Fluid flow induces RANKL expression in primary murine calvarial osteoblasts, *J Cell Biochem* 98:1271-1283, 2006.
138. Ren Y, Maltha JC, Kuijpers-Jagtman AM: Optimum force magnitude for orthodontic tooth movement: a systematic literature review, *Angle Orthod* 73:86-92, 2003.
139. Ren Y, Maltha JC, Van't Hof MA, Kuipers-Jagtman AM: Optimum force magnitude for orthodontic tooth movement: a mathematic model, *Am J Orthod Dentofacial Orthop* 125:71-77, 2004.

CHAPTER 27

Orthodontic Root Resorption

Gregory J. King

Root resorption is a common problem associated with orthodontic treatment. Minor and clinically insignificant amounts of root resorption occur frequently. In some rare cases, however, the extent of orthodontically related root resorption can be severe enough to jeopardize the prognosis for the teeth involved (Fig. 27-1). This chapter discusses the following topics related to orthodontic root resorption: (1) clinical and biological background; (2) epidemiology; (3) risk factors; and (4) prediction, early detection, and treatment.

CLINICAL AND BIOLOGICAL BACKGROUND OF ROOT RESORPTION

Whether occurring in the pulp chamber or on the root surface, root resorption is almost always associated with a healing response to some type of insult. Injured tissue is removed in preparation for the reparative phase of wound healing.[1] The mechanism controlling this reparative process currently is not well understood, but newer evidence suggests that the mechanism may be similar to that controlling bone remodeling.

In bone remodeling the *receptor activator of nuclear factor kappa B* (NF-κB) ligand (RANKL), found on the osteoblast stromal cells, binds to RANK, located on the osteoclast precursor cells, to stimulate osteoclast numbers and activities. *Osteoprotegerin* (OPG) is a circulating molecule that acts as a decoy receptor that binds to RANKL, thereby preventing the genesis of osteoclasts. The relative concentration of the stimulator and inhibitor is a common signaling mechanism that controls osteoclasts and bone remodeling in response to most stimulators. As with other stromal cells, periodontal ligament (PDL) cells and cementoblasts possess RANKL, suggesting that they also may be able to control odontoclastogenesis and root resorption in response to stimulation by parathyroid hormone–related protein (PTHrp).[2,3] Some investigators have suggested that antiresorption factors may reside in both the PDL and the pulp, and if these are impaired by injury, root resorption can occur.[1] Current evidence suggests that such a mechanism may exist in the form of OPG, but that the ultimate control of root resorption may reside in a combination of both inhibition and stimulation of odontoclasts. The clinical observation that endodontically treated teeth are more resistant to orthodontic root resorption suggests that pulpal cells also may play a role in this control.[4]

The most common classification of external root resorption categorizes the sites in ascending order of the severity of associated trauma.[1] The mildest form, *surface* root resorption, is characterized by cemental cratering that can extend into the dentin. These sites are usually adjacent to focal injuries in the PDL, the most common being the hyalinization lesions that occur at compression sites during orthodontic tooth movement. *Inflammatory* root resorption is the next order of severity. Involved sites are adjacent to inflammatory lesions and may be related to orthodontic tooth movement, but usually these are related to more extensive injuries of traumatic or endodontic origin. The response to the most severe types of injuries, including tooth displacement, avulsion, and reimplantation, manifests as replacement resorption. The radiographic picture of replacement resorption is characterized by root resorption, with the crater being repaired by bone. This type of resorption is often progressive and, because the PDL space is lost, results in ankylosis of the tooth.[5]

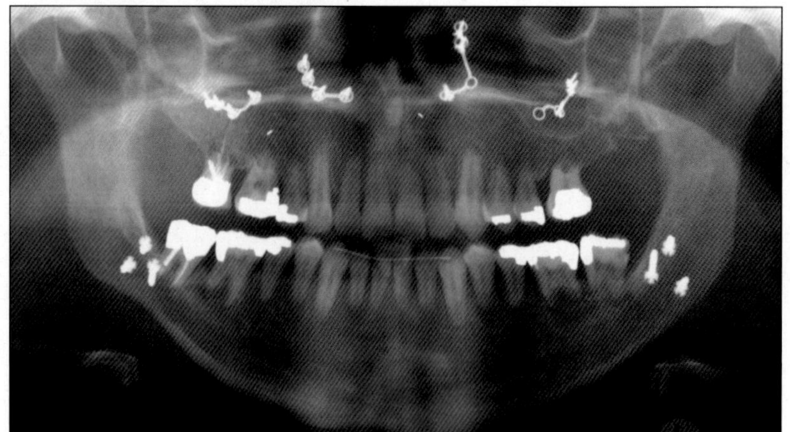

Fig. 27-1 Posttreatment radiograph of a patient who was highly susceptible to external apical root resorption (EARR).

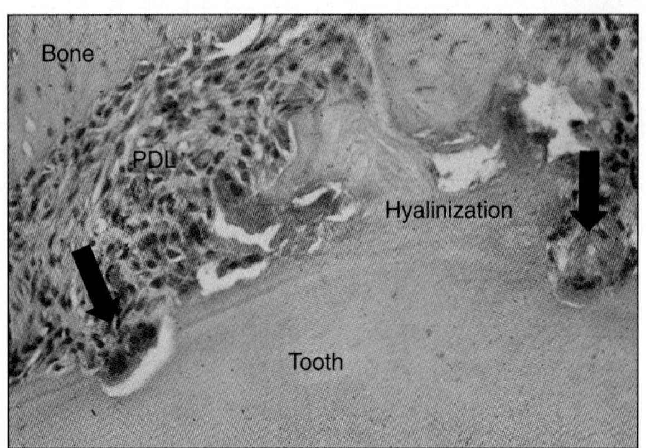

Fig. 27-2 Periodontal ligament *(PDL)* necrosis ("hyalinization") showing peripheral resorption, especially at the root surface *(arrows)*.

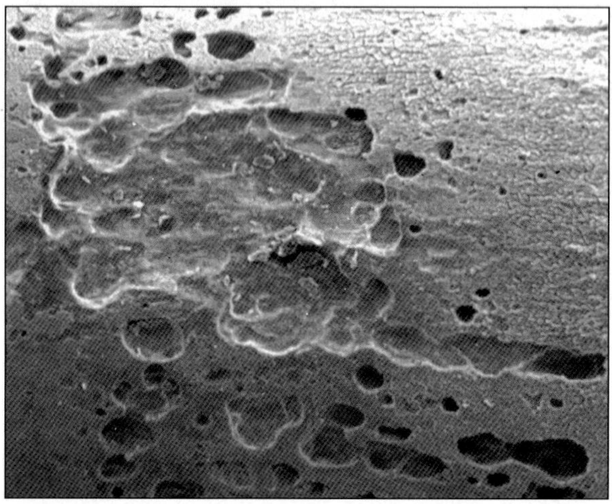

Fig. 27-3 Scanning electron micrograph of orthodontic root resorption adjacent to periodontal ligament necrosis.

The pathogenesis of orthodontic root resorption has been well described through animal models and initiates at sites of compression.[6] Orthodontic appliances produce sustained pressure that exceeds the pressure in the PDL arterioles. This results in their occlusion and the necrosis of the PDL served by them. These necrotic lesions, known as "hyalinizations" because of their histological resemblance to hyaline cartilage, have been well described and consist of cells with pyknotic nuclei, as well as fragmented PDL fibers. Adjacent arterioles compensate by becoming engorged, and the lesions are removed at the periphery by various resorptive cells, including macrophages, osteoclasts, and cementoclasts.[7] Surface root resorption results from this peripheral removal at the tooth surface[8,9] (Figs. 27-2 and 27-3).

This process is progressive until the necrotic lesions are removed, finally permitting the tooth to move. Presumably, if new PDL necrotic lesions were generated at the same site after movement or reactivation of the appliance, progression of the root resorption would continue. This is consistent with the clinical impression that, in the absence of other inflammatory lesions, the progression of orthodontic root resorption ceases when orthodontic treatment ceases. It also may explain why patients with long durations of treatment or those requiring significant root movements are at risk for more extensive root resorption lesions; most likely these types of treatments require more appliance activations with greater risk of focal necroses in the PDL.[10,11]

Only limited healing potential exists once a root resorption lesion has been created. Most cemental craters can repair completely with secondary cementum,[12] but loss of root length or gross changes in root morphology do not entirely repair. Instead, restoration of these larger lesions does not proceed beyond their becoming lined with secondary cementum.

The most common radiographic image of orthodontic root resorption is loss of root length from the apex. Because of the prevalence of this clinical picture, the descriptive term *external apical root resorption* (EARR) has begun to appear in the root resorption literature. If the histological evidence links orthodontic root resorption to sites of compression, one must ask, "Why is apical root resorption so common?" Several possible explanations exist. First, root apices are common sites of compression in modern orthodontic mechanical approaches, including tipping, torque, and intrusion. Second, tooth structure is minimal at the root apex, which means these sites are more prone to morphological change with less loss of tissue. Third, standard radiographs easily visualize the root apex but not root loss from the lateral root surface because much (on buccal and lingual aspects) is not visible. However, autopsy sections from orthodontic patients and sections prepared from extracted premolars with orthodontic treatment clearly demonstrate that resorption sites are not found exclusively at the apex.[13]

The sequelae of orthodontic root resorption range from being clinically insignificant or minor to severe enough to jeopardize the longevity of the dentition. Cases of minor root loss (<2 mm) are common and have no clinical consequences. However, persistent tooth mobility is a risk in teeth that lose significant root length.[14] Therefore close follow-up of those teeth is indicated to prevent loss of crestal alveolar bone height. There are no good data on the prevalence of actual tooth loss as a result of severe orthodontic root resorption, but anecdotal clinical reports suggest this outcome is extremely rare.

EPIDEMIOLOGY

The prevalence of EARR varies among the different tooth types. Maxillary central incisors are most commonly affected.[10,11] The reasons for this finding are not well understood. It is possible that the morphological or biological composition of these teeth make them highly prone to root loss or that they more often require orthodontic mechanics that put them at risk. Certainly the latter is likely considering that Class II and III malocclusions represent significant problems requiring orthodontic treatment, often with greater root movements and higher torquing forces to correct overjets. Maxillary incisors also may be more prone to lateral traumatic forces from mastication, putting them at risk for root loss before and during orthodontic treatment.

The prevalence of EARR in nonorthodontic patients is low (1%-2%)[15,16] and is probably related to minor traumatic lesions or occlusal interferences. By contrast, the prevalence in orthodontic patients has been reported as high as 70%,[17] strongly suggesting that the minor periodontal ligament (PDL) trauma associated with orthodontic treatment is a significant contributing factor. Most orthodontic patients experience clinically insignificant EARR (<2 mm). However, 2% to 5% experience greater than 5 mm of loss in root length.[18,19]

Therefore most orthodontic patients who experience root shortening do not have clinically significant sequelae. The important subpopulation of orthodontic patients is the 2% to 5% who do experience enough root loss to constitute a clinical problem. Because modern orthodontic appliances and approaches are similar, it is difficult to see how these patients are experiencing unusual orthodontic treatments that alone are causing greater root loss. Assuming this is the case, it follows that the patients who experience severe EARR are more susceptible to the minor PDL traumas associated with orthodontic treatment caused by host, not environmental, factors.

RISK FACTORS

Orthodontic root resorption is a multifactorial condition with wide variation in occurrence and severity.[20] The list of risk factors for EARR is therefore extensive. For clarity of discussion, these can be broadly categorized as "environmental" factors or "host" factors (e.g., dental, genetic, dietary/hormonal, immunological).

Environmental Factors

All the environmental factors are associated with trauma to the PDL. The trauma can be gross, as with accidents that result in tooth displacement and avulsion with reimplantation. Tooth transplantation, also with a high prevalence of root resorption, can be considered in this category of gross trauma.[1] Subtler PDL trauma might result from occlusal interferences during mastication, but this risk apparently has not been assessed.

Orthodontic treatment also may be viewed as a limited type of PDL trauma. All environmental risk factors associated with aspects of orthodontic treatment seem to represent approaches that increase the likelihood of increased trauma to the PDL, including duration of treatment, amount of root movement, extraction treatment, and force magnitude.

Interestingly, gender, a factor without an obvious relationship to increased PDL trauma, does not seem to be associated with increased risk of EARR.[10,11,17]

Host Factors

The host factors that place patients at risk for EARR have been examined extensively because the epidemiological evidence would seem to suggest that a small percentage of people who experience severe root loss are unusually susceptible to the minor PDL trauma that accompanies routine orthodontic treatment. Dental anomalies have received the most attention.

Dental anomalies

The suggestion has been made that patients with generalized tooth anomalies, including ectopic eruption, impactions, crown shape anomalies, and agenesis, are more prone to EARR.[21] Others have reported no differences in mean root resorption between patients with and without dental anomalies, and none of the individual anomalies appears to be a risk factor.[22,23] Certain types of unusual root morphology do seem to be significant for EARR, however, with narrow, pointed roots more at risk and blunter roots somewhat resistant.[24,25]

Ectopic eruption is a risk factor for EARR, with proximity to the dental follicle the primary reason (Fig. 27-4, *A*). Resorption of neighboring permanent teeth during eruption

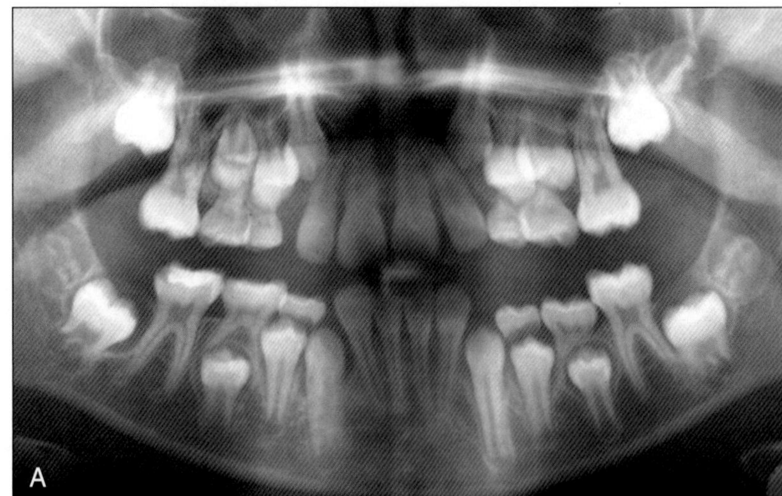

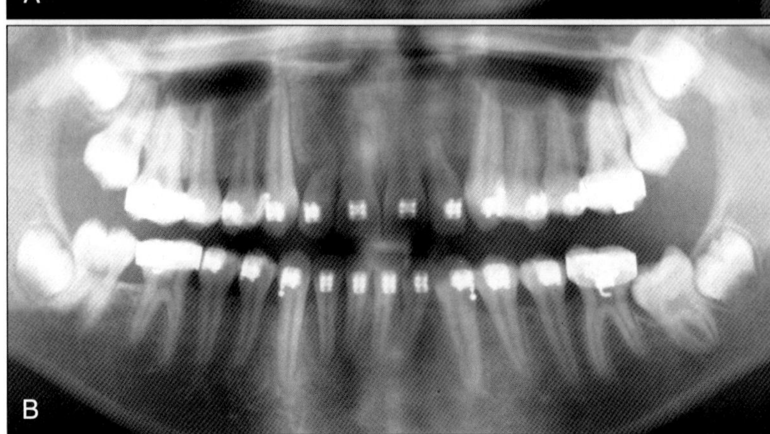

Fig. 27-4 **A,** Severe root resorption of maxillary lateral incisors caused by proximity to the erupting canine dental follicles. **B,** After orthodontic treatment.

is most likely an effect of the physical contact between the erupting tooth and the adjacent tooth and the characteristic cellular activity in the tissues at the contact points.[26] Current biological evidence indicates that the dental follicle adjacent to the erupting tooth crown attracts pre-osteoclasts with CSF1 and activates them through the RANK/RANKL/OPG mechanism previously described.[27] This mechanism is presumably the means by which erupting permanent teeth remove alveolar bone and deciduous root during the process of normal eruption. In all likelihood, the resorptive potential of the dental follicle, not pressure, causes the type of root resorption associated with ectopic eruption.

Commencing orthodontic treatment before the completion of root formation has often been suggested as increasing the likelihood of root shortening. Surprisingly, studies have shown that roots treated before the completion of root formation become longer by the end of treatment, whereas those closer to root completion at the start of treatment become shorter.[28] This finding suggests that routine orthodontic treatment has little or no effect on the completion of root formation.

Genetic factors

Genetics appears to be a potent host risk factor for EARR, with heritability estimates averaging 50%, with some teeth significantly greater.[29,30] This is supported by the observation that certain ethnic groups are at higher risk for EARR than others. Asians have a low risk, followed by Caucasians, with Hispanics experiencing the most root resorption.[10] Again, if the main source of EARR were the trauma associated with orthodontic mechanics, one would not expect ethnic differences, with little reason to postulate different modes of treatment across ethnicities.

Although not well understood, the genetic mechanism controlling EARR may involve heterogeneities of the genes that control bone resorption, such as interleukin-1 beta (IL-1β) and tumor necrosis factor alpha (TNF-α).[30-32] Studies seem to suggest an inverse relationship between bone resorption and root resorption, with the orthodontic movement through less dense bone being protective for root resorption.

Dietary and hormonal mechanisms

Some have implicated diet and hormones in the prevalence of EARR. The calciotropic hormones—parathyroid hormone (PTH), calcitonin, and vitamin D—as well as dietary calcium, appear to have some impact on root resorption, suggesting that hormonal mechanisms reducing alveolar bone density may be protective.[33] Others have concluded that stimulation of bone resorption may lead to greater root resorption.[34] Clearly, a better understanding is needed of the relationship between bone-remodeling activity and root resorption. This could produce studies aimed at much needed therapies and approaches to prediction of those at risk for EARR.

A second hormonal mechanism related to root resorption involves thyroid hormone (TH). The suggestion has been made that TH may be protective and that administration of low doses of TH may protect the root surface during orthodontic treatment.[35]

Immunodeficiency states

Immunological mechanisms may play a role in the process of root resorption. Patients with allergies have a slightly higher prevalence of root resorption, but this is not statistically significant.[36,37]

Enhanced traumatic root resorption in a mouse model was shown to coincide with a decline in naturally occurring serum antibody levels to autologous dentin, suggesting that immunodeficiency states may present risks for EARR.[38] This idea gains support from the observations that cats infected with feline immunodeficiency virus experience higher levels of spontaneous root resorption[39] and patients with the rare immunodeficiency known as hyper-IgE syndrome have a very high prevalence (~72% in one sample) of the previously unrecognized feature of failure or delay in the shedding of primary teeth caused by lack of root resorption.[40]

PREDICTION, EARLY DETECTION, AND TREATMENT

Predicting patients who are at risk for severe root resorption should be the initial focus of any screening methodology. Once the 2% to 5% of the population with high susceptibility can be easily and reliably identified, orthodontists could counsel them and plan treatment accordingly. Future estimations of susceptibility to EARR will likely involve some form of genetic analysis. With the availability of the human genome, powerful molecular methods to simultaneously monitor the relative activities of thousands of genes, and inbred strains of animals with specific genes "knocked out" or amplified, genetic screening seems to be imminent and may be a reality within a decade.

Early detection of root resorption for those at risk is also essential. Anticipating root resorption after oral trauma or during orthodontic treatment has involved radiographic monitoring. Clinicians have exploited subtle radiographic clues to detect early development of EARR,[41] but these require frequent exposures and are not entirely reliable.[42] Advances in imaging technologies will provide opportunities to make major leaps forward in this area. Three-dimensional computed tomography (CT) and magnetic resonance imaging (MRI) approaches are now commonly available. These should allow clinicians to more reliably monitor tooth roots in susceptible patients with greater precision.

The development of biochemical approaches also offers the promise of accurate and noninvasive monitoring of the status of the roots during treatment. Once marker molecules that are specific to the tooth root or the process of root resorption have been identified, means to monitor their presence in the circulation or gingival crevicular fluid should make this approach viable.[43]

Treatment approaches to EARR fall into two categories: alteration in treatment and administration of drugs. The former is much more feasible today, but the latter should become increasingly more common. Alteration in strategies may include deciding not to treat the patient or certain teeth, limiting the exposure of certain teeth to force, or limiting treatment objectives.

Most pharmacological approaches have limited value during orthodontic treatment because they also inhibit tooth movement. Bisphosphonate treatment has proved useful after orthodontic treatment because it has direct effects on osteoclasts,[44] although it may increase the risk of osteonecrosis of the jaws. Calcitonin and TH administration also have been shown to suppress root resorption in animals.[34,35]

CONCLUSION

The inverse relationship between alveolar bone density and root resorption needs to be clarified because it may be used to decouple the rate of tooth movement from the risk of root resorption.

REFERENCES

1. Andreasen JO, Andreasen FM: Root resorption following traumatic dental injuries, *Proc Finn Dent Soc* 88(Suppl 1):95-114, 1992.
2. Boabaid F, Berry JE, Koh AJ, et al: The role of parathyroid hormone–related protein in the regulation of osteoclastogenesis by cementoblasts, *J Periodontol* 75:1247-1254, 2004.
3. Fukushima H, Jimi E, Kajiya H, et al: Parathyroid-hormone-related protein induces expression of receptor activator of NF-κB ligand in human periodontal ligament cells via a cAMP/protein kinase A–independent pathway, *J Dent Res* 84:329-334, 2005.
4. Mirabella AD, Artun J: Risk factors for apical root resorption of maxillary anterior teeth in adult orthodontic patients, *Am J Orthod Dentofacial Orthop* 108:48-55, 1995.
5. Majorana A, Bardellini E, Conti G, et al: Root resorption in dental trauma: 45 cases followed for 5 years, *Dent Traumatol* 19:262-265, 2003.
6. Brudvik P, Rygh P: The initial phase of orthodontic root resorption incident to local compression of the periodontal ligament, *Eur J Orthod* 15:249-263, 1993.
7. Brudvik P, Rygh P: The repair of orthodontic root resorption: an ultrastructural study, *Eur J Orthod* 17:189-198, 1995.
8. Brudvik P, Rygh P: Multi-nucleated cells remove the main hyalinized tissue and start resorption of adjacent root surfaces, *Eur J Orthod* 16:265-273, 1994.
9. Brudvik P, Rygh P: Root resorption beneath the main hyalinized zone, *Eur J Orthod* 16:249-263, 1994.
10. Sameshima GT, Sinclair PM: Predicting and preventing root resorption. Part I. Diagnostic factors, *Am J Orthod Dentofacial Orthop* 119:505-510, 2001.

11. Sameshima GT, Sinclair PM: Predicting and preventing root resorption. Part II. Treatment factors, *Am J Orthod Dentofacial Orthop* 119:511-515, 2001.
12. Owman-Moll P, Kurol J: The early reparative process of orthodontically induced root resorption in adolescents: location and type of tissue, *Eur J Orthod* 20:727-732, 1998.
13. Casa MA, Faltin RM, Faltin K, et al: Root resorptions in upper first premolars after application of continuous torque moment: intra-individual study, *J Orofac Orthop* 62:285-295, 2001.
14. Levander E, Malmgren O: Long-term follow-up of maxillary incisors with severe apical root resorption, *Eur J Orthod* 22:85-92, 2000.
15. Harris EF, Kineret SE, Tolley EA: A heritable component for external apical root resorption in patients treated orthodontically, *Am J Orthod Dentofacial Orthop* 111:301-309, 1997.
16. Lupi JE, Handelman CS, Sadowsky C: Prevalence and severity of apical root resorption and alveolar bone loss in orthodontically treated adults, *Am J Orthod Dentofacial Orthop* 109:28-37, 1996.
17. Brin I, Tulloch JF, Koroluk L, Philips C: External apical root resorption in Class II malocclusion: a retrospective review of 1- versus 2-phase treatment, *Am J Orthod Dentofacial Orthop* 124:151-156, 2003.
18. Killiany DM: Root resorption caused by orthodontic treatment: an evidence-based review of literature, *Semin Orthod* 5:128-133, 1999.
19. Taithongchai R, Sookkorn K, Killiany DM: Facial and dentoalveolar structure and the prediction of apical root shortening, *Am J Orthod Dentofacial Orthop* 110:296-302, 1996.
20. Vlaskalic V, Boyd RL, Baumrind S: Etiology and sequelae of root resorption, *Semin Orthod* 4:124-131, 1998.
21. Kjaer I: Morphological characteristics of dentitions developing excessive root resorption during orthodontic treatment, *Eur J Orthod* 17:25-34, 1995.
22. Lee RY, Artun J, Alonzo TA: Are dental anomalies risk factors for apical root resorption in orthodontic patients? *Am J Orthod Dentofacial Orthop* 116:187-195, 1999.
23. Kook YA, Park S, Sameshima GT: Peg-shaped and small lateral incisors not at higher risk for root resorption, *Am J Orthod Dentofacial Orthop* 123:253-258, 2003.
24. Sameshima GT, Sinclair PM: Characteristics of patients with severe root resorption, *Orthod Craniofac Res* 7:108-114, 2004.
25. Mirabella AD, Artun J: Risk factors for apical root resorption of maxillary anterior teeth in adult orthodontic patients, *Am J Orthod Dentofacial Orthop* 108:48-55, 1995.
26. Ericson S, Bjerklin K, Falahat B: Does the canine dental follicle cause resorption of permanent incisor roots? A computed tomographic study of erupting maxillary canines, *Angle Orthod* 72:95-104, 2002.
27. Marks SC Jr, Schroeder HE: Tooth eruption: theories and facts, *Anat Rec* 245:374-393, 1996.
28. Mavragani M, Boe OE, Wisth PJ, Selvig KA: Changes in root length during orthodontic treatment: advantages for immature teeth, *Eur J Orthod* 24:91-97, 2002.
29. Harris EF, Kineret SE, Tolley EA: A heritable component for external apical root resorption in patients treated orthodontically, *Am J Orthod Dentofacial Orthop* 111:301-309, 1997.
30. Hartsfield JK Jr, Everett ET, Al-Qawasmi RA: Genetic factors in external apical root resorption and orthodontic treatment, *Crit Rev Oral Biol Med* 15:115-122, 2004.
31. Al-Qawasmi RA, Hartsfield JK, Hartsfield JK Jr, et al: Root resorption associated with orthodontic force in IL-1β knockout mouse, *J Musculoskelet Neuronal Interact* 4:383-385, 2004.
32. Al-Qawasmi RA, Hartsfield JK Jr, Everett ET, et al: Genetic predisposition to external apical root resorption in orthodontic patients: linkage of chromosome-18 marker, *J Dent Res* 82:356-360, 2003.
33. Goldie RS, King GJ: Root resorption and tooth movement in orthodontically treated, calcium-deficient, and lactating rats, *Am J Orthod* 85:424-430, 1984.
34. Takada K, Kajiya H, Fukushima H, et al: Calcitonin in human odontoclasts regulates root resorption activity via protein kinase A, *J Bone Miner Metab* 22:12-18, 2004.
35. Vazquez-Landaverde LA, Rojas-Huidobro R, Alonso Gallegos-Corona M, Aceves C: Periodontal 5′-deiodination on forced-induced root resorption: the protective effect of thyroid hormone administration, *Eur J Orthod* 24:363-369, 2002.
36. Owman-Moll P, Kurol J: Root resorption after orthodontic treatment in high- and low-risk patients: analysis of allergy as a possible predisposing factor, *Eur J Orthod* 22:657-663, 2000.
37. McNab S, Battistutta D, Taverne A, Symons AL: External apical root resorption of posterior teeth in asthmatics after orthodontic treatment, *Am J Orthod Dentofacial Orthop* 116:545-551, 1999.
38. Wheeler TT, Stroup SE: Traumatic root resorption in dentine-immunized mice, *Am J Orthod Dentofacial Orthop* 103:352-357, 1993.
39. Hofmann-Lehmann R, Berger M, Sigrist B, et al: Feline immunodeficiency virus (FIV) infection leads to increased incidence of feline odontoclastic resorptive lesions (FORL), *Vet Immunol Immunopathol* 65:299-308, 1998.
40. Grimbacher B, Holland SM, Gallin JI, et al: Hyper-IgE syndrome with recurrent infections: an autosomal dominant multisystem disorder, *N Engl J Med* 340:692-702, 1999.
41. Cohen S, Blanco L, Berman LH: Early radiographic diagnosis of inflammatory root resorption, *Gen Dent* 51:235-240, 2003.
42. Levander E, Bajka R, Malmgren O: Early radiographic diagnosis of apical root resorption during orthodontic treatment: a study of maxillary incisors, *Eur J Orthod* 20:57-63, 1998.
43. Mah J, Prasad N: Dentine phosphoproteins in gingival crevicular fluid during root resorption, *Eur J Orthod* 26:25-30, 2004.
44. Igarashi K, Adachi H, Mitani H, Shinoda H: Inhibitory effect of the topical administration of a bisphosphonate (risedronate) on root resorption incident to orthodontic tooth movement in rats, *J Dent Res* 75:1644-1649, 1996.

CHAPTER 28

Restoration of Oral and Craniofacial Defects by Stem Cells and Bioengineering Approaches

■ *Jin Y. Kim, Candice Zemnick, and Jeremy J. Mao*

The face distinguishes one human being from another. Through evolution, the human face is highly individualized compared with most other species. The facial tissues and organs are arguably the most complex in the human body, accommodating multiple functions of vision, hearing, smell, taste, touch, mastication, swallowing, and breathing. The face is a portal for the "inner self," a source of self-recognition and attraction.

The face is considered to be harmonious if there is a high degree of symmetry between the left and right sides. When disfigurement of the face occurs from trauma, tumors, chronic diseases, or congenital deformities, the physical and psychosocial effects can be extremely detrimental. In 2000 the U.S. Surgeon General's Report on Oral Health stated that a serious facial and oral disfigurement "may undermine self-image and self-esteem, discourage normal social interaction, and lead to chronic stress and depression as well as to incurring great financial cost." Furthermore, facial and oral disfigurement "may interfere with vital functions such as breathing, eating, swallowing, and speaking. The burden of disease restricts activities in school, work, and home, and often significantly diminishes the quality of life."

Several medical and dental specialties, including dentistry, orthodontics, maxillofacial prosthetics, prosthodontics, plastic and reconstructive surgery, ear-nose-throat surgery, and oral/maxillofacial surgery are devoted to the reconstruction of facial disfigurement. Sometimes, the complexity and diversity of the involved tissue phenotypes of dental, oral, and craniofacial defects require a multidisciplinary approach for reconstruction.

This chapter discusses the major clinical challenges in craniofacial reconstruction, outlines current clinical management approaches, and identifies emerging approaches in tissue engineering and stem cell biology toward biologically based reconstruction of dental, oral, and craniofacial defects. Because of limited space, only selected topics in oral and craniofacial diseases and biologically based reconstruction are discussed. The reader is referred to several insightful and more specialized reviews that have recently been published.[1-8]

CLINICAL NEEDS FOR CRANIOFACIAL BONE AND SOFT TISSUE RECONSTRUCTION

Trauma/Injuries

According to the Centers for Disease Control and Prevention (CDC), more than 5 million individuals were admitted to the emergency department for facial trauma in 2005 in the United States.[9] Facial trauma is considered any injury to the face, including skin lacerations, soft tissue injuries, obstruction to the nasal cavity or sinuses, damage to the orbital sockets, and fracture to the jawbone and teeth.

One of the common causes of oral and craniofacial trauma in children is playground-related injuries (Table 28-1). Emergency departments in the United States treat more than 200,000 playground injuries each year for children age 14 years or younger.[10] The total cost of treating these injuries is estimated at $1.2 billion.[11]

Among the elderly population, falls are the leading cause of injury deaths and the most common cause of injuries and hospital admissions for trauma (Table 28-1). In the United States, one of every three persons age 65 years or older falls each year. The total cost of treating all fall injuries for this age group in 1994 was $27 billion. In 2002, almost 13,000 people age 65 and older died of fall-related injuries. As the number of people over age 65 rises from 31 million in 1990 to 68 million by 2040 in the United States, the cost of fall

TABLE 28-1

Facial Trauma in Young and Elderly Populations, United States (Annual)

Age	Causes	Incidence (million)	Cost (billions)
14 and younger	Playground injuries	0.2	$1.2
65 and older	Falls	1	$27

Data from Office of Technology Assessment, US Congress: *Risks to students in school,* Washington, DC, 1995, US Government Printing Office; and Englander F, Hodson TJ, Terregrossa RA: *J Forensic Sci* 41:733-746, 1996.

injuries is expected to increase to $44 billion (in current dollars).[12] Although the frequency of facial injuries from falling is not high, even a small fraction of fall-related facial injuries can carry a significant cost.

According to the 2005 report of the American Society of Plastic Surgeons, reconstructive surgeries performed for trauma-related injuries (e.g., animal bite, burn care, laceration repair, maxillofacial surgery, scar revision) make up 13% of all reconstructive surgeries performed in the United States. Even though this report does not provide the statistics for facial trauma reconstruction, the economic consequence of facial trauma is significant because facial reconstruction often requires multiple surgeries.

Congenital Deformations

Cleft lip/palate

According to the National Center on Birth Defects and Developmental Disabilities, a division of the CDC, cleft lip/palate occurs in one of every 700 to 1000 live births and is the most common congenital malformations of the head and neck region. A cleft results from the failure of fusion of parts of the lip and/or palate during the early months of prenatal development. The etiology of cleft lip/palate is multifactorial, including genetic defects, nutritional deficiencies, maternal hypoxia, alcohol ingestion, and drug use. Certain medications during the first trimester of pregnancy may contribute to clefts.[13]

Unilateral cleft lip, with or without cleft palate, is one of the most common birth defects in humans and is genetically distinct from isolated cleft palate.[14,15] Relatively few candidate genes have been linked to nonsyndromic cleft lip/palate,[16] although the genetic contribution to nonsyndromic orofacial clefts has been estimated at 20% to 50%.[17] Unilateral cleft lip and palate occurs more commonly in males and more frequently on the left side. Patients with isolated cleft lip may also have a cleft of the anterior part of the maxillary alveolar process. Bilateral clefts and isolated clefts of the lip and palate are not uncommon. Other facial clefts also occur, much less frequently, involving the orbits, zygoma, and commissures of the lip clefts.[13]

TABLE 28-2

Number of Reconstructive Surgeries for Congenital Craniofacial Defects, United States, 2005

Surgery	Number
Birth defect reconstruction	32,000
Cleft lip/palate surgeries	19,000

Data from American Society of Plastic Surgeons, 2005.

The goals of cleft lip/palate therapy are to restore function and improve esthetics. These difficult tasks require multiple interventions and careful coordination between different specialties. The craniofacial team usually consists of oral and maxillofacial surgeon, plastic surgeon, speech pathologist, pediatrician, pediatric dentist, orthodontist, otolaryngologist, and maxillofacial prosthodontist. Other critical members usually include nurses, feeding specialists, psychologists, geneticists, and a social worker.

The American Society of Plastic Surgeons reports that a total of 32,000 birth-defect reconstruction surgeries were performed in 2005, almost 19,000 of which were cleft lip/palate surgeries (Table 28-2). One of the surgical guidelines is the "rule of 10s" before the lip repair. The infant weighs at least 10 pounds, has 10 mg/dL of hemoglobin, and is at least 10 weeks of age. The rule of 10s decreases the risk for anesthetic complications while allowing the doctors to perform additional tests to evaluate for cardiac, pulmonary, or renal abnormalities. Palate repair is usually performed in a single stage at 9 to 18 months of age to promote proper speech development. Additional surgical and dental procedures (orthognathic surgery, bone grafting, orthodontic treatment, pediatric dentistry, prosthodontic treatment) and nondental therapies (additional revision plastic surgery, speech therapy, swallowing therapy) are sometimes needed to address esthetic and functional concerns.

Craniosynostosis

Craniosynostosis, the premature fusion of cranial sutures, is another common craniofacial birth defect, occurring in one of every 2500 live births.[18,19] Premature fusion of one or more cranial sutures prevents subsequent cranial growth surrounding the fused cranial sutures while inducing excessive growth at patent sutures. The net result is craniofacial deformities. Craniosynostosis leads to abnormally high intracranial pressure, impaired cerebral blood flow, airway obstruction, impaired vision and hearing, learning difficulties, and adverse psychological effects.[20] Surgical intervention is currently the only way to relieve intracranial pressure and reshape disfigured skull bones.

Tumors: Oral and Head and Neck Cancers

Each year in the United States, approximately 30,000 people are newly diagnosed with oral and pharyngeal cancer[21]

TABLE 28-3

Estimated New Cancer Cases and Deaths from Oropharyngeal Cancer, United States

Oral Cavity and Pharynx	Estimated New Cases	Estimated Deaths
Tongue	9,040	1,780
Mouth	10,230	1,870
Pharynx	8,950	2,110
Other oral cavity	2,770	1,670
TOTAL	30,990	7,430
Male	20,180	
Female	10,810	

Data from American Cancer Society: *Cancer facts and figures,* 2006.

(Table 28-3). Worldwide, approximately 350,000 to 400,000 oral cancer cases are reported each year, although these undoubtedly represent a fraction of all oral cancer cases. Although oral cancer only accounts for 2% to 4% of all cancers diagnosed annually in the United States, the survival rates of oral cancers are among the lowest of major cancers, according to the CDC. Only half of individuals diagnosed with oral cancers survive 5 years after diagnosis. In contrast to other cancers, such as breast, colorectal, and prostate, the overall U.S. survival rate from oropharyngeal cancer has not improved in the past 16 years.[22] Oral cancer is twice as common in males as females, which is much different from the 5:1 male/female ratio about 40 years ago. Increased tobacco use among women is the main reason for the increases in oral cancer rates. Age is also a factor; 95% of oral cancers occur among persons older than 40, with 60 years the average age at diagnosis.[23]

Resection of oral cancer frequently results in severe disfigurement. The reconstruction of hard and soft tissues of the facial and oral structures is usually a demanding task. One of the key difficulties in reconstruction surgeries of oral cancer is shortage of tissue. Squamous cell carcinoma is the most common malignancy of the oral cavity, but minor salivary gland tumors, primary bone tumors, and tumors of dental origin also occur, with margins greater than 1 cm required to achieve disease control and wide, clear margins.[24]

Chronic Diseases: Temporomandibular Joint Disorders

The National Institute of Dental and Craniofacial Research (NIDCR) of the National Institutes of Health (NIH) states that more than 10 million people in the United States have temporomandibular joint (TMJ) disorders, or jaw joint problems, at any given time. The total direct and indirect cost of TMJ-related disorders is unclear, but the CDC reports that the total cost of arthritis and other rheumatic conditions in the United States in 1997 was $86.2 billion.[25] TMJ disorders include degenerative joint disease, which encompasses a variety of symptoms, including pain in the TMJ region, "joint noise," and limitation of jaw motion.[26] Severely affected patients often endure excruciating pain in everyday activities such as eating, yawning, and talking. In many patients the symptoms may be relieved by a combination of pain control medications, resting the jaw, adopting a soft diet, and applying heat to the muscles. If these conservative techniques are not effective, a clinician may have to consider more invasive procedures that involve replacing the jaw joints with artificial implants.

CURRENT CLINICAL APPROACHES IN RECONSTRUCTION OF CRANIOFACIAL DEFECTS

A wide range of the technical approaches are used to reconstruct disfigured dental, oral, and craniofacial structures including soft tissue grafting and bone grafting by means of autografts, allografts, and xenografts.[27-29] Despite various levels of clinical success, these procedures are limited by donor site morbidity, limited tissue supply, immune rejection, and potential transmission of pathogens.[30-32] Improved surgical reconstructive techniques include pedicled flaps and microvascular free-tissue transfers of composite flaps that can be designed to compensate for both hard and soft tissue deficits. These improved methods still necessitate significant morbidity, however, and the outcome of true form and function is still compromised.

Scientists and clinicians have also explored the field of *growth factor therapy* for treating patients with osseous defects.[33] However, the limitations of growth factor therapy include rapid denaturation and diffusion of the factor, high cost, and potential toxicity.

In 2005, French surgeons performed the first face transplant for a female patient whose face was disfigured by dog attack. The risks of chronic immunosuppression, malignancy, and infection are the major downfall to this risky procedure.[34] Face transplantation is also ethically controversial.[35]

Maxillofacial *prosthetics* are used to restore extraoral and intraoral defects and often represent the least invasive approach. Currently, a myriad of maxillofacial prostheses are used in patients with defects resulting from cancer, trauma, or congenital anomalies. However, retention and stability of a large prosthesis may be difficult. Prosthetic devices can be combined with and can complement flap reconstruction. Microvascular free flaps have several benefits, as well as contraindications. Previous radiation therapy, previous neck surgery, ligation of the facial artery, and other insulting factors decrease the chance of flap survival. Difficulties in preserving rerouting and reimplanting arteries and salivary ducts need to be addressed. Donor site morbidity includes flap reliability, risk of nerve palsy, sensory deficits or intolerances, motor weakness, accessibility, functional impairment, and cosmetic issues.[36-38] Patient occupation may preclude the use of certain donor sites. Tissues that are unhealthy, hair bearing, or in esthetic zones limit potential site selection and outcome. Donor tissue cannot be harvested from sites where this will aggravate facial asymmetry and distort or disrupt overall facial dynamics.

Reconstruction of Tongue Defects

The tongue plays a vital role in speech, swallowing, and mastication and is intimately related to the mandible, dentition, neck, and larynx. Most tongue defects result from surgically resected carcinomas, although traumatic defects are not uncommon after gunshot wounds.

Partial glossectomy reconstruction

Common procedures and flaps for anterior oral tongue reconstruction include primary closure and secondary reepithelialization for smaller defects. Larger defects are restored by allografts, autografts, and regional myocutaneous flaps. For more substantial defects, free-tissue fasciocutaneous transfers from the radial forearm, lateral arm and thigh, and scapula and abdominal free flaps are used for partial to near-total glossectomies. Prosthodontic treatment for partial glossectomies is necessary only when the patient experiences difficulty in speaking or managing a food bolus. Either a palatal or a mandibular augmentation prosthesis may be fabricated. The function of the augmentation prosthesis is to fill the volume deficiency between the remaining tongue and the mandible and palate.

Ventral tongue and floor of mouth reconstruction

The floor of the mouth is the second most common defect after the tongue. Tumor size and characteristics will determine the extent of the resection and type of reconstruction modality. Full-thickness grafts from areas of redundant tissue and split-thickness grafts from areas such as the lateral thigh can be used. Survival of the graft relies on neovascularization, and therefore the recipient bed and the graft must be in good condition and rendered immobile to promote capillary neogenesis. Radiated tissue represents a poor recipient bed, and grafts are contraindicated or likely to fail. Platysma myocutaneous flap can also be used, especially if the defect is continuous with the neck.[39]

For extensive soft tissue reconstruction in the oral cavity, the radial forearm free flap has become immensely popular because it can be shaped to approximate most defects and contains healthy vascular supply with venous outflow. The *radial forearm free flap* (RFFF) provides thin, pliable, and predominantly hairless tissue with reliable vascularity.[40,41] Overall success rate is reported to be 97%.[42] The volar tissue provides large pedicles with nerve anastomosis. Closure of the donor site is accomplished using a split-thickness skin graft. The potential for morbidity of the donor site, the extended operative time, and technical expertise required in free-tissue reconstruction should be weighed during evaluation.

Reconstruction of base of tongue and total glossectomy defects

In almost 70% of oropharyngeal cancers, the base of the tongue is involved.[43] Five-year survival rates for stage 1 and 2 disease remain at 80%.[44] Early-stage tumors are treated by surgery or radiation. Reconstruction is difficult because of inherently compromised tissue. Local control with combined-modality treatment is higher, at 60%. Small to partial base-of-tongue defects can involve primary closure to fasciocutaneous (radial, ulnar, and lateral arm) or myocutaneous pedicled flap (pectoralis major). Subtotal to total glossectomy defects can be addressed with an array of these flaps, including those from the latissimus dorsi, anterolateral thigh, and scapular areas.

Resection of any part of the tongue affects deglutition (swallowing function), articulation (speech intelligibility), and aspiration (airway protection) and compromises motor and sensory function. Functional tongue reconstruction has remained a challenge because of the complex motor function involved in normal deglutition and articulation. Although some current reconstruction techniques employ motor innervation, little if any coordinated muscle function results from these methods. Donor site morbidity, prolonged surgery, and limited collaborative resources may preclude the preferential treatment with microvascular free flaps. Current tongue flaps may severely compromise tongue mobility and thus speech and swallowing.

Defects of Buccal Mucosa and Salivary Ducts

Reconstructive options for the buccal mucosa and salivary ducts usually involve the use of split-thickness skin grafts. These grafts have low patient donor site morbidity but can experience significant graft contracture and scar band formation at the mucosal junction. The use of acellular human collagen matrix (Alloderm, Lifecell Corporation, Branchburg, N.J.) has also been described for the reconstruction of mucosal defects.[45] Preserving the elasticity of the buccal mucosa is advantageous because large scar bands may significantly hinder jaw opening, mastication, and mobilization of the food bolus.

The most common reconstructive method for buccal mucosa is the RFFF, with a success rate of up to 95%.[46] However, the deficiencies of RFFF include the lengthy recovery time, rehabilitation of the forearm, and high demand for microvascular expertise. Other free-tissue transfers are possible using the lateral arm, latissimus dorsi, rectus abdominus, and lateral thigh to fill in buccal defects that may arise from resection of the buccinator muscle and buccal fat, which leads to hollowing of the midface if left unreconstructed.

Hard Palate Reconstruction

The hard palate is essential to separating the oral cavity from the nasal and sinus cavities, thus allowing proper phonation and articulation, as well as breathing and chewing. Hard palate defects result in the oral cavity, maxillary sinus, and nasal cavity becoming one confluent chamber. Maxillofacial prostheses have a primary role in reconstruction of palatal defects by obturating the cavity, sealing the palate, and providing dentition. Prosthetic intervention, when desired, should occur at surgery, and surgical enhancements can maximize the prosthetic outcome and patient acceptance.

To maximize retention and stability of the prosthesis, as much of the hard palate and dentition as possible should be retained. The premaxillary region enhances stability and support and is extremely important in minimizing the fulcrum of prosthesis into the defect and, if preserved, reduces the collapse of the facial form and postoperative contracture. The medial margin of the defect should be covered with palatal mucosa for added tolerance and stability. Similarly, a split-thickness skin graft is recommended to cover the denuded surfaces of the cheek to reduce healing time, prevent the migration of respiratory epithelium, and allow for a keratinized denture-bearing surface. A lateral scar band will occur at the junction of the skin graft with the remaining buccal mucosa, attributed to providing retention through an anatomical undercut. A split-thickness skin graft can also be applied to the sinus walls, thus providing additional area for retention and reducing mucus production. In larger defects, removal of the inferior turbinate is also recommended to allow for the medial wall of the obturator bulb to extend into the nasal cavity.[47,48] The additional height counters rotation of the prosthesis during function.

A surgical obturator should be provided immediately at resection to act as a matrix for the surgical dressing and permit speech and swallowing postoperatively, often eliminating the need for a nasogastric tube. In addition, the obturator prevents oral contamination of the surgical site while psychologically assisting the patient by restoring normal palatal contours. Screws, sutures, or ligature wire can be used initially to secure the prosthesis. An interim obturator is delivered 1 week later and can be customized to enhance stability, retention, and esthetics. After the resected area has stabilized (6-12 months later), a final obturator prosthesis is fabricated.

Various pedicled autogenous tissues have been described to correct palatal defects but may be limited by the lack of tissue bulk, length of vascular pedicle, and need for multiple stages of reconstruction to achieve the final result. Alternatively, microvascular free-tissue transfer offers adequate amounts of bone and soft tissue bulk that can be transferred in a single-stage procedure. Various free-tissue transfers, including myocutaneous, myofacial, and osteocutaneous flaps, can be used for reconstruction of the palate and midface. The radial forearm, latissumus dorsi, rectus abdominus, scapular, fibular, and iliac crest flaps are most often used.[49]

The thin, pliable tissue characteristics of the RFFF allow the palate to be sealed and to serve as a potential surface for dentures. In addition, the radial bone can be used to recreate the maxillary arch and can support osseointegrated implants.[50] Radial bone can reconstruct the premaxillary area and thus help support the upper lip and nasal base. The scapular osteocutaneous flap has the advantage of a soft tissue component that can be rotated around adequate vascularized bone and can support implants. This is especially advantageous in the edentulous patient who requires a dental prosthesis. The fibular free flap and the iliac crest free flap tissue transfers have been shown to have an adequate column of bone to support osseointegrated implants.[51-53]

Surgical reconstruction of large defects may fail to reproduce palatal contour, which adversely affects bolus control and speech. Also, bulky flaps may prevent placement of an intraoral prosthesis.

Reconstruction of Cleft Lip/Palate

Complex congenital deformities such as cleft lip and palate have significant physical and psychological effects and require multidisciplinary management. Timing of repair and reconstructive options depend on severity and extent of the deformity, consideration of speech development, facial growth, psychological effects, and safety of anesthesia. Various palatoplasty approaches have been described, including two-flap palatoplasty for complete unilateral and bilateral clefts, three-flap palatoplasty for incomplete clefts, and double-reversing Z-plasty for submucosal clefts and incomplete secondary palate clefts.

Although plastic surgery has made great advances in the area of cleft surgery, surgical repair cannot alone solve the multiple problems encountered with the deformities that result from cleft lip and palate. Creation of an esthetically acceptable columnella and the deformity of nasal cartilages are especially difficult. Prosthetic intervention with a *presurgical nasoalveolar molding device* (PNAM) addresses these problems using an intraoral plate and nasal extension that dynamically repositions the deformed nasal cartilages and alveolar processes while lengthening the deficient columnella.[54,55] Continual modifications to this appliance ameliorate the initial cleft nasal deformity and can eliminate the need for surgical correction of the columnella while minimizing the extent of scarring of the oronasal complex. Possible disadvantages of the PNAM include soft tissue breakdown when forces exceed tissue tolerances. Success of the appliance is based on parental compliance and dedicated, consistent, and proper use of the device. When used in conjunction with a modified surgical approach, the PNAM allows for a single initial surgical procedure to address the lip-nose-alveolar complex and its deformity, and it decreases the number of future corrective surgeries.

For cleft palate patients who have not been surgically treated, the anterior nasal communication is addressed using an obturator, as previously described. Often a patient with an unrestored cleft palate presents with complicated occlusion issues, including an undesirable maxillomandibular relationship. Teeth adjacent to the defect may be compromised because of poor bone quality and should be splinted for preservation. The patient requires fabrication of a removable partial denture or a complete denture prosthesis that will simultaneously repair the defect, restore the continuity to the premaxilla, ensure occlusal function, and create an esthetic appearance.

EMERGING APPROACHES: STEM CELLS AND TISSUE ENGINEERING

Oral and craniofacial defects have a high demand for multiple tissue phenotypes and frequently present with many complex issues for reconstruction. Current approaches for facial reconstruction are limited by several intrinsic deficiencies. For example, autologous tissue grafts necessitate donor site morbidity; prostheses do not integrate with host tissues; and allogeneic and other grafts are associated with immune incompatibility and potential pathogen transmission. Clinicians and scientists have attempted to restore facial defects with the patient's own stem cells in approaches that minimize current deficiencies such as donor site morbidity, immunorejection, pathogen transmission, and suboptimal repair. Recent studies have demonstrated the proof of the principle of using stem cells in the reconstruction of dental, oral, and craniofacial defects.[2,4]

Large-scale tissue-engineering research, in craniofacial or other areas, began in the early 1990s after the discovery of stem cells that not only can self-renew, but also are capable of differentiating into multiple cell lineages. So far, substantial advances have been made in tissue engineering because of advances in seemingly unrelated disciplines, including cell and molecular biology, polymer chemistry, molecular genetics, materials science, robotics, and mechanical engineering, converged into the self-assembling field of tissue engineering.[56,57]

Stem Cells

The complex three-dimensional form of the face arises from the growth and fusion of several embryonic *primordia.* The middle and upper regions of the face are derived from the frontonasal process, the cheeks and upper portion of the jaw from the paired maxillary primordia, and the lower aspects of the jaw from the mandibular primordia. These primordia are populated by mesenchymal cells that are multipotent and capable of differentiating into osteoblasts, chondrocytes, adipocytes, and fibroblasts.[3,58-60] Mesenchymal cells are derivatives of embryonic stem cells, a few hundred cells of the inner mass of the blastocyst. Embryonic stem cells differentiate into neural crest cells that in turn migrate to form facial primordia.[61,62]

What is the difference between the mesenchymal cells and the mesenchymal *stem* cells (MSCs)? Although there is no clear answer, the following conjecture is provided on the basis of fragmented experimental evidence. The MSC is likely the product of an asymmetrical division of mesenchymal cell. While one offspring cell differentiates toward an end-stage cell, the other cell replicates into an offspring mesenchymal cell. On completion of morphogenesis, the residual offsprings of mesenchymal cells probably continue to reside in various craniofacial tissues and retain their status as stem cells, capable of self-renewal and differentiation into multiple progeny. In the adult, MSCs maintain physiologically necessary tissue turnover and, with injury or disease, differentiate to enable tissue regeneration.[3,4]

Mesenchymal stem cells have been experimentally differentiated into virtually all mesenchymal or connective tissue lineages.[3,58-60] In many cases, MSCs have also been used to generate craniofacial structures in vivo that their prenatal predecessors, mesenchymal cells, are capable of generating during development. Figure 28-1 provides an example to demonstrate that human MSCs have been differentiated into chondrocytes, osteoblasts, and adipocytes, three cell lineages that form the bulk of craniofacial tissue phenotypes. To engineer a functional biological structure, cells must be instructed to differentiate and to synthesize the appropriate extracellular matrix molecules in the overall shape and dimensions of the diseased or missing tissues or organs.[2] Biomimetic scaffolds are frequently needed to enable cell growth and differentiation in an environment previously unfamiliar to biologists or engineers. Craniofacial structures offer complex and, in many cases, unique challenges when engineered.

Bioengineered Replacement of the Temporomandibular Joint

Because many people have joint diseases such as osteoarthritis and rheumatoid arthritis, considerable effort has been made to regenerate TMJ structures (Fig. 28-2). Regeneration of a mandibular condyle represents a substantial challenge because the mandibular joint, as with other joints, consists of stratified layers of cartilage and bone. Progress has been made in regenerating a human-sized mandibular condyle using MSCs[1,3,63,64] (Fig. 28-3).

To regenerate mandibular condyle, rat or human MSCs were first isolated from bone marrow and exposed separately to chondrogenic or osteogenic supplemented culture medium.[1,30] Polyethylene glycol diacrylate (PEGDA) was dissolved in phosphate-buffered saline (PBS) with a biocompatible ultraviolet photoinitiator. MSC-derived cells were encapsulated in PEGDA hydrogel into a negative mold of an adult human cadaver mandibular condyle in two stratified but integrated layers. This construct was implanted in the dorsum of immunodeficient mice for up to 12 weeks. When 20×10^6 cells/mL was used, the tissue-engineered mandibular joint condyles retained the shape and dimensions of the cadaver mandibular condyle. The chondrogenic and osteogenic portions remained in their respective layers.[63] The chondrogenic layer was positively stained by chondrogenic marker, safranin O, and contained type II collagen. In the deep layer, near the interface between cartilaginous and osseous layers, hypertrophic chondrocytes were characterized by the expression of type X collagen. In contrast, only the osteogenic markers, such as osteopontin and osteonectin, stained the osseous layer. Most importantly, there was mutual infiltration of the cartilaginous and osseous components into each other's territory that resembled mandibular condyle.

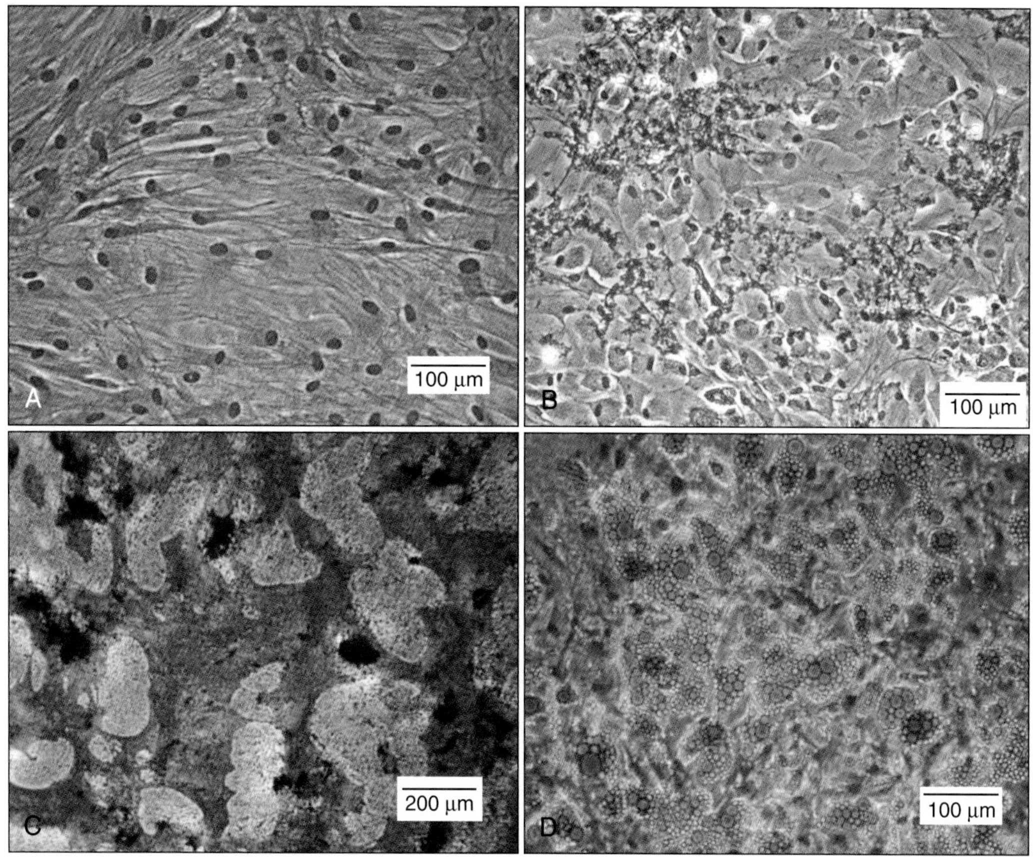

Fig. 28-1 **A,** Human mesenchymal stem cells (MSCs) isolated from anonymous adult human bone marrow donor after culture expansion on hematoxylin and eosin (H&E) staining. Further enrichment of MSCs can be accomplished by positive selection using cell surface markers, including STRO-1, CD 133 (prominin, AC133), p75LNGFR (p75, low-affinity nerve growth factor receptor), CD29, CD44, CD90, CD105, *c-kit,* SH2 (CD105), SH3, SH4 (CD73), CD71, CD 106, CD120a, CD124, and HLA-DR or negative selection. **B,** Chondrocytes derived from human MSCs showing positive staining to Alcian blue. **C,** Osteoblasts derived from human MSCs showing positive von Kossa staining for calcium deposition *(black)* and active alkaline phosphatase enzyme *(red).* **D,** Adipocytes derived from human MSCs showing positive Oil Red-O staining of intracellular lipids. Additional molecular and genetic markers can be used to further characterize MSC-derived chondrocytes, osteoblasts, and adipocytes. (From Marion NW, Mao JJ: *Methods Enzymol* 420:339-361, 2006.)

Dental Tissue Engineering: Dentin and Periodontal Ligament Regeneration

Cells with properties of adult stem cells have been isolated from dental pulp, exfoliated deciduous teeth, and periodontal ligament (PDL).[65-68] After confirming that *dental pulp stem cells* (DPSCs) differentiate into multiple lineages, their capacity to form dentin-like structures was studied following in vivo implantation.[69] *Stem cells from human exfoliated deciduous teeth* (SHED) have also been differentiated into odontoblast-like cells, which in turn produced small, dentin-like structures.[68]

Isolated stem cells from human PDL have been shown to regenerate cementum/PDL-like structures that resemble the native PDL as a thin layer of cementum and interfaced with dense collagen fibers, similar to Sharpey's fibers.[70] The potential to reconstruct periodontal tissue defects[8,71] and periodontal attachment structures in vivo[72-76] has been studied using transplanted periodontal stem cells. Cementoblasts have a marked ability to induce mineralization in an ex vivo model[77] and in vivo with periodontal wounds.[78] Bone marrow–derived MSCs transplanted into periodontal osseous defects are capable of regenerating periodontal tissue in furcation defects.[79]

Regeneration of the periodontium not only is meaningful in the field of periodontology, but also has implications in orthodontics, oral surgery, and prosthodontics. By repairing periodontal defects, orthodontists and oral surgeons can place temporary anchorage devices and dental implants to improve anchorage for orthodontic movement and restore missing teeth, respectively. Also, improving bony defects in the mouth will allow orthodontists to position the teeth

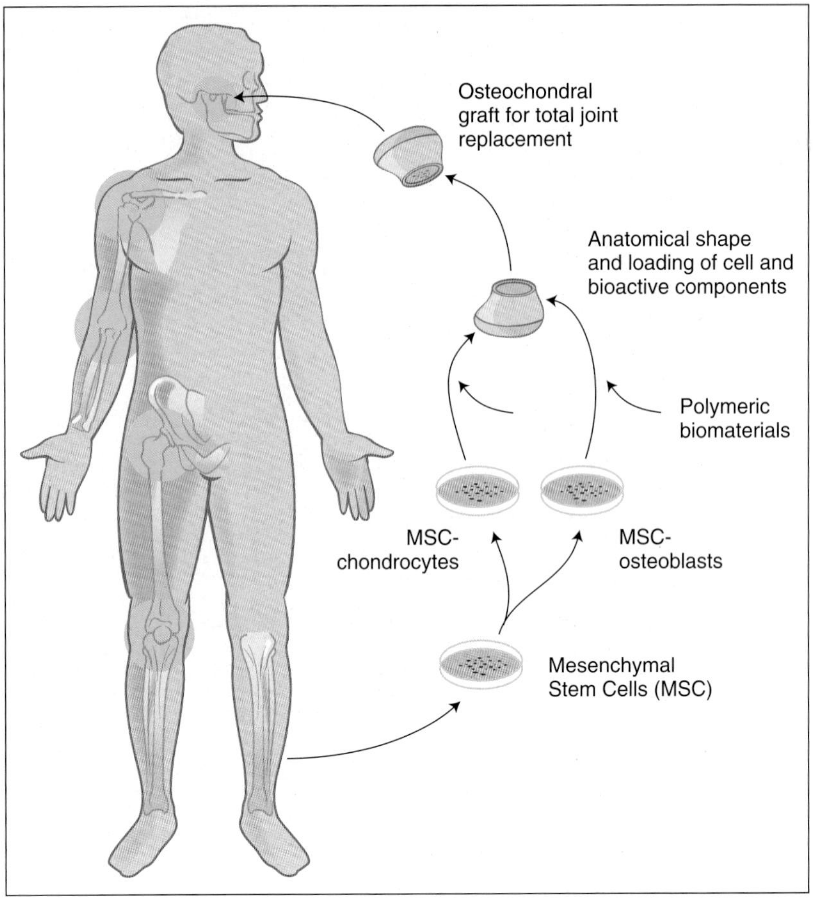

Fig. 28-2 Autologous, MSC-based tissue-engineering therapy for total joint replacement. Progenitor cells such as MSCs are isolated from the bone marrow or other connective sources (e.g., adipose tissue), culture-expanded, and/or differentiated ex vivo toward chondrocytes and osteoblasts. Cells are seeded in biocompatible materials shaped into the anatomical structures of the synovial joint condyle and implanted in vivo. Preliminary proof-of-concept studies have been reported. (Redrawn from Marion NW, Mao JJ: *Methods Enzymol* 420:339-361, 2006.)

into sites where it was not possible without regenerative therapy.

Craniofacial Bone Engineering

The most common surgical approaches for reconstructing craniofacial bone defects include autogenous bone, allogeneic materials, and prosthetic compounds such as metal and plastic.[80-86] Despite certain levels of clinical success, each of these strategies has major limitations, such as donor site morbidity, rejection, infection, and device failure.

Stem cell–based strategies for craniofacial bone reconstruction may overcome these deficiencies. *Adipose-derived mesenchymal cells* (AMCs) are multipotent and capable of differentiation into muscle, bone, and cartilage cells.[86-90] AMCs have been isolated through lipoaspirate.[89-91] The AMCs were seeded in apatite-coated polylactic co-glycolic acid (PLGA) scaffolds and implanted in the surgically created, critical-size calvarial defects, and they induced new bone formation similar to bone marrow–derived MSCs or osteoblasts.[86]

Radiation therapy is a common procedure for oral cancer patients. Irradiation severely affects bone marrow stroma, remodeling, and fracture healing.[92,93] Another adverse effect of radiation therapy is increased apoptosis and compromised vascularization, which complicates reconstructive surgery.[94,95] To promote bone formation in irradiated sites, recombinant human bone morphogenetic protein-2 (BMP-2)–treated hydroxyapatite disks were effective in regenerating bone, although healing was incomplete.[96] A combination of pedicle muscle flap with BMP-3 treatment was effective in bone regeneration in irradiated sites, suggesting the need for a well-vascularized recipient bed and an adequate population of responsive osteogenic cells.[97] Bone formation by transplanted bone marrow stromal cells is enhanced by the concurrent administration of anabolic doses of parathyroid hormone.[98] Another side effect of irradiation therapy for malignant head and neck cancer patients is xerostomia, or dry mouth. Preliminary results of salivary gland regeneration have been reported using primary human salivary cells to form acinar gland–like structures that express amylase.[99,100]

CONCLUSION

Defects of the face are common and particularly detrimental to the psychosocial well-being of patients. Current treatment approaches have used the patient's own tissues, allogeneic grafts, or synthetic implants. As a shift of paradigm, craniofacial tissue engineering aims to replace defects with cells capable of developing into the relevant tissues. An increasing number of proof-of-concept studies, including those

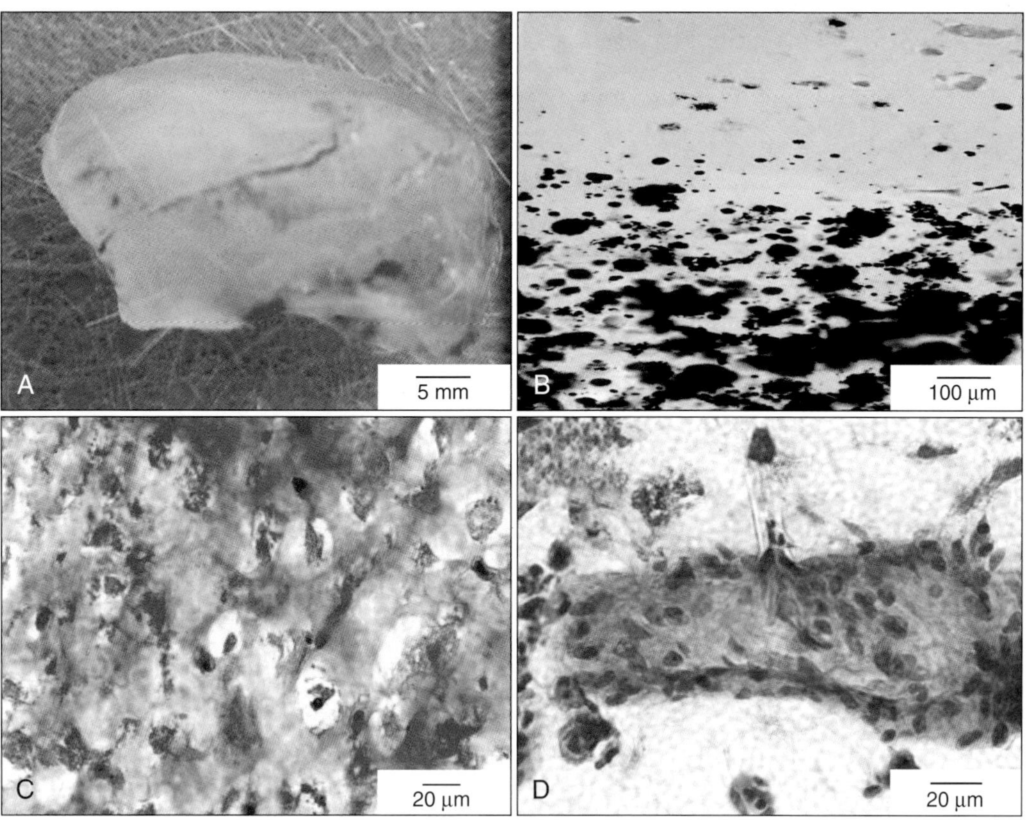

Fig. 28-3 Engineered neogenesis of human-shaped mandibular condyle from MSCs. **A,** Harvested osteochondral construct retained the shape and dimension of the cadaver human mandibular condyle after in vivo implantation. *Scale bar:* 5 mm. **B,** Von Kossa–stained section showing the interface between stratified chondral and osseous layers. Multiple mineralization nodules are present in the osseous layer (lower half of photomicrograph), but absent in the chondral layer. **C,** Positive safranin O staining of the chondrogenic layer indicates the synthesis of abundant glycosaminoglycans. **D,** H&E-stained section of the osteogenic layer showing a representative osseous island-like structure consisting of MSC-differentiated osteoblast-like cells on the surface and in the center. (μm = micron.) (From Mao JJ, Giannobile WV, Helms JA, et al: *J Dent Res* 85:966-979, 2006.)

described in this chapter, have identified the feasibility of "growing" craniofacial tissues and organs in vivo. This effort of cell-based craniofacial reconstruction represents an unprecedented approach in biomedical research, requiring a synthesis of engineering, biology, and genetics. By definition, craniofacial reconstruction requires multidisciplinary and interdisciplinary approaches. Despite the remarkable progress of craniofacial tissue engineering within less than 10 years since its inception, the following important issues still must be addressed for the field to continue moving forward.

- What are the optimal sources of cells for craniofacial regeneration?
- Are these sources derived from bone marrow, adipose tissue, teeth, or other sites?
- How do we design and fabricate scaffolds that accommodate the complex and often multiple tissue phenotypes of the dental, oral, and craniofacial structures?

For the field of orthodontics, possible changes may include biologically derived periodontium, including single or multiple elements, such as PDL, cementum/alveolar bone, tissue-engineered TMJ, and cell-based bone grafts for congenital anomalies such as cleft palate. Also, orthodontics specialty students must become involved in cell-based approaches of dental, oral, and craniofacial regeneration. The impact of cell-based craniofacial reconstruction on the practice of orthodontics is expected to be substantial.

ACKNOWLEDGMENTS

This chapter is dedicated to Dr. Ram Nanda, for his commitment to orthodontics education and research. We thank Dr. Ravi Nanda and Dr. Sunil Kapila for providing the opportunity to participate in this highly meritorious effort. We are grateful to Sarah Kennedy for technical assistance. We appreciate the administrative assistance from Richard

Abbott and Janina Acloque. This research was supported by NIH grants DE15391 and EB006261 to J.J.M.

References

1. Alhadlaq A, Mao JJ: Tissue-engineered neogenesis of human-shaped mandibular condyle from rat mesenchymal stem cells, *J Dent Res* 82:951-956, 2003.
2. Rahaman MN, Mao JJ: Stem cell–based composite tissue constructs for regenerative medicine, *Biotechnol Bioeng* 91:261-284, 2005.
3. Marion NW, Mao JJ: Mesenchymal stem cells and tissue engineering, *Methods Enzymol* 420:339-361, 2006.
4. Mao JJ, Giannobile WV, Helms JA, et al: Craniofacial tissue engineering by stem cells, *J Dent Res* 85:966-979, 2006.
5. Garcia-Godoy F, Murray PE: Status and potential commercial impact of stem cell–based treatments on dental and craniofacial regeneration, *Stem Cells Dev* 15:881-887, 2006.
6. Robey PG, Bianco P: The use of adult stem cells in rebuilding the human face, *J Am Dent Assoc* 137:961-972, 2006.
7. Yen AH, Sharpe PT: Regeneration of teeth using stem cell-based tissue engineering, *Expert Opin Biol Ther* 6:9-16, 2006.
8. Risbud MV, Shapiro IM: Stem cells in craniofacial and dental tissue engineering, *Orthod Craniofac Res* 8:54-59, 2005.
9. Centers for Disease Control and Prevention, Atlanta, 2006, CDC.
10. Tinsworth D, McDonald J: *Injuries and deaths associated with children's playground equipment* (special study), Washington, DC, 2001, US Consumer Product Safety Commission.
11. Office of Technology Assessment, US Congress: Risks to students in school, Washington, DC, 1995, US Government Printing Office.
12. Englander F, Hodson TJ, Terregrossa RA: Economic dimensions of slip and fall injuries, *J Forensic Sci* 41:733-746, 1996.
13. Management of the child with cleft lip and palate, *AAOMS Surg Update* 20(1), 2006.
14. Bear JC: A genetic study of facial clefting in Northern England, *Clin Genet* 9:277-284, 1976.
15. Fraser FC: Animal models for craniofacial disorders, *Prog Clin Biol Res* 46:1-23, 1980.
16. Schutte BC, Murray JC: The many faces and factors of orofacial clefts, *Hum Mol Genet* 8:1853-1859, 1999.
17. Wyszynsky DF et al: Genetics of nonsyndromic oral clefts revisited, *Cleft Palate Craniofac J* 33:406-417, 1996.
18. Hunter AGW, Rudd NL: Craniosynostosis. I. Sagittal synostosis: its genetics and associated clinical findings in 214 patients who lacked involvement of the coronal suture(s), *Teratology* 14:185-194, 1976.
19. Lajeune E, Le Merrer M, Bonaiti-Pellie C, et al: Genetic study of scaphonephaly, *Am J Med Genet* 62:282-285, 1996.
20. Wilkie AOM, Morriss-Kay GM, Jones EY, Heath JK: Functions of fibroblasts growth factors and their receptors, *Curr Biol* 5:500-507, 1995.
21. Greenlee RT, Hill-Harmon MB, Murray T, Thun M: Cancer statistics, 2001, *CA Cancer J Clin* 51:15-36, 2001.
22. Mashberg A, Samit A: Early diagnosis of asymptomatic oral and oropharyngeal squamous cancers, *CA Cancer J Clin* 45:328-351, 1995.
23. Silverman S Jr: *Oral cancer*, ed 4, Hamilton, Ontario, 1998, American Cancer Society.
24. Palme CE, Gullane PJ: Principles and history of oral cavity reconstruction. In Day TA, Girod DA, editors: *Oral cavity reconstruction,* New York, 2006, Taylor and Francis Group, p 2.
25. Yelin E, Cisternas MG, Pasta DJ, et al: Medical care expenditures and earnings losses of persons with arthritis and other rheumatic conditions in the United States in 1997: total and incremental estimates, *Arthritis Rheum* 50:2317-2326, 2004.
26. Okeson JP: *Management of temporomandibular disorders and occlusion*, ed 4, St. Louis, 1996, Mosby-Year Book.
27. Bugbee WD: Fresh osteochondral allografts, *J Knee Surg* 15:191-195, 2002.
28. Jakob RP, Franz T, Gautier E, Manil-Verlet P: Autologous osteochondral grafting in the knee: indication, results, and reflections, *Clin Orthop* 401:170-184, 2002.
29. Tom JA, Rodeo SA: Soft tissue allografts for knee reconstruction in sports medicine, *Clin Orthop* 402:135-136, 2002.
30. Alhadlaq A, Elisseeff JH, Hong L, et al: Adult stem cell driven genesis of human-shaped articular condyle, *Ann Biomed Eng* 32:911-923, 2004.
31. Buckwalter JA: Articular cartilage injuries, *Clin Orthop* 402:21-37, 2002.
32. Hagody L, Feczko P, Bartha L, et al: Mosaicplasty for the treatment of articular defects of the knee and ankle, *Clin Orthop* 391(Suppl): S328-S336, 2002.
33. Bruder SP, Jaiswal N, Ricalton NS, et al: Mesenchymal stem cells in osteobiology and applied bone regeneration, *Clin Orthop* 355:S247-S256, 1998.
34. Robertson JA: Face transplants: enriching the debate, *Am J Bioeth* 4:32-33, 2004.
35. Preminger BA, Fins JJ: Face transplantation: an extraordinary case with lessons for ordinary practice, *Plast Reconstr Surg* 118:1073-1074, 2006.
36. Richardson D, Fischer SE, Vaughan ED, Brown JS: Radial forearm flap donor-site complications and morbidity: a prospective study, *Plast Reconstr Surg* 99:109-115, 1997.
37. Schoeller T, Otto A, Wechselberger G, Lille S: Radial forearm flap donor-site complications and morbidity, *Plast Reconstr Surg* 101:874-875, 1998.
38. Skoner JM, Bascom DA, Cohen JI, et al: Short-term functional donor morbidity after radial forearm fasciocutaneous free flap harvest, *Laryngoscope* 113:2091-2094, 2003.
39. Futrell JW, Johns ME, Edgerton MT, et al: Platysma myocutaneous flap for intraoral reconstruction, *Am J Surg* 136:504-507, 1978.
40. Yang GF, Chen PJ, Gao YZ, et al: Forearm free skin flap transplantation: a report of 56 cases, *Br J Plast Surg* 50:162-165, 1997.
41. Soutar DS, Scheker LR, Tanner NS, McGregor IA: The radial forearm flap: a versatile method for intra-oral reconstruction, *Br J Plast Surg* 36:1-8, 1983.
42. Evans GR, Schusterman MA, Kroll SS, et al: The radial forearm free flap for head and neck reconstruction: a review, *Am J Surg* 168:446-450, 1994.
43. Wax MK, Smith DS: Reconstruction of the base of tongue and total glossectomy defects. In Day TA, Girod DA, editors: *Oral cavity reconstruction,* New York, 2006, Taylor and Francis Group, p 223.
44. Prince S, Bailey BM: Squamous carcinoma of the tongue: review, *Br J Oral Maxillofac Surg* 37:164-174, 1999.

45. Rhee PH, Friedman CD, Ridge JA, Kusiak J: The use of processed allograft dermal matrix for intraoral resurfacing: an alternative to split-thickness skin grafts, *Arch Otolaryngol Head Neck Surg* 124:1201-1204, 1998.
46. Haughey BH, Wilson E, Kluwe L, et al: Free flap reconstruction of the head and neck: analysis of 241 cases, *Otolaryngol Head Neck Surg* 125:10-17, 2001.
47. Curtis TA, Beumer J 3rd: Restoration of acquired hard palate defects. In Beumer J 3rd, Curtis TA, Marunick MT, editors: *Maxillofacial rehabilitation: prosthodontic and surgical considerations,* St Louis, 1996, Ishiyaku EuroAmerica, pp 233-237.
48. Jacob RF: Clinical management of the edentulous maxillectomy patient. In Taylor TD, editor: *Clinical maxillofacial prosthetics,* Chicago, 2000, Quintessence, pp 85-87.
49. Wadsworth JT, Futran N: Hard palate reconstruction. In Day TA, Girod DA, editors: *Oral cavity reconstruction,* New York, 2006, Taylor and Francis Group, p 255.
50. Cordiero PG, Bacilious N, Schantz S, Spiro R: The radial forearm osteocutaneous "sandwich" free flap for reconstruction of the bilateral subtotal maxillectomy defect, *Ann Plast Surg* 40:397-402, 1998.
51. Sadove RC, Powell LA: Simultaneous maxillary and mandibular reconstruction with one free osteocutaneous flap, *Plast Reconstr Surg* 92:141-146, 1993.
52. Nakayama B, Matsuura H, Ishihara O, et al: Functional reconstruction of a bilateral maxillectomy defect using a fibular osteocutaneous flap with osseointegrated implants, *Plast Reconstr Surg* 96:1201-1204, 1993.
53. Anthony JP, Foster RD, Sharma AB, et al: Reconstruction of a complex midfacial defect with the folded fibular free flap and osseointegrated implants, *Ann Plast Surg* 37:204-210, 1996.
54. Grayson BH, Santiago PE, Brecht LE, Cutting CB: Presurgical nasoalveolar molding in infants with cleft lip and palate, *Cleft Palate Craniofac J* 36:486-498, 1999.
55. Bennun RD, Figueroa AA: Dynamic presurgical nasal remodeling in patients with unilateral and bilateral cleft lip and palate: modification of the original technique, *Cleft Palate Craniofac J* 43:639-648, 2006.
56. Nerem RM: Cellular engineering, *Ann Biomed Eng* 19:529-545, 1991.
57. Langer R, Vacanti P: Tissue engineering, *Science* 260:920-926, 1993.
58. Caplan AI: Mesenchymal stem cells, *J Orthop Res* 9:641-650, 1991.
59. Pittenger MF, Mackay AM, Beck SC, et al: Multi-lineage potential of adult human mesenchymal stem cells, *Science* 284:143-147, 1999.
60. Alhadlaq A, Mao JJ: Mesenchymal stem cells: isolation and therapeutics, *Stem Cells Dev* 13:436-448, 2004.
61. Noden DM: The role of the neural crest in patterning of avian cranial skeletal, connective, and muscle tissues, *Dev Biol* 96(1):144-165, 1983.
62. Couly GF, Coltey PM, Le Douarin NM: The triple origin of skull in higher vertebrates: a study in quail-chick chimeras, *Development* 117:409-429, 1993.
63. Alhadlaq A, Mao JJ: Tissue engineered osteochondral constructs in the shape of an articular condyle, *J Bone Joint Surg Am* 87:936-944, 2005.
64. Troken A, Mao JJ: Cell density in TMJ tissue engineering. Articular cartilage tissue engineering (special issue), *J Eng Med,* 2007 (in press).
65. Gronthos S, Mankani M, Brahim J, et al: Postnatal human dental pulp stem cells (DPSCs) in vitro and in vivo, *Proc Natl Acad Sci USA* 97:13625-13630, 2000.
66. Shi S, Robey PG, Gronthos S: Comparison of human dental pulp and bone marrow stromal stem cells by cDNA microarray analysis, *Bone* 29:532-539, 2001.
67. Batouli S, Miura M, Brahim J, et al: Comparison of stem-cell-mediated osteogenesis and dentinogenesis, *J Dent Res* 82:976-981, 2003.
68. Miura M, Gronthos S, Zhao M, et al: SHED: stem cells from human exfoliated deciduous teeth, *Proc Natl Acad Sci USA* 100:5807-5812, 2003.
69. Shi S, Gronthos S: Perivascular niche of postnatal mesenchymal stem cells in human bone marrow and dental pulp, *J Bone Miner Res* 18:696-704, 2003.
70. Seo BM, Miura M, Gronthos S, et al: Investigation of multipotent postnatal stem cells from human periodontal ligament, *Lancet* 364:149-155, 2004.
71. Thesleff I, Tummers M: Stem cells and tissue engineering: prospects for regenerating tissues in dental practice, *Med Princ Pract* 12(Suppl 1):43-50, 2003.
72. Lekic PC, Rajshankar D, Chen H, et al: Transplantation of labeled periodontal ligament cells promotes regeneration of alveolar bone, *Anat Rec* 262:193-202, 2001.
73. Dogan A, Ozdemir A, Kubar A, Oygur T: Healing of artificial fenestration defects by seeding of fibroblast-like cells derived from regenerated periodontal ligament in a god: a preliminary study, *Tissue Eng* 9:1189-1196, 2003.
74. Nakahara T, Nakamura T, Tobayashi E, et al: In situ tissue engineering of periodontal tissues by seeding with periodontal ligament–derived cells, *Tissue Eng* 10:537-544, 2004.
75. Akizuki T, Oda S, Komaki M, et al: Application of periodontal ligament cell sheet for periodontal regeneration: a pilot study in beagle dogs, *J Periodont Res* 40:245-251, 2005.
76. Hasegawa M, Yamato M, Kikushi A, et al: Human periodontal ligament cell sheets can regenerate periodontal ligament tissue in an athymic rat model, *Tissue Eng* 11:469-478, 2005.
77. Jin QM, Anusaksathien O, Webb SA, et al: Gene therapy of bone morphogenetic protein for periodontal tissue engineering, *J Periodontol* 74:202-213, 2003.
78. Zhao M, Jin Q, Berry JE, et al: Cementoblast delivery for periodontal tissue engineering, *J Periodontol* 75:154-161, 2004.
79. Kawaguchi H, Hirachi A, Hasegawa N, et al: Enhancement of periodontal tissue regeneration by transplantation of bone marrow mesenchymal stem cells, *J Periodontol* 75:1281-1287, 2004.
80. Marchac D: Split-rib grafts in craniofacial surgery, *Plast Reconstr Surg* 69:566-567, 1982.
81. Shenaq SM: Reconstruction of complex cranial and craniofacial defects utilizing iliac crest–internal oblique microsurgical free flap, *Microsurgery* 9:154-158, 1998.
82. Goodrich JT, Argamaso R, Hall CD: Split-thickness bone graft in complex craniofacial reconstructions, *Pediatr Neurosurg* 18:195-201, 1992.
83. Nicholson JW: Glass-ionomers in medicine and dentistry, *Proc Inst Mech Eng H* 212:121-126, 1998.
84. Rah DK: Art of replacing craniofacial bone defects, *Yonsei Med J* 41:756-765, 2000.
85. Bruens ML, Pieterman H, de Wijn JR, Vaandrager JM: Porous polymethylmethacrylate as bone substitute in the craniofacial area, *J Cranofac Surg* 14:63-68, 2003.

86. Cowan CM, Shi YY, Aalami OO, et al: Adipose-derived adult stromal cells heal critical-size mouse calvarial defects, *Nat Biotechnol* 22:560-567, 2004.
87. Gimble JM, Builak F: Differentiation potential of adipose-derived adult stem (ADAS) cells, *Curr Top Dev Biol* 58:137-160, 2003.
88. Hicok KC, Du Laney TV, Zhou YS, et al: Human adipose-derived adult stem cells produce osteoid in vivo, *Tissue Eng* 10:371-380, 2004.
89. Zuk PA, Zhu M, Mizuno H, et al: Multilineage cells from human adipose tissue: implications for cell-based therapies, *Tissue Eng* 7:211-228, 2001.
90. Zuk PA, Zhu M, Ashjian P, et al: Human adipose tissue is a source of multipotent stem cells, *Mol Biol Cell* 13:4279-4295, 2002.
91. De Ugarte DA, Morizono K, Elbarbary A, et al: Comparison of multi-lineage cells from human adipose tissue and bone marrow, *Cells Tissues Organs* 174:101-109, 2003.
92. Mitchell MJ, Logan PM: Radiation-induced changes in bone, *Radiographics* 18:1125-1136, 1998.
93. Spear MA, Dupuy DE, Park JJ, et al: Tolerance of autologous and allogeneic bone grafts to therapeutic radiation in humans, *Int J Radiat Oncol Biol Phys* 45:1275-1280, 1999.
94. Okunieff P, Mester M, Wang J, et al: In vivo radioprotective effects of angiogenic growth factors on the small bowel of C3H mice, *Radiat Res* 150:204-211, 1998.
95. Okunieff P, Wang X, Rubin P, et al: Radiation-induced changes in bone perfusion and angiogenesis, *Int J Radiat Oncol Biol Phys* 42:885-889, 1998.
96. Wurzler KK, DeWeese TL, Sebald W, Reddi AH: Radiation-induced impairment of bone healing can be overcome by recombinant human bone morphogenetic protein-2, *J Craniofac Surg* 9:131-137, 1998.
97. Khouri RK, Brown DM, Koudsi B, et al: Repair of calvarial defects with flap tissue: role of bone morphogenetic proteins and competent responding tissues, *Plast Reconstr Surg* 98:103-109, 1996.
98. Schneider A, Taboas JM, McCauley LK, Krebsbach PH: Skeletal homeostasis in tissue-engineered bone, *J Orthop Res* 21:859-864, 2003.
99. Bücheler M, Wirz C, Schütz A, et al: Tissue engineering of human salivary gland organoids, *Acta Otolaryngol* 122:541-545, 2002.
100. Joraku A, Sullivan CA, Yoo JJ, et al: Tissue engineering of functional salivary gland tissue, *Laryngoscope* 115:244-248, 2005.

INDEX

Page numbers followed by f indicate figure(s); t, table(s); b, box(es).

N

O

Q

R

S

U

V